The Behavioral Neuroscience of Tinnitus

The Behavioral Neuroscience of Tinnitus

Editor: Justin Bailey

MURPHY & MOORE
www.murphy-moorepublishing.com

www.murphy-moorepublishing.com

MURPHY & MOORE

Cataloging-in-Publication Data

The behavioral neuroscience of tinnitus / edited by Justin Bailey.
p. cm.
Includes bibliographical references and index.
ISBN 978-1-63987-770-6
1. Tinnitus. 2. Hearing disorders. 3. Tinnitus--Etiology. 4. Symptoms.
5. Tinnitus--Treatment. I. Bailey, Justin.
RF293.8 .T56 2023
617.8--dc23

Murphy & Moore Publishing
1 Rockefeller Plaza,
New York City,
NY 10020, USA

ISBN 978-1-63987-770-6

Contents

Preface

Tinnitus is a condition characterized by hearing hissing, ringing, whistling, buzzing, chirping or other sounds in the absence of any external sound. It may affect one or both the ears. The level of the noise can vary and it can be either constant or intermittent. There are commonly two types of tinnitus, categorized into objective tinnitus and subjective tinnitus. The sound of tinnitus experienced by people is frequently linked to hearing loss. It is also linked to changes in neural synchrony, neuronal transfer functions and tonotopic organization, as well as changes in neuronal hypoactivity or hyperactivity. The diagnosis of tinnitus is typically based on the individual's description. It can also be diagnosed through an audiogram, otolaryngological examination and neurological examination. Tinnitus is mainly treated with talk therapy, hearing aids and sound therapy. This book provides comprehensive insights into the neuroscience of tinnitus. Its extensive content provides the readers with a thorough understanding of the medical condition.

This book unites the global concepts and researches in an organized manner for a comprehensive understanding of the subject. It is a ripe text for all researchers, students, scientists or anyone else who is interested in acquiring a better knowledge of this dynamic field.

I extend my sincere thanks to the contributors for such eloquent research chapters. Finally, I thank my family for being a source of support and help.

Editor

1

Is the effect of tinnitus on auditory steady-state response amplitude mediated by attention?

Eugen Diesch[1]*, Martin Andermann[2] and Andre Rupp[2]

[1] *Department of Clinical and Cognitive Neuroscience, Central Institute of Mental Health, Medical Faculty Mannheim, Heidelberg University, Mannheim, Germany*
[2] *Department of Neurology, Section of Biomagnetism, University Hospital Heidelberg, Heidelberg, Germany*

***Correspondence:**
Eugen Diesch, Department of Clinical and Cognitive Neuroscience Central Institute of Mental Health, Medical Faculty Mannheim, Heidelberg University, Square J5, D-68159 Mannheim, Germany. e-mail: eugen.diesch@zi-mannheim.de

Objectives: Auditory steady-state response (ASSR) amplitude enhancement effects have been reported in tinnitus patients. As ASSR amplitude is also enhanced by attention, the effect of tinnitus on ASSR amplitude could be interpreted as an effect of attention mediated by tinnitus. As N1 attention effects are significantly larger than those on the ASSR, if the effect of tinnitus on ASSR amplitude were due to attention, there should be similar amplitude enhancement effects in tinnitus for the N1 component of the auditory-evoked response. **Methods:** MEG recordings which were previously examined for the ASSR (Diesch et al., 2010a) were analyzed with respect to the N1m component. Like the ASSR previously, the N1m was analyzed in the source domain (source space projection). Stimuli were amplitude-modulated (AM) tones with one of three carrier frequencies matching the tinnitus frequency or a surrogate frequency 1½ octave above the audiometric edge frequency in controls, the audiometric edge frequency, and a frequency below the audiometric edge. Single AM-tones were presented in a single condition and superpositions of three AM-tones differing in carrier and modulation frequency in a composite condition. **Results:** In the earlier ASSR study (Diesch et al., 2010a), the ASSR amplitude in tinnitus patients, but not in controls, was significantly larger in the (surrogate) tinnitus condition than in the edge condition. Patients showed less evidence than controls of reciprocal inhibition of component ASSR responses in the composite condition. In the present study, N1m amplitudes elicited by stimuli located at the audiometric edge and at the (surrogate) tinnitus frequency were smaller than N1m amplitudes elicited by sub-edge tones both in patients and controls. The relationship of the N1m response in the composite condition to the N1m response in the single condition indicated that reciprocal inhibition among component N1m responses was reduced in patients compared against controls. **Conclusions:** In the present study, no evidence was found for an N1-amplitude enhancement effect in tinnitus. Compared to controls, reciprocal inhibition is reduced in tinnitus patients. Thus, as there is no effect on N1m that could potentially be attributed to attention, it seems unlikely that the enhancement effect of tinnitus on ASSR amplitude could be accounted for in terms of attention induced by tinnitus.

Keywords: tinnitus, auditory cortex, hyperexcitability, attention

INTRODUCTION

In previous studies it has been found that the amplitude of the magnetically recorded auditory steady-state response (ASSR) is enhanced for frequencies in the tinnitus frequency region (Diesch et al., 2004, 2010a,b). This enhancement effect may extend to nearby frequencies below this region (Diesch et al., 2004; Wienbruch et al., 2006). The ASSR may be elicited by trains of clicks and tone pips or by beats and sinusoidally amplitude-modulated (AM) tones. The source of the ASSR has been localized to the primary auditory cortex in the medial partition of Heschl's gyrus (Mäkelä and Hari, 1987; Gutschalk et al., 1999; Ross et al., 2000, 2002; Schoonhoven et al., 2003). Amplitude enhancement in tinnitus of stimulus-driven activity in the afferent auditory pathway may be interpreted to reflect the workings of gain control mechanisms inherent in the functioning of the subcortical auditory nuclei and the auditory cortex (Salvi et al., 2000; Syka, 2002; Eggermont and Roberts, 2004; Parra and Pearlmutter, 2007; Sun et al., 2009; Norena, 2010). However, because ASSR amplitude is also enhanced by attention (Ross et al., 2004; Bidet-Caulet et al., 2007; Gander et al., 2007, 2010; Müller et al., 2009), the effect of tinnitus on ASSR amplitude could in principle be an effect of attention in disguise. Those affected by tinnitus may direct attention to the auditory modality, to the ear affected by tinnitus, or even to the frequency or frequency range optimally corresponding to the equivalent tinnitus frequency or the dominant frequencies of the tinnitus spectrum. The two hypotheses are similar in that amplitude enhancement by attention of stimulus-evoked neural activity in the auditory pathway may be conceptualized in terms of attention-driven gain adjustment (Hillyard et al., 1998; Winkowski and Knudsen,

2006; Fritz et al., 2007; Winkowski and Knudsen, 2008). They differ in that the gain control hypothesis proper posits a modular autoregulatory process within the afferent auditory pathway while the gain-adjustment-by-attention hypothesis postulates that sensory activity is amplified by an interactive top-down process.

Not only the ASSR, but also several components of the transient auditory-evoked response, among them the auditory N1, are modulated by attention (Näätänen, 1992). The N1 component of the auditory-evoked potential and its magnetic counterpart, the N1m, occurs with a latency of approximately 100 ms in response to stimulus onset, stimulus offset, and stimulus change (Näätänen and Picton, 1987). The N1(m) receives contributions from the primary auditory cortex (Steinschneider et al., 1994), but the gravitational center of the N1(m) source has been localized to an auditory belt area in the planum temporale posterior to Heschl's gyrus (Pantev et al., 1995; Lütkenhöner and Steinsträter, 1998; Godey et al., 2001). While not much is known about attention effects on the offset and the change N1(m), there is ample evidence that the onset N1(m) shows attention enhancement effects (electrical: Hillyard et al., 1973; Picton and Hillyard, 1974), magnetic: (Arthur et al., 1991; Rif et al., 1991; Woldorff et al., 1993; Fujiwara et al., 1998). Moreover, N1 attention enhancement effects are significantly larger than ASSR attention enhancement effects (Okamoto et al., 2011). Thus, if the effect of tinnitus on ASSR amplitude were actually due to attention, similar, if not larger, amplitude enhancement effects should be found for the N1(m) component of the auditory-evoked response.

Previous studies on the N1 in tinnitus that reported tinnitus-related amplitude decrease rather than amplitude increase (e.g., Jacobson et al., 1991; Colding-Jorgensen et al., 1992; Jacobson and McCaslin, 2003; Walpurger et al., 2003) do not necessarily provide evidence against the attention hypothesis, as 1000 Hz sine tones exclusively were used as stimuli, whereas for most individuals affected the dominant tinnitus frequency is above 1000 Hz. Norena et al. (1999) also presented 1000 Hz tones and reported an increase of the slope of the N1 amplitude-level function in tinnitus patients and Kadner et al. (2002) obtained a steeper N1 amplitude-level function in tinnitus patients for tonal stimuli at the tinnitus frequency than for stimuli at lower frequencies. Thus, there remains a possibility that the N1 amplitude show attention-related enhancement effects mediated by tinnitus, especially with tonal stimuli close to the tinnitus frequency.

Here, we examine the N1m responses in a data-set that we have studied previously for the ASSR. Specifically, we look at N1m amplitude enhancement effects in tinnitus. If these were absent, it would seem unlikely that the tinnitus-associated ASSR amplitude enhancement effects observed previously (Diesch et al., 2004, 2010a,b) are mediated by attention[1]. Secondly, we compare the amplitude of the N1m elicited by composite stimuli to the linear superposition sum of the amplitudes of the N1m responses elicited by the individual component stimuli. The frequency bands of the auditory system are not independent, but rather constitute a multi-stage lateral, or reciprocal, inhibiton network (Shamma and Symmes, 1985; Müller and Scheich, 1988; Vater et al., 1992; Rhode and Greenberg, 1994; Suga, 1995; Sutter et al., 1999; Jen et al., 2002; Kopp-Scheinpflug et al., 2002). In the auditory cortex, integration of thalamocortical and intracortical inputs occurs over a range that spans a large proportion of the audible spectrum (Schulze and Langner, 1999; Kaur et al., 2004; Metherate et al., 2005). Attention affects sensory processing not only by increasing the gain, but also by increasing the selectivity of the receptive fields of single units (Fritz et al., 2007) and neural populations (Okamoto et al., 2007; Kauramäki et al., 2007; Neelon et al., 2011). Top-down control of reciprocal inhibition may be the mechanism or one of the mechanisms by means of which this increase of selectivity is accomplished. If it were, a putative tinnitus-related effect of attention on N1m amplitude should reduce the ratio of N1m response amplitude to composite to the superposition sum of N1m response amplitudes to component stimuli.

MATERIALS AND METHODS

MEG recordings of auditory-evoked responses that were previously examined for the ASSR (Diesch et al., 2010a) were analyzed with regard to the N1m component. Patients were included in the study if their tinnitus had lasted for six months or longer and featured a dominant tonal or quasi-tonal component that an equivalent tinnitus frequency of at least 1000 Hz could be determined for. Controls did not present with tinnitus. Both patients and controls were selected only if they showed some high-frequency hearing loss above an audiometric edge, where the audiometric edge was defined as that point on the frequency axis at which the hearing loss function exhibited its largest downward slope. Thirty-six subjects, 18 tinnitus patients and 18 healthy controls, participated in the original study. Subjects gave written informed consent following procedures approved by the ethics committee of the University of Heidelberg. Because musicians exhibit larger auditory-evoked response amplitudes and, therefore, deliver better signal-to-noise ratios than non-musicians when presented with spectrally complex sounds (Pantev et al., 1998a; Kuriki et al., 2006), half of the participants, eight of the patients and 10 of the controls, were selected to be musicians. Participants were assigned to the musician group if either they worked as professional musicians or earned a score of 25 or higher on the Advanced Measures of Music Audiation (AMMA) test (Gordon, 1989, 1998), or both. Thus, there were four groups, musicians with tinnitus (group MT, $n = 8$, mean age = 44.4 years, SD = 12.7, range: 21–63), non-musicians with tinnitus (group NT, $n = 10$, mean age = 51.4 years, SD = 11.0, range: 21–58), musicians without tinnitus (group MN, $N = 10$, mean age = 36.1 years, SD = 11.3, range: 21–52), and non-musicians without tinnitus (group NN, $n = 8$, mean age = 44.3 years, SD = 13.7, range: 23–58). The groups did not differ significantly in sex and handedness, but tinnitus patients were marginally older than healthy controls [$F_{(3,32)} = 2.68$, $p < 0.07$]. Patients and controls did not significantly differ in musicality. As a result of the

[1]Following the logic laid out by Okamoto et al. (2011), the sustained field could also have been examined. We were prevented from doing this because an analog highpass filter with a cutoff frequency of 0.03 Hz was used in the original recording. Extraction and analysis of the sustained field require DC recordings.

selection procedure, musicians had higher AMMA scores than non-musicians [$F_{(1,28)} = 64.5, p < 0.0001$].

The absolute threshold of hearing was obtained for 12 tonal frequencies between 125 Hz and 15 kHz (**Figure 1**). Summary indices of hearing loss both in the stimulated and the non-stimulated ear were determined by computing averages across frequencies, i.e., from 125 Hz to 746 Hz for low frequency and from 1183 Hz to 15 kHz for high frequency hearing loss. The equivalent tonal frequency of the tinnitus was determined using a recursive two-interval forced-choice procedure, with pure tones presented in both of the intervals, which has proven a reliable measure of tinnitus frequency (Henry and Meikle, 2000; Henry et al., 2000). The tinnitus minimum masking level (TMML) was determined as the difference between the level that was just sufficient for masking the tinnitus and the threshold level at which the masker was just audible by using a narrow-band (0.7 critical bands) "low-noise noise" (Kohlrausch et al., 1997; Dau et al., 1999) masker the center frequency of which was equated with the tinnitus frequency. The German version of the Tinnitus Questionnaire (Hallam et al., 1988; Hallam, 1996) published by Goebel and Hiller (1994, 1998) with its subscales of tinnitus intrusiveness, cognitive and emotional distress, auditory and perceptual diffculties, somatic complaints, and sleep disturbances was used to measure tinnitus severity.

Hearing loss (**Figure 1**) was more pronounced for patients than controls both for low [125...746 Hz: $F_{(1,32)} = 6.7$, $p < 0.02$] and for high frequencies [1.18...15 kHz: $F_{(1,32)} = 10.6$, $p < 0.005$]. For high frequencies, the stimulated ear was significantly worse than the non-stimulated ear [$F_{(1,32)} = 8.28$, $p < 0.01$]. Musicality and its interactions were not significant. Audiometric edge frequency did not differ significantly between patients and controls or musicians and non-musicians. Musicians with tinnituss did not differ from non-musicians with tinnitus with regard to tinnitus frequency, TMML, the tinnitus questionnaire total score, and the tinnitus questionnaire subscale scores.

The stimuli for the MEG-study were AM sine tones with a duration of 8192 ms, 20 ms onset and offset cosine ramps, and a modulation depth of 100%. The offset-to-onset inter-stimulus interval was allowed to vary randomly between 800 and 1200 ms. There were three individually adjusted carrier frequencies matching the tinnitus frequency in patients and the "surrogate tinnitus frequency" 1½ octaves above the audiometric edge frequency in controls (tinnitus condition: T), the audiometric edge frequency (edge condition: E), and a frequency 1½ octaves below

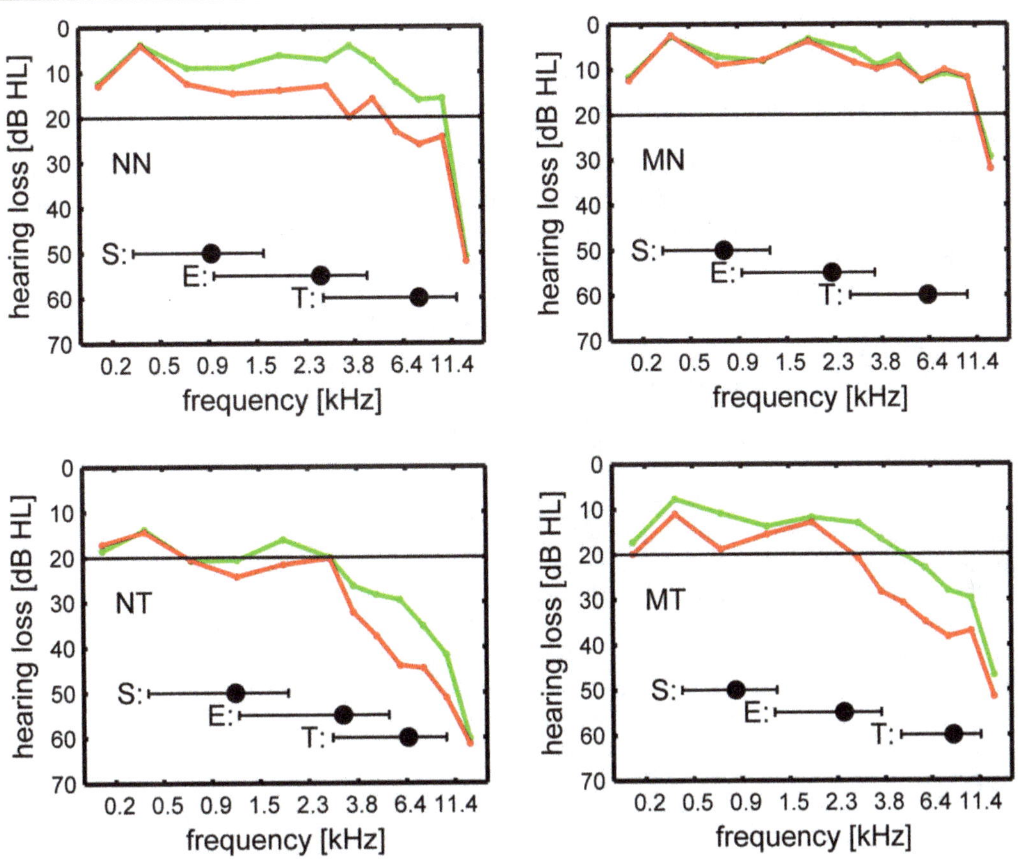

FIGURE 1 | Hearing loss, in dB HL, in the stimulated ear (red line) and the non-stimulated ear (green line). The inset bars show mean and standard deviation of the individually adjusted stimulus carrier frequencies for the sub-edge condition (S), the edge condition (E), and the (surrogate) tinnitus condition (T). NN: non-musicians without tinnitus, MN: musicians without tinnitus, NT: non-musicians with tinnitus, MT: musicians with tinnitus.

the audiometric edge (sub-edge condition: S). There were three modulation frequencies set to 38.6, 40.6, and 42.6 Hz (conditions 38, 40, and 42). All possible combinations of carrier and modulation frequencies occurred equally often both in a single tone (S38, S40, S42, E38, E40, E42, T38, T40, T42) and a composite tone condition (S38_E40_T42, S40_E42_T38, S42_E38_T40). Composite tones were created through linear superposition of single tones.

With regard to composite tones, there is an important difference between the ASSR and the N1m. Single tones elicited an ASSR with a frequency equal to the stimulus modulation rate. As to be expected (Lins and Picton, 1995; Lins et al., 1996; John et al., 1998; Fujiki et al., 2002; Kaneko et al., 2003), composite tones elicited three simultaneous SSRs with frequencies equal to the three stimulus modulation rates that were extracted separately using appropriate bandpass filters (Diesch et al., 2010a). Both single and composite tones elicited an N1m. However, it is not possible to decompose the composite tones N1m into component responses that one could attribute to the component tones. As a consequence, putative reciprocal inhibition among component N1m responses cannot be measured in the way that reciprocal inhibition between multiple ASSR components can be measured. For the ASSR, the amplitudes of the component responses in the composite stimulus condition may be compared to the respective same-modulation rate response in the single stimulus condition, with amplitude reduction in the composite stimulus condition indicating reciprocal inhibition and amplitude enhancement indicating reciprocal facilitation (Diesch et al., 2010a). For the N1m, one has to find an estimate of the composite stimulus condition N1m amplitude free of putative reciprocal inhibition or facilitation effects. An estimate may be obtained by computing the source amplitude of the equivalent current source fitted to the linear superposition of the field distributions accounted for by the single stimulus condition N1m sources which, in turn, may be approximated by simply computing the sum of the single stimulus condition N1m source amplitudes (Diesch and Luce, 1997).

The neuromagnetic field was recorded with a 122-channel gradiometer (Neuromag, Helsinki, Finland). The analog signal was lowpass-filtered (330 Hz), highpass-filtered (0.03 Hz), and digitized with a digitization rate of 1000 Hz. The stimuli were delivered monaurally through a plastic tube to the ear with the larger amount of hearing loss above 1 kHz. The stimulus presentation sequence was randomized. The stimulus level was set to 50 dB sensation level (dB SL), measured with the participant seated under the dewar, both for single tone stimuli and composite tone component stimuli. The stimulus level was lowered, if the resulting level of the composite stimuli was uncomfortable to the participant or the extent of the hearing loss was such that the limits of the transmission system were reached. The minimum stimulus level used was 35 dB SL. The stimulus level was lowered for four participants of group NT (3 × 35, 40 dB SL), three participants of group MT (2 × 35, 40 dB SL), and one participant of group NN (40 dB SL). However, for any one participant the same stimulus level (re sensation level) was used throughout. Due to their more pronounced high frequency hearing loss, the need to lower the stimulus level arose more frequently for tinnitus patients than for controls. Stimuli were equated re sensation level rather than in perceived loudness, because both ASSR and N1m amplitudes were intended to be studied as indicators of auditory system gain.

In accordance with the earlier ASSR analysis (Diesch et al., 2010a), the N1m was analyzed in the source domain using source space projection. To obtain the requisite spatial projection filter, the raw MEG signal was highpass-filtered at 1 Hz and lowpass-filtered at 30 Hz. Epochs of 500 ms duration including a 200 ms prestimulus baseline interval were extracted from the continuous data. Epochs exceeding 3000 fT/cm in amplitude were discarded. A grand average was computed across all stimulus conditions. Dipole source analysis was conducted using the BESA Ver. 5.2 software (MEGIS Software GmbH, Munich, Germany). A source model with two equivalent current dipoles, one in either hemisphere, was selected. Source fits were deemed acceptable if the equivalent sources were located in the supratemporal plane and the residual variance was 15% or less. The average residual variance obtained was 8.9% (SD = 3.73). Because of a bad source fit resulting from low signal amplitude one of the NT group participants was excluded from the N1m analysis. Following Hämälainen et al. (1993) and Robinson (1989), the unfiltered raw data were projected into the source domain, with the dipoles of the source model being used as the spatial projection filter. This resulted in two continuous source domain data streams representing activity of the auditory cortices of the left and the right hemisphere at the locations of the N1m sources. **Figure 2** illustrates the outcome of the application of the source space projection filter, not to the raw data, however, but to the grand average that was computed across all stimulus conditions.

The source domain time series were exported to MATLAB for further analysis. The exported continuous source domain data were highpass-filtered (1 Hz), lowpass-filtered (30 Hz), and selectively averaged with hemisphere and stimulus type, i.e., the three carrier frequencies of the single stimulus condition and the

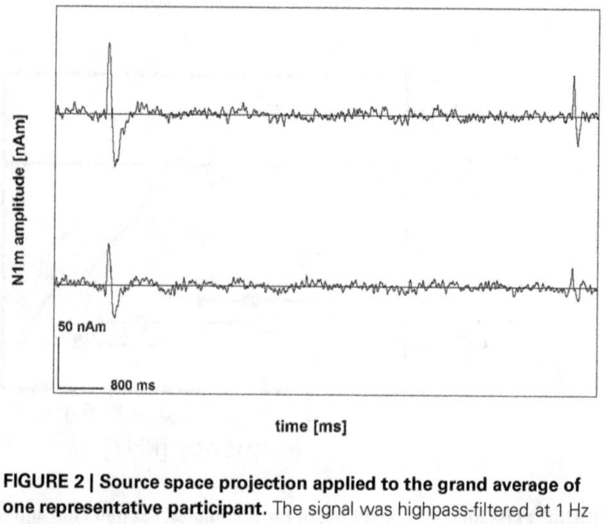

FIGURE 2 | Source space projection applied to the grand average of one representative participant. The signal was highpass-filtered at 1 Hz and lowpass-filtered at 30 Hz and exhibits prominent onset and offset N1m deflections.

composite stimuli of the composite stimulus condition, as conditions for epochs of 500 ms duration. The modulation rate conditions were pooled in the averaging process. The epochs included a 200 ms pre-stimulus baseline interval. The N1m response peak was determined as the amplitude maximum within an analysis windows extending from 80 ms to 140 ms re-stimulus onset.

The N1m reciprocal inhibition ratio was defined as the ratio of source amplitude in the composite stimulus condition and the linear superposition sum of the source amplitudes in the three single stimulus conditions. Thus, larger reciprocal inhibition ratios indicate smaller amounts of reciprocal inhibition. The single stimulus condition N1m source amplitude data were submitted to a multivariate analysis of variance (SPSS GLM) with source amplitude as the dependent variable, hemisphere and tonal frequency as repeated measurement factors, and tinnitus status and musicality as grouping factors. Analysis of the data from the composite stimulus condition and of the reciprocal inhibition ratios was done accordingly, with hemisphere as a repeated measurement factor and tinnitus status and musicality as grouping factors.

RESULTS

In the single stimulus condition, there were two statistically significant main effects of N1m source amplitude, hemisphere [$T^2_{(1, 31)} = 0.879$, $p < 0.0005$] and tonal frequency [$T^2_{(2, 30)} = 1.021$, $p < 0.0005$]. The mean N1m source amplitude, across tonal frequencies, was larger in the contralateral (42.0 nAm) than in the ipsilateral hemisphere (30.5 nAm). Averaged across hemispheres, N1m amplitude was largest in the sub-edge condition (42.3 nAm), intermediate in the edge condition (35.0 nAm), and smallest in the (surrogate) tinnitus condition (31.4 nAm). The same pattern was shown by tinnitus patients and healthy controls both in the contra- and the ipsilateral hemisphere (**Figure 3A**). The difference between tinnitus patients and controls did not attain significance and neither did the grouping factor of musicality or any of the interactions. When the analysis was rerun with age and low and high frequency hearing loss in the stimulated and the non-stimulated ear as covariates, the effect of frequency was preserved [$T^2_{(2, 23)} = 0.45$, $p < 0.02$], but the effect of hemisphere was not [$T^2_{(1, 24)} = 0.15$, n.s.]. However, the interaction of musicality and hemisphere attained significance [$T^2_{(1, 24)} = 0.19$, $p < 0.05$]. The difference between contra- and ipsilateral hemisphere was larger for musicians than for non-musicians.

On the face of it and in accordance with Colding-Jorgensen et al. (1992); Jacobson et al. (1991); Jacobson and McCaslin (2003); and Walpurger et al. (2003); mean N1m source amplitude was smaller for patients than controls (**Figure 3A**), but the difference failed to attain significance, possibly because of the use of individually adjusted tonal stimulus frequencies which may have generated additional between-subject variance. After two outliers with exceptionally large N1m amplitudes were removed from the group of musicians without tinnitus and the analysis was rerun using a hierarchical sum-of-squares decomposition approach (SPSS GLM SSTYPES = 1) which adjusted every term of the ANOVA model for the log of the individual audiometric edge frequency, not only the main effects of hemisphere [$T^2_{(1, 25)} = 1.18$, $p < 0.0005$] and frequency [$T^2_{(2, 24)} = 1.16$, $p < 0.0005$], but also the interactions between tinnitus status and musicality [$F_{(1, 25)} = 7.69$, $p < 0.01$], tinnitus status and hemisphere [$T^2_{(1, 25)} = 0.21$, $p < 0.05$], and tinnitus status, hemisphere, and frequency [$T^2_{(2, 24)} = 0.31$, $p < 0.05$] attained significance. The difference between patients and controls was larger for non-musicians than musicians and larger for the ipsilateral than for the contralateral hemisphere, especially in the sub-edge condition. Simple effects testing revealed that patients showed marginally smaller N1m amplitudes than controls among non-musicians [$F_{(1, 25)} = 3.80$, $p < 0.07$], for the ipsilateral hemisphere [$F_{(1, 25)} = 4.95$, $p < 0.05$], and for the sub-edge condition within the ipsilateral hemisphere [$F_{(1, 25)} = 9.73$, $p < 0.005$].

In the composite stimulus condition, the effects of hemisphere and musicality were statistically significant. N1m source amplitude was larger in the contralateral than in the ipsilateral hemisphere [$T^2_{(1, 31)} = 1.159$, $p < 0.0005$] and larger in musicians than in non-musicians [$F_{(1, 31)} = 4.578$, $p < 0.05$]. The musicality-by-hemisphere interaction was marginally significant [$T^2_{(1, 31)} = 0.133$, $p < 0.06$]. The hemisphere difference was marginally larger for musicians (cH: 88.0 nAm, iH: 59.8 nAm) than non-musicians (cH: 55.1 nAm, iH: 40.5 nAm).

Tinnitus patients and healthy controls differed with regard to N1m reciprocal inhibition. The N1m reciprocal inhibition score, i.e., the ratio of source amplitude in the composite stimulus condition and the superposition sum of the source amplitudes in the three single stimulus conditions, was significantly larger in patients than in healthy controls [$F_{(1, 31)} = 8.9$, $p < 0.01$]. Thus, the patients showed less reciprocal inhibition than the controls (**Figure 3B**). The factors of musicality and hemisphere and all the possible interactions they were part of did not attain significance.

For comparison, **Figure 3C** shows single tone ASSR amplitudes and composite tone ASSR component amplitudes (Diesch et al., 2010a). In patients, ASSR amplitude was significantly larger in the tinnitus than in the edge condition [$F_{(1, 34)} = 5.7$, $p < 0.025$]. In controls, ASSR amplitude was significantly smaller in the edge [$F_{(1, 34)} = 20.2$, $p < 0.005$] and the surrogate tinnitus condition [$F_{(1, 34)} = 4.8$, $p < 0.05$] than in the sub-edge condition. There were significant interactions of mode of presentation (single, composite) and tinnitus status [$F_{(1, 32)} = 10.5$, $p < 0.005$] and mode of presentation, carrier frequency, and tinnitus status [$T^2_{(2, 31)} = 0.35$, $p < 0.01$]. Inspection of the interactions shows that, except for the edge condition, ASSR amplitude was larger in the composite than in the single presentation condition in patients. Throughout, ASSR amplitude was smaller for the composite than the single condition in controls. The composite condition amplitude reduction in the edge condition was larger for controls than for patients.

DISCUSSION

When single tones were presented, the N1m source amplitude was larger in the hemisphere contralatersal than in the hemisphere ipsilateral to the stimulated ear. This laterality effect is in agreement with previous N1m findings (Pantev et al., 1998b). N1m amplitude was largest for sub-edge tonal frequencies, intermediate for edge frequencies, and smallest for (surrogate) tinnitus

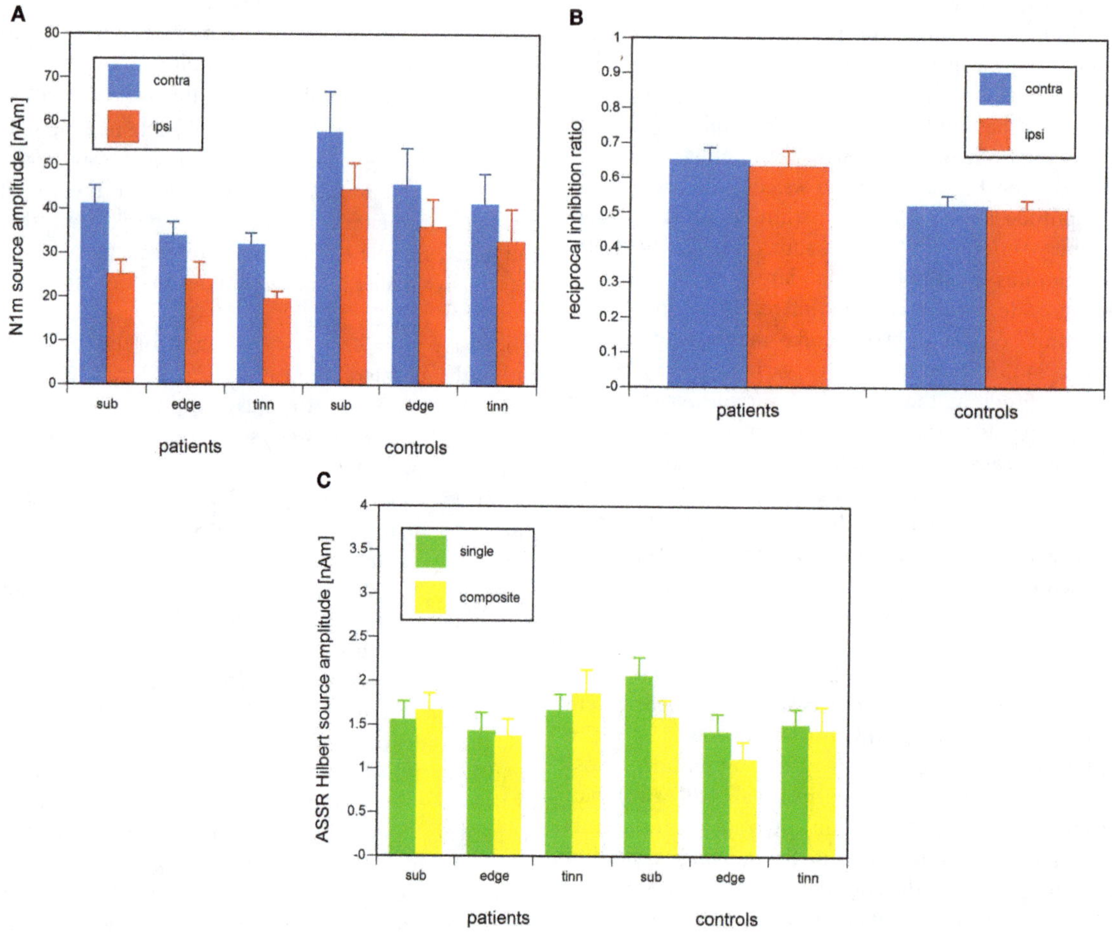

FIGURE 3 | (A) N1m source amplitude in the single stimulus condition for the contra- and the ipsilateral hemisphere, relative to the stimulated ear, in tinnitus patients and healthy controls for the tonal frequency conditions of sub-edge frequency, edge frequency, and (surrogate) tinnitus frequency. The error bars represent the standard error of measurement. **(B)** The reciprocal inhibition ratio, i.e., the ratio of source amplitude in the composite stimulus condition and the linear superposition sum of the source amplitudes in the three single stimulus conditions, in the contra- and the ipsilateral hemisphere, relative to the stimulated ear, of tinnitus patients, and healthy controls. The error bars represent the standard error of measurement. **(C)** Sub-edge, edge, and (surrogate) tinnitus single and composite stimulus condition ASSR source amplitude in tinnitus patients and healthy controls [as reported in Diesch et al. (2010a)]. The error bars represent the standard error of measurement.

frequencies. This is in agreement with the observation that, above approximately 1000 Hz, N1m amplitude decreases as a function of frequency (Pantev et al., 1995; Fujioka et al., 2002; Gabriel et al., 2004). These findings were preserved when age and hearing loss were entered as covariates into the analysis. N1m source amplitude was not larger in tinnitus patients than in healthy controls in any of the tonal frequency conditions, the (surrogate) tinnitus frequency included. If anything, N1m source amplitude was smaller for patients than controls, but this apparent difference, which is in agreement with previous reports on the amplitude of the N1 in tinnitus (Jacobson et al., 1991; Colding-Jorgensen et al., 1992; Jacobson and McCaslin, 2003; Walpurger et al., 2003), did not attain statistical significance as a main effect. This may be due to the additional between-subject variance generated by the individual adjustment of stimulus carrier frequencies. Simple effects testing after inclusion of the audiometric edge frequency into the ANOVA model showed that, among non-musicians, for the hemisphere ipsilateral to the stimulated ear, and for the sub-edge frequency within the ipsilateral hemisphere, patients exhibited smaller N1m amplitudes than controls. This partially accords with the findings of Colding-Jorgensen et al. (1992); Jacobson et al. (1991); Jacobson and McCaslin (2003); and Walpurger et al. (2003); and it is tempting to interpret it in terms of a refractory state that the tinnitus signal may produce for the N1m generator according to Jacobson and McCaslin (2003). However, the difference between patients and controls was largest in the sub-edge condition within the ipsilateral hemisphere, not the (surrogate) tinnitus condition. It could also be the result of the fact that stimulus level had to be lowered below 50 dB SL more often for patients than for controls.

As in the single stimulus condition, in the composite stimulus condition the N1m amplitude was larger in the hemisphere contralateral than in the hemisphere ipsilateral to the stimulated ear. While this difference was not significant in the single stimulus condition, N1m amplitude was larger in musicians than in non-musicians in the composite stimulus condition. This finding corresponds to previous reports concerning the processing of spectrally complex stimuli in musicians (Pantev et al., 1998a; Kuriki et al., 2006; Baumann et al., 2008; but see Schneider et al., 2002 and Lütkenhöner et al., 2006 for evidence to the contrary).

Qualitatively, the pattern of N1m source amplitude findings in patients and controls matches the one for ASSR source amplitude in controls obtained in earlier studies. In Diesch et al. (2010a), ASSR source amplitude in controls was smaller in the edge and the surrogate tinnitus frequency conditions than in the sub-edge condition and the edge and the surrogate tinnitus frequency condition did not differ significantly. However, in tinnitus patients, ASSR source amplitude was significantly larger in the tinnitus condition than in the edge condition. ASSR amplitude is affected by attention (Ross et al., 2004; Bidet-Caulet et al., 2007; Gander et al., 2007, 2010; Müller et al., 2009) and the perception of tinnitus and activity enhancement effects associated with tinnitus have frequently been interpreted in terms of attentional processes (Newman et al., 1997; Cuny et al., 2004; Zenner et al., 2006; Searchfield et al., 2007; Knobel and Sanchez, 2008; Gu et al., 2010; Rauschecker et al., 2010). Accordingly, it seems important to come to a conclusion on the the ASSR enhancement effect in tinnitus. Given that N1m attention enhancement effects are significantly larger than ASSR attention enhancement effects in healthy controls (Okamoto et al., 2011), if the ASSR amplitude enhancement effect in tinnitus were an effect of attention, an amplitude enhancement effects should also be found for the N1m. However, in the current study, the amplitude enhancement effect was conspicuously absent from the N1m source amplitude data. This renders it unlikely that the enhancement effect of tinnitus on ASSR amplitude is due to top-down effect of attention and strengthens the hypothesis of autoregulatory gain control being inherent to the functioning of the subcortical nuclei of the afferent auditory pathway and the primary and non-primary auditory cortex fields.

The finding that the N1m reciprocal inhibition score was significantly larger in patients than in healthy controls indicates that reciprocal inhibition was reduced in patients and structurally matches earlier ASSR findings. Diesch et al. (2010a) studied the ASSR to single AM tones and the ASSR to superpositions of three AM-tones differing in carrier and modulation frequency. Modulation frequency-specific ASSR components were recovered by bandpass filtering. Compared to the response to single AM-tones, ASSR components in the composite stimulus condition were reduced in amplitude in healthy controls, but increased in tinnitus patients. In controls, multiple response components seemed to reciprocally inhibit one another, but in tinnitus patients there seemed to be reciprocal facilitation.

It may be argued that the reduction of reciprocal inhibition in tinnitus provides further evidence against the attention hypothesis. Attention affects sensory processing not only by increasing the gain, but also by increasing the selectivity of single unit receptive fields (Fritz et al., 2007) and of the response of populations of single units (Okamoto et al., 2007; Kauramäki et al., 2007; Neelon et al., 2011). As reciprocal inhibition among parallel sensory input streams is capable of sharpening the distinctiveness of each of them, the top-down control of reciprocal inhibition may be one of the mechanisms of attention. The reduction of reciprocal inhibition shown by tinnitus patients both with respect to the ASSR and the N1m is the opposite of what would be expected under the hypothesis of attention-directed modulation of sensory input streams.

The conclusion that attention does not account for the ASSR enhancement effect in tinnitus does not mean that there are no effects of tinnitus on attention and cognitive performance and no role of attention in tinnitus development and maintenance. Stroop paradigm, auditory working memory, and divided attention studies have provided evidence for attention and performance deficits in tinnitus patients (Andersson et al., 2000; Rossiter et al., 2006; Stevens et al., 2007) that suggests that tinnitus may curtail the focussing of attention on external stimuli. Neither does it mean that attention could not be involved in the plastic changes that generate gain change and activity enhancement effects in the primary afferent auditory pathway and the auditory cortex. The patients investigated in the present study on N1m amplitude and in the Diesch et al. (2010a) study on ASSR amplitude represented a chronic condition, with a reported mean duration of the tinnitus since its onset of 13 years, six months. While attention does not seem to account for tinnitus-related ASSR amplitude enhancement in this population, it is possible that this may be an altogether different matter in a population of acute patients. At least some forms of training-induced cortical plasticity (Polley et al., 2006; Fahle, 2009) may require top-down attentional control. This may also be true of the neuroplasticity that is induced by cochlear lesions and may result in tinnitus (Zenner et al., 2006).

ACKNOWLEDGMENTS

This research was supported by a grant of the Deutsche Forschungsgemeinschaft to Eugen Diesch and Andre Rupp (Di497/3-2). We would like to thank the reviewers of an earlier version of this paper for their insightful and constructive comments.

REFERENCES

Andersson, G., Eriksson, J., Lundh, L. G., and Lyttkens, L. (2000). Tinnitus and cognitive interference: a stroop paradigm study. *J. Speech Lang. Hear. Res.* 43, 1168–1173.

Arthur, D. L., Lewis, P. S., Medvick, P. A., and Flynn, E. R. (1991). A neuromagnetic study of selective auditory attention. *Electroencephalogr. Clin. Neurophysiol.* 78, 348–360.

Baumann, S., Meyer, M., and Jancke, L. (2008). Enhancement of auditory-evoked potentials in musicians reflects an influence of expertise but not selective attention. *J. Cogn. Neurosci.* 20, 2238–2249.

Bidet-Caulet, A., Fischer, C., Besle, J., Aguera, P. E., Giard, M. H., and Bertrand, O. (2007). Effects of selective attention on the electrophysiological representation of concurrent sounds in the human auditory cortex. *J. Neurosci.* 27, 9252–9261.

Colding-Jorgensen, E., Lauritzen, M., Johnsen, N. J., Mikkelsen, K. B., and Saermark, K. (1992). On the evidence of auditory evoked magnetic fields as an objective measure of tinnitus. *Electroencephalogr. Clin. Neurophysiol.* 83, 322–327.

Cuny, C., Norena, A., El Massioui, F., and Chery-Croze, S. (2004). Reduced attention shift in response to auditory changes in subjects with tinnitus. *Audiol. Neurootol.* 9, 294–302.

Dau, T., Verhey, J., and Kohlrausch, A. (1999). Intrinsic envelope fluctuations and modulation-detection thresholds for narrow-band noise carriers. *J. Acoust. Soc. Am.* 106, 2752–2760.

Diesch, E., Andermann, M., Flor, H., and Rupp, A. (2010a). Interaction among the components of multiple auditory steady-state responses: enhancement in tinnitus patients, inhibition in controls. *Neuroscience* 167, 540–553.

Diesch, E., Andermann, M., Flor, H., and Rupp, A. (2010b). Functional and structural aspects of tinnitus-related enhancement and suppression of auditory cortex activity. *Neuroimage* 50, 1545–1559.

Diesch, E., and Luce, T. (1997). Magnetic fields elicited by tones and vowel formants reveal tonotopy and nonlinear summation of cortical activation. *Psychophysiology* 34, 501–510.

Diesch, E., Struve, M., Rupp, A., Ritter, S., Hulse, M., and Flor, H. (2004). Enhancement of steady-state auditory evoked magnetic fields in tinnitus. *Eur. J. Neurosci.* 19, 1093–1104.

Eggermont, J. J., and Roberts, L. E. (2004). The neuroscience of tinnitus. *Trends Neurosci.* 27, 676–682.

Fahle, M. (2009). Perceptual learning and sensomotor flexibility: cortical plasticity under attentional control? *Philos. Trans. R. Soc. Lond. B Biol. Sci.* 364, 313–319.

Fritz, J. B., Elhilali, M., David, S. V., and Shamma, S. A. (2007). Auditory attention–focusing the searchlight on sound. *Curr. Opin. Neurobiol.* 17, 437–455.

Fujiki, N., Jousmaki, V., and Hari, R. (2002). Neuromagnetic responses to frequency-tagged sounds: a new method to follow inputs from each ear to the human auditory cortex during binaural hearing. *J. Neurosci.* 22, RC205.

Fujioka, T., Kakigi, R., Gunji, A., and Takeshima, Y. (2002). The auditory evoked magnetic fields to very high frequency tones. *Neuroscience* 112, 367–381.

Fujiwara, N., Nagamine, T., Imai, M., Tanaka, T., and Shibasaki, H. (1998). Role of the primary auditory cortex in auditory selective attention studied by whole-head neuromagnetometer. *Brain Res. Cogn. Brain Res.* 7, 99–109.

Gabriel, D., Veuillet, E., Ragot, R., Schwartz, D., Ducorps, A., Norena, A., Durrant, J. D., Bonmartin, A., Cotton, F., and Collet, L. (2004). Effect of stimulus frequency and stimulation site on the N1m response of the human auditory cortex. *Hear. Res.* 197, 55–64.

Gander, P. E., Bosnyak, D. J., and Roberts, L. E. (2010). Evidence for modality-specific but not frequency-specific modulation of human primary auditory cortex by attention. *Hear. Res.* 268, 213–226.

Gander, P. E., Bosnyak, D. J., Wolek, R., and Roberts, L. E. (2007). Modulation of the 40-Hz auditory steady-state response by attention during acoustic training. *Int. Congr. Ser.* 1300, 37–40.

Godey, B., Schwartz, D., de Graaf, J. B., Chauvel, P., and Liegeois-Chauvel, C. (2001). Neuromagnetic source localization of auditory evoked fields and intracerebral evoked potentials: a comparison of data in the same patients. *Clin. Neurophysiol.* 112, 1850–1859.

Goebel, G., and Hiller, W. (1994). The tinnitus questionnaire. A standard instrument for grading the degree of tinnitus. Results of a multicenter study with the tinnitus questionnaire. *HNO* 42, 166–172.

Goebel, G., and Hiller, W. (1998). *Der Tinnitus-Fragebogen.* Göttingen: Hogrefe.

Gordon, E. (1989). *Advanced Measures of Music Audiation.* Chicago, IL: GIA Publications.

Gordon, E. (1998). *Introduction to Research and the Psychology of Music.* Chicago, IL: GIA Publications.

Gu, J. W., Halpin, C. F., Nam, E. C., Levine, R. A., and Melcher, J. R. (2010). Tinnitus, diminished sound-level tolerance, and elevated auditory activity in humans with clinically normal hearing sensitivity. *J. Neurophysiol.* 104, 3361–3370.

Gutschalk, A., Mase, R., Roth, R., Ille, N., Rupp, A., Hähnel, S., Picton, T. W., and Scherg, M. (1999). Deconvolution of 40 Hz steady-state fields reveals two overlapping source activities of the human auditory cortex. *Clin. Neurophysiol.* 110, 856–868.

Hämälainen, M., Hari, R., Ilmoniemi, R., Knuutila, J., and Lounasmaa, O. V. (1993). Magnetoencephalography – theory, instrumentation, and applications to noninvasive studies of the working human brain. *Rev. Mod. Phys.* 65, 413–497.

Hallam, R. S. (1996). *Manual of the Tinnitus Questionnaire (TQ).* London, UK: Psychological Corporation.

Hallam, R. S., Jakes, S. C., and Hinchcliffe, R. (1988). Cognitive variables in tinnitus annoyance. *Br. J. Clin. Psychol.* 27(Pt 3), 213–222.

Henry, J. A., Fausti, S. A., Flick, C. L., Helt, W. J., and Ellingson, R. M. (2000). Computer-automated clinical technique for tinnitus quantification. *Am. J. Audiol.* 9, 36–49.

Henry, J. A., and Meikle, M. B. (2000). Psychoacoustic measures of tinnitus. *J. Am. Acad. Audiol.* 11, 138–155.

Hillyard, S. A., Hink, R. F., Schwent, V. L., and Picton, T. W. (1973). Electrical signs of selective attention in the human brain. *Science* 182, 177–180.

Hillyard, S. A., Vogel, E. K., and Luck, S. J. (1998). Sensory gain control (amplification) as a mechanism of selective attention: electrophysiological and neuroimaging evidence [In Process Citation]. *Philos. Trans. R. Soc. Lond. B Biol. Sci.* 353, 1257–1270.

Jacobson, G. P., Ahmad, B. K., Moran, J., Newman, C. W., Tepley, N., and Wharton, J. (1991). Auditory evoked cortical magnetic field (M100-M200) measurements in tinnitus and normal groups. *Hear. Res.* 56, 44–52.

Jacobson, G. P., and McCaslin, D. L. (2003). A reexamination of the long latency N1 response in patients with tinnitus. *J. Am. Acad. Audiol.* 14, 393–400.

Jen, P. H., Chen, Q. C., and Wu, F. J. (2002). Interaction between excitation and inhibition affects frequency tuning curve, response size and latency of neurons in the auditory cortex of the big brown bat, *Eptesicus fuscus*. *Hear. Res.* 174, 281–289.

John, M. S., Lins, O. G., Boucher, B. L., and Picton, T. W. (1998). Multiple auditory steady-state responses (MASTER): stimulus and recording parameters. *Audiology* 37, 59–82.

Kadner, A., Viirre, E., Wester, D. C., Walsh, S. F., Hestenes, J., Vankov, A., and Pineda, J. A. (2002). Lateral inhibition in the auditory cortex: an EEG index of tinnitus? *Neuroreport* 13, 443–446.

Kaneko, K., Fujiki, N., and Hari, R. (2003). Binaural interaction in the human auditory cortex revealed by neuromagnetic frequency tagging: no effect of stimulus intensity. *Hear. Res.* 183, 1–6.

Kaur, S., Lazar, R., and Metherate, R. (2004). Intracortical pathways determine breadth of subthreshold frequency receptive fields in primary auditory cortex. *J. Neurophysiol.* 91, 2551–2567.

Kauramäki, J., Jaaskelainen, I. P., and Sams, M. (2007). Selective attention increases both gain and feature selectivity of the human auditory cortex. *PLoS ONE* 2:e909. doi: 10.1371/journal.pone.0000909

Knobel, K. A., and Sanchez, T. G. (2008). Influence of silence and attention on tinnitus perception. *Otolaryngol. Head Neck Surg.* 138, 18–22.

Kohlrausch, A., Fassel, R., van der Heijden, M., Kortekaas, R., van de Par, S., Oxenham, A., and Püschel, D. (1997). Detection of tones in low-noise noise: further evidence for the role of envelope fluctuations. *Acustica Acta Acustica* 83, 659–669.

Kopp-Scheinpflug, C., Dehmel, S., Dorrscheidt, G. J., and Rubsamen, R. (2002). Interaction of excitation and inhibition in anteroventral cochlear nucleus neurons that receive large endbulb synaptic endings. *J. Neurosci.* 22, 11004–11018.

Kuriki, S., Kanda, S., and Hirata, Y. (2006). Effects of musical experience on different components of MEG responses elicited by sequential piano-tones and chords. *J. Neurosci.* 26, 4046–4053.

Lins, O. G., and Picton, T. W. (1995). Auditory steady-state responses to multiple simultaneous stimuli. *Electroencephalogr. Clin. Neurophysiol.* 96, 420–432.

Lins, O. G., Picton, T. W., Boucher, B. L., Durieux-Smith, A., Champagne, S. C., Moran, L. M., Perez-Abalo, M. C., Martin, V., and Savio, G. (1996). Frequency-specific audiometry using steady-state responses. *Ear Hear.* 17, 81–96.

Lütkenhöner, B., Seither-Preisler, A., and Seither, S. (2006). Piano tones evoke stronger magnetic fields than pure tones or noise, both in musicians and non-musicians. *Neuroimage* 30, 927–937.

Lütkenhöner, B., and Steinsträter, O. (1998). High-precision neuromagnetic study of the functional organization of the human auditory cortex. *Audiol. Neurootol.* 3, 191–213.

Mäkelä, J. P., and Hari, R. (1987). Evidence for cortical origin of the 40 Hz auditory evoked response in man. *Electroencephalogr. Clin. Neurophysiol.* 66, 539–546.

Metherate, R., Kaur, S., Kawai, H., Lazar, R., Liang, K., and Rose, H. J. (2005). Spectral integration in auditory cortex: mechanisms and modulation. *Hear. Res.* 206, 146–158.

Müller, C. M., and Scheich, H. (1988). Contribution of GABAergic inhibition to the response characteristics of auditory units in the avian forebrain. *J. Neurophysiol.* 59, 1673–1689.

Müller, N., Schlee, W., Hartmann, T., Lorenz, I., and Weisz, N. (2009). Top-down modulation of the auditory steady-state response in a task-switch paradigm. *Front. Hum. Neurosci.* 3:1. doi: 10.3389/neuro.09.001.2009

Näätänen, R. (1992). *Attention and Brain Function.* Hillsdale, NJ: Erlbaum.

Näätänen, R., and Picton, T. (1987). The N1 wave of the human electric and magnetic response to sound: a review and an analysis of the component structure. *Psychophysiology* 24, 375–425.

Neelon, M. F., Williams, J., and Garell, P. C. (2011). Elastic attention: enhanced, then sharpened response to auditory input as attentional load increases. *Front. Hum. Neurosci.* 5:41. doi: 10.3389/fnhum.2011.00041

Newman, C. W., Wharton, J. A., and Jacobson, G. P. (1997). Self-focused and somatic attention in patients with tinnitus. *J. Am. Acad. Audiol.* 8, 143–149.

Norena, A., Cransac, H., and Chery-Croze, S. (1999). Towards an objectification by classification of tinnitus. *Clin. Neurophysiol.* 110, 666–675.

Norena, A. J. (2010). An integrative model of tinnitus based on a central gain controlling neural sensitivity. *Neurosci. Biobehav. Rev.* 35, 1089–1109.

Okamoto, H., Stracke, H., Bermudez, P., and Pantev, C. (2011). Sound processing hierarchy within human auditory cortex. *J. Cogn. Neurosci.* 23, 1855–1863.

Okamoto, H., Stracke, H., Wolters, C. H., Schmael, F., and Pantev, C. (2007). Attention improves population-level frequency tuning in human auditory cortex. *J. Neurosci.* 27, 10383–10390.

Pantev, C., Bertrand, O., Eulitz, C., Verkindt, C., Hampson, S., Schuierer, G., and Elbert, T. (1995). Specific tonotopic organizations of different areas of the human auditory cortex revealed by simultaneous magnetic and electric recordings. *Electroencephalogr. Clin. Neurophysiol.* 94, 26–40.

Pantev, C., Oostenveld, R., Engelien, A., Ross, B., Roberts, L. E., and Hoke, M. (1998a). Increased auditory cortical representation in musicians. *Nature* 392, 811–814.

Pantev, C., Ross, B., Berg, P., Elbert, T., and Rockstroh, B. (1998b). Study of the human auditory cortices using a whole-head magnetometer: left vs. right hemisphere and ipsilateral vs. contralateral stimulation. *Audiol. Neurootol.* 3, 183–190.

Parra, L. C., and Pearlmutter, B. A. (2007). Illusory percepts from auditory adaptation. *J. Acoust. Soc. Am.* 121, 1632–1641.

Picton, T. W., and Hillyard, S. A. (1974). Human auditory evoked potentials. II. Effects of attention. *Electroencephalogr. Clin. Neurophysiol.* 36, 191–199.

Polley, D. B., Steinberg, E. E., and Merzenich, M. M. (2006). Perceptual learning directs auditory cortical map reorganization through top-down influences. *J. Neurosci.* 26, 4970–4982.

Rauschecker, J. P., Leaver, A. M., and Muhlau, M. (2010). Tuning out the noise: limbic-auditory interactions in tinnitus. *Neuron* 66, 819–826.

Rhode, W. S., and Greenberg, S. (1994). Encoding of amplitude modulation in the cochlear nucleus of the cat. *J. Neurophysiol.* 71, 1797–1825.

Rif, J., Hari, R., Hamalainen, M. S., and Sams, M. (1991). Auditory attention affects two different areas in the human supratemporal cortex. *Electroencephalogr. Clin. Neurophysiol.* 79, 464–472.

Robinson, S. E. (1989). "Theory and properties of lead field synthesis analysis," in *Advances in Biomagnetism,* eds S. J. Williamson, M. Hoke, G. Stroink, and M. Kotani (New York, NY: Plenum Press), 599–602.

Ross, B., Borgmann, C., Draganova, R., Roberts, L. E., and Pantev, C. (2000). A high-precision magnetoencephalographic study of human auditory steady-state responses to amplitude-modulated tones. *J. Acoust. Soc. Am.* 108, 679–691.

Ross, B., Picton, T. W., Herdman, A. T., and Pantev, C. (2004). The effect of attention on the auditory steady-state response. *Neurol. Clin. Neurophysiol.* 2004, 22.

Ross, B., Picton, T. W., and Pantev, C. (2002). Temporal integration in the human auditory cortex as represented by the development of the steady-state magnetic field. *Hear. Res.* 165, 68–84.

Rossiter, S., Stevens, C., and Walker, G. (2006). Tinnitus and its effect on working memory and attention. *J. Speech Lang. Hear. Res.* 49, 150–160.

Salvi, R. J., Wang, J., and Ding, D. (2000). Auditory plasticity and hyperactivity following cochlear damage. *Hear. Res.* 147, 261–274.

Shamma, S. A., and Symmes, D. (1985). Patterns of inhibition in auditory cortical cells in awake squirrel monkeys. *Hear. Res.* 19, 1–13.

Schneider, P., Scherg, M., Dosch, H. G., Specht, H. J., Gutschalk, A., and Rupp, A. (2002). Morphology of Heschl's gyrus reflects enhanced activation in the auditory cortex of musicians. *Nat. Neurosci.* 5, 688–694.

Schoonhoven, R., Boden, C. J., Verbunt, J. P., and de Munck, J. C. (2003). A whole head MEG study of the amplitude-modulation-following response: phase coherence, group delay and dipole source analysis. *Clin. Neurophysiol.* 114, 2096–2106.

Schulze, H., and Langner, G. (1999). Auditory cortical responses to amplitude modulations with spectra above frequency receptive fields: evidence for wide spectral integration. *J. Comp. Physiol. A* 185, 493–508.

Searchfield, G. D., Morrison-Low, J., and Wise, K. (2007). Object identification and attention training for treating tinnitus. *Prog. Brain Res.* 166, 441–460.

Steinschneider, M., Schroeder, C. E., Arezzo, J. C., and Vaughan, H. G. Jr. (1994). Speech-evoked activity in primary auditory cortex: effects of voice onset time. *Electroencephalogr. Clin. Neurophysiol.* 92, 30–43.

Stevens, C., Walker, G., Boyer, M., and Gallagher, M. (2007). Severe tinnitus and its effect on selective and divided attention. *Int. J. Audiol.* 46, 208–216.

Suga, N. (1995). Sharpening of frequency tuning by inhibition in the central auditory system: tribute to Yasuji Katsuki. *Neurosci. Res.* 21, 287–299.

Sun, W., Lu, J., Stolzberg, D., Gray, L., Deng, A., Lobarinas, E., and Salvi, R. J. (2009). Salicylate increases the gain of the central auditory system. *Neuroscience* 159, 325–334.

Sutter, M. L., Schreiner, C. E., McLean, M., O'connor, K. N., and Loftus, W. C. (1999). Organization of inhibitory frequency receptive fields in cat primary auditory cortex. *J. Neurophysiol.* 82, 2358–2371.

Syka, J. (2002). Plastic changes in the central auditory system after hearing loss, restoration of function, and during learning. *Physiol. Rev.* 82, 601–636.

Vater, M., Habbicht, H., Kossl, M., and Grothe, B. (1992). The functional role of GABA and glycine in monaural and binaural processing in the inferior colliculus of horseshoe bats. *J. Comp. Physiol. A* 171, 541–553.

Walpurger, V., Hebing-Lennartz, G., Denecke, H., and Pietrowsky, R. (2003). Habituation deficit in auditory event-related potentials in tinnitus complainers. *Hear. Res.* 181, 57–64.

Wienbruch, C., Paul, I., Weisz, N., Elbert, T., and Roberts, L. E. (2006). Frequency organization of the 40-Hz auditory steady-state response in normal hearing and in tinnitus. *Neuroimage* 33, 180–194.

Winkowski, D. E., and Knudsen, E. I. (2006). Top-down gain control of the auditory space map by gaze control circuitry in the barn owl. *Nature* 439, 336–339.

Winkowski, D. E., and Knudsen, E. I. (2008). Distinct mechanisms for top-down control of neural gain and sensitivity in the owl optic tectum. *Neuron* 60, 698–708.

Woldorff, M. G., Gallen, C. C., Hampson, S. A., Hillyard, S. A., Pantev, C., Sobel, D., and Bloom, F. E. (1993). Modulation of early sensory processing in human auditory cortex during auditory selective attention. *Proc. Natl. Acad. Sci. U.S.A.* 90, 8722–8726.

Zenner, H. P., Pfister, M., and Birbaumer, N. (2006). Tinnitus sensitization: sensory and psychophysiological aspects of a new pathway of acquired centralization of chronic tinnitus. *Otol. Neurotol.* 27, 1054–1063.

2

Can temporal repetitive transcranial magnetic stimulation be enhanced by targeting affective components of tinnitus with frontal rTMS?

Peter Michael Kreuzer[1]*, Michael Landgrebe[1], Martin Schecklmann[1], Timm B. Poeppl[1], Veronika Vielsmeier[2], Goeran Hajak[1,3], Tobias Kleinjung[2,4] and Berthold Langguth[1]

[1] Department of Psychiatry and Psychotherapy, University of Regensburg, Regensburg, Germany
[2] Department of Otolaryngology, University of Regensburg, Regensburg, Germany
[3] Department of Psychiatry, Psychosomatic Medicine and Psychotherapy, Bezirkskrankenhaus Bamberg, Bamberg, Germany
[4] Department of Otolaryngology, University of Zurich, Zurich, Switzerland

Correspondence:
Peter Michael Kreuzer, Department of Psychiatry and Psychotherapy, University of Regensburg; Universitaetsstr. 84, 93053 Regensburg, Germany.
e-mail: peter.kreuzer@medbo.de

Objectives: Low-frequency repetitive transcranial magnetic stimulation (rTMS) of the temporal cortex has been investigated as a new treatment tool for chronic tinnitus during the last years and has shown moderate efficacy. However, there is growing evidence that tinnitus is not a pathology of a specific brain region, but rather the result of network dysfunction involving both auditory and non-auditory brain regions. In functional imaging studies the right dorsolateral prefrontal cortex has been identified as an important hub in tinnitus related networks and has been shown to particularly reflect the affective components of tinnitus. Based on these findings we aimed to investigate whether the effects of left low-frequency rTMS can be enhanced by antecedent right prefrontal low-frequency rTMS. **Study Design:** Fifty-six patients were randomized to receive either low-frequency left temporal rTMS or a combination of low-frequency right prefrontal followed by low-frequency left temporal rTMS. The change of the tinnitus questionnaire (TQ) score was the primary outcome, secondary outcome parameters included the Tinnitus Handicap Inventory, numeric rating scales, and the Beck Depression Inventory. The study is registered in clinicaltrials.gov (NCT01261949). **Results:** Directly after therapy there was a significant improvement of the TQ-score in both groups. Comparison of both groups revealed a trend toward more pronounced effects for the combined group (effect size: Cohen's $d = 0.176$), but this effect did not reach significance. A persistent trend toward better efficacy was also observed in all other outcome criteria. **Conclusion:** Additional stimulation of the right prefrontal cortex seems to be a promising strategy for enhancing TMS effects over the temporal cortex. These results further support the involvement of the right DLPFC in the pathophysiology of tinnitus. The small effect size might be due to the study design comparing the protocol to an active control condition.

Keywords: chronic tinnitus, dorsolateral prefrontal cortex, limbic system, transcranial magnetic stimulation, rTMS, neuromodulation

INTRODUCTION

Subjective tinnitus is characterized by the perception of sound or noise in the absence of an objective physical sound source (Moller, 2003). There is convincing evidence from functional imaging (Crippa et al., 2010; Lanting et al., 2010) and neurophysiologic studies (Weisz et al., 2007a,b) that tinnitus is related to abnormal functioning of the central auditory system (Moller, 2003). Based on these findings repetitive transcranial magnetic stimulation (rTMS) of the temporal and temporoparietal cortex has been proposed as a potential treatment for chronic tinnitus (Eichhammer et al., 2003).

Transcranial magnetic stimulation (TMS) is a non-invasive tool for inducing electric currents in the brain (Hallett, 2000). Fast oscillating magnetic fields created by a strong electric current circulating within a coil, penetrate the skull and result in depolarization of superficial cortical neurons (Ridding and Rothwell, 2007). rTMS can induce alterations of neuronal activity that outlast the actual stimulation period for a considerable amount of time (Hallett, 2000). Therefore, this technique has gained increasing attention as a potential clinical tool for the treatment of different neuropsychiatric disorders. Although the direct effects of the magnetic field are limited to directly stimulated superficial brain areas (Siebner et al., 2003), indirect effects can also occur in functionally connected remote areas (Hallett, 2000; Siebner et al., 2000). Such remote stimulation effects have also been demonstrated in thalamic regions after temporal rTMS by using voxel-based morphometry (May et al., 2007).

Several clinical studies consistently showed a reduction of tinnitus severity after repeated 1 Hz rTMS applied to the temporal cortex, whereas sham treatment had no effect (Kleinjung et al., 2005; Plewnia et al., 2007; Rossi et al., 2007; Smith et al., 2007). However, treatment results are burdened by only moderate improvement and high inter-individual variability indicating the need for optimization strategies.

As hypothesized already more than 20 years ago (Jastreboff, 1990) and confirmed by recent neuroimaging findings, tinnitus is related to (i) abnormal activity in both auditory and non-auditory brain regions (Lanting et al., 2009; Leaver et al., 2011) and to (ii) abnormal functional connectivity between these regions (Schlee et al., 2008, 2009a,b; De Ridder et al., 2011). In these studies the right dorsolateral prefrontal cortex has been identified as an important hub (Schlee et al., 2008, 2009a,b; Vanneste et al., 2010a). It has been hypothesized that this area might especially be related to the affective components of tinnitus (Vanneste et al., 2010a; De Ridder et al., 2011; Langguth et al., 2011). It has even been speculated that based on the emotional relevance, involved limbic and paralimbic structures may effectively switch the perceived signal on and off (Rauschecker et al., 2010).

This is in line with electrophysiological studies that demonstrated the relevance of dysfunctional top-down inhibitory mechanisms originating in the prefrontal lobe for tinnitus generation (Norena et al., 1999). The critical relevance of the DLPFC for tinnitus annoyance has been affirmed by recent studies that demonstrated symptom reduction after bifrontal tDCS (Vanneste et al., 2010b; Frank et al., 2011). Furthermore, it has been shown that rTMS over the DLPFC is apt to modulate the activity in functionally connected central limbic pathways such as the anterior cingulated cortex (Paus et al., 2001). Modulation of neuronal activity in the anterior cingulate, parahippocampus, and auditory cortex has also been reported in tinnitus patients after transcranial direct current stimulation of the prefrontal cortex (Vanneste and De Ridder, 2011).

A further rationale for low-frequency stimulation of the right DLPFC derives from affective research. Frontal asymmetry is known to influence emotion regulation and the emotional reaction to sensory stimuli (Davidson, 1992; Schmidt and Hanslmayr, 2009). It has also been shown that low-frequency rTMS of the right DLPFC exerts antidepressant effects of similar magnitude like high frequency rTMS of the left DLPC, which is conventionally applied in depressive disorders (Schutter, 2010).

Based on these data and the right lateralized alterations of frontal cortex activity in tinnitus patients (Schlee et al., 2008) we hypothesized that low-frequency rTMS of the right DLPFC might enhance treatment effects of low-frequency rTMS in tinnitus patients and compared the combined prefrontal and temporal rTMS therapy in tinnitus patients with the standard procedure of temporal rTMS.

PATIENTS AND METHODS

Fifty-six patients with chronic unilateral or bilateral tinnitus were enrolled in the study after having given written informed consent. The study has been registered with clinicaltrials.gov (http://clinicaltrials.gov/ct2/show/NCT01261949), was approved by the local ethics committee and performed according to the declarations of Helsinki. All patients suffered from disturbing tinnitus and had tried several standard treatment modalities such as cognitive behavioral therapy, hearing aids, white-noise generators, vasodilators, or antidepressants in the past. Normal middle ear status was demonstrated by tympanometry, stapedius reflex tests, and otoscopy. Patients with a history of seizures, a suspected diagnosis of organic brain damage, as well as patients with cardiac pacemakers, mobile metal implants, or implanted medication pumps were excluded. Sample characteristics are provided in **Table 1**. All data in the text and table is given as mean ± SD. rTMS was applied with the use of a Medtronic system with a figure-8 coil (Cool B-65 Butterfly; Medtronic, Minneapolis, MN, USA). Patients were enrolled in the study on a Monday and received stimulation on 10 subsequent working days. Patients were randomly assigned to one of two treatment protocols. One protocol (standard protocol) consisted of 2000 stimuli at a frequency of 1 Hz and an intensity of 110% resting motor threshold (RMT) over the left auditory cortex. In the second treatment protocol (combined protocol), low-frequency stimulation (1000 stimuli, 1 Hz, 110% motor threshold) applied to the right DLPFC preceded left temporal stimulation (1000 Stimuli, 1 Hz, 110% RMT). Thus, the total number of applied stimuli per session was identical for both groups. Stimulation was administered over the right DLPC and the left temporal cortex regardless of handedness or tinnitus laterality (Kleinjung et al., 2007b, 2008). The handle of the coil was pointing upward. Thus, the induced current in the brain was directed approximately perpendicular to the location of the superior temporal gyrus. During treatment the coil was held with a mechanical arm. In the combined stimulation group, the TMS coil was localized over the right DLPFC according to a standard algorithm by moving the coil from the optimal position for stimulation of the left abductor minimi 6 cm in the anterior direction and transferring this spot to the contralateral hemisphere in respect of the distance to the sagittal axis of the skull (George

Table 1 | Clinical and demographic characteristics (mean ± SD).

	1 Hz	1/1 Hz	T/χ^2	df	p
Age	46.5 ± 14.9	51.1 ± 13.9	1.196	54	0.237
Preceding treatments	2.5 ± 0.95	2.9 ± 0.56	2.063	53	0.044
Tinnitus duration (in months)	81.8 ± 78.0	109.6 ± 129.9	0.968	52	0.337
Gender (male/female)	23/7	19/7	0.096	1	0.757
Tinnitus laterality (right/left/both)	2/3/22	1/7/14	3,235	2	0.198
THI total score at baseline	41.5 ± 19.7	39.6 ± 22.4	−0.328	54	0.744
BDI total score at baseline	8.9 ± 7.7	6.9 ± 5.6	−1.103	54	0.275
TQ total score at baseline	39.5 ± 17.7	35.9 ± 17.1	−0.774	54	0.442
Audiogram (average from 125 Hz to 8 kHz of both ears)	20.8 ± 14.0	25.5 ± 17.8	0.650	54	0.519

et al., 1995). The RMT was determined over the left motor cortex for the right abductor digiti minimi and defined as the lowest intensity at which at least four of eight consecutive MEPs were 50 mV in amplitude while the muscle being investigated was at rest. Tinnitus severity was assessed before treatment (baseline), at the end of treatment (week 2), and during a certain follow-up period after rTMS treatment (week 4 and week 12). Tinnitus assessments included the German versions of the tinnitus questionnaire (TQ; Goebel and Hiller, 1994), the Tinnitus Handicap Inventory (Kleinjung et al., 2007a), the Beck Depression Inventory (Beck and Steer, 1984), several tinnitus numeric rating scales (loudness, discomfort, annoyance, distractibility, unpleasantness; Landgrebe et al., 2010), and a quality of life scale (WHOQOL-BREF; Murphy et al., 2000).

STATISTICAL ANALYSIS

The data analysis was based on data of the Tinnitus Research Initiative Database. Data management was conducted according to the Data Handling Plan (TRI-DHP V07, May 9th, 2011). Data analysis was conducted according to the Standard Operating Procedure (TRI-SA V01, May 9th, 2011), thereby following a study-specific Statistical Analysis Plan (SAP-003, May 18th, 2011) that was written according to the SAP template (TRI-SAP V01, May 12th, 2011). All documents are to be found under http://database.tinnitusresearch.org/.

The statistical analysis was performed on an intention-to-treat basis including all patients who participated in at least one measurement time point using a last observation carried forward or backward approach. Primary outcome was the change in TQ scores from baseline to week 2. For this purpose, we conducted an analysis of variance (ANOVA) with the within-subjects factor time (baseline vs. week 2) and the between-subjects factor group (combined vs. temporal group). Secondary outcome measures and exploratory analyses included chi-square tests for the variables group and treatment response which was defined as amelioration of at least 5 points in the TQ. We pooled the group of responders and non-responders of both treatments and compared them in regard to demographic and clinical characteristics with chi-square and t-tests. Furthermore, we compared baseline corrected TQ scores (week 2 minus baseline) between the treatment groups with Student's t-tests. In addition, we again conducted an ANOVA with the factor group (between-subjects factor) and time (within-subjects factor), this time including five measurement time points (screening, baseline, week 2, week 4, and week 12). This ANOVA was also computed for all other secondary outcome parameters (i.e., THI, BDI, and WHOQoL-BREF). Furthermore, we compared baseline corrected TQ scores (week 2 minus baseline; week 4 minus baseline) between the treatment groups. The statistical threshold for alpha error was set at 0.05. The analysis of secondary outcome parameters followed an exploratory approach, without corrections for multiple comparisons.

RESULTS

Both stimulation protocols were well tolerated, and all patients except one completed the treatment. This patient (combined stimulation group) refused further stimulation after day 3 because she feared a possible deterioration of the symptoms. A total of seven patients (including the one mentioned before) did not complete the course of the study (not shown up for follow-up-visit without giving further explanation). Three of them were treated in the combined stimulation group, four in the conventional group. Transient mild to moderate headache and feelings of twitching muscles at the stimulation site were reported as side effects. Serious adverse or side effects were not observed.

Primary outcome analysis indicated a significant change over time for both groups as indicated by a significant main effect of time ($F = 6.1$; df $= 1.54$; $p = 0.017$), but no group differences (main effect of group: $F = 0.8$; df $= 1.54$; $p = 0.375$; interaction effect time by group $F = 0.434$; df $= 1.54$; $p = 0.513$).

Response rate was comparable between groups (combined: 40%; temporal: 37%; $\chi^2 = 0.1$; df $= 1$; $p = 0.800$). Effect sizes were near zero for the non-responder groups (combined: $d = 0.085$; temporal: $d = 0.104$) and medium to high for the responder groups (combined: $d = 0.700$; temporal: $d = 0.454$). Contrasts between these groups indicated no significant differences for age, gender, tinnitus laterality, duration, and hearing loss. We only found an effect for the change in TQ and THI from screening to baseline for the non-responder group in contrast to the responder group of the combined treatment (TQ: $T = 2.156$; df $= 24$; $p = 0.041$; THI: $T = 3.675$; df $= 24$; $p = 0.001$), i.e., there was a reduction of questionnaire scores from screening to baseline for the non-responder (TQ: -5.2 ± 11.7; THI: -5.6 ± 7.7) and an increase for the responder group (TQ: 3.5 ± 6.1; THI: 5.8 ± 8.0).

Comparable to the primary outcome analysis, ANOVAs with five time points for TQ, THI, and BDI indicated significant main effects of time (all $Fs > 2.3$; df $= 4.212$; all $ps < 0.065$) and neither significant effects of group (all $Fs < 2.6$; df $= 1.53$; all $ps > 0.115$) nor time by group (all $Fs < 0.9$; df $= 4.216$; all $ps > 0.462$). *Post hoc* tests indicated an amelioration of symptoms after beginning of treatment and a return to baseline levels during the last follow-up (see **Figure 1**), i.e., tinnitus scores were significantly bettered for week 2 and week 4 in contrast to screening, baseline and follow-up.

Baseline corrected group contrasts (week 2 minus baseline; week 4 minus baseline) indicated no significant differences for week 2 (all $ps > 0.265$) and week 4 (all $ps > 0.088$) for TQ, THI, and BDI. Range of effect sizes were between 0.168 and 0.461 (0.176 for primary outcome analysis) indicating more pronounced improvement for the combined group in contrast to the temporal group for all variables.

DISCUSSION

The main finding of this trial is that additional low-frequency stimulation of the right DLPFC failed to significantly improve the effects of low-frequency temporal stimulation in the treatment of tinnitus. However, on a descriptive level the combined treatment protocol yielded better results in all assessment instruments that have been applied. Primary outcome analysis showed an effect size of 0.176 (group contrast in week 2) indicating a small effect according to Cohen (1988). Thus, the effect size was

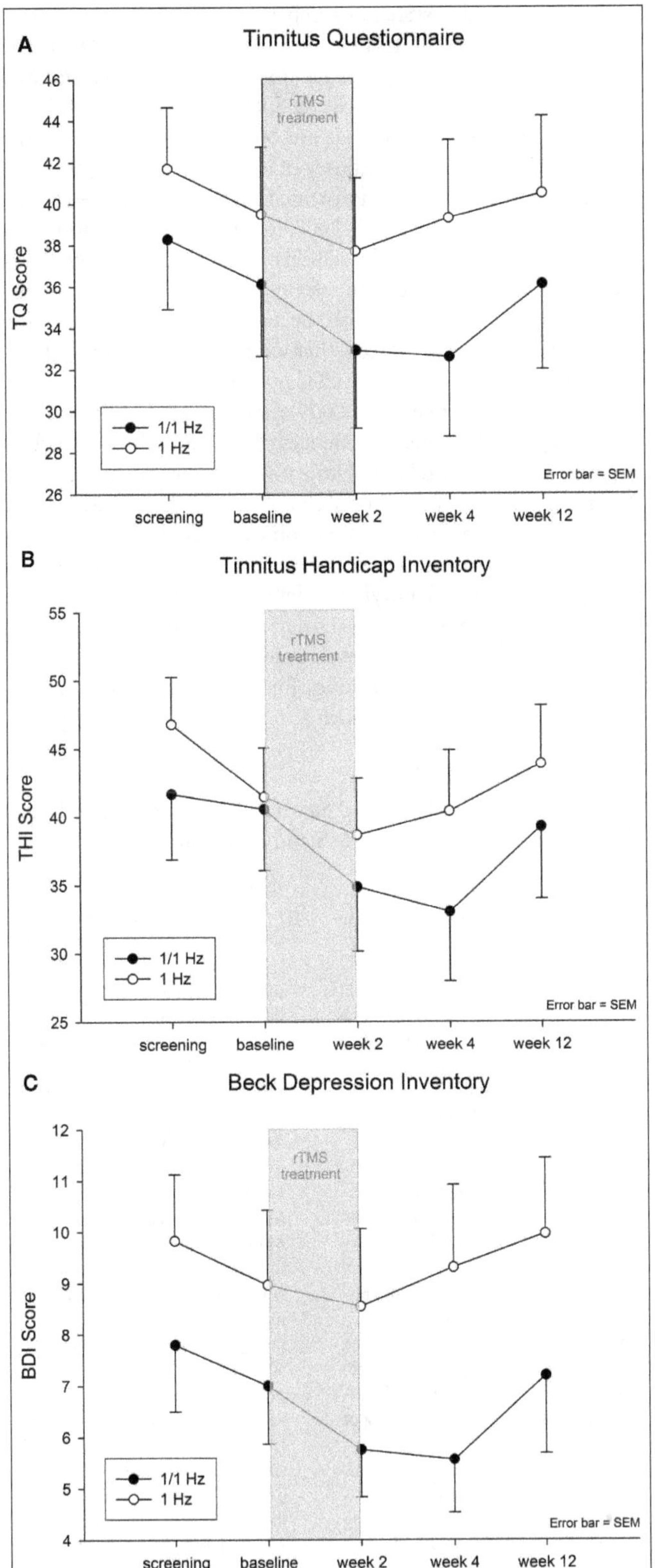

FIGURE 1 | (A) Tinnitus Questionnaire Score (TQ; mean ± SEM), **(B)** Tinnitus Handicap Inventory (THI; mean ± SEM), and **(C)** Beck Depression Inventory (BDI; mean ± SEM).

smaller than expected resulting in limited power and the failure to demonstrate significant effects. In this context it should be noted that significant improvement after rTMS was observed in both stimulation groups. The effect size for responders from temporal stimulation was medium ($d = 0.45$) for the responders from the combined stimulation protocol high ($d = 0.70$) according to Cohen (1988). Interestingly, the responder group differed significantly from non-responders in the change of THI and TQ scores from screening to baseline (non-responders: mean effect −4 TQ/7 THI points; responders: mean effect +2 TQ/THI points). This might be interpreted as a hint for the induction of homeostatic effects by TMS (Siebner et al., 2004). Further analysis did not reveal any differences between responders and non-responders in respect to gender, age, tinnitus duration, laterality, number of previous treatments, hearing loss, numeric rating scales, and values (screening/baseline) for THI, BDI, and TQ.

A further important finding was the decrease of mean baseline values for TQ, THI (for the 1/1-Hz group), and BDI from screening to baseline. This effect was similar in both stimulation groups and may have several reasons. First screening scores are based on completion of the TQ at home before the first consultation in our tinnitus clinic. The examination and consultation in the tinnitus clinic, which also involves counseling, may have resulted in the reduction of the tinnitus scores. Alternatively the improvement can be interpreted as an anticipation effect. Similar effects were observed in patients enrolled in waiting list control groups (Hesser et al., 2011).

Facing the fact that the combined stimulation group has been compared to an actively treated control group [that has undergone an already established standard treatment protocol (Kleinjung et al., 2005; Plewnia et al., 2007; Rossi et al., 2007; Smith et al., 2007)] it would be a bit too early to draw the conclusion that the small effect sizes might not possibly reflect clinically relevant changes especially taking into consideration the much higher effect sizes of the responder group. Even if this pilot study might have been designed with limited power presumptions, the results suggest at least that the applied combined study protocol did prove to be non-inferior in comparison to the established stimulation pattern of 1 Hz to temporal targets.

In this study all patients received rTMS over the left temporal cortex and in the combined group additionally over the right DLPFC. For both targets it remains a matter of debate, whether a more individualized strategy may not be more efficient. For the temporal cortex there are conflicting results whether stimulation ipsi- or contra-lateral to the perceived tinnitus laterality is more efficient (Frank et al., 2010; Khedr et al., 2010). We chose left temporal stimulation in all patients for better comparison with previous studies that investigated enhancement strategies for rTMS (Kleinjung et al., 2008, 2011; Langguth et al., 2008). With respect to frontal stimulation individualized targeting based on function imaging data revealed conflicting results as well (Kimbrell et al., 1999; Herwig et al., 2003) and more consistent antidepressant efficacy has been reported for low-frequency rTMS over the right DLPFC independent from imaging data (Schutter, 2010).

There is growing evidence from many recent neuroimaging studies that the influence of non-auditory brain structures may have been underestimated in the pathophysiology of chronic tinnitus in the past. A study investigating long-range connectivity of brain areas in patients suffering from chronic tinnitus by means of magnetoencephalography detected mainly the prefrontal cortex and the orbitofrontal region as hubs in tinnitus related networks (Schlee et al., 2009b). Moreover with increasing tinnitus duration non-auditory areas seem to gain importance in tinnitus related networks in comparison to auditory areas (Schlee et al., 2009b). But not only the DLPFC and neighboring regions seem to be of decisive relevance; also the left hippocampus (Landgrebe et al., 2009), parahippocampus (Lockwood et al., 1998; Schecklmann et al., 2011), the anterior (Plewnia et al., 2007) and posterior cingulate cortex (Vanneste et al., 2010a; Schecklmann et al., 2011), the temporoparietal junction (=auditory association area; Shulman, 1995; Giraud et al., 1999; Lockwood et al., 1999; Gardner et al., 2002), the dorsolateral prefrontal cortex (Mirz et al., 2000; Voisin et al., 2006), and the cerebellum (Lanting et al., 2009) have consistently been shown to exert functional influence in chronic tinnitus.

Possibly other rTMS techniques with different target locations, frequencies, and stimulation protocols (e.g., burst protocols; Arfeller et al., 2009; Kleinjung and Langguth, 2009) might represent promising approaches. Very recently a new rTMS coil, the so-called double-cone-coil with increased stimulation depth in the brain, has been introduced. Based on the use of this device it has been shown that a direct modulating influence of rTMS can be exerted to the limbic system, namely the anterior cingulate cortex (Hayward et al., 2007). In first clinical trials this new technique has been proven to be safe and its application is feasible and well tolerated (personal communication S Vanneste and D de Ridder).

Even if the present study has not been placebo controlled, the results further support the efficacy of low-frequency rTMS for the treatment of tinnitus as demonstrated in previous studies (Kleinjung et al., 2005; Plewnia et al., 2007; Rossi et al., 2007; Smith et al., 2007). The inter-individual variability has been high in both treatment groups, highlighting the relevance of a more individualized treatment approach. The limited accuracy of the coil positioning procedure over the DLPFC together with the large anatomic inter-individual variability of the DLPFC in Brodman Area 9 and Brodman Area 46 (Herbsman et al., 2009) may play a role in this context as well as potential genetic influences on neuromodulatory effects as proposed for the BDNF polymorphisms (Cheeran et al., 2008). It has been shown that clinical characteristics have only limited value for predicting treatment outcome (Frank et al., 2010). Neuroimaging such as electro- or magnet-encephalography may be more promising for identifying patients who may respond well on specific stimulation protocols (Lorenz et al., 2010; Vanneste et al., 2011). This may lead to the development of individualized multi-site-rTMS-stimulation techniques for the treatment of tinnitus, but also in other indications such as depression or chronic pain.

ACKNOWLEDGMENTS

We thank Helene Niebling and Sandra Pfluegl for their technical assistance in administering rTMS and collecting data.

REFERENCES

Arfeller, C., Vonthein, R., Plontke, S. K., and Plewnia, C. (2009). Efficacy and safety of bilateral continuous theta burst stimulation (cTBS) for the treatment of chronic tinnitus: design of a three-armed randomized controlled trial. *Trials* 10, 74.

Beck, A. T., and Steer, R. A. (1984). Internal consistencies of the original and revised Beck Depression Inventory. *J. Clin. Psychol.* 40, 1365–1367.

Cheeran, B., Talelli, P., Mori, F., Koch, G., Suppa, A., Edwards, M., Houlden, H., Bhatia, K., Greenwood, R., and Rothwell, J. C. (2008). A common polymorphism in the brain-derived neurotrophic factor gene (BDNF) modulates human cortical plasticity and the response to rTMS. *J. Physiol. (Lond.)* 586, 5717–5725.

Cohen, J. (1988). *Statistical Power for the Behavioral Sciences.* Hillsdale, NJ: Erlbaum.

Crippa, A., Lanting, C. P., Van Dijk, P., and Roerdink, J. B. (2010). A diffusion tensor imaging study on the auditory system and tinnitus. *Open. Neuroimag. J.* 4, 16–25.

Davidson, R. J. (1992). Anterior cerebral asymmetry and the nature of emotion. *Brain Cogn.* 20, 125–151.

De Ridder, D., Elgoyhen, A. B., Romo, R., and Langguth, B. (2011). Phantom percepts: tinnitus and pain as persisting aversive memory networks. *Proc. Natl. Acad. Sci. U.S.A.* 108, 8075–8080.

Eichhammer, P., Langguth, B., Marienhagen, J., Kleinjung, T., and Hajak, G. (2003). Neuronavigated repetitive transcranial magnetic stimulation in patients with tinnitus: a short case series. *Biol. Psychiatry* 54, 862–865.

Frank, E., Schecklmann, M., Landgrebe, M., Burger, J., Kreuzer, P., Poeppl, T. B., Kleinjung, T., Hajak, G., and Langguth, B. (2011). Treatment of chronic tinnitus with repeated sessions of prefrontal transcranial direct current stimulation: outcomes from an open-label pilot study. *J. Neurol.* doi: 10.1007/s00415-011-6189-4. [Epub ahead of print].

Frank, G., Kleinjung, T., Landgrebe, M., Vielsmeier, V., Steffenhagen, C., Burger, J., Frank, E., Vollberg, G., Hajak, G., and Langguth, B. (2010). Left temporal low-frequency rTMS for the treatment of tinnitus: clinical predictors of treatment outcome – a retrospective study. *Eur. J. Neurol.* 17, 951–956.

Gardner, A., Pagani, M., Jacobsson, H., Lindberg, G., Larsson, S. A., Wagner, A., and Hallstrom, T. (2002). Differences in resting state regional cerebral blood flow assessed with 99mTc-HMPAO SPECT and brain atlas matching between depressed patients with and without tinnitus. *Nucl. Med. Commun.* 23, 429–439.

George, M. S., Wassermann, E. M., Williams, W. A., Callahan, A., Ketter, T. A., Basser, P., Hallett, M., and Post, R. M. (1995). Daily repetitive transcranial magnetic stimulation (rTMS) improves mood in depression. *Neuroreport* 6, 1853–1856.

Giraud, A. L., Chery-Croze, S., Fischer, G., Fischer, C., Vighetto, A., Gregoire, M. C., Lavenne, F., and Collet, L. (1999). A selective imaging of tinnitus. *Neuroreport* 10, 1–5.

Goebel, G., and Hiller, W. (1994). The tinnitus questionnaire. A standard instrument for grading the degree of tinnitus. Results of a multicenter study with the tinnitus questionnaire. *HNO* 42, 166–172.

Hallett, M. (2000). Transcranial magnetic stimulation and the human brain. *Nature* 406, 147–150.

Hayward, G., Mehta, M. A., Harmer, C., Spinks, T. J., Grasby, P. M., and Goodwin, G. M. (2007). Exploring the physiological effects of double-cone coil TMS over the medial frontal cortex on the anterior cingulate cortex: an H2(15)O PET study. *Eur. J. Neurosci.* 25, 2224–2233.

Herbsman, T., Avery, D., Ramsey, D., Holtzheimer, P., Wadjik, C., Hardaway, F., Haynor, D., George, M. S., and Nahas, Z. (2009). More lateral and anterior prefrontal coil location is associated with better repetitive transcranial magnetic stimulation antidepressant response. *Biol. Psychiatry* 66, 509–515.

Herwig, U., Abler, B., Schonfeldt-Lecuona, C., Wunderlich, A., Grothe, J., Spitzer, M., and Walter, H. (2003). Verbal storage in a premotor-parietal network: evidence from fMRI-guided magnetic stimulation. *Neuroimage* 20, 1032–1041.

Hesser, H., Weise, C., Rief, W., and Andersson, G. (2011). The effect of waiting: a meta-analysis of wait-list control groups in trials for tinnitus distress. *J. Psychosom. Res.* 70, 378–384.

Jastreboff, P. J. (1990). Phantom auditory perception (tinnitus): mechanisms of generation and perception. *Neurosci. Res.* 8, 221–254.

Khedr, E. M., Abo-Elfetoh, N., Rothwell, J. C., El-Atar, A., Sayed, E., and Khalifa, H. (2010). Contralateral versus ipsilateral rTMS of temporoparietal cortex for the treatment of chronic unilateral tinnitus: comparative study. *Eur. J. Neurol.* 17, 976–983.

Kimbrell, T. A., Little, J. T., Dunn, R. T., Frye, M. A., Greenberg, B. D., Wassermann, E. M., Repella, J. D., Danielson, A. L., Willis, M. W., Benson, B. E., Speer, A. M., Osuch, E., George, M. S., and Post, R. M. (1999). Frequency dependence of antidepressant response to left prefrontal repetitive transcranial magnetic stimulation (rTMS) as a function of baseline cerebral glucose metabolism. *Biol. Psychiatry* 46, 1603–1613.

Kleinjung, T., Eichhammer, P., Landgrebe, M., Sand, P., Hajak, G., Steffens, T., Strutz, J., and Langguth, B. (2008). Combined temporal and prefrontal transcranial magnetic stimulation for tinnitus treatment: a pilot study. *Otolaryngol. Head Neck Surg.* 138, 497–501.

Kleinjung, T., Eichhammer, P., Langguth, B., Jacob, P., Marienhagen, J., Hajak, G., Wolf, S. R., and Strutz, J. (2005). Long-term effects of repetitive transcranial magnetic stimulation (rTMS) in patients with chronic tinnitus. *Otolaryngol. Head Neck Surg.* 132, 566–569.

Kleinjung, T., Fischer, B., Langguth, B., Sand, P., Hajak, G., Dvorakova, J., and Eichhammer, P. (2007a). Validation of the German-version Tinnitus Handicap Inventory (THI). *Psychiatr. Prax.* 34, 140–142.

Kleinjung, T., Steffens, T., Sand, P., Murthum, T., Hajak, G., Strutz, J., Langguth, B., and Eichhammer, P. (2007b). Which tinnitus patients benefit from transcranial magnetic stimulation? *Otolaryngol. Head Neck Surg.* 137, 589–595.

Kleinjung, T., and Langguth, B. (2009). Strategies for enhancement of transcranial magnetic stimulation effects in tinnitus patients. *Int. Tinnitus J.* 15, 154–160.

Kleinjung, T., Steffens, T., Landgrebe, M., Vielsmeier, V., Frank, E., Burger, J., Strutz, J., Hajak, G., and Langguth, B. (2011). Repetitive transcranial magnetic stimulation for tinnitus treatment: no enhancement by the dopamine and noradrenaline reuptake inhibitor bupropion. *Brain Stimul.* 4, 65–70.

Landgrebe, M., Langguth, B., Rosengarth, K., Braun, S., Koch, A., Kleinjung, T., May, A., De Ridder, D., and Hajak, G. (2009). Structural brain changes in tinnitus: grey matter decrease in auditory and non-auditory brain areas. *Neuroimage* 46, 213–218.

Landgrebe, M., Zeman, F., Koller, M., Eberl, Y., Mohr, M., Reiter, J., Staudinger, S., Hajak, G., and Langguth, B. (2010). The Tinnitus Research Initiative (TRI) database: a new approach for delineation of tinnitus subtypes and generation of predictors for treatment outcome. *BMC Med. Inform. Decis. Mak.* 10, 42. doi: 10.1186/1472-6947-10-42

Langguth, B., Kleinjung, T., Frank, E., Landgrebe, M., Sand, P., Dvorakova, J., Frick, U., Eichhammer, P., and Hajak, G. (2008). High-frequency priming stimulation does not enhance the effect of low-frequency rTMS in the treatment of tinnitus. *Exp. Brain Res.* 184, 587–591.

Langguth, B., Landgrebe, M., Kleinjung, T., Sand, G. P., and Hajak, G. (2011). Tinnitus and depression. *World J. Biol. Psychiatry* 12, 489–500.

Lanting, C. P., De Kleine, E., Eppinga, R. N., and Van Dijk, P. (2010). Neural correlates of human somatosensory integration in tinnitus. *Hear. Res.* 267, 78–88.

Lanting, C. P., De Kleine, E., and Van Dijk, P. (2009). Neural activity underlying tinnitus generation: results from PET and fMRI. *Hear. Res.* 255, 1–13.

Leaver, A. M., Renier, L., Chevillet, M. A., Morgan, S., Kim, H. J., and Rauschecker, J. P. (2011). Dysregulation of limbic and auditory networks in tinnitus. *Neuron* 69, 33–43.

Lockwood, A. H., Salvi, R. J., Burkard, R. F., Galantowicz, P. J., Coad, M. L., and Wack, D. S. (1999). Neuroanatomy of tinnitus. *Scand. Audiol. Suppl.* 51, 47–52.

Lockwood, A. H., Salvi, R. J., Coad, M. L., Towsley, M. L., Wack, D. S., and Murphy, B. W. (1998). The functional neuroanatomy of tinnitus: evidence for limbic system links and neural plasticity. *Neurology* 50, 114–120.

Lorenz, I., Muller, N., Schlee, W., Langguth, B., and Weisz, N. (2010). Short-term effects of single repetitive TMS sessions on auditory evoked activity in patients with chronic tinnitus. *J. Neurophysiol.* 104, 1497–1505.

May, A., Hajak, G., Ganssbauer, S., Steffens, T., Langguth, B., Kleinjung, T., and Eichhammer, P. (2007). Structural brain alterations following 5 days of intervention: dynamic aspects of neuroplasticity. *Cereb. Cortex* 17, 205–210.

Mirz, F., Gjedde, A., Ishizu, K., and Pedersen, C. B. (2000). Cortical networks subserving the perception of tinnitus – a PET study. *Acta Otolaryngol. Suppl.* 543, 241–243.

Moller, A. R. (2003). Pathophysiology of tinnitus. *Otolaryngol. Clin. North Am.* 36, 249–266, v–vi.

Murphy, B., Herrman, H., Hawthorne, G., Pinzone, T., and Evert, H. (2000). *Australian WHOQoL Instruments: User's Manual and Interpretation Guide.* Melbourne: Australian WHOQol Field Study Centre.

Norena, A., Cransac, H., and Chery-Croze, S. (1999). Towards an objectification by classification of tinnitus. *Clin. Neurophysiol.* 110, 666–675.

Paus, T., Castro-Alamancos, M. A., and Petrides, M. (2001). Cortico-cortical connectivity of the human mid-dorsolateral frontal cortex and its modulation by repetitive transcranial magnetic stimulation. *Eur. J. Neurosci.* 14, 1405–1411.

Plewnia, C., Reimold, M., Najib, A., Reischl, G., Plontke, S. K., and Gerloff, C. (2007). Moderate therapeutic efficacy of positron emission tomography-navigated repetitive transcranial magnetic stimulation for chronic tinnitus: a randomised, controlled pilot study. *J. Neurol. Neurosurg. Psychiatr.* 78, 152–156.

Rauschecker, J. P., Leaver, A. M., and Muhlau, M. (2010). Tuning out the noise: limbic-auditory interactions in tinnitus. *Neuron* 66, 819–826.

Ridding, M. C., and Rothwell, J. C. (2007). Is there a future for therapeutic use of transcranial magnetic stimulation? *Nat. Rev. Neurosci.* 8, 559–567.

Rossi, S., De Capua, A., Ulivelli, M., Bartalini, S., Falzarano, V., Filippone, G., and Passero, S. (2007). Effects of repetitive transcranial magnetic stimulation on chronic tinnitus: a randomised, crossover, double blind, placebo controlled study. *J. Neurol. Neurosurg. Psychiatr.* 78, 857–863.

Schecklmann, M., Landgrebe, M., Poeppl, T., Kreuzer, P., Maenner, P., Marienhagen, J., Wack, D., Kleinjung, T., Hajak, G., and Langguth, B. (2011). Neuronal correlates of tinnitus duration and distress: a positron emission tomography study. *Hum. Brain Mapp.* doi: 10.1002/hbm.21426. [Epub ahead of print].

Schlee, W., Hartmann, T., Langguth, B., and Weisz, N. (2009a). Abnormal resting-state cortical coupling in chronic tinnitus. *BMC Neurosci.* 10, 11. doi: 10.1186/1471-2202-10-11

Schlee, W., Mueller, N., Hartmann, T., Keil, J., Lorenz, I., and Weisz, N. (2009b). Mapping cortical hubs in tinnitus. *BMC Biol.* 7, 80. doi: 10.1186/1741-7007-7-80

Schlee, W., Weisz, N., Bertrand, O., Hartmann, T., and Elbert, T. (2008). Using auditory steady state responses to outline the functional connectivity in the tinnitus brain. *PLoS ONE* 3, e3720. doi: 10.1371/journal.pone.0003720

Schmidt, B., and Hanslmayr, S. (2009). Resting frontal EEG alpha-asymmetry predicts the evaluation of affective musical stimuli. *Neurosci. Lett.* 460, 237–240.

Schutter, D. J. (2010). Quantitative review of the efficacy of slow-frequency magnetic brain stimulation in major depressive disorder. *Psychol. Med.* 40, 1789–1795.

Shulman, A. (1995). A final common pathway for tinnitus – the medial temporal lobe system. *Int. Tinnitus J.* 1, 115–126.

Siebner, H. R., Filipovic, S. R., Rowe, J. B., Cordivari, C., Gerschlager, W., Rothwell, J. C., Frackowiak, R. S., and Bhatia, K. P. (2003). Patients with focal arm dystonia have increased sensitivity to slow-frequency repetitive TMS of the dorsal premotor cortex. *Brain* 126, 2710–2725.

Siebner, H. R., Lang, N., Rizzo, V., Nitsche, M. A., Paulus, W., Lemon, R. N., and Rothwell, J. C. (2004). Preconditioning of low-frequency repetitive transcranial magnetic stimulation with transcranial direct current stimulation: evidence for homeostatic plasticity in the human motor cortex. *J. Neurosci.* 24, 3379–3385.

Siebner, H. R., Peller, M., Willoch, F., Minoshima, S., Boecker, H., Auer, C., Drzezga, A., Conrad, B., and Bartenstein, P. (2000). Lasting cortical activation after repetitive TMS of the motor cortex: a glucose metabolic study. *Neurology* 54, 956–963.

Smith, J. A., Mennemeier, M., Bartel, T., Chelette, K. C., Kimbrell, T., Triggs, W., and Dornhoffer, J. L. (2007). Repetitive transcranial magnetic stimulation for tinnitus: a pilot study. *Laryngoscope* 117, 529–534.

Vanneste, S., and De Ridder, D. (2011). Bifrontal transcranial direct current stimulation modulates tinnitus intensity and tinnitus-distress-related brain activity. *Eur. J. Neurosci.* 34, 605–614.

Vanneste, S., Focquaert, F., Van De Heyning, P., and De Ridder, D. (2011). Different resting state brain activity and functional connectivity in patients who respond and not respond to bifrontal tDCS for tinnitus suppression. *Exp. Brain Res.* 210, 217–227.

Vanneste, S., Plazier, M., Der Loo, E., De Heyning, P. V., Congedo, M., and De Ridder, D. (2010a). The neural correlates of tinnitus-related distress. *Neuroimage* 52, 470–480.

Vanneste, S., Plazier, M., Ost, J., Van Der Loo, E., Van De Heyning, P., and De Ridder, D. (2010b). Bilateral dorsolateral prefrontal cortex modulation for tinnitus by transcranial direct current stimulation: a preliminary clinical study. *Exp. Brain Res.* 202, 779–785.

Voisin, J., Bidet-Caulet, A., Bertrand, O., and Fonlupt, P. (2006). Listening in silence activates auditory areas: a functional magnetic resonance imaging study. *J. Neurosci.* 26, 273–278.

Weisz, N., Dohrmann, K., and Elbert, T. (2007a). The relevance of spontaneous activity for the coding of the tinnitus sensation. *Prog. Brain Res.* 166, 61–70.

Weisz, N., Muller, S., Schlee, W., Dohrmann, K., Hartmann, T., and Elbert, T. (2007b). The neural code of auditory phantom perception. *J. Neurosci.* 27, 1479–1484.

3

Cortico-limbic morphology separates tinnitus from tinnitus distress

Amber M. Leaver[1], Anna Seydell-Greenwald[1], Ted K. Turesky[1], Susan Morgan[2], Hung J. Kim[3] and Josef P. Rauschecker[1]*

[1] *Department of Neuroscience, Georgetown University Medical Center, Washington, DC, USA*
[2] *Division of Audiology, Georgetown University Hospital, Washington, DC, USA*
[3] *Department of Otolaryngology, Georgetown University Hospital, Washington, DC, USA*

Correspondence:
Josef P. Rauschecker, Department of Neuroscience, Georgetown University Medical Center, 3970 Reservoir Rd NW, Washington, DC 20057, USA.
e-mail: rauschej@georgetown.edu

Tinnitus is a common auditory disorder characterized by a chronic ringing or buzzing "in the ear." Despite the auditory-perceptual nature of this disorder, a growing number of studies have reported neuroanatomical differences in tinnitus patients outside the auditory-perceptual system. Some have used this evidence to characterize chronic tinnitus as dysregulation of the auditory system, either resulting from inefficient inhibitory control or through the formation of aversive associations with tinnitus. It remains unclear, however, whether these "non-auditory" anatomical markers of tinnitus are related to the tinnitus signal itself, or merely to negative emotional reactions to tinnitus (i.e., tinnitus distress). In the current study, we used anatomical MRI to identify neural markers of tinnitus, and measured their relationship to a variety of tinnitus characteristics and other factors often linked to tinnitus, such as hearing loss, depression, anxiety, and noise sensitivity. In a new cohort of participants, we confirmed that people with chronic tinnitus exhibit reduced gray matter in ventromedial prefrontal cortex (vmPFC) compared to controls matched for age and hearing loss. This effect was driven by reduced cortical surface area, and was not related to tinnitus distress, symptoms of depression or anxiety, noise sensitivity, or other factors. Instead, tinnitus distress was positively correlated with cortical thickness in the anterior insula in tinnitus patients, while symptoms of anxiety and depression were negatively correlated with cortical thickness in subcallosal anterior cingulate cortex (scACC) across all groups. Tinnitus patients also exhibited increased gyrification of dorsomedial prefrontal cortex (dmPFC), which was more severe in those patients with constant (vs. intermittent) tinnitus awareness. Our data suggest that the neural systems associated with chronic tinnitus are different from those involved in aversive or distressed reactions to tinnitus.

Keywords: tinnitus, anatomical MRI, medial prefrontal cortex, subcallosal anterior cingulate

INTRODUCTION

Tinnitus pathophysiology is typically thought to involve damage at one or more sites along peripheral and/or central auditory pathways; however, auditory system damage alone does not seem to be sufficient to cause chronic tinnitus. Indeed, a growing body of evidence suggests a relationship between tinnitus and other parts of the brain, both in the form of atypical function and anatomy (Shulman et al., 1995; Lockwood et al., 1998; Mirz et al., 2000; Lowry et al., 2004; Mühlau et al., 2006; Landgrebe et al., 2009; Schlee et al., 2009; Cheung and Larson, 2010; Leaver et al., 2011). Correspondingly, a number of models of tinnitus argue that non-auditory-perceptual networks are necessary components of tinnitus pathophysiology (Jastreboff, 1990; Møller, 2003; Mühlau et al., 2006; Rauschecker et al., 2010; De Ridder et al., 2011).

Of particular relevance is the limbic system, parts of which have been shown to be affected in tinnitus across several studies (Shulman et al., 1995; Lockwood et al., 1998; Mirz et al., 2000; Lowry et al., 2004; Mühlau et al., 2006; Landgrebe et al., 2009; Cheung and Larson, 2010; Leaver et al., 2011). Our previous work has identified an area of reduced gray matter (GM) in the ventromedial prefrontal cortices (vmPFC) of tinnitus patients using voxel-based morphometry (VBM) (Mühlau et al., 2006; Leaver et al., 2011). Based on these findings, we proposed that chronic tinnitus is caused by failure of the vmPFC-network to suppress aberrant activity in the auditory system (Mühlau et al., 2006; Rauschecker et al., 2010). This hypothesis is consistent with the role the vmPFC and associated structures play in the evaluation of many types of stimuli (Kable and Glimcher, 2009), and characterizes tinnitus as a problem of "noise cancellation."

However, alternative explanations remain. Previous work in mood disorders consistently identifies reduced GM in vmPFC and subcallosal anterior cingulate (scACC) in individuals suffering from clinical depression and anxiety (Drevets et al., 1997; Mayberg, 1997; Koenigs and Grafman, 2009). Also, tinnitus itself can be associated with stress and negative mood (Sullivan et al.,

1988; Folmer et al., 1999; Dobie, 2003). Some theories of tinnitus pathophysiology argue that negative emotional reactions to tinnitus are necessary for the disorder to become chronic (Jastreboff, 1990; De Ridder et al., 2011). If aversive reactions to tinnitus are necessary components of tinnitus pathophysiology, one might expect a positive relationship between the severity of: (1) the auditory-perceptual characteristics of tinnitus, like loudness or awareness (i.e., the amount of time patients are aware of their tinnitus), (2) the patient's suffering and/or the presence of concomitant mood disorders or symptoms, and (3) reductions in vmPFC gray matter or other markers of tinnitus. On the other hand, if vmPFC can affect the gain of tinnitus independent of any emotional reaction (Mühlau et al., 2006; Rauschecker et al., 2010), one would expect reductions in vmPFC gray matter to be related to the auditory-perceptual characteristics of tinnitus, but not its aversiveness or symptoms of depression or anxiety.

Furthermore, due to the inherent limitations of VBM analyses used in previous studies (Mühlau et al., 2006; Landgrebe et al., 2009; Husain et al., 2011; Leaver et al., 2011), the exact nature of this anatomical anomaly in vmPFC and other anatomical markers of tinnitus are unknown. Decreases in cortical thickness, surface area, and gyrification (i.e., curvature or folding) could, in theory, all lead to similar VBM effects (Hutton et al., 2009). In addition, variability in these morphological features across individuals is likely to have different genetic origins and, correspondingly, cellular bases (Panizzon et al., 2009). Thus, going beyond the indirect measures of tissue volume that VBM offers should yield a more detailed picture of tinnitus pathophysiology.

In the current study, we used magnetic resonance imaging (MRI) to identify neuroanatomical correlates of tinnitus, and their relationship to tinnitus characteristics, tinnitus distress, and other factors. In a new cohort of participants, we first measured GM volume using volume-based methods (i.e., VBM). Turning to more sophisticated morphometric techniques, we sought to pinpoint the morphological basis of GM volume reductions using surface-based analyses. Finally, we attempted to determine whether vmPFC morphology reflected tinnitus distress, consistent with the typical view of the limbic system (Jastreboff, 1990; Møller, 2003; De Ridder et al., 2011), or whether vmPFC correlated with auditory-perceptual characteristics of tinnitus, consistent with our model (Mühlau et al., 2006; Rauschecker et al., 2010). By using a series of detailed questionnaires, we also measured the relationship between tinnitus symptoms and non-tinnitus factors like hearing loss, depression, and anxiety.

METHODS

PARTICIPANTS

Forty-four volunteers (23 tinnitus patients, 21 controls) gave informed consent to participate in this study according to procedures of the Institutional Review Board at Georgetown University. Participants were recruited such that the two groups would be matched by age and sex, and standard MRI safety considerations were used as exclusion criteria. Tinnitus patients ranged in age from 23 to 66 years; control participants ranged from 27 to 67 years of age. Detailed characteristics of these groups can be found in **Table 1**.

Table 1 | Participant characteristics.

	Patients	Controls
N	23	21
Age (years)	47.4 (2.9)	49.0 (2.6)
Sex (female, male)	11, 12	13, 8
Mean hearing loss (dB)	31.1 (2.8)	23.4 (2.5)
Loudness discomfort levels (dB)*	87.1 (2.2)	93.7 (1.6)
Noise sensitivity ratings (5-point scale)*	2.0 (0.2)	0.4 (0.1)
Depression score (PHQ9, 27 max score)**	4.7 (1.0)	2.5 (0.6)
Anxiety score (GAD7, 21 max score)**	4.7 (1.0)	2.5 (0.7)
History of mood disorder or medications (yes, no)	6, 17	3, 18
History of closed-head injury (yes, no)	4, 19	3, 18

Note: Mean values or counts are given where appropriate; numerical values in parentheses indicate standard error.

**Scores were normalized and combined to form combined Noise Sensitivity Scores.*

***Measures were summed to form combined scores.*

AUDIOMETRY

Audiometric testing assessed pure-tone thresholds in all participants at the Division of Audiology at Georgetown University (**Figure 1**). Pure tones ranging from 250 Hz to 20 kHz were presented to each ear at increasing intensities until the threshold of detection was reached. The "standard" clinical audiogram tests frequencies from 250 Hz to 8 kHz; we tested additional frequencies above 8 kHz to create an "extended" audiogram for each subject. A conservative "normal" hearing range included thresholds below 20 dB Hearing Level (HL). Thresholds between 20 and 40 dB HL were considered a mild loss, 40–60 dB HL was considered moderate, and 60–90 dB HL severe. Thresholds above 90 dB HL were considered profound. Only two participants (1 tinnitus, 1 control) exhibited profound hearing loss in the standard frequency range (i.e., ≤8 kHz), at a single frequency, 8 kHz. Chi-squared analyses indicated no significant difference in the proportion of tinnitus patients and controls with normal, mild, moderate, severe, or profound loss in the standard audiogram (≤8 kHz: $X^2_{(4)} = 6.5, p = 0.17$) or extended audiogram (>8 kHz: $X^2_{(4)} = 3.98,\ p = 0.41$). Therefore, only the mean hearing loss across the entire audiogram for both ears was considered for further analysis.

Noise sensitivity was tested using Loudness Discomfort Levels (LDLs) and a rating scale included in the Tinnitus Sample Case History Questionnaire (TSCHQ) (Langguth et al., 2007). During LDL assessment, pure tones of various frequencies were presented to both ears with increasing amplitude until the subject indicated an undesirable degree of discomfort. Frequencies tested included a 1 kHz standard and three others dependent on the subject's audiogram. Stimulation was aborted at 100 or 105 dB HL, so stimuli did not overlap with the entire normal range of LDLs (Morgan et al., 1974). Therefore, LDL scores were combined with a noise sensitivity rating score to yield a combined noise sensitivity measure. Both tinnitus patients and control participants used a 5-point scale to answer the following question from the TSCHQ: *Do you have a problem tolerating sounds because they often seem much too loud? That is, do you often experience sounds which other*

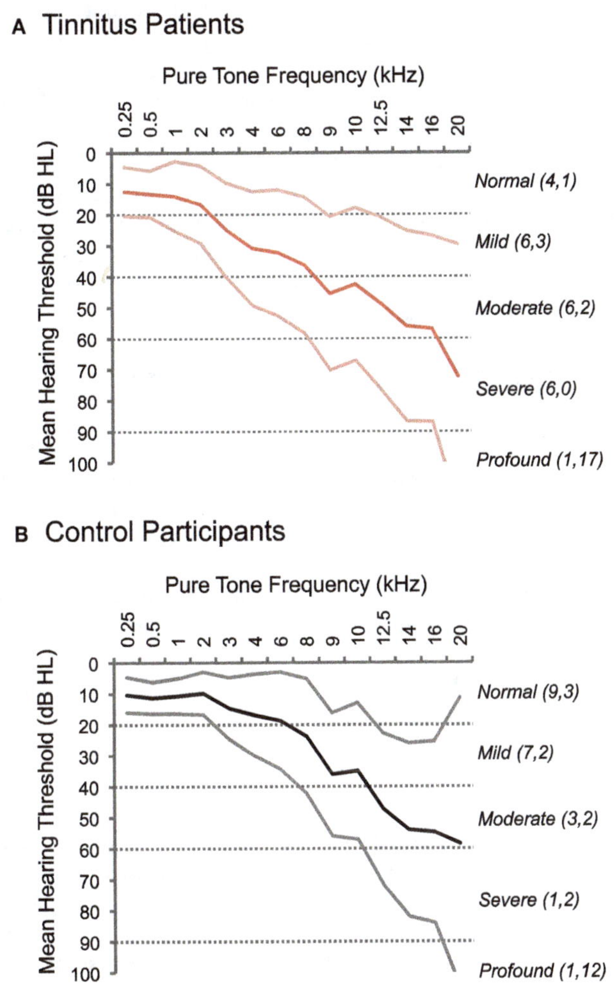

FIGURE 1 | Hearing thresholds in tinnitus patients and controls. The results of pure-tone audiometry are plotted for tinnitus patients **(A)** and control participants **(B)**. Thresholds in dB Hearing Level (HL) are displayed on the y-axis, and test frequencies are plotted on the x-axis, including standard audiogram frequencies up to 8 kHz and extended test frequencies >8 kHz. Thick lines indicate the mean threshold; thinner lines indicate standard error above and below the mean. Dotted lines delineate ranges of normal (≤20 dB HL), mild (20–40 dB HL), moderate (40–60 dB HL), severe (60–90 dB HL), and profound (>90 dB HL) hearing loss. The number of participants with maximum hearing loss in at least one frequency is indicated for each category in parentheses on the right, separately for standard (first number) and extended (second number) ranges of test frequencies.

people around you find quite comfortable as too loud or hurtful? (0 = never; 1 = rarely; 2 = sometimes; 3 = usually; 4 = always). To compute the combined score, mean LDLs and noise sensitivity ratings were each normalized (0–1) and summed. Thus, a combined score of 0 indicated minimal noise sensitivity (i.e., LDL score = 100 dB HL and rating score of 0) and 2 indicated maximal noise sensitivity (i.e., LDL score = 0 dB HL and rating score of 4).

Tinnitus patients had experienced tinnitus for at least 4 months [mean (SD) = 12.5 (17.6) years], and reported no history of clinical hyperacusis or phonophobia. Best frequency-match to dominant tinnitus pitch was typically high [mean (SD) = 4,612 (3,073) Hz], and most reported bilateral tinnitus ($n = 18$). The reported etiology of tinnitus was variable and included change in hearing due to loud noise exposure or other factors ($n = 7$), combined hearing change and head trauma (2), ear or sinus infection (4), unknown or unspecified causes (8), and other factors (2). Tinnitus patients completed two questionnaires related to tinnitus, including the Tinnitus Handicap Inventory (THI) to measure tinnitus impact or distress (Newman et al., 1996) and the TSCHQ to assess tinnitus characteristics. We used three individual questions from the TSCHQ in our analyses. One question measured perceived sensitivity to noise as described above. The other two questions assessed auditory-perceptual characteristics of tinnitus, including the perceived loudness of tinnitus and the percentage of time patients were typically aware of their tinnitus throughout the day (i.e., "awareness"). The latter two questions are worded as follows: (1) *Describe the loudness of your tinnitus using a scale from 1 to 100,* and (2) *What percentage of your total awake time, over the last month, have you been aware of your tinnitus? For example, 100% would indicate that you were aware of your tinnitus all the time, and 25% would indicate that you were aware of your tinnitus one fourth of the time.*

NEUROLOGICAL HISTORY AND QUESTIONNAIRES

Participants reported aspects of their medical history during MRI safety screening and the TSCHQ, including history of minor closed-head injury, mood disorder, and current use of neuromodulatory medications. This information is reported in **Table 1**. A subset of participants reported either a history of mood disorder or current use of neuromodulatory medications (six tinnitus patients, three controls). Of these participants, five reported history of mood disorder (three tinnitus, two control), including depression (two tinnitus, two control), anxiety (two tinnitus), and mild bipolar disorder (one tinnitus). Five participants (four tinnitus, one control) were taking neuromodulatory medication at the time of the study, including GABA agonists or analogues (three patients, one control) and drugs targeting the serotonin system (two patients). These participants were singled out for further analyses.

Participants completed three questionnaires designed to assess symptoms of depression and anxiety: PHQ9 [Patient Health Questionnaire 9, depression; (Kroenke et al., 2001)], GAD7 [Generalized Anxiety Disorder; (Spitzer et al., 2006)], HADS [Hospital Anxiety and Depression Scale (Zigmond and Snaith, 1983)]. The depression and anxiety subscales of the HADS inventory were highly correlated with the PHQ9 and GAD7, respectively ($r = 0.77$, $t_{(42)} = 7.92$, $p < 0.0001$, and $r = 0.85$, $t_{(42)} = 10.33$, $p < 0.0001$), and are not discussed further. Depression and anxiety scores were also highly intercorrelated (PHQ9 × GAD: $r = 0.81$, $t_{(42)} = 8.92$, $p < 0.0001$); therefore, PHQ9 and GAD7 measures were summed to create a combined depression and anxiety score for each participant to be used in subsequent analyses.

STATISTICAL ANALYSIS OF AUDIOMETRIC AND QUESTIONNAIRE DATA

Data acquired during the audiological exam and on questionnaires were analyzed using Matlab's Statistics Toolbox

(*Mathworks*). Student's t-tests assessed differences between group means on these measures. Equal variance was assumed between groups for those characteristics that were deliberately matched during recruitment (i.e., age), and unequal variance was assumed for all other tests (i.e., mean hearing loss, combined noise sensitivity scores, combined depression and anxiety scores). Chi-squared tests were used to assess differences between groups on categorical data (i.e., sex, history of head injury, history of mood disorder or neuromodulatory medication). Correction for multiple tests was implemented using Bonferroni's method, by dividing alpha by the total number of tests (t or Chi-squared) performed (7). Relationships between tinnitus symptoms and other patient characteristics were tested using multiple linear regression; no post hoc corrections were applied.

IMAGE ACQUISITION

Images were acquired using a 3.0 Tesla Siemens TIM Trio scanner. A high-resolution anatomical scan (MPRAGE) was performed for each subject, using a sequence that optimizes image contrast between white and gray matter. MPRAGE parameters were as follows: TR = 2530 ms, TE = 3.5 ms, inversion time = 1100 ms, flip angle = 7°, 176 sagittal slices, matrix size $256 \times 256\,\text{mm}^2$, $1 \times 1 \times 1\,\text{mm}^3$ resolution.

IMAGE PROCESSING AND ANALYSIS: VOLUME-BASED MORPHOMETRY

Volumetric analyses were done using VBM in SPM8 (*Wellcome Trust Centre for Neuroimaging*) using the DARTEL (Diffeomorphic Anatomical Registration Through Exponentiated Lie Algebra; Ashburner, 2007) toolbox. Images were first corrected for inhomogeneities in intensity, and segmented by tissue type using tissue probability templates native to SPM8 (International Consortium for Brain Mapping, www.loni.ucla.edu/ICBM). Study-specific templates were then created using GM images from all subjects. GM images were aligned to this study-specific template, warped to MNI space, and modulated to reflect the amount of deformation applied during normalization (i.e., Jacobian scaling). Images were smoothed with a $6\,\text{mm}^3$ FWHM Gaussian kernel, and corrected for total GM volume using proportional scaling. Resulting images were thresholded at 0.20 probability of tissue classification prior to statistical analyses. Between-groups comparisons were conducted voxel-wise across the entire brain, with compensation for unequal variance between groups (i.e., "non-sphericity" correction). Peak MNI coordinates are reported.

Morphometric techniques that rely on tissue segmentation, like VBM, may not be optimal for assessing subcortical structures containing multiple types of tissue (i.e., both white and gray matter) (Ashburner and Friston, 2000). Therefore, additional volumetric analyses of subcortical structures were performed using Freesurfer software version 1.313.2.6 (www.surfer.nmr.mgh.harvard.edu). Images were first corrected for intensity bias and normalized into MNI space. Subcortical structures in these images were identified with an automated procedure that estimates the probability of structure-classification based on prior templates in which those structures were manually identified (Fischl et al., 2002). Subcortical structures identified using this method include the thalamus, caudate, putamen, globus pallidus, nucleus accumbens, amygdala, and hippocampus. Once segmented, the total volume of these structures was calculated in each hemisphere. Because results were similar in each hemisphere, volumes for both hemispheres were summed for statistical analyses reported here. Between-groups differences in total volume were assessed for each structure with Student's t-tests assuming unequal variance, using the percentage of total subcortical volume as the dependent measure. Because no tests survived a Bonferroni-correction for the number of t-tests performed (7), uncorrected p-values are reported.

IMAGE PROCESSING AND ANALYSIS: SURFACE-BASED MORPHOMETRY

Surface-based analyses were done using Freesurfer. In an automated procedure, images were corrected for intensity bias, and segmented into cortical gray and white matter to reconstruct gray and white matter surfaces. Reconstructed surfaces were inflated, sphere-ized, and aligned with Freesurfer's template average. Automated segmentation of the cortex failed in one tinnitus patient; this participant's data was excluded from surface-based analyses.

For each point (i.e., vertex) on the successfully reconstructed surfaces, values were calculated for pial surface area, thickness, volume (the product of surface area and thickness), and gyrification (i.e., curvature). These data were smoothed in surface-space using a $10\,\text{mm}^2$ FWHM Gaussian kernel. A larger kernel is desirable here because smoothing is more likely to occur within tissue type (i.e., gray matter). Between-groups comparisons (i.e., controls > patients) and correlation analyses were conducted vertex-wise across the entire cortex using the general linear model (GLM). Data were not corrected for head size because: (1) significant clusters obtained from the GLM were not correlated with head size and (2) including, e.g., total gray matter volume as a "nuisance" covariate in the GLM did not qualitatively affect the results (data not shown). Peak MNI coordinates are reported.

Region-of-interest (ROI) analyses were also performed. All ROI analyses used the average value (surface area, thickness, or gyrification) for all vertices within the ROI patch as the dependent measure. ROI analyses included t-tests (Student's t) with unequal variance assumed between groups, ANCOVA analyses (group × relevant covariate), and correlation analyses (Pearson's r).

In those regions exhibiting reductions in GM volume in tinnitus patients compared to controls in the whole-head, surface-based analyses, ROI analyses were performed to determine whether volume differences could be explained by differences in surface area, thickness, gyrification, or some combination of these factors. One-tailed t-tests were used here, because, for example, a reduction in gray matter in tinnitus patients would be unlikely to be accompanied by increased cortical thickness. Bonferroni-corrections were applied for the total number of ROI tests (12).

To determine whether non-tinnitus factors affected anatomical differences identified between tinnitus patients and controls, we conducted ROI ANCOVAs, using the morphological feature that best described "volume" differences in each ROI (surface area, thickness, or gyrification). ANCOVAs allowed us to measure differences between groups while statistically controlling for the effects of three separate covariates: mean hearing loss, combined depression and anxiety scores, or combined noise sensitivity scores. T-statistics on the between-groups differences are reported with one-tailed significance values as above, and Bonferroni-adjustments were made for the number of tests in each ROI (3).

ROI analyses also measured the relationship between tinnitus characteristics and cortical morphology in those regions exhibiting significant differences between tinnitus patients and controls. Tinnitus characteristics tested included the number of years since tinnitus onset, tinnitus loudness ratings, the percentage of time patients reported being aware of their tinnitus, and total THI score (i.e., tinnitus distress). One-tailed tests were performed, as we hypothesized that tinnitus patients with more severe symptoms (e.g., louder tinnitus) would exhibit morphology less like controls. Because no tests survived a Bonferroni-correction for the number of correlation tests performed (4 per ROI), uncorrected p-values are reported.

RESULTS

RELATIONSHIPS BETWEEN TINNITUS, TINNITUS SYMPTOMS, AND "NON-TINNITUS" FACTORS

In order to determine whether chronic tinnitus was concomitant with other non-tinnitus factors, we compared tinnitus patients and controls in a variety of measures (**Table 1**). Tinnitus patients were deliberately matched by age and sex during recruitment; the groups did not differ on these dimensions (age: $t_{(42)} = 0.39$, $p_{corr} = 1$; sex: $X^2_{(1)} = 0.35$, $p_{corr} = 1$). Tinnitus patients also did not differ from controls in mean hearing loss ($t_{(42)} = 2.11$, $p_{corr} = 0.14$) or depression and anxiety scores ($t_{(35)} = 2.02$, $p_{corr} = 0.18$; depression and anxiety scores were highly intercorrelated and thus combined). The proportion of people reporting lifetime incidence of depression, anxiety, or mood-targeting medications did not differ between groups ($X^2_{(1)} = 0.33$, $p_{corr} = 1$), nor did the incidence of head injury differ between groups ($X^2_{(1)} = 0.79$, $p_{corr} = 1$). Tinnitus patients did score significantly higher in noise sensitivity scores ($t_{(35)} = 6.26$, $p_{corr} = 0.04 \times 10^{-6}$), despite the absence of clinical diagnosis of hyperacusis. Although this indicates a heightened sensitivity to noise on average, many patients overlapped with the range of noise sensitivity scores in controls. Thus, the presence of tinnitus in these patients cannot be fully explained by any of these factors alone.

We also assessed the extent to which the severity of tinnitus can be predicted by other factors, using regression analyses to target two symptoms: tinnitus distress and tinnitus loudness. Tinnitus distress was best predicted by combined depression and anxiety scores ($r = 0.71$, $t_{(17)} = 3.13$, $p = 0.006$). No other factor explained a significant amount of variance in tinnitus distress, including mean hearing loss ($r = 0.14$, $t_{(17)} = 1.41$, $p = 0.18$), noise sensitivity ($r = 0.39$, $t_{(17)} = -0.43$, $p = 0.67$), percent time aware of tinnitus ($r = 0.54$, $t_{(17)} = 0.85$, $p = 0.41$), or tinnitus loudness ($r = 0.31$, $t_{(17)} = 0.40$, $p = 0.70$).

Tinnitus loudness was not significantly related to combined depression and anxiety scores ($r = 0.23$, $t_{(17)} = -1.33$, $p = 0.20$) or tinnitus distress ($r = 0.31$, $t_{(17)} = 0.40$, $p = 0.70$). Instead, the perceived loudness of tinnitus was best predicted by the amount of time patients reported being aware of their tinnitus ($r = 0.56$, $t_{(17)} = 2.39$, $p = 0.03$), and to a lesser extent noise sensitivity scores ($r = 0.48$, $t_{(17)} = 2.15$, $p = 0.05$). Degree of hearing loss was also not a good predictor of tinnitus loudness ($r = 0.05$, $t_{(17)} = 0.53$, $p = 0.60$). These data suggest that the severity of the auditory-perceptual symptoms of tinnitus (e.g., loudness) cannot be explained by ongoing emotional or distressed reactions to tinnitus, and are consistent with previous reports (Hiller and Goebel, 2006).

TINNITUS-RELATED DIFFERENCES IN CORTICAL ANATOMY

Using a single-voxel DARTEL-VBM analysis across the entire brain, we identified regions with significantly different GM volume in tinnitus patients as compared to controls ($p < 0.002$, $k > 3.0\ mm^3$; **Figure 2**). Tinnitus patients exhibited significantly less GM volume in ventromedial prefrontal cortex (vmPFC) compared to control participants (MNI coordinates X,Y,Z = 2, 21, –15). Additional GM reductions were identified in dorsomedial prefrontal cortex (dmPFC; MNI coordinates X,Y,Z = 2, 38, 39) and left supramarginal gyrus (SMG; MNI coordinates X,Y,Z = 59, –40, 24) adjacent to posterior auditory cortex. Tinnitus patients did not show greater GM volume than controls in any part of the brain at our chosen threshold.

These tinnitus-related reductions in GM volume were confirmed using a different approach targeting the entire cortical

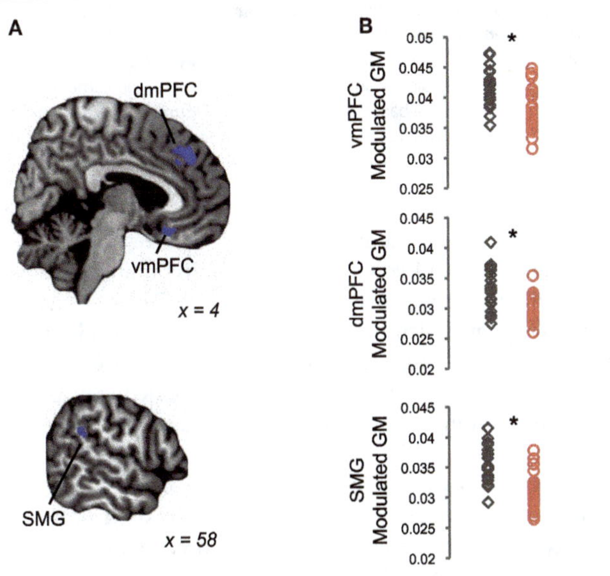

FIGURE 2 | Reductions in gray matter in tinnitus, using a volume-based analysis. (A) Tinnitus patients showed reduced GM volume in ventromedial prefrontal cortex (vmPFC), dorsomedial prefrontal cortex (dmPFC), and supramarginal gyrus (SMG), as compared to control participants in a whole-brain voxel-based morphometry (VBM) analysis (blue). Statistical maps of between-groups differences are shown on parasagittal slices through single-subject template anatomy; the X-dimension in MNI space is displayed for each view. **(B)** Plots show mean modulated GM values in each cluster shown in **(A)** for each tinnitus patient (red) and control participant (gray). Asterisks indicate a significant difference between groups, as assessed by the whole-brain analysis in **(A)**.

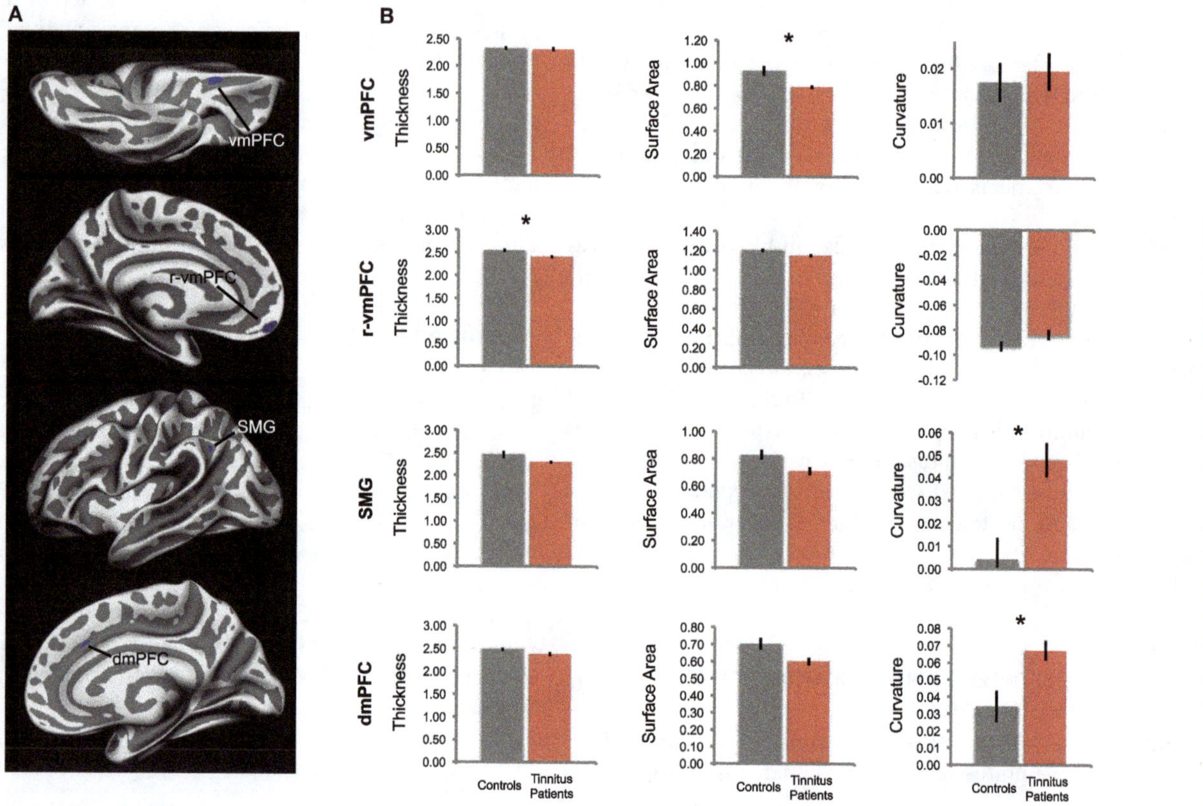

FIGURE 3 | Differences in cortical morphology in tinnitus, in a surface-based analysis. (A) Tinnitus-related reductions in GM volume are confirmed in a single-vertex analysis across the entire cortical surface. Tinnitus patients had significantly smaller GM volumes in the same areas identified in the volume-based analysis shown in **Figure 1**, vmPFC, dmPFC, and SMG, as well as an additional cluster in rostral vmPFC (r-vmPFC). **(B)** For each cluster in **(A)**, the mean values of morphological features are plotted, including cortical thickness, surface area, and gyrification (curvature) for each group. For gyrification, positive values indicate sulci, negative values indicate gyri. Tinnitus patients are plotted in red; control participants are plotted in gray. Error bars represent standard error, and asterisks denote significant difference between groups ($p_{corr} < 0.05$).

surface (i.e., a surface-based analysis in Freesurfer). Again, significantly less GM volume was detected in tinnitus patients in left vmPFC in the olfactory sulcus, right dmPFC in the outer bank of the cingulate sulcus, and left SMG ($p < 0.005$; **Figure 3A**). An additional left vmPFC region also exhibited less GM volume in tinnitus patients than controls but was located rostral to the one identified during volume-based analysis, which was near the frontal pole (r-vmPFC).

Reduced GM volume in tinnitus patients could be explained by smaller surface area, thinner cortex, decreased gyrification, or some combination of these factors. Therefore, we used ROI analyses to assess the morphometric origin of volume differences in these four areas (**Figure 3B**). In posterior vmPFC, volume reductions were best explained by a reduction in cortical surface area ($t_{(25)} = 3.22$, $p_{corr} = 0.02$). Cortical thickness and gyrification were not different in this region between groups ($t_{(39)} = 0.38$, $p_{corr} = 1$; $t_{(41)} = -0.41$, $p_{corr} = 1$).

In SMG, cortical thickness and surface area did not differ between groups ($t_{(28)} = 2.00$, $p_{corr} = 0.33$; $t_{(39)} = 2.53$, $p_{corr} = 0.09$); instead, gyrification differed between groups ($t_{(38)} = -3.61$, $p_{corr} = 0.005$). Specifically, the sulcus on which the ROI was located was deeper in tinnitus patients than controls (positive values indicate sulci, negative values indicate gyri). Similarly, the volume difference in dmPFC is again best explained by differences in sulcal depth ($t_{(34)} = -3.00$, $p_{corr} = 0.03$); cortical thickness and surface area did not differ in dmPFC ($t_{(40)} = 1.85$, $p_{corr} = 0.43$; $t_{(34)} = 2.54$, $p_{corr} = 0.10$). These differences in gyrification in SMG and dmPFC were associated with a trend toward corresponding reduction in surface area ($p_{corr} = 0.09$ and $p_{corr} = 0.10$, respectively), consistent with the idea that deeper sulci typically contain less cortical tissue than other parts of the cortical surface (Fischl and Dale, 2000).

In rostral vmPFC, cortex was thinner in tinnitus patients than in controls ($t_{(41)} = 2.89$, $p_{corr} = 0.04$). No significant differences were indicated in gyrification ($t_{(41)} = -1.65$, $p_{corr} = 0.64$) or surface area ($t_{(41)} = 2.33$, $p_{corr} = 0.15$) in this region.

TINNITUS-RELATED DIFFERENCES IN SUBCORTICAL ANATOMY

The volume of subcortical structures, including the thalamus, caudate, putamen, globus pallidus, nucleus accumbens, amygdala, and hippocampus, did not differ between tinnitus patients and controls (**Table 2**). There was a trend toward increased volume in the left hippocampus of tinnitus patients ($t_{(39)} = 1.90$, $p = 0.07$), but this difference was not statistically significant.

Table 2 | Volume of subcortical structures in tinnitus patients and control participants.

	Patients (mean, sd)	Controls (mean, sd)	Statistics (t, p)
Thalamus	3.97 (0.33)	3.91 (0.31)	−0.06, 0.54
Caudate	2.12 (0.23)	2.08 (0.23)	−0.07, 0.53
Putamen	3.03 (0.33)	3.01 (0.36)	−0.17, 0.86
Globus pallidus	1.01 (0.09)	0.96 (0.12)	−1.57, 0.13
Nucleus accumbens	0.31 (0.03)	0.31 (0.04)	−0.09, 0.93
Amygdala	0.87 (0.08)	0.85 (0.08)	−0.99, 0.34
Hippocampus	2.23 (0.18)	2.18 (0.17)	−1.06, 0.31

Note: Volume measures displayed are the percent of total subcortical volume. Statistics reflect the result of t tests, unequal variance assumed.

CORTICAL DIFFERENCES IN TINNITUS AND THEIR RELATIONSHIPS TO NON-TINNITUS FACTORS

Next, we sought to determine whether non-tinnitus factors affected anatomical differences we identified between tinnitus patients and controls (**Figure 4**). In the regions of interest (ROIs) defined above, we performed ANCOVAs using the morphological feature that best described "volume" differences in those regions (i.e., surface area for vmPFC, thickness in rostral vmPFC, and gyrification for SMG and dmPFC). Differences were measured between groups while statistically controlling for the potential influence of three separate covariates: mean hearing loss, combined depression and anxiety scores, and combined noise sensitivity scores.

In vmPFC, morphological differences observed between tinnitus patients and controls were not driven by non-tinnitus factors. Differences between these groups in vmPFC were significant when controlling for the influence of hearing loss ($t_{(39)} = 2.98$, $p_{corr} = 0.008$), noise sensitivity ($t_{(36)} = 2.27$, $p_{corr} = 0.04$), and combined depression and anxiety scores ($t_{(39)} = 3.21$, $p_{corr} = 0.004$). Differences in surface area in vmPFC are thus likely to be related to the presence of tinnitus, and not other factors.

In dmPFC, there was a non-significant trend toward a difference between groups when controlling for noise sensitivity ($t_{(36)} = 2.03$, $p_{corr} = 0.08$). After correcting for an outlier (>3 SD below patients' mean), the tinnitus-related difference in morphology was indeed significant ($t_{(35)} = 2.30$, $p_{corr} = 0.04$). Hearing loss and depression/anxiety scores did not influence the difference between groups in dmPFC ($t_{(38)} = 3.39$, $p_{corr} = 0.003$ and $t_{(38)} = 3.38$, $p_{corr} = 0.003$, respectively).

In SMG and rostral vmPFC, between-groups differences were not driven by hearing loss or depression/anxiety scores, but were influenced by noise sensitivity. In SMG, differences between tinnitus patients and controls were not significant when statistically controlling for noise sensitivity scores ($t_{(36)} = 1.44$, $p_{corr} = 0.24$). In addition, there was an overall trend toward a positive correlation between noise sensitivity and SMG curvature in both groups ($F_{(1, 36)} = 2.09$, $p = 0.16$). This indicates that the difference in gyrification we identified between tinnitus patients and controls in SMG may be due to differences in noise sensitivity between these participants. In ROI analyses including mean hearing loss and depression/anxiety scores as "nuisance" covariates, between-groups differences were significant ($t_{(39)} = 3.86$, $p_{corr} = 0.0006$ and $t_{(39)} = 3.12$, $p_{corr} = 0.005$, respectively).

A similar pattern was observed in rostral vmPFC, in which differences in cortical thickness between tinnitus patients and controls were not significant when taking noise sensitivity scores into account ($t_{(36)} = 0.76$, $p_{corr} = 0.68$). Noise sensitivity scores were also modestly correlated with cortical thickness in this region ($F_{(1, 36)} = 2.87$, $p = 0.10$). Differences between groups were significant in analyses controlling for mean hearing loss and depression/anxiety scores in rostral vmPFC ($t_{(39)} = 2.57$, $p_{corr} = 0.02$ and $t_{(39)} = 2.57$, $p_{corr} = 0.02$, respectively).

TINNITUS CHARACTERISTICS AND BRAIN ANATOMY

The previous analysis identified two areas of the brain with significant anatomical differences between tinnitus patients and controls when controlling for non-tinnitus factors: vmPFC and dmPFC. ROI analyses in these two areas determined whether their morphology related to the severity of tinnitus distress or other symptoms (**Figure 5**). In dmPFC, a significant positive correlation was present with the percentage of time participants were aware of their tinnitus ($p = 0.02$, after removal of outlier described above). Thus, patients with deeper sulci reported being aware of their tinnitus more often than those with dmPFC gyrificiation similar to control participants. A modest negative correlation was also indicated between vmPFC surface area and tinnitus loudness ($p = 0.06$), such that those patients with the highest loudness ratings also exhibited the greatest reductions in cortical surface area. No other correlations were significant ($p > 0.05$).

Correlations between cortical morphology (thickness, surface area, and gyrification) and tinnitus characteristics were also measured across the entire brain ($p < 0.0005$, $k > 70$ vertices; **Figure 6**). Tinnitus distress was positively correlated with cortical thickness in anterior insula (aIns). Percent of time patients reported being aware of their tinnitus positively correlated with STG thickness and SMG surface area. There was an additional area in the postcentral gyrus (PCG) that showed a positive correlation between cortical thickness and duration since the onset of tinnitus. No area in the brain exhibited correlations between tinnitus loudness ratings and whole-brain morphology.

In a post hoc ROI analysis, cortical thickness in aIns was positively correlated with combined depression and anxiety scores in patients ($r = 0.78$, $p < 0.0001$). However, this relationship was not present in controls ($r = -0.16$, $p = 0.50$).

DEPRESSION AND ANXIETY

We also assessed the relationship between cortical anatomy and measures of anxiety and depression across the whole brain using the surface-based approach. We looked specifically for negative correlations between depression and anxiety and cortical thickness, in light of previous evidence linking these disorders to cortical volume reductions in scACC. Indeed, we saw a negative correlation between combined depression and anxiety scores (see Methods) and cortical thickness in scACC, when combining data

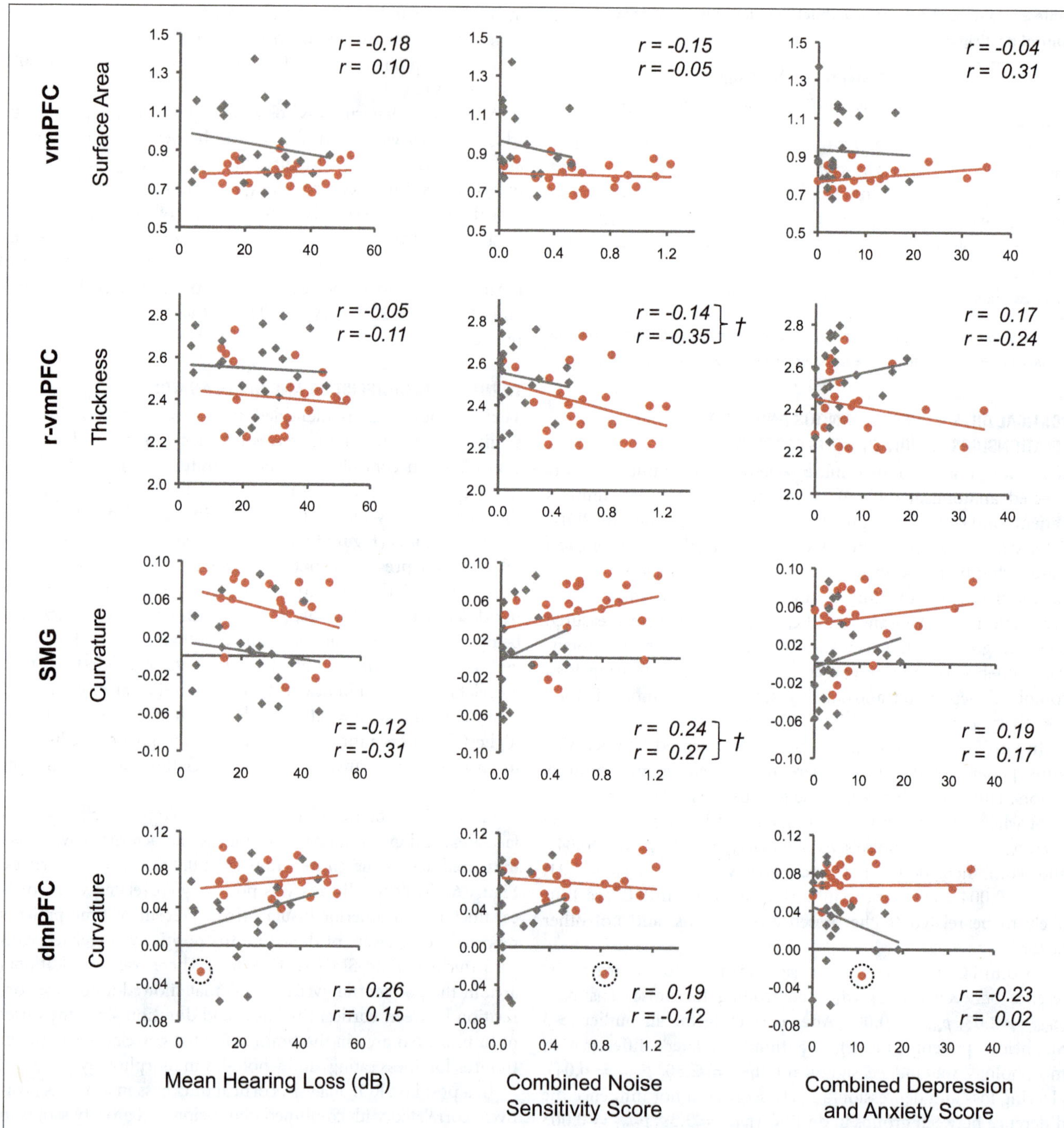

FIGURE 4 | Tinnitus-related cortical morphology and non-tinnitus factors. Scatterplots show the relationship between morphological features that best explain differences between tinnitus patients and controls in posterior vmPFC, rostral vmPFC, dmPFC, and SMG, and non-tinnitus factors. The mean value is plotted for each tinnitus patient (red) and control (gray) in each cluster, against mean hearing loss (left), noise sensitivity (middle), and combined depression and anxiety scores (right). Regression lines are plotted for each group, and insets display corresponding Pearson's *r* values for patients (red) and controls (black). Crosses (†) mark those plots for which ANCOVA analysis failed to find a difference between groups, and also indicated moderate correlation between morphological features and non-tinnitus factors. An outlier with dmPFC curvature >3 SD below the mean of tinnitus patients is encircled with a dashed line.

from both tinnitus patients and controls ($p < 0.005$; **Figure 7**; MNI coordinates $X,Y,Z = 6, 24, -8$; $k = 12\ \text{mm}^2$). An additional cluster was identified in dorsal ACC (MNI coordinates $X,Y,Z = 6, 14, 32$; $k = 19\ \text{mm}^2$).

DISCUSSION

In our structural MRI study, we identified morphological markers of tinnitus, and assessed the relationship between these markers and various tinnitus characteristics and non-tinnitus factors

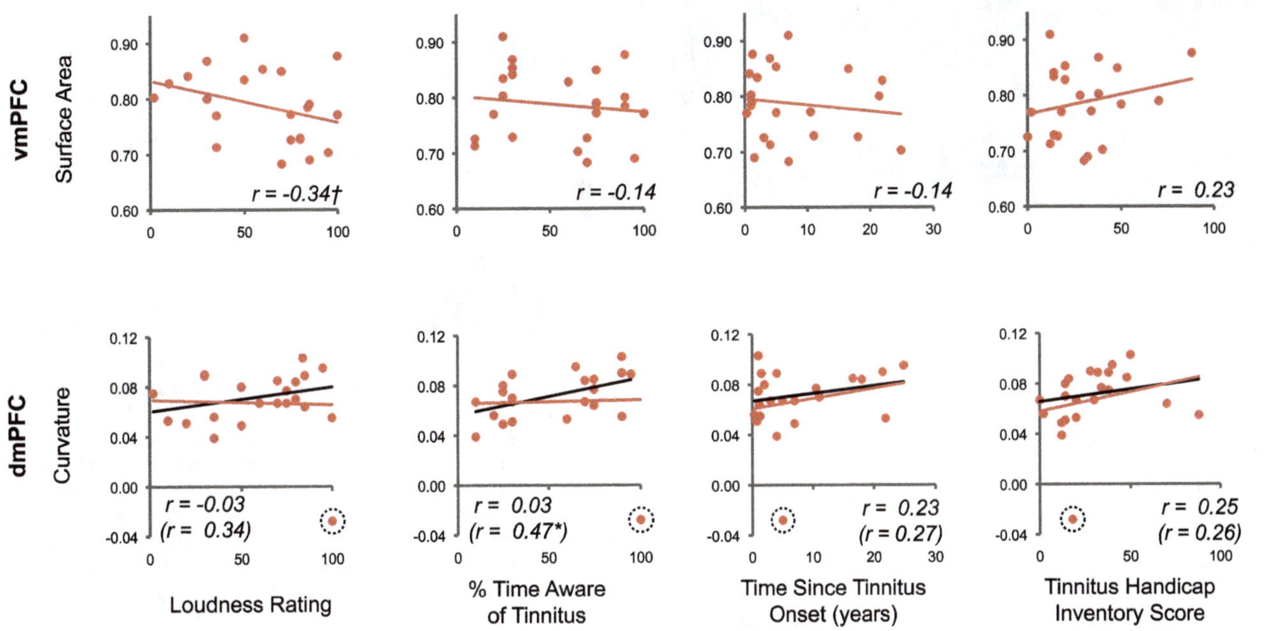

FIGURE 5 | Relationship between tinnitus severity and anatomical markers of tinnitus. For those clusters exhibiting a robust anatomical difference between tinnitus patients and controls, the relationship between morphological features and tinnitus characteristics are shown. Values for each subject are plotted, with corresponding regression lines and Pearson's *r* values. A modest negative correlation was indicated between vmPFC surface area and tinnitus loudness (†$p = 0.06$, one-tailed test). A significant correlation was also apparent between dmPFC curvature and the percentage of time patients reported being aware of their tinnitus after removal of a statistical outlier (*$p = 0.02$, one-tailed test). Black regression lines and *r* statistics in parentheses reflect the results of correlation analyses performed after removing this outlier.

linked to tinnitus like depression, anxiety, and noise sensitivity. We confirmed the association between tinnitus and reduced GM in vmPFC in an entirely new set of subjects, and identified a new tinnitus-related effect in dmPFC. These morphological differences in vmPFC and dmPFC were not affected by non-tinnitus factors or tinnitus distress, but seem to be related to auditory-perceptual characteristics of tinnitus. Tinnitus distress, on the other hand, was linked to variability in cortical thickness in the anterior insula, while depression and anxiety scores predicted cortical thickness in scACC in both tinnitus patients and controls. In addition, we report that noise sensitivity may be related to anatomy in SMG and rostral vmPFC. Taken together, our data suggest that the neural systems related to the tinnitus perception itself are distinct from those affected by tinnitus distress, mood disorders, and noise sensitivity. We take this to mean that aversive or affective reactions to the tinnitus percept may not be necessary for chronic tinnitus to develop, although future research is needed to directly address causality. Regardless, the possibility that the perceptual characteristics of tinnitus are separable from ongoing affective reactions should be considered in current models of tinnitus pathophysiology and in approaches to treatment.

THE ROLE OF MIDLINE FRONTAL CORTEX IN TINNITUS

In a subregion of vmPFC, we identified GM reductions in a third group of tinnitus patients, providing confirmation of our previous studies (Mühlau et al., 2006; Leaver et al., 2011). We also presented two additional novel findings in the current paper regarding vmPFC morphology. First, we showed that the anatomical anomaly (i.e., GM reduction) in vmPFC of tinnitus patients is due to a reduction in cortical surface area, not cortical thinning or gyrification. Methods used in previous studies have been unable to examine morphology in such detail (Mühlau et al., 2006; Landgrebe et al., 2009; Husain et al., 2011; Leaver et al., 2011; Mahoney et al., 2011). In addition, we demonstrated that reduced gray matter in vmPFC is not correlated with depression, anxiety, or tinnitus distress, suggesting that GM reductions in vmPFC are not likely to be caused by the aversiveness of tinnitus or stress caused by the disorder. Instead, morphology in this area was modestly correlated with the perceptual loudness of the tinnitus sensation, indicating that vmPFC is related to the perception of tinnitus and is thus part of the gating system postulated previously (Rauschecker et al., 2010).

Because the relationship between midline frontal areas and affect is well documented (Drevets et al., 1997; Mayberg, 1997; Koenigs and Grafman, 2009), it was important to show that tinnitus-related effects in vmPFC were not due to, for example, cell death resulting from prolonged exposure to an aversive sound (i.e., tinnitus). If ongoing emotional reactions to tinnitus caused GM loss in vmPFC, one would expect the severity of that loss to correlate with how annoyed or bothered each patient was by his or her tinnitus, or perhaps with the amount of time since the onset of the disorder. We found neither of these to be true. The morphology of this subregion of vmPFC seems to have no bearing on ongoing negative or emotional reactions to tinnitus.

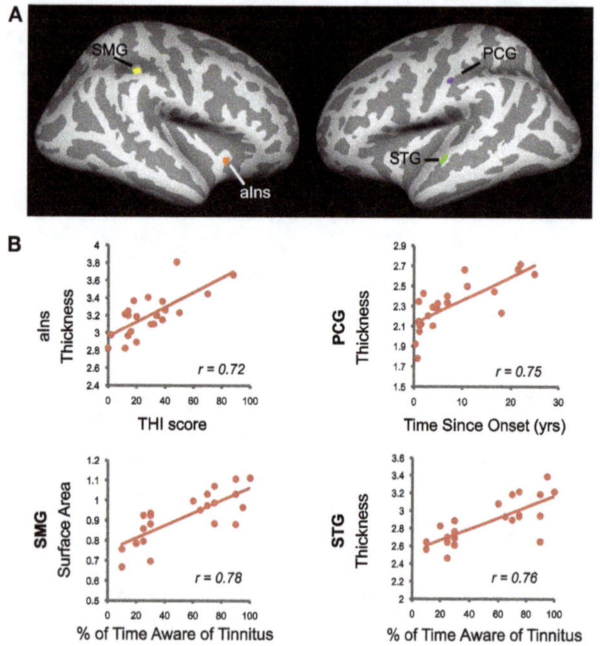

FIGURE 6 | Tinnitus characteristics and cortical anatomy. (A) Correlations between cortical morphology and tinnitus characteristics are displayed on the cortical surface. Positive correlation between tinnitus distress and cortical thickness in anterior insula (aIns) is shown in orange. Positive correlations between the percentage of time patients reported being aware of their tinnitus were present in two areas: supramarginal gyrus (SMG) surface area in yellow and superior temporal gyrus (STG) thickness in green. A purple cluster indicates a positive correlation between time since tinnitus onset and cortical thickness in postcentral gyrus (PCG). **(B)** Scatterplots show mean data for the clusters identified in **(A)**. Values are indicated for each tinnitus patient, with regression lines and Pearson's *r* values shown.

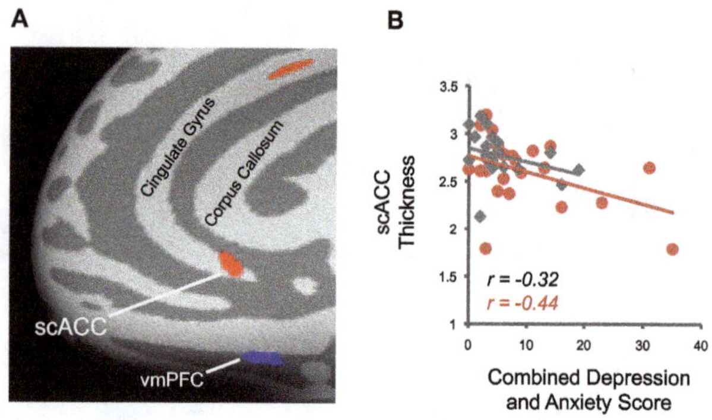

FIGURE 7 | Relationship between depression and anxiety and cortical thickness. (A) Right subcallosal anterior cingulate cortex (scACC) and dorsal anterior cingulate cortex exhibited a negative relationship between combined depression and anxiety scores and cortical thickness (red). The mirrored location of reduced gray matter volume in tinnitus patients in left vmPFC (**Figure 3A**, top panel) is also displayed for reference (blue), illustrating the spatial dissociation of the two effects. The inflated surface was rotated from the medial aspect of the brain along the y-axis so that all clusters are within view. **(B)** Data from the scACC cluster shown in **(A)** is plotted for each tinnitus patient (red) and control (gray). Regression lines and Pearson's *r* values for each group are displayed, which show the negative relationship between depression/anxiety scores and cortical morphology in this region.

We did identify a relationship between symptoms of anxiety and depression (as measured by questionnaire) and cortical thickness in scACC, close to but clearly separate from tinnitus-related reductions in vmPFC surface area. The scACC has been implicated in mood disorders (Drevets et al., 1997; Mayberg, 1997; Hamani et al., 2011), and is a target of deep brain stimulation treatment for major depression (Lozano et al., 2008). Tinnitus itself is sometimes comorbid with depression (Sullivan et al., 1988; Folmer et al., 1999; Dobie, 2003; Robinson et al., 2008), and even our own behavioral data indicated a (non-significant) tendency for tinnitus patients to score higher on measures of depression and anxiety (uncorrected $p = 0.06$; **Table 1**). However, this correlation between scACC thickness and symptoms of depression and anxiety was present in both tinnitus patients and controls, and there was no difference between groups in cortical thickness in this area. Thus, these data suggest a dissociation between midline frontal areas affected in depression from those affected in tinnitus perception. The extent to which the pathophysiology of depression overlaps with that of anxiety and other mood disorders is an ongoing area of research (e.g., Savitz and Drevets, 2009) and may be informative in future studies of tinnitus and tinnitus-related suffering.

Although midline frontal cortex as a whole might be involved in both affective processing and tinnitus (De Ridder et al., 2011), our data indicate a spatial dissociation within this region between tinnitus-related (vmPFC) and mood-related (scACC) effects (**Figure 7A**). This underscores the importance of appreciating the rich functional heterogeneity within midline frontal cortex (Ongür et al., 2003) when examining the functional and structural effects of tinnitus in this part of the brain. All VBM studies of tinnitus thus far have used comparable imaging parameters, including voxel resolution, and smoothing (Mühlau et al., 2006; Landgrebe et al., 2009; Husain et al., 2011; Leaver et al., 2011; Mahoney et al., 2011); however, most of these studies have not distinguished between tinnitus, tinnitus distress, and negative mood. Our current data indicate that tinnitus research that does not measure symptoms of anxiety and depression as well as tinnitus may run the risk of not unraveling tinnitus-related effects in vmPFC (Landgrebe et al., 2009; Husain et al., 2011; Mahoney et al., 2011), or conflating the latter with mood-related effects in scACC (Mühlau et al., 2006; Leaver et al., 2011).

Indeed, we identified an additional midline structure, dmPFC, which showed tinnitus-related effects complementary to those seen in vmPFC. As in vmPFC, morphological differences in dmPFC were not affected by depression, anxiety, or tinnitus distress. Instead, dmPFC morphology, characterized as a difference in cortical curvature, was related to an auditory-perceptual characteristic of tinnitus—awareness, or the proportion of time patients were aware of their tinnitus. This suggests that these two areas may play complementary roles in tinnitus. To the best of our knowledge, these findings in dmPFC are novel, and may result from superior image-alignment afforded by the methods used in the current study (i.e., DARTEL-VBM and cortex-based alignment in Freesurfer). Future studies delineating the respective roles of these regions in tinnitus will contribute to the ongoing debate regarding the differential function of dorsal and ventral regions of medial frontal cortex in other domains (Steele and Lawrie, 2004; Etkin et al., 2011; Shackman et al., 2011).

What causes these morphological differences in midline frontal cortex between tinnitus patients and controls remains to be determined. In terms of timing, our data suggest two hypotheses: that the relative size (and cellular make-up) of vmPFC is determined prior to tinnitus onset, or that GM loss in vmPFC occurs soon after the onset of the disorder. In our data, GM levels in vmPFC and dmPFC were the same whether patients had tinnitus for their entire lives or only 4–6 months (**Figure 5**); longitudinal studies could capture morphological changes over the first few months of tinnitus onset to determine which hypothesis is correct. Apart from timing, there are several possible causes for tinnitus-related differences in vmPFC, which are not mutually exclusive. Genetic factors may determine vmPFC size from birth, or they may cause midline frontal regions to be more vulnerable to stressors or lesions. Environmental factors like chronic stress, depression, or mechanical injuries may also cause cell loss in vmPFC or connected midline structures, or may make the area more susceptible to damage. Indeed, mechanical injuries, such as head trauma or blast injury, can specifically affect ventral frontal regions (Mattson and Levin, 1990; Fujiwara et al., 2008). In theory, damage to a single subregion may also affect other parts of the midline and orbital frontal system, as these areas are richly interconnected (Ongür and Price, 2000). In addition to longitudinal studies to determine timing, histological studies would be useful in determining the cellular bases of tinnitus-related differences in midline frontal cortex. So, although stressful life events or depression may be one way of damaging or over-working this system and causing chronic tinnitus (e.g., combined with sensorineural hearing loss), we argue that it is only one of many ways that the vmPFC-network can be compromised in tinnitus pathophysiology.

Overall, our data are consistent with the idea that midline frontal areas are involved in regulating interoceptive functions, including bodily sensations like pain (Kuchinad et al., 2007), emotions (Drevets et al., 1997; Mayberg, 1997), or even unwanted thoughts or actions (Floresco et al., 2009). In the context of tinnitus, we propose that an "intact" vmPFC is able to suppress aberrant thalamocortical activity in the auditory system (e.g., tinnitus), through its "driver" inputs to inhibitory neurons in the subsection of the reticular nucleus near auditory thalamus (Zikopoulos and Barbas, 2006). If vmPFC is compromised, this circuit is less efficient in regulating unwanted activity, and tinnitus persists (Mühlau et al., 2006; Rauschecker et al., 2010). In the model we propose, a negative or emotional reaction to tinnitus is not necessary for the disorder to become chronic, though stress and negative affect can clearly have modulatory effects on these circuits.

TINNITUS DISTRESS AND CORTICAL MORPHOLOGY

Tinnitus can be debilitating, but there is also variability in the degree to which tinnitus affects each patient's quality of life (Heller, 2003; Eggermont and Roberts, 2004). Our behavioral data indicate that the auditory-perceptual symptoms of tinnitus (e.g., perceived loudness or awareness) are not good predictors of tinnitus distress. Correspondingly, those areas of the brain showing tinnitus-related differences in morphology in our study (i.e., vmPFC, dmPFC) do not seem to be affected by tinnitus distress. Instead, a separation seems to exist between those parts of the brain mediating tinnitus, and those meditating the emotional or stress reaction to tinnitus. Specifically, we saw that the severity of tinnitus distress was correlated with cortical thickness in the anterior insula (aIns). Several studies have implicated aIns in pain (DaSilva et al., 2008), stress (Choi et al., 2011; Dannlowski et al., 2012), mood disorders (Mayberg et al., 1999), and tinnitus distress (van der Loo et al., 2011), suggesting it may be involved in mediating the visceral sensations associated with stress and negative affect.

In our data, aIns thickness was also positively correlated with depression and anxiety scores in patients, but not in controls. This may indicate that aIns plays a role in affective reactions specific to tinnitus or other "interoceptive" phenomena (Craig, 2003) not experienced by controls, or that some tinnitus patients process stress or negative affect differently. However, the range of depression and anxiety scores in the current study was limited, and scores for the great majority of participants fell below the cutoff for potential clinical significance. Studies that include a wider range of participants, perhaps including those with clinically diagnosed depression, or who are more severely distressed by their tinnitus, may be better able to address whether some tinnitus patients process stress and negative affect in a unique way.

RELATIONSHIP BETWEEN TINNITUS AND NOISE SENSITIVITY

Pathological noise sensitivity, or "hyperacusis," is often comorbid with tinnitus (Goldstein and Shulman, 1996; Salvi et al., 2000). Although our participants reported having no history of hyperacusis, our behavioral data support the idea that tinnitus patients tend to be more sensitive to noise overall. The neural basis of clinical hyperacusis is not well understood, but a few human imaging studies report a dissociation between involvement of subcortical auditory structures in hyperacusis and auditory cortex in tinnitus (Gu et al., 2010; Mahoney et al., 2011). Indeed, many studies show auditory cortex hyperactivity in tinnitus (Lockwood et al., 1998; Giraud et al., 1999; Reyes et al., 2002; Plewnia et al., 2007; Leaver et al., 2011), and the current study found a significant relationship between tinnitus awareness and cortical thickness in part of auditory cortex (STG), complementing previous reports of tinnitus-related GM reductions in auditory cortex (Schneider et al., 2009). These previous studies indicate a separation within the auditory system between sites of tinnitus (cortical) and hyperacusis (subcortical), the latter affecting basic gain-control mechanisms (Gu et al., 2010).

With regard to noise sensitivity in our current study, we also found a modest relationship between SMG and rostral vmPFC morphology and combined noise sensitivity scores. Morphology in these regions (curvature in SMG and thickness in r-vmPFC) appeared to differ between groups; however, this effect was actually driven by differences in noise sensitivity scores between groups. It is unclear whether these neuroanatomical differences are specific to individuals with comorbid tinnitus and hyperacusis, or whether we might find similar morphological differences in SMG and rostral vmPFC in people with hyperacusis but no tinnitus. Studies specifically designed to address these issues are needed, particularly those including patients with hyperacusis (Gu et al., 2010; Mahoney et al., 2011). Considering the influence of noise sensitivity in tinnitus research (and vice versa) is clearly important.

TINNITUS AND ATTENTION

The site of tinnitus-related morphological differences we reported in SMG in the current study (MNI coordinates $X,Y,Z = 59, -40, 24$) is very close to a region of posterior auditory cortex that exhibited hyperactivity in tinnitus patients in our previous study [MNI coordinates of largest cluster $X,Y,Z = 56, -40, 15$; (Leaver et al., 2011)]. In our previous study, we postulated that this hyperactivity reflected the attempt by patients to separate their tinnitus sound from experimental stimuli in order to complete the task. In everyday situations, the SMG (and other parts of posterior parietal cortex) is involved in the attentional modulation of sensory stimuli (Corbetta and Shulman, 2002, 2011). Adjacent posterior auditory cortex has been shown to be recruited in tasks requiring the separation of competing auditory signals (Zatorre et al., 2002; Alain et al., 2005; Wilson et al., 2007; Wong et al., 2008), often called the "cocktail party problem." Under this assumption, the relationship between right SMG surface area and tinnitus awareness could be explained by inter-individual variability in the capacity to separate meaningful sounds from background noise. In other words, patients with larger (or use-dependent increases in) SMG surface area may be better able to incorporate tinnitus into (relatively) unattended background noise, allowing them to focus on relevant sounds with more success. Indeed, many studies have reported increased activity in posterior auditory cortex in tinnitus (Lockwood et al., 1998; Giraud et al., 1999; Reyes et al., 2002). So, although the role of posterior auditory cortex and adjacent parietal areas as a whole is likely to be more complex (Griffiths and Warren, 2002; Rauschecker and Scott, 2009), these areas are very likely to play a role in the attentional modulation of tinnitus as well.

INTERPRETING OF VARIABILITY IN CORTICAL THICKNESS, SURFACE AREA, AND GYRIFICATION

Surface-based methods like the ones used here are able to measure morphology in greater detail than volumetric analyses. For example, both surface area and thickness can contribute to the overall volume of cortex, and areas with greater local gyrification are likely to have greater cortical volume (i.e., more gyri = greater surface area = more gray matter). Because these morphological features can have different genetic origins (Panizzon et al., 2009; Winkler et al., 2010; Eyler et al., 2011), precise knowledge of morphological anomalies in clinical populations can increase our understanding of the cellular bases of these anomalies and can serve as a better complement to post mortem histological studies.

However, there is evidence that brain morphology can change with use-dependent experience (May and Gaser, 2006) and age (Good et al., 2001; Hutton et al., 2009) as well. Thus, neuromorphological effects, as reported here, can have multiple interpretations based on genetics and/or experience. Moreover, it is unclear whether a change in cell number due to experience or cell death would be more likely to affect thickness, surface area, or both. Cortical thickness and surface area both tend to decrease with age (Hutton et al., 2009; Lemaitre et al., 2012), suggesting that atrophy can affect both these neuro-morphological features (even if age is unlikely to play a role in the current study). Indeed, we hypothesized that morphology in some parts of the brain may change progressively in relation to tinnitus onset in the current study; however, we only saw one such effect in an area between the postcentral and angular gyri. This could be evidence of use-dependent increases in cell number in this area, though the exact interpretation is unclear. Longitudinal research, both within the context of tinnitus and without, is needed to better understand the effects of plasticity on brain morphology.

CONCLUSIONS: IMPLICATIONS FOR MODELS OF TINNITUS PATHOPHYSIOLOGY

Overall, the present data support the hypothesis that parts of the limbic system play a central role in tinnitus pathophysiology beyond a mere reaction to the tinnitus sound. Specifically, we argue that chronic tinnitus is caused by failure of the vmPFC-network to suppress unwanted activity in the auditory system (Mühlau et al., 2006; Rauschecker et al., 2010). This model is supported by evidence of GM reductions in vmPFC in three independent samples of participants [(Mühlau et al., 2006; Leaver et al., 2011) and the present study], in addition to anomalous activity in this network (Schlee et al., 2009; Leaver et al., 2011; Schecklmann et al., 2011). Furthermore, separate neural systems seem to mediate the tinnitus percept itself and the emotional reaction to tinnitus. Our data showed that the severity of tinnitus distress predicted cortical thickness in aIns, and symptoms of anxiety and depression correlated with scACC thickness; neither of these correlations was present in vmPFC. Note too that morphology in aIns and scACC did not differ between tinnitus patients and controls. Chronic tinnitus may not be caused, as some have argued, by forming negative associations with tinnitus. Stress and negative affect can certainly exacerbate tinnitus (Sullivan et al., 1988; Folmer et al., 1999; Dobie, 2003), but our data suggest that stress and negative affect are not necessary components of chronic tinnitus. The simple fact that not all tinnitus patients are distressed by their tinnitus suggests that models predicated on distress are unlikely to truly capture the disorder. If the neuroanatomical bases of tinnitus-related suffering and negative affect are indeed separable from those mediating the tinnitus signal itself, this underscores the importance of addressing both systems when developing treatment programs for tinnitus (Jastreboff, 2007).

ACKNOWLEDGMENTS

We wish to thank Sylke-Monina Chowdhury and Brannon Green for their technical assistance. This work was funded by the National Institutes of Health (RC1-DC010720 to Josef P. Rauschecker).

REFERENCES

Alain, C., Reinke, K., McDonald, K. L., Chau, W., Tam, F., Pacurar, A., and Graham, S. (2005). Left thalamo-cortical network implicated in successful speech separation and identification. *Neuroimage* 26, 592–599.

Ashburner, J. (2007). A fast diffeomorphic image registration algorithm. *Neuroimage* 38, 95–113.

Ashburner, J., and Friston, K. J. (2000). Voxel-based morphometry–the methods. *Neuroimage* 11, 805–821.

Cheung, S. W., and Larson, P. S. (2010). Tinnitus modulation by deep brain stimulation in locus of caudate neurons (area LC). *Neuroscience* 169, 1768–1778.

Choi, J. M., Padmala, S., and Pessoa, L. (2011). Impact of state anxiety on the interaction between threat monitoring and cognition. *Neuroimage* 59, 1912–1923.

Corbetta, M., and Shulman, G. L. (2002). Control of goal-directed and stimulus-driven attention in the brain. *Nat. Rev. Neurosci.* 3, 201–215.

Corbetta, M., and Shulman, G. L. (2011). Spatial neglect and attention networks. *Annu. Rev. Neurosci.* 34, 569–599.

Craig, A. D. (2003). Interoception: the sense of the physiological condition of the body. *Curr. Opin. Neurobiol.* 13, 500–505.

DaSilva, A. F., Becerra, L., Pendse, G., Chizh, B., Tully, S., and Borsook, D. (2008). Colocalized structural and functional changes in the cortex of patients with trigeminal neuropathic pain. *PLoS One* 3:e3396. doi: 10.1371/journal.pone.0003396

Dannlowski, U., Stuhrmann, A., Beutelmann, V., Zwanzger, P., Lenzen, T., Grotegerd, D., Domschke, K., Hohoff, C., Ohrmann, P., Bauer, J., Lindner, C., Postert, C., Konrad, C., Arolt, V., Heindel, W., Suslow, T., and Kugel, H. (2012). Limbic scars: long-term consequences of childhood maltreatment revealed by functional and structural magnetic resonance imaging. *Biol. Psychiatry* 71, 286–293.

De Ridder, D., Elgoyhen, A. B., Romo, R., and Langguth, B. (2011). Phantom percepts: tinnitus and pain as persisting aversive memory networks. *Proc. Natl. Acad. Sci. U.S.A.* 108, 8075–8080.

Dobie, R. A. (2003). Depression and tinnitus. *Otolaryngol. Clin. North Am.* 36, 383–388.

Drevets, W. C., Price, J. L., Simpson, J. R. Jr., Todd, R. D., Reich, T., Vannier, M., and Raichle, M. E. (1997). Subgenual prefrontal cortex abnormalities in mood disorders. *Nature* 386, 824–827.

Eggermont, J. J., and Roberts, L. E. (2004). The neuroscience of tinnitus. *Trends Neurosci.* 27, 676–682.

Etkin, A., Egner, T., and Kalisch, R. (2011). Emotional processing in anterior cingulate and medial prefrontal cortex. *Trends Cogn. Sci.* 15, 85–93.

Eyler, L. T., Prom-Wormley, E., Panizzon, M. S., Kaup, A. R., Fennema-Notestine, C., Neale, M. C., Jernigan, T. L., Fischl, B., Franz, C. E., Lyons, M. J., Grant, M., Stevens, A., Pacheco, J., Perry, M. E., Schmitt, J. E., Seidman, L. J., Thermenos, H. W., Tsuang, M. T., Chen, C. H., Thompson, W. K., Jak, A., Dale, A. M., and Kremen, W. S. (2011). Genetic and environmental contributions to regional cortical surface area in humans: a magnetic resonance imaging twin study. *Cereb. Cortex* 21, 2313–2321.

Fischl, B., and Dale, A. M. (2000). Measuring the thickness of the human cerebral cortex from magnetic resonance images. *Proc. Natl. Acad. Sci. U.S.A.* 97, 11050–11055.

Fischl, B., Salat, D. H., Busa, E., Albert, M., Dieterich, M., Haselgrove, C., van der Kouwe, A., Killiany, R., Kennedy, D., Klaveness, S., Montillo, A., Makris, N., Rosen, B., and Dale, A. M. (2002). Whole brain segmentation: automated labeling of neuroanatomical structures in the human brain. *Neuron* 33, 341–355.

Floresco, S. B., Zhang, Y., and Enomoto, T. (2009). Neural circuits subserving behavioral flexibility and their relevance to schizophrenia. *Behav. Brain Res.* 204, 396–409.

Folmer, R. L., Griest, S. E., Meikle, M. B., and Martin, W. H. (1999). Tinnitus severity, loudness, and depression. *Otolaryngol. Head Neck Surg.* 121, 48–51.

Fujiwara, E., Schwartz, M. L., Gao, F., Black, S. E., and Levine, B. (2008). Ventral frontal cortex functions and quantified MRI in traumatic brain injury. *Neuropsychologia* 46, 461–474.

Giraud, A. L., Chery-Croze, S., Fischer, G., Fischer, C., Vighetto, A., Gregoire, M. C., Lavenne, F., and Collet, L. (1999). A selective imaging of tinnitus. *Neuroreport* 10, 1–5.

Goldstein, B., and Shulman, A. (1996). Tinnitus-hyperacusis and the loudness discomfort level test-A preliminary report. *Int. Tinnitus J.* 2, 83–89.

Good, C. D., Johnsrude, I. S., Ashburner, J., Henson, R. N., Friston, K. J., and Frackowiak, R. S. (2001). A voxel-based morphometric study of ageing in 465 normal adult human brains. *Neuroimage* 14, 21–36.

Griffiths, T. D., and Warren, J. D. (2002). The planum temporale as a computational hub. *Trends Neurosci.* 25, 348–353.

Gu, J. W., Halpin, C. F., Nam, E. C., Levine, R. A., and Melcher, J. R. (2010). Tinnitus, diminished sound-level tolerance, and elevated auditory activity in humans with clinically normal hearing sensitivity. *J. Neurophysiol.* 104, 3361–3370.

Hamani, C., Mayberg, H., Stone, S., Laxton, A., Haber, S., and Lozano, A. M. (2011). The subcallosal cingulate gyrus in the context of major depression. *Biol. Psychiatry* 69, 301–308.

Heller, A. J. (2003). Classification and epidemiology of tinnitus. *Otolaryngol. Clin. North Am.* 36, 239–248.

Hiller, W., and Goebel, G. (2006). Factors influencing tinnitus loudness and annoyance. *Arch. Otolaryngol. Head Neck Surg.* 132, 1323–1330.

Husain, F. T., Medina, R. E., Davis, C. W., Szymko-Bennett, Y., Simonyan, K., Pajor, N. M., and Horwitz, B. (2011). Neuroanatomical changes due to hearing loss and chronic tinnitus: a combined VBM and DTI study. *Brain Res.* 1369, 74–88.

Hutton, C., Draganski, B., Ashburner, J., and Weiskopf, N. (2009). A comparison between voxel-based cortical thickness and voxel-based morphometry in normal aging. *Neuroimage* 48, 371–380.

Jastreboff, P. J. (1990). Phantom auditory perception (tinnitus): mechanisms of generation and perception. *Neurosci. Res.* 8, 221–254.

Jastreboff, P. J. (2007). Tinnitus retraining therapy. *Prog. Brain Res.* 166, 415–423.

Kable, J. W., and Glimcher, P. W. (2009). The neurobiology of decision: consensus and controversy. *Neuron* 63, 733–745.

Koenigs, M., and Grafman, J. (2009). The functional neuroanatomy of depression: distinct roles for ventromedial and dorsolateral prefrontal cortex. *Behav. Brain Res.* 201, 239–243.

Kroenke, K., Spitzer, R. L., and Williams, J. B. (2001). The PHQ-9: validity of a brief depression severity measure. *J. Gen. Intern. Med.* 16, 606–613.

Kuchinad, A., Schweinhardt, P., Seminowicz, D. A., Wood, P. B., Chizh, B. A., and Bushnell, M. C. (2007). Accelerated brain gray matter loss in fibromyalgia patients: premature aging of the brain? *J. Neurosci.* 27, 4004–4007.

Landgrebe, M., Langguth, B., Rosengarth, K., Braun, S., Koch, A., Kleinjung, T., May, A., De Ridder, D., and Hajak, G. (2009). Structural brain changes in tinnitus: grey matter decrease in auditory and non-auditory brain areas. *Neuroimage* 46, 213–218.

Langguth, B., Goodey, R., Azevedo, A., Bjorne, A., Cacace, A., Crocetti, A., Del Bo, L., De Ridder, D., Diges, I., Elbert, T., Flor, H., Herraiz, C., Ganz Sanchez, T., Eichhammer, P., Figueiredo, R., Hajak, G., Kleinjung, T., Landgrebe, M., Londero, A., Lainez, M. J., Mazzoli, M., Meikle, M. B., Melcher, J., Rauschecker, J. P., Sand, P. G., Struve, M., Van de Heyning, P., Van Dijk, P., and Vergara, R. (2007). Consensus for tinnitus patient assessment and treatment outcome measurement: tinnitus research initiative meeting, Regensburg, July 2006. *Prog. Brain Res.* 166, 525–536.

Leaver, A. M., Renier, L., Chevillet, M. A., Morgan, S., Kim, H. J., and Rauschecker, J. P. (2011). Dysregulation of limbic and auditory networks in tinnitus. *Neuron* 69, 33–43.

Lemaitre, H., Goldman, A. L., Sambataro, F., Verchinski, B. A., Meyer-Lindenberg, A., Weinberger, D. R., and Mattay, V. S. (2012). Normal age-related brain morphometric changes: nonuniformity across cortical thickness, surface area and gray matter volume? *Neurobiol. Aging* 33, 617e1–617e9.

Lockwood, A. H., Salvi, R. J., Coad, M. L., Towsley, M. L., Wack, D. S., and Murphy, B. W. (1998). The functional neuroanatomy of tinnitus: evidence for limbic system links and neural plasticity. *Neurology* 50, 114–120.

Lowry, L. D., Eisenman, L. M., and Saunders, J. C. (2004). An absence of tinnitus. *Otol. Neurotol.* 25, 474–478.

Lozano, A. M., Mayberg, H. S., Giacobbe, P., Hamani, C., Craddock, R. C., and Kennedy, S. H. (2008). Subcallosal cingulate gyrus deep brain stimulation for treatment-resistant depression. *Biol. Psychiatry* 64, 461–467.

Mahoney, C. J., Rohrer, J. D., Goll, J. C., Fox, N. C., Rossor, M. N., and Warren, J. D. (2011). Structural neuroanatomy of tinnitus and hyperacusis in semantic dementia.

J. Neurol. Neurosurg. Psychiatry 82, 1274–1278.

Mattson, A. J., and Levin, H. S. (1990). Frontal lobe dysfunction following closed head injury. A review of the literature. *J. Nerv. Ment. Dis.* 178, 282–291.

May, A., and Gaser, C. (2006). Magnetic resonance-based morphometry: a window into structural plasticity of the brain. *Curr. Opin. Neurol.* 19, 407–411.

Mayberg, H. S. (1997). Limbic-cortical dysregulation: a proposed model of depression. *J. Neuropsychiatry Clin. Neurosci.* 9, 471–481.

Mayberg, H. S., Liotti, M., Brannan, S. K., McGinnis, S., Mahurin, R. K., Jerabek, P. A., Silva, J. A., Tekell, J. L., Martin, C. C., Lancaster, J. L., and Fox, P. T. (1999). Reciprocal limbic-cortical function and negative mood: converging PET findings in depression and normal sadness. *Am. J. Psychiatry* 156, 675–682.

Mirz, F., Gjedde, A., Ishizu, K., and Pedersen, C. B. (2000). Cortical networks subserving the perception of tinnitus–a PET study. *Acta Otolaryngol.* 543, 241–243.

Morgan, D. E., Wilson, R. H., and Dirks, D. D. (1974). Loudness discomfort level: selected methods and stimuli. *J. Acoust. Soc. Am.* 56, 577–581.

Møller, A. R. (2003). Pathophysiology of tinnitus. *Otolaryngol. Clin. North Am.* 36, 249–266.

Mühlau, M., Rauschecker, J. P., Oestreicher, E., Gaser, C., Röttinger, M., Wohlschläger, A. M., Simon, F., Etgen, T., Conrad, B., and Sander, D. (2006). Structural brain changes in tinnitus. *Cereb. Cortex* 16, 1283–1288.

Newman, C. W., Jacobson, G. P., and Spitzer, J. B. (1996). Development of the Tinnitus Handicap Inventory. *Arch. Otolaryngol. Head Neck Surg.* 122, 143–148.

Ongür, D., Ferry, A. T., and Price, J. L. (2003). Architectonic subdivision of the human orbital and medial prefrontal cortex. *J. Comp. Neurol.* 460, 425–449.

Ongür, D., and Price, J. L. (2000). The organization of networks within the orbital and medial prefrontal cortex of rats, monkeys and humans. *Cereb. Cortex* 10, 206–219.

Panizzon, M. S., Fennema-Notestine, C., Eyler, L. T., Jernigan, T. L., Prom-Wormley, E., Neale, M., Jacobson, K., Lyons, M. J., Grant, M. D., Franz, C. E., Xian, H., Tsuang, M., Fischl, B., Seidman, L., Dale, A., and Kremen, W. S. (2009). Distinct genetic influences on cortical surface area and cortical thickness. *Cereb. Cortex* 19, 2728–2735.

Plewnia, C., Reimold, M., Najib, A., Brehm, B., Reischl, G., Plontke, S. K., and Gerloff, C. (2007). Dose-dependent attenuation of auditory phantom perception (tinnitus) by PET-guided repetitive transcranial magnetic stimulation. *Hum. Brain Mapp.* 28, 238–246.

Rauschecker, J. P., Leaver, A. M., and Mühlau, M. (2010). Tuning out the noise: limbic-auditory interactions in tinnitus. *Neuron* 66, 819–826.

Rauschecker, J. P., and Scott, S. K. (2009). Maps and streams in the auditory cortex: nonhuman primates illuminate human speech processing. *Nat. Neurosci.* 12, 718–724.

Reyes, S. A., Salvi, R. J., Burkard, R. F., Coad, M. L., Wack, D. S., Galantowicz, P. J., and Lockwood, A. H. (2002). Brain imaging of the effects of lidocaine on tinnitus. *Hear. Res.* 171, 43–50.

Robinson, S. K., Viirre, E. S., Bailey, K. A., Kindermann, S., Minassian, A. L., Goldin, P. R., Pedrelli, P., Harris, J. P., and McQuaid, J. R. (2008). A randomized controlled trial of cognitive-behavior therapy for tinnitus. *Int. Tinnitus J.* 14, 119–126.

Salvi, R. J., Wang, J., and Ding, D. (2000). Auditory plasticity and hyperactivity following cochlear damage. *Hear. Res.* 147, 261–274.

Savitz, J., and Drevets, W. C. (2009). Bipolar and major depressive disorder: neuroimaging the developmental-degenerative divide. *Neurosci. Biobehav. Rev.* 33, 699–771.

Schecklmann, M., Landgrebe, M., Poeppl, T. B., Kreuzer, P., Männer, P., Marienhagen, J., Wack, D. S., Kleinjung, T., Hajak, G., and Langguth, B. (2011). Neural correlates of tinnitus duration and Distress: a positron emission tomography study. *Hum. Brain Mapp.* doi: 10.1002/hbm.21426. [Epub ahead of print]

Schlee, W., Mueller, N., Hartmann, T., Keil, J., Lorenz, I., and Weisz, N. (2009). Mapping cortical hubs in tinnitus. *BMC Biol.* 7, 80.

Schneider, P., Andermann, M., Wengenroth, M., Goebel, R., Flor, H., Rupp, A., and Diesch, E. (2009). Reduced volume of Heschl's gyrus in tinnitus. *Neuroimage* 45, 927–939.

Shackman, A. J., Salomons, T. V., Slagter, H. A., Fox, A. S., Winter, J. J., and Davidson, R. J. (2011). The integration of negative affect, pain and cognitive control in the cingulate cortex. *Nat. Rev. Neurosci.* 12, 154–167.

Shulman, A., Strashun, A. M., Afriyie, M., Aronson, F., Abel, W., and Goldstein, B. (1995). SPECT imaging of brain and tinnitus-neurotologic/neurologic implications. *Int. Tinnitus J.* 1, 13–29.

Spitzer, R. L., Kroenke, K., Williams, J. B., and Lowe, B. (2006). A brief measure for assessing generalized anxiety disorder: the GAD-7. *Arch. Intern. Med.* 166, 1092–1097.

Steele, J. D., and Lawrie, S. M. (2004). Segregation of cognitive and emotional function in the prefrontal cortex: a stereotactic meta-analysis. *Neuroimage* 21, 868–875.

Sullivan, M. D., Katon, W., Dobie, R., Sakai, C., Russo, J., and Harrop-Griffiths, J. (1988). Disabling tinnitus. *Association with affective disorder. Gen. Hosp. Psychiatry* 10, 285–291.

van der Loo, E., Congedo, M., Vanneste, S., De Heyning, P. V., and De Ridder, D. (2011). Insular lateralization in tinnitus distress. *Auton. Neurosci.* 165, 191–194.

Wilson, E. C., Melcher, J. R., Micheyl, C., Gutschalk, A., and Oxenham, A. J. (2007). Cortical FMRI activation to sequences of tones alternating in frequency: relationship to perceived rate and streaming. *J. Neurophysiol.* 97, 2230–2238.

Winkler, A. M., Kochunov, P., Blangero, J., Almasy, L., Zilles, K., Fox, P. T., Duggirala, R., and Glahn, D. C. (2010). Cortical thickness or grey matter volume? The importance of selecting the phenotype for imaging genetics studies. *Neuroimage* 53, 1135–1146.

Wong, P. C., Uppunda, A. K., Parrish, T. B., and Dhar, S. (2008). Cortical mechanisms of speech perception in noise. *J. Speech Lang. Hear. Res.* 51, 1026–1041.

Zatorre, R. J., Bouffard, M., Ahad, P., and Belin, P. (2002). Where is "where" in the human auditory cortex? *Nat. Neurosci.* 5, 905–909.

Zigmond, A. S., and Snaith, R. P. (1983). The hospital anxiety and depression scale. *Acta Psychiatr. Scand.* 67, 361–370.

Zikopoulos, B., and Barbas, H. (2006). Prefrontal projections to the thalamic reticular nucleus form a unique circuit for attentional mechanisms. *J. Neurosci.* 26, 7348–7361.

4

Resequencing of the auxiliary $GABA_B$ receptor subunit gene *KCTD12* in chronic tinnitus

P. G. Sand[1]*, B. Langguth[1], J. Itzhacki[2], A. Bauer[2], S. Geis[2], Z. E. Cárdenas-Conejo[2], V. Pimentel[2] and T. Kleinjung[3,4]

[1] *Department of Psychiatry, University of Regensburg, Regensburg, Germany*
[2] *Experimental and Clinical Neurosciences Graduate Program, University of Regensburg, Regensburg, Germany*
[3] *Department of Otorhinolaryngology, University of Regensburg, Regensburg, Germany*
[4] *Department of Otorhinolaryngology, University of Zurich, Zurich, Switzerland*

Correspondence:
P. G. Sand, Department of Psychiatry, University of Regensburg, Universitaetsstrasse 84, 93053 Regensburg, Germany.
e-mail: philipp.sand@klinik.uni-regensburg.de

Tinnitus is a common and often incapacitating hearing disorder marked by the perception of phantom sounds. Susceptibility factors remain largely unknown but $GABA_B$ receptor signaling has long been implicated in the response to treatment and, putatively, in the etiology of the disorder. We hypothesized that variation in KCTD12, the gene encoding an auxiliary subunit of $GABA_B$ receptors, could help to predict the risk of developing tinnitus. Ninety-five Caucasian outpatients with a diagnosis of chronic tinnitus were systematically screened for mutations in the KCTD12 open reading frame and the adjacent 3′ untranslated region by Sanger sequencing. Allele frequencies were determined for 14 known variants of which three (rs73237446, rs34544607, and rs41287030) were polymorphic. When allele frequencies were compared to data from a large reference population of European ancestry, rs34544607 was associated with tinnitus ($p = 0.04$). However, KCTD12 genotype did not predict tinnitus severity ($p = 0.52$) and the association with rs34544607 was weakened after screening 50 additional cases ($p = 0.07$). Pending replication in a larger cohort, KCTD12 may act as a risk modifier in chronic tinnitus. Issues that are yet to be addressed include the effects of neighboring variants, e.g., in the KCTD12 gene regulatory region, plus interactions with variants of $GABA_{B1}$ and $GABA_{B2}$.

Keywords: KCTD12, association analysis, tinnitus, cortical inhibition

INTRODUCTION

Tinnitus is an unpleasant and often agonizing condition marked by the phantom perception of sound. According to recent epidemiological estimates, 25% of the US general populations are affected with one in three subjects reporting daily tinnitus (Shargorodsky et al., 2010). While there is evidence of a genetic susceptibility to tinnitus (Sand, 2011), a complex mode of inheritance suggests the presence of multiple risk genes, and comparatively small effect sizes for any single risk allele. Heritability estimates vary from 0.11 to 0.39 (Petersen et al., 2002; Kvestad et al., 2010). Owing to the lack of linkage studies, the search for candidate genes in primary tinnitus is hypothesis-driven. A well-established theoretical framework for tinnitus has been provided by the disruption of $GABA_B$ receptor signaling in animal models (Szczepaniak and Møller, 1995, 1996) that may explain altered cortical inhibition in patients (Eichhammer et al., 2004). More recently, a key role for $GABA_B$ receptors has been confirmed by the effects of receptor agonists on tinnitus symptomatology (Zheng et al., 2012), renewing the interest in controlled clinical trials (Westerberg et al., 1996). In the light of these developments, further characterization of the $GABA_B$ receptor complex is advocated, including the genes encoding the respective receptor structures.

An auxiliary subunit that associates tightly with the carboxy terminus of $GABA_{B2}$ receptors is KCTD12 (also known as PFET1 or BTB/POZ domain-containing protein), a potassium channel tetramerization domain-containing protein (Bartoi et al., 2010). Coassembly of KCTD12 and $GABA_{B2}$ changes the properties of the $GABA_{B(1,2)}$ core receptor by increasing agonist potency, by altering G-protein signaling, and by promoting desensitization (Schwenk et al., 2010). Effects on the pharmacology and the kinetics of $GABA_B$ receptors occur in various cochlear cell classes, e.g., in type I fibrocytes of the spiral ligament and in type I vestibular hair cells (Resendes et al., 2004). Knockdown of the KCTD12 ortholog *right on* leads to improper neuronal differentiation in the zebrafish auditory pathway (Kuo, 2005). Unlike other KCTD proteins, however, KCTD12 is also widely expressed in the adult mammalian brain (Metz et al., 2011) and, therefore, likely to act beyond early periods of maturation. KCTD12 is encoded by an intronless gene on human chr13q21 for which only limited data are presently available in hearing disorders. To determine the impact of this candidate gene on chronic tinnitus, we systematically screened the entire open reading frame for genetic variants, and compared observed allele frequencies to published reference data.

MATERIALS AND METHODS

In 95 German outpatients (67 men and 28 women, age 50.6 ± 12.1 years, mean ± SD) consulting for chronic tinnitus, the diagnosis was confirmed by a detailed neurootological examination including otoscopy, stapedius reflexes, middle ear pressure measurements, and pure tone audiometry. For the present study, only patients with subjective tinnitus were included. Tinnitus severity was assessed by the Tinnitus Questionnnaire (TQ) (Goebel and Hiller, 1994). An additional 50 subjects with chronic tinnitus (40 men and 10 women, age 49.3 ± 11.3 years, mean ± SD) formed an extension sample and underwent the same diagnostic workup as outlined above. All participants were Cauacasians and a majority originated from the Upper Palatinate region of Bavaria. All provided informed consent and the study was approved by the local ethics committee at the University of Regensburg.

Genomic DNA was extracted from lymphocytes using standard procedures prior to amplification of the *KCTD12* open reading frame and adjacent 3′ sequence by PCR. Briefly, two overlapping amplicons of 438 bp (a) and 819 bp (b) were generated using the following primer pairs: 5′-CGG TTG CAG CTC CTG AGT-3′ (forward, a), 5′-AGC TCT GGC AGC TCG AAG TA-3′ (reverse, a), 5′-CTC GTG CTG CCC GAC TAC TT-3′ (forward, b) and 5′-GAC AGG TCT CAC CCA GCT AC-3′ (reverse, b). PCR products were purified with ExoSAP-IT (GE Healthcare, Freiburg, Germany) for Sanger sequencing, and for the identification of variants against the human genome reference (Genome Reference Consortium Build 37, February 2009 release). In the extension sample, only amplicon b was sequenced. Multiple sequence alignments were conducted with DNA Dynamo 1.0 (Blue Tractor Software, UK). Linkage disequilibrium and conformity with Hardy–Weinberg equilibrium was measured with HaploView 4.2 (Barrett et al., 2005). PS V2.1.15 (Dupont and Plummer, 1990) was used for power simulations. *KCTD12* allele frequencies from a large reference population of European ancestry (NHLBI GO Exome Sequencing Project, ESP) were retrieved with the Exome Variant Server (URL: http://evs.gs.washington.edu/EVS/). ESP allele frequency data were compared to the frequencies observed in tinnitus using Fisher's exact tests. *T*-tests were employed to compare self-reported tinnitus severity in carriers and non-carriers of the minor *KCTD12* alleles. STATA 8.0 (Stata Corporation, College Station, TX, USA) was used for descriptive statistics. The Shapiro–Wilk statistic served to test the null hypothesis of normally distributed TQ scores. The level of statistical significance was set at $p < 0.05$. All p-values are uncorrected for multiple testing.

For estimating the functionality of confirmed sequence variants, evolutionary conservation in primates was assessed with a phylogenetic hidden Markov model-based method, phastCons, that describes the process of DNA substitution at each site in a genome and the way this process changes from one site to the next (Siepel et al., 2005). Computational annotations of SNP function (Xu and Taylor, 2009) were obtained from the SNPinfo WebServer (URL: http://snpinfo.niehs.nih.gov/snpfunc.htm, accessed Dec. 2011). *In silico* predictions of structural effects at the amino acid level were based on information from homologous proteins using metaPrDOS at default parameters (Ishida and Kinoshita, 2008).

RESULTS

We confirmed the existence of two coding variants, F87F (rs73237446) and T178T (rs34544607), plus one previously described, non-coding variant in the gene's 3′ UTR (rs41287030) at heterozygosities of 0.01, 0.10, and 0.02, respectively. All genotype distributions conformed to the Hardy–Weinberg

Table 1 | Allele frequencies for the *KCTD12* sequence screened in subjects with chronic tinnitus as compared to frequencies in a large control population.

dbSNP ID	chr13 position	Major>minor alleles[a]	Variant amino acid	MAF in chronic tinnitus (2N)[b]	MAF in controls (2N)[c]	*p*
rs141180437	77,460,118	C>T	P56S	0.0000 (190)	0.0000 (6972)	n.s.
rs116710456	77,460,080	G>A	Q68Q	0.0000 (190)	0.0003 (6858)	n.s.
rs143013358	77,460,078	C>T	P69L	0.0000 (190)	0.0000 (6844)	n.s.
rs694997	77,460,068	G>A	L72L	0.0000 (190)	0.0003 (6872)	n.s.
rs146434030	77,460,065	C>A	A73A	0.0000 (190)	0.0000 (6894)	n.s.
rs73237446	77,460,023	C>T	F87F	0.0053 (190)	0.0089 (6890)	n.s.
rs141477426	77,460,015	G>A	R90H	0.0000 (190)	0.0001 (6858)	n.s.
rs144225285	77,459,981	C>T	L101L	0.0000 (190)	0.0000 (6756)	n.s.
rs34544607	77,459,750	G>C	T178T	0.0458 (262)	0.0263 (5058)	0.07
rs139291676	77,459,507	C>T	P259P	0.0000 (262)	0.0000 (7018)	n.s.
rs151278314	77,459,394	C>T	T297M	0.0000 (262)	0.0000 (7020)	n.s.
rs142368706	77,459,383	G>A	A301T	0.0000 (262)	0.0000 (7020)	n.s.
rs140689403	77,459,359	A>G	S309G	0.0000 (262)	0.0001 (7020)	n.s.
rs41287030	77,459,221	C>T	–	0.0076 (262)	–	–

Fisher's exact tests were used to address allelic association.

[a] *Nucleobases on the transcribed strand.*

[b] *Call rates of 85% were achieved in the first round of screening amplicon b.*

[c] *Reference population of European ancestry from the NHLBI GO Exome Sequencing Project.*

MAF, minor allele frequency.

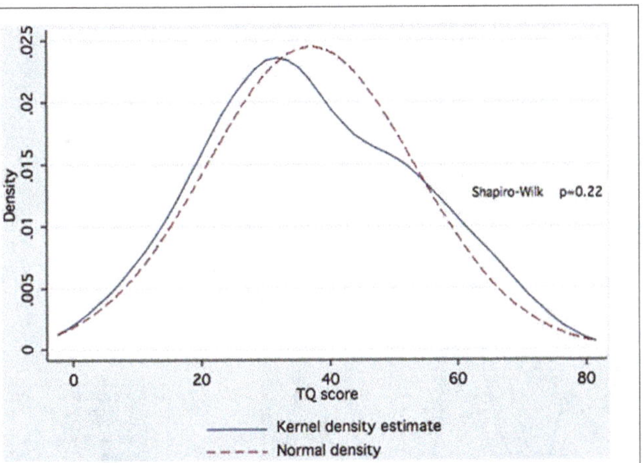

FIGURE 1 | Distribution of TQ scores in 144 subjects with chronic tinnitus does not deviate from the expected Gaussian curve ($p = 0.22$).

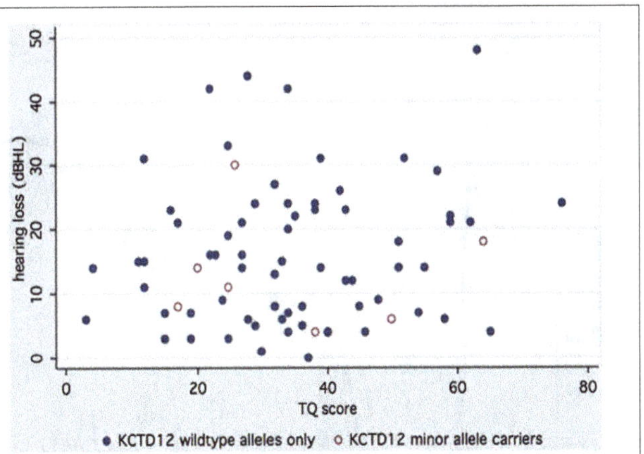

FIGURE 2 | Stratification of TQ scores by hearing loss and KCTD12 minor allele carrier status. Open circles indicate T178T carriers, filled circles indicate homozygous carriers of wildtype alleles. The degree of hearing loss is expressed as the binaural pure tone average involving air conduction across seven test frequencies (0.125, 0.25, 0.5, 1, 2, 4, and 8 kHz).

equilibrium ($p > 0.75$). No novel sequence variants emerged and 11 *KCTD12* variants listed in dbSNP were absent from our sample (rs141180437, rs116710456, rs143013358, rs694997, rs146434030, rs141477426, rs144225285, rs139291676, rs151278314, rs142368706, and rs140689403, **Table 1**). When allele frequencies in subjects with chronic tinnitus were compared to reference frequencies from a large control population of European ancestry, an increased prevalence of the minor allele was noted for T178T (0.0494 vs. 0.0263, $p = 0.04$). To put this finding into perspective, the original screening sample was augmented by 100 chromosomes from a second set of patients, whereupon the MAF in cases dropped to 0.0458 for rs34544607, weakening the association with tinnitus ($p = 0.07$). Power simulations, based on the entire sample of patients diagnosed with chronic tinnitus and on ESP control data, indicated that we should expect a statistical power of >80% to detect a susceptibility factor with an allelic relative risk of >1.77 for the T178T variant. The number of tinnitus cases needed to reach this power was estimated at 363.

We next examined whether *KCTD12* variants could serve as predictors of tinnitus severity. Overall, TQ scores followed a Gaussian distribution (**Figure 1**) and averaged 37.1 ± 16.3 (mean $\pm$ SD) out of 84 points ($N = 144$). By this measure, tinnitus was rated mild (0–30 points) in 55 subjects (38.2%), moderate (31–46 points) in 46 subjects (31.9%), severe (47–59 points) in 29 subjects (20.1%), and extreme (60–84 points) in 14 subjects (9.7%). There was no significant difference in mean TQ scores or in the degree of concomitant hearing loss between carriers and non-carriers of the minor allele at rs34544607 ($p = 0.52$ and $p = 0.48$, respectively, *t*-test, **Figure 2**). A positive family history of tinnitus in first-degree relatives did not predict rs34544607 genotype ($p = 0.67$, Fisher's exact test). As we encountered only one carrier of rs73237446, and only two carriers of rs41287030, the interplay of these substitutions with tinnitus severity, hearing loss, or with a family history of tinnitus could not be fully judged.

Using the degree of evolutionary conservation as a surrogate parameter of functionality, both rs73237446 and rs34544607 scored high on the comparative genomics scale (**Figure 3**).

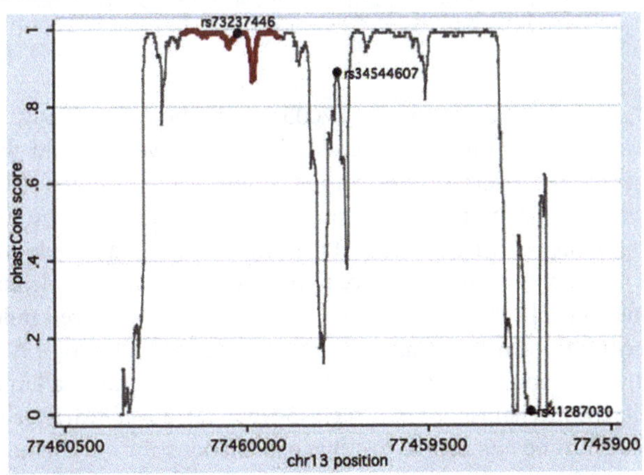

FIGURE 3 | Comparative genomic analysis of the *KCTD12* sequence screened. Only confirmed variants are shown. F87F (rs73237446) and T178T (rs34544607) map to regions (*x*-axis) highly conserved in primates. Conservation scores (*y*-axis) for the potassium channel tetramerization domain (delimited by residues 36 and 125) are plotted in red.

Further *in silico* analyses confirmed that rs73237446 maps to the potassium channel tetramerization domain (**Figure 3**) whereas residue 178, encoded by rs34544607, maps to a disordered region of KCTD12 (**Figure 4**) which may affect the molecular recognition of proteins and DNA. The non-coding variant rs41287030 is only poorly conserved among primates but could have acquired a functional role in the recent past. Thus, rs41287030 would appear to alter a micro RNA binding site and may thereby inhibit protein translation (see the corresponding SNPinfo entry for prediction results).

DISCUSSION

Screening of the *KCTD12* ORF in chronic tinnitus extends preliminary results on genomic variation as obtained from 88 subjects

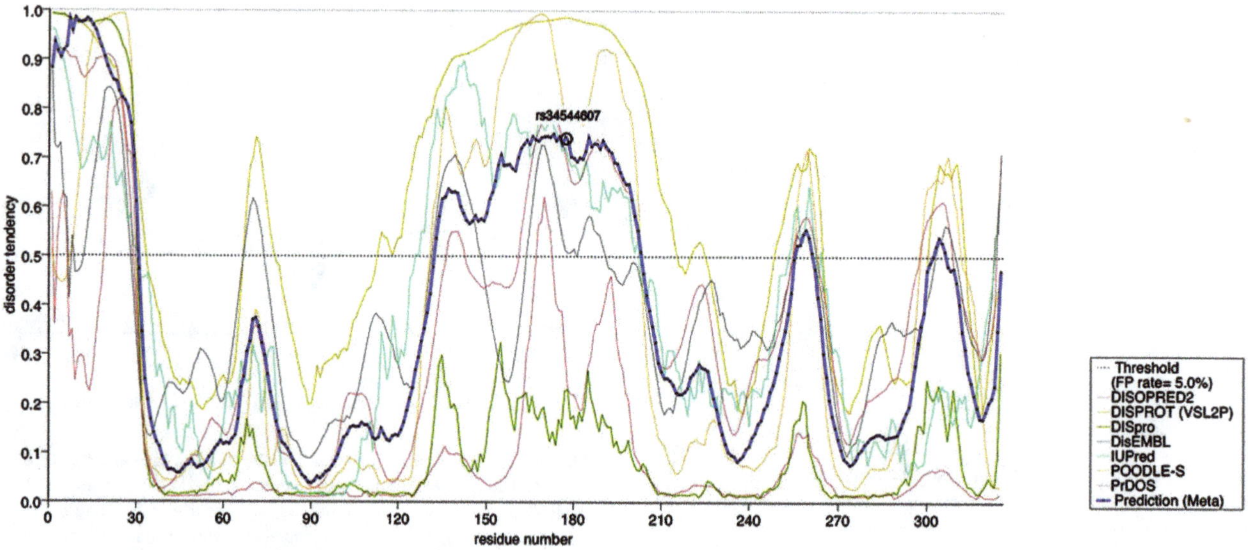

FIGURE 4 | *In silico* structural analysis of the KCTD12 protein. KCTD12 residues are plotted on the *x*-axis. Eight prediction scores on the *y*-axis (see legend) are combined using metaPrDOS to locate disordered regions based on homologies with other proteins (blue line). T178T (rs34544607) maps to a relative maximum, i.e., a region that may affect interactions with other proteins or DNA. A default false positive (FP) threshold of 5% was applied.

with congenital deafness (Kuo, 2005). As in the earlier study, no novel sequence variants were identified. However, a trend was observed for association of chronic tinnitus with a highly conserved, synonymous substitution, rs34544607. The relevance of this finding is unclear in view of the moderately sized sample and the use of an external reference population. It is conceivable that some control subjects from the ESP may have experienced mild, subclinical forms of tinnitus, increasing the likelihood of a type II error. Pending replication of this association trend at a larger scale, the mechanism by which rs34544607 can affect hearing also remains to be elucidated. Possible explanations for synonymous mutations' functionality are offered by interference with RNA processing, or by changes in translation kinetics that affect protein folding (Sauna and Kimchi-Sarfaty, 2011). Phenotypically, rs34544607 carriers may be indistinguishable from other subjects unless treated with baclofen or another GABAB receptor agonist. If rs34544607 truly impacts on $GABA_B$ signaling, we should expect electrophysiological measures of cortical inhibition to discriminate between carriers and non-carriers. Electrophysiological data (motor threshold, short-interval intracortical inhibition, intracortical facilitation, and cortical silent period) were available only in a subset of our sample and did not suggest a major effect. The degree of hearing loss did not predict rs34544607 carrier status but further stratification by etiology (noise-induced vs. congenital) is recommended in future studies. With regard to rs41287030, the current lack of publicly available control data and a MAF < 0.01 in tinnitus subjects call for a re-examination in a larger population of affecteds and controls in order to test for a possible association with the phenotype.

Taken together, the present results implicate genetic variation in a $GABA_B$ receptor auxiliary subunit as a possible risk modifier in chronic tinnitus. More research is also invited to address *KCTD12* promoter variants, and to explore the interaction with variants in genes encoding other elements of the receptor complex, e.g., $GABA_{B1}$ and $GABA_{B2}$ proteins.

ACKNOWLEDGMENTS

We gratefully acknowledge support by the German Research Foundation and the Open Access Publishing Fund of the University of Regensburg.

REFERENCES

Barrett, J. C., Fry, B., Maller, J., and Daly, M. J. (2005). Haploview: analysis and visualization of LD and haplotype maps. *Bioinformatics* 21, 263–265.

Bartoi, T., Rigbolt, K. T., Du, D., Köhr, G., Blagoev, B., and Kornau, H. C. (2010). $GABA_B$ receptor constituents revealed by tandem affinity purification from transgenic mice. *J. Biol. Chem.* 285, 20625–20633.

Dupont, W. D., and Plummer, W. D. Jr. (1990). Power and sample size calculations. A review and computer program. *Control. Clin. Trials* 11, 116–128.

Eichhammer, P., Langguth, B., Zowe, M., Kleinjung, T., Jacob, P., Sand, P., and Hajak, G. (2004). $GABA_B$-associated neuropsychiatric disorders. *Psychiatr. Prax.* 31(Suppl. 1), S44–S46.

Goebel, G., and Hiller, W. (1994). The tinnitus questionnaire. A standard instrument for grading the degree of tinnitus. Results of a multicenter study with the tinnitus questionnaire. *HNO* 42, 166–172.

Ishida, T., and Kinoshita, K. (2008). Prediction of disordered regions in proteins based on the meta approach. *Bioinformatics* 24, 1344–1348.

Kuo, S. F. (2005). *Characterization of KCTD12/PFET1, an Intronless Gene with Predominant Fetal Expression.* PhD dissertation. Harvard-MIT Division of Health Sciences and Technology.

Kvestad, E., Czajkowski, N., Engdahl, B., Hoffman, H. J., and Tambs, K. (2010). Low heritability of tinnitus: results from the second Nord-Trøndelag health study. *Arch. Otolaryngol. Head Neck Surg.* 136, 178–182.

Metz, M., Gassmann, M., Fakler, B., Schaeren-Wiemers, N., and Bettler, B. (2011). Distribution of the auxiliary $GABA_B$ receptor subunits KCTD8 12, 12b, and 16 in the mouse brain. *J. Comp. Neurol.* 519, 1435–1454.

Petersen, H. C., Andersen, T., Frederiksen, H., Hoffman, H. J., and Christensen, K. (2002). The heritability of tinnitus: a twin study. *Poster presented at: Nordic Epidemiology Congress; June 9–12, 2002.* Aarhus, Denmark.

Resendes, B. L., Kuo, S. F., Robertson, N. G., Giersch, A. B., Honrubia, D., Ohara, O., Adams, J. C., and Morton, C. C. (2004). Isolation from cochlea of a novel human intronless gene with predominant fetal expression. *J. Assoc. Res. Otolaryngol.* 5, 185–202.

Sand, P. G. (2011). "Genetic risk factors in chronic tinnitus," in *Textbook of Tinnitus,* eds A. R. Møller, B. Langguth, D. DeRidder, and T. Kleinjung (New York, NY: Springer), 47–50.

Sauna, Z. E., and Kimchi-Sarfaty, C. (2011). Understanding the contribution of synonymous mutations to human disease. *Nat. Rev. Genet.* 12, 683–691.

Schwenk, J., Metz, M., Zolles, G., Turecek, R., Fritzius, T., Bildl, W., Tarusawa, E., Kulik, A., Unger, A., Ivankova, K., Seddik, R., Tiao, J. Y., Rajalu, M., Trojanova, J., Rohde, V., Gassmann, M., Schulte, U., Fakler, B., and Bettler, B. (2010). Native GABA(B) receptors are heteromultimers with a family of auxiliary subunits. *Nature* 465, 231–235.

Shargorodsky, J., Curhan, G. C., and Farwell, W. R. (2010). Prevalence and characteristics of tinnitus among US adults. *Am. J. Med.* 123, 711–718.

Siepel, A., Bejerano, G., Pedersen, J. S., Hinrichs, A. S., Hou, M., Rosenbloom, K., Clawson, H., Spieth, J., Hillier, L. W., Richards, S., Weinstock, G. M., Wilson, R. K., Gibbs, R. A., Kent, W. J., Miller, W., and Haussler, D. (2005). Evolutionarily conserved elements in vertebrate, insect, worm, and yeast genomes. *Genome Res.* 15, 1034–1050.

Szczepaniak, W. S., and Møller, A. R. (1995). Effects of L-baclofen and D-baclofen on the auditory system: a study of click-evoked potentials from the inferior colliculus in the rat. *Ann. Otol. Rhinol. Laryngol.* 104, 399–404.

Szczepaniak, W. S., and Møller, A. R. (1996). Effects of (-)-baclofen, clonazepam, and diazepam on tone exposure-induced hyperexcitability of the inferior colliculus in the rat: possible therapeutic implications for pharmacological management of tinnitus and hyperacusis. *Hear. Res.* 97, 46–53.

Westerberg, B. D., Roberson, J. B. Jr., and Stach, B. A. (1996). A double-blind placebo-controlled trial of baclofen in the treatment of tinnitus. *Am. J. Otol.* 17, 896–903.

Xu, Z., and Taylor, J. A. (2009). SNPinfo: integrating GWAS and candidate gene information into functional SNP selection for genetic association studies. *Nucleic Acids Res.* 37, W600–W605.

Zheng, Y., Vagal, S., McNamara, E., Darlington, C. L., and Smith, P. F. (2012). A dose-response analysis of the effects of L-baclofen on chronic tinnitus caused by acoustic trauma in rats. *Neuropharmacology* 62, 940–946.

5

Salicylate toxicity model of tinnitus

Daniel Stolzberg*, Richard J. Salvi and Brian L. Allman

Center for Hearing and Deafness, University at Buffalo, The State University of New York, Buffalo, NY, USA

****Correspondence:***
Daniel Stolzberg, Center for Hearing and Deafness, University at Buffalo, The State University of New York, 137 Cary Hall, Buffalo, NY 14214, USA.
e-mail: djs32@buffalo.edu

Salicylate, the active component of the common drug aspirin, has mild analgesic, antipyretic, and anti-inflammatory effects at moderate doses. At higher doses, however, salicylate temporarily induces moderate hearing loss and the perception of a high-pitch ringing in humans and animals. This phantom perception of sound known as tinnitus is qualitatively similar to the persistent subjective tinnitus induced by high-level noise exposure, ototoxic drugs, or aging, which affects ~14% of the general population. For over a quarter century, auditory scientists have used the salicylate toxicity model to investigate candidate biochemical and neurophysiological mechanisms underlying phantom sound perception. In this review, we summarize some of the intriguing biochemical and physiological effects associated with salicylate-induced tinnitus, some of which occur in the periphery and others in the central nervous system. The relevance and general utility of the salicylate toxicity model in understanding phantom sound perception in general are discussed.

Keywords: salicylate, aspirin, tinnitus, hearing loss, auditory dysfunction, animal models

INTRODUCTION

Subjective tinnitus is characterized by the perception of a sound in the absence of an acoustic source in the environment. A recent health census in the United States indicated approximately 50 million adults report having experienced tinnitus and 16 million experience it frequently (Shargorodsky et al., 2010).

Although the cochlea is responsible for transducing acoustic signals into neural activity, it is becoming clear that the brain is capable of generating neural activity of its own within the auditory pathway leading to tinnitus perception. Subjective tinnitus is primarily associated with sensorineural hearing loss (Norena et al., 2002; Weisz et al., 2006) which may be the consequence of loud noises, ototoxic drugs, or aging. While noise exposure is likely the most common trigger of tinnitus (Axelsson and Sandh, 1985), several ototoxic drugs are known to cause tinnitus in humans and animals. Among these are the chemotherapeutics such as cisplatin (Bokemeyer et al., 1998; Rachel et al., 2002), the antimalarial drug quinine (Kenmochi and Eggermont, 1997; Ochi and Eggermont, 1997; Eggermont and Kenmochi, 1998; Lobarinas et al., 2006; Ralli et al., 2010), and salicylate, the active component of the non-steroidal anti-inflammatory drug aspirin (Cazals, 2000). At therapeutic doses salicylate has mild analgesic, anti-inflammatory, and antipyretic effects and is commonly used for minor headaches and traditionally for rheumatic arthritis. At high doses, however, salicylate causes temporary hearing loss and reversible tinnitus, while hyperventilation, vertigo, confusion, hemorrhaging, or death may result from extremely high doses (Graham and Parker, 1948; Rauschka et al., 2007).

Since the establishment of a behavioral model of salicylate-induced tinnitus in rats (Jastreboff et al., 1988a,b), the drug has been used in various animal species to investigate the biological mechanisms of tinnitus generation. Although the mechanisms of tinnitus induction by salicylate may differ from those caused by other hearing disorders, salicylate-induced tinnitus has several distinct advantages over other methods of tinnitus induction such as acute noise trauma. Two such advantages are the rapid induction and reversibility of salicylate-induced tinnitus. Following oral consumption or systemic injection of the drug, tinnitus presents within minutes and subsides within 72 h of the final dose (Mongan et al., 1973). Interestingly, in a study by Mongan et al. (1973), it was found that the majority of humans with preexisting hearing loss (~68%) did not report tinnitus despite very high blood serum levels of salicylate. In rats, induction of tinnitus by systemic administration of salicylate was found to be highly reliable with proper dosing (Lobarinas et al., 2006), whereas noise trauma has a much more variable success of tinnitus induction (Kraus et al., 2010).

Salicylate has several well-established effects on cochlear function; however, more recent experiments have highlighted the drug's direct modulation of neural activity in the brain. The cochlear and central effects of salicylate should come as no surprise since the drug rapidly enters cochlear perilymph and cerebrospinal fluid simultaneously (Jastreboff et al., 1986). The widespread distribution of the drug adds to the complexity of understanding the mechanisms that are directly responsible for salicylate-induced tinnitus. Here we review some critical features of the salicylate toxicity model of tinnitus. We begin with a discussion of salicylate's primary effects in the cochlea, followed by its modulation of neurotransmitter systems and neural activity within the brain. Insights gained from the salicylate model of tinnitus continue to inform researchers about the potential mechanisms that lead to tinnitus perception.

COCHLEAR EFFECTS

Salicylate ototoxicity differs from most ototoxic drugs in that hearing loss and tinnitus normally subside within 1–3 days following cessation of treatment (Myers and Bernstein, 1965). Several independent effects of salicylate on the peripheral auditory system have been identified, each of which likely contribute to some aspect of the resulting hearing loss (summarized in **Figure 1**). Furthermore, salicylate-induced tinnitus has been hypothesized by some groups to be generated by altered cochlear activity and transmitted with fidelity to the central auditory system.

There exists a strong linear correlation between plasma levels of unbound salicylate and the extent of decreased auditory sensitivity (Day et al., 1989) reaching asymptote at a threshold of ~40 dB elevation despite increased dosing (Myers and Bernstein, 1965; McFadden and Plattsmier, 1984); however, the relationship of blood plasma salicylate levels to the presence of tinnitus is much less predictable (Mongan et al., 1973; Halla et al., 1991). This threshold shift can be accounted for by dysfunction of the outer hair cell (OHC) active response to sound. Otoacoustic emissions (OAEs) are acoustic signals generated by the electromotile OHCs and serve to improve sensitivity and sharpen frequency selectivity. Sound evoked OAEs, especially distortion product OAEs (DPOAE), are reduced in humans and animals at low to moderate stimulus levels during salicylate toxicity (Wier et al., 1988; Kujawa et al., 1992; Fitzgerald et al., 1993; Guitton et al., 2003; Ruel et al., 2008; Ralli et al., 2010; Stolzberg et al., 2011). *In vitro*, salicylate alters membrane conductance and the shape of OHCs (Douek et al., 1983; Shehata et al., 1991). Subsequent experiments showed that salicylate acts as a competitive antagonist for the chloride anion binding site of prestin (Oliver et al., 2001), the motor protein of OHCs, resulting in inhibition of OHC motility (Kakehata and Santos-Sacchi, 1996; Zheng et al., 2000).

Recently, we reported that acute systemic salicylate treatment in ketamine/xylazine anesthetized rats (300 mg/kg sodium salicylate, i.p.) suppresses high and low frequency DPOAEs to a greater extent than at middle frequencies (Stolzberg et al., 2011). Interestingly, the region of greatest sensitivity following salicylate corresponded to the behaviorally estimated pitch of tinnitus in rats (Yang et al., 2007; Kizawa et al., 2010).

The active generation of a sound within the cochlea by spontaneous OAEs (SOAEs) was an early hypothesis pointing to a peripheral generator of tinnitus (Wilson, 1980). SOAEs can be measured in ~38% of the population (Wier et al., 1984); however, most people with SOAEs do not have tinnitus. Conversely, SOAEs are absent in many people with tinnitus (Zurek, 1981). Salicylate treatment reduces or abolishes SOAEs in humans (McFadden and Plattsmier, 1984; Wier et al., 1988). Thus, SOAEs are unlikely to be a generator of the tinnitus signal.

Other measures of cochlear function, such as the cochlear microphonic (CM) and summating potential (SP), have been evaluated following local or systemic salicylate administration. The CM is an electrical signal that reflects the net flow of ionic currents alternating across cellular membranes in response to a periodic sound stimulus such as a tone. The CM, therefore, provides a gross index of the permeability of primarily OHCs of the inner ear. The CM has been shown to be unaffected in guinea pigs following cochlear perfusion of salicylate in response to 10 kHz tones (Puel et al., 1990), but increased in response to 1 kHz tones (Fitzgerald et al., 1993). Fitzgerald et al. (1993) attributed the different results of the two studies to the choice of stimulus frequency. The SP is a measure of the direct-current response of hair cells to sound recorded from the round window of the cochlea and most likely reflects both IHC and OHC function (Durrant et al., 1998). Cochlear perfusion of salicylate did not have an effect on SP in guinea pigs (Puel et al., 1990).

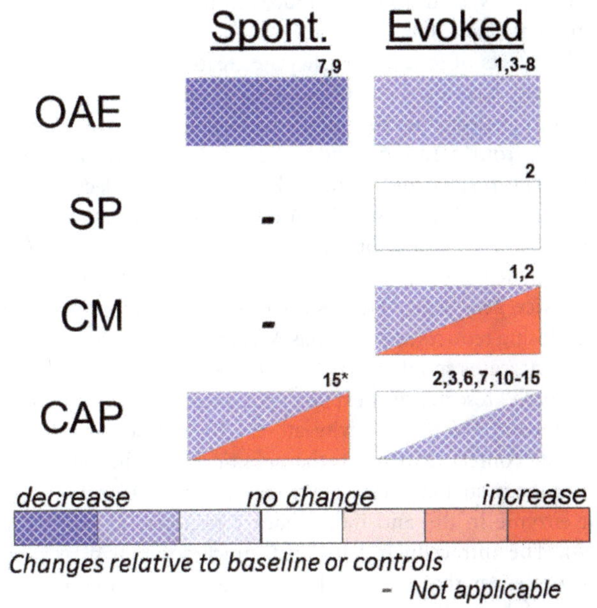

FIGURE 1 | Effects of systemic or cochlear perfusion of salicylate on spontaneous (Spont.) or sound-evoked (Evoked) cochlear measures. OAE, otoacoustic emissions; SP, summating potential; CM, cochlear microphonic; CAP, compound action potential. 1. Fitzgerald et al. (1993); 2. Puel et al. (1990); 3. Stolzberg et al. (2011); 4. Ruel et al. (2008); 5. Ralli et al. (2010); 6. Guitton et al. (2003); 7. Wier et al. (1988); 8. Janssen et al. (2000); 9. McFadden and Plattsmier (1984); 10. Muller et al. (2003); 11. Didier et al. (1993); 12. Silverstein et al. (1967); 13. Guitton et al. (2005); 14. Chen et al. (2010); 15. Cazals et al. (1998) (*spontaneous cochleoneural activity was decreased immediately after injection and increased on longer timescale; see text).

Auditory nerve (AN) fiber recordings following systemic salicylate administration have yielded variable results, most likely attributable to differential effects of moderate versus high dosing levels. In cats, Evans and Borerwe (1982) observed a significant increase in spontaneous firing rates following a high dose of sodium salicylate (400 mg/kg i.v.) in a subpopulation of AN fibers with baseline high spontaneous rate. This dose is extremely high for the cat since a slightly lower dose (350 mg/kg i.p.) has been reported to result in hyperventilation and death (Silverstein et al., 1967). In contrast, AN fibers in gerbils showed a small, yet significant, decrease in spontaneous firing rates in fibers with low characteristic frequencies (CFs) and no change in fibers with high CFs following a moderate dose of salicylate (200 mg/kg i.p. salicylic acid) (Muller et al., 2003). Kumagai (1992) reported that a high systemic dose (400 mg/kg i.v. sodium salicylate) significantly increased AN spontaneous firing rates in guinea pigs, whereas spontaneous firing rates were not affected by the low systemic dose (200 mg/kg i.v. sodium salicylate). The lower dose of salicylate, although it did not alter spontaneous activity in guinea pig AN, is sufficient to induce tinnitus-like behavior in rats (Lobarinas et al., 2006).

The effects of long-term salicylate treatment on spontaneous AN activity have also been investigated for changes in the average spectrum of electrophysiological cochleoneural activity (ASECA) recorded from a round window of guinea pigs (Cazals et al., 1998). The magnitude of the ASECA measure reflects spontaneous activity of the AN. ASECA decreased following the initial treatment of salicylate, but increased from baseline levels after approximately 1 week of treatments (200 mg/kg sodium salicylate, i.m., twice per diem). The results from this study indicate that acute dosing reduces spontaneous AN activity, whereas long-term dosing increases spontaneous AN activity.

Recently, research has explored the mechanisms of increased spontaneous AN fiber activity at very high doses of salicylate. Salicylate confers many of its therapeutic effects through inhibition of the inducible form of cyclooxygenase, COX-2, an important enzyme in the anti-inflammatory response of cells (Vane, 1998). The intracellular fatty acid, arachidonic acid, is a second messenger that is cleaved by the COX-2 enzyme, resulting in the synthesis of prostaglandins. The presence of arachidonic acid in high concentrations is known to potentiate *N*-Methyl-D-aspartate (NMDA) ionic currents in spiral ganglion neurons (Miller et al., 1992). Peng et al. (2003) showed salicylate does indeed potentiate NMDA currents in isolated pre-hearing postnatal mouse spiral ganglion cells. Ruel et al. (2008) further demonstrated that salicylate potentiated NMDA currents in AN afferent terminals by increasing available arachidonic acid. In addition, perilymphatic perfusion of a high concentration of salicylate (5 mM) increased AN spontaneous firing rates (Ruel et al., 2008). The same group (Guitton et al., 2005) demonstrated that blockade of NMDA channels prevented rats from developing salicylate-induced tinnitus, supporting their hypothesis that tinnitus is generated within the cochlea. In the study by Ruel et al. (2008), increased spontaneous firing rates of AN fibers was proposed to underlie tinnitus generation; however, the NMDA currents driving increased AN firing rates may only occur at extremely high concentrations of salicylate, far above those sufficient to induce tinnitus. In fact, the 5 mM sodium salicylate used in this study was the peak concentration measured in guinea pig perilymph following systemic treatment with 460 mg/kg (Jastreboff et al., 1986), a dose well above that sufficient to induce behavioral evidence of tinnitus in animals (Lobarinas et al., 2006). Indeed, Ruel et al. (2008) indicated in their report that 1 mM sodium salicylate failed to elicit detectable NMDA currents in spiral ganglion neurons. Thus, some of the reported effects of salicylate in the cochlea likely occur only at very high concentrations and may not be directly involved in tinnitus generation *per se*, but may play a role in determining the quality of the tinnitus percept. Anecdotal evidence suggests that at extremely high dose levels of aspirin alters the perception of tinnitus from reasonably tonal to cricket-like (see discussion in McFadden et al., 1984). It is plausible that a cricket-like perception may result from increased spontaneous AN activity.

Overall, salicylate's effects in the cochlea following systemic administration manifest as a reduction of sound-driven activity, primarily due to the reduction of OHC electromotility. Furthermore, at doses sufficient to induce tinnitus in animals, salicylate does not seem to significantly increase spontaneous AN activity. Taken together, the evidence from the literature seems to argue against AN hyperactivity as the direct cause of tinnitus; therefore, the cochlea is not likely generating the tinnitus signal. Moreover, a purely cochlear model of tinnitus generation is problematic because spontaneous activity is always present in the AN (Walsh et al., 1972) but does not normally cause tinnitus perception. While spontaneous AN activity is important for the encoding of acoustic signals (Koerber et al., 1966; Liberman and Kiang, 1978), the brain is normally capable of tuning out peripheral spontaneous activity unrelated to acoustic stimulation; i.e., most people do not experience tinnitus despite having spontaneous AN activity. Based on anatomical and electrophysiological studies of the brain in animal models of tinnitus, the following sections provide compelling evidence for a central contribution to salicylate-induced phantom sound perception.

CENTRAL EFFECTS

Salicylate clearly decreases the sensitivity of the sensory epithelium to sound and may modulate the rate of spontaneous AN transmission; however, there is also strong evidence that the drug directly modulates neurotransmission in the brain. An early study in human subjects provided evidence that the perception of tinnitus most often precedes self-reported hearing loss (Mongan et al., 1973). Since salicylate is delivered to both the perilymph and cerebrospinal fluid (Jastreboff et al., 1986), the report that tinnitus perception precedes self-reported hearing loss may indicate that the brain is more sensitive to the presence of salicylate than the cochlea. Furthermore, as discussed below, salicylate has been found to directly modulate inhibitory neurotransmission in the brain which may facilitate the rapidity at which phantom sound is experienced following systemic administration of the drug. The decreased cochlear sensitivity and/or alterations in spontaneous firing rates in the AN may serve more to determine the tinnitus pitch, whereas salicylate's direct effects on the brain act to generate and/or permit spurious neural activity to reach awareness.

IDENTIFYING KEY BRAIN REGIONS

Cytological markers of neural activity have been observed in several auditory and non-auditory brain regions in salicylate-induced tinnitus (**Figure 2**). The earliest studies used radioactive glucose, [^{14}C]2-deoxyglucose (2-DG) (Kauer et al., 1982; Wallhausser-Franke et al., 1996); whereas more recent studies have utilized immunolabeling of the immediate early gene *c-fos* (Wallhausser-Franke, 1997; Wallhausser-Franke et al., 2003; Wu et al., 2003), which is up-regulated in response to increased neural activity. Chronic systemic salicylate treatment at a dose known to induce behavioral evidence of tinnitus in gerbils resulted in reduced 2-DG uptake in the inferior colliculus (IC), particularly in the high-frequency responsive region, while increased uptake was observed in the auditory cortex (AC), as compared to saline controls (Wallhausser-Franke et al., 1996). In subsequent studies, small increases in c-fos were observed following acute systemic salicylate treatment (350 mg/kg i.p., sufficient to induce tinnitus) in the dorsal cochlear nucleus (dCN) and the dorsal division of the medial geniculate body (dMGB), but not in ventral

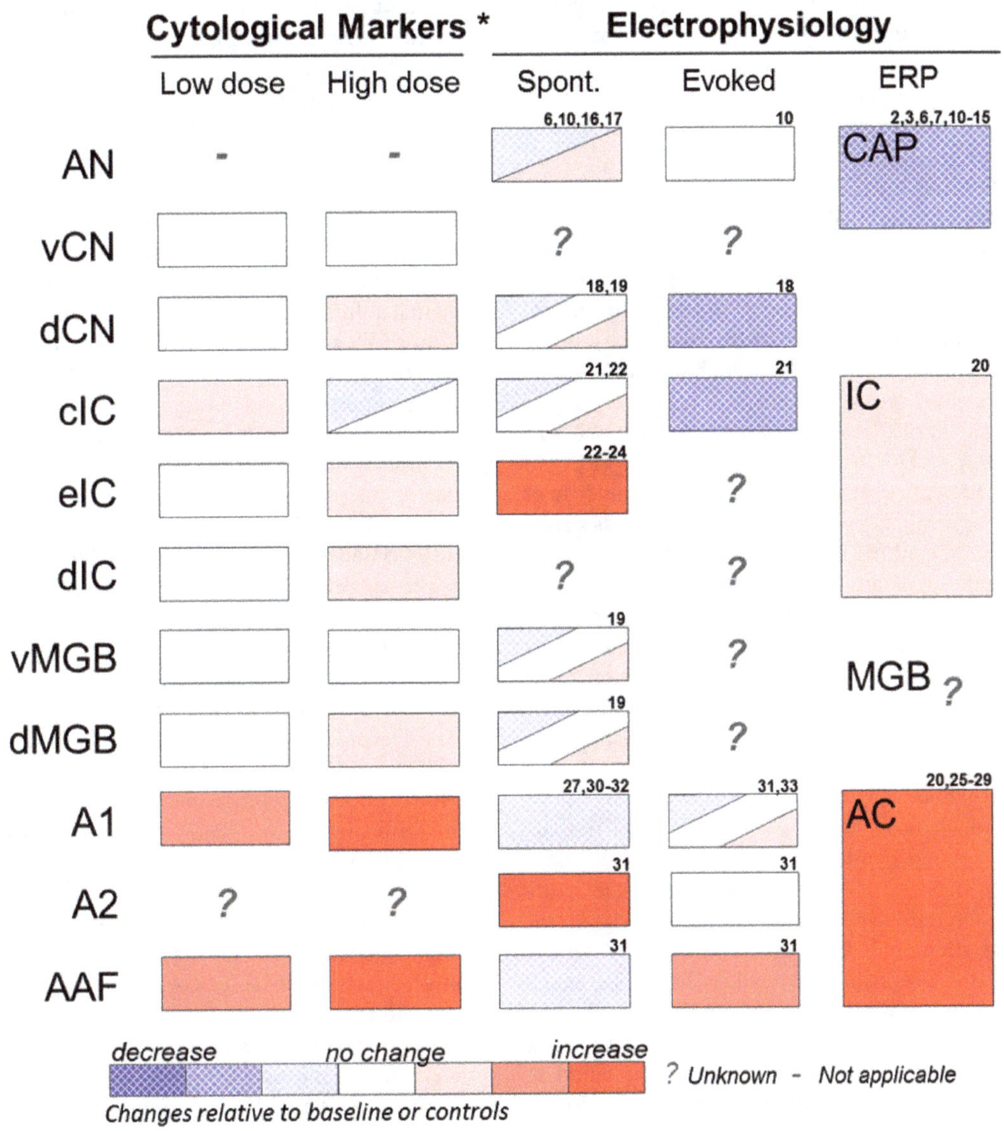

FIGURE 2 | Summary of effects of salicylate on various auditory structures. Cytological studies include results from 2-DG and fos-IR imaging studies (see Section "Identifying Key Brain Regions") and were performed at low (50 mg/kg i.p.) or high (350 mg/kg i.p.) acute doses of salicylate. Electrophysiology recordings were performed at various moderate to high salicylate doses. Results are from studies using *in vivo* extracellular recordings or *in vitro* extracellular or patch clamp recordings (see Section "Electrophysiology"). AN, auditory nerve; vCN, ventral cochlear nucleus; dCN, dorsal cochlear nucleus; cIC, central nucleus of the inferior colliculus; eIC, external nucleus of the inferior colliculus; dIC, dorsal nucleus of the inferior colliculus; vMGB, ventral portion of the medial geniculate body; dMGB, dorsal portion of the medial geniculate body; A1, primary auditory cortex; A2, secondary auditory cortex; AAF, anterior auditory field. Spont, single unit or multiunit spontaneous firing rates; Evoked, sound-evoked single unit or multiunit firing rates; ERP, sound-evoked response field potential; CAP, compound action potential of the cochlea; IC, inferior colliculus response potential; MGB, medial geniculate response potential; AC, auditory cortex response potential. *Represents acute effects of salicylate treatment (Wallhausser-Franke, 1997; Wallhausser-Franke et al., 2003). 2. Puel et al. (1990); 3. Stolzberg et al. (2011); 6. Guitton et al. (2003); 7. Wier et al. (1988); 8. Janssen et al. (2000); 9. McFadden and Plattsmier (1984); 10. Muller et al. (2003); 11. Didier et al. (1993); 12. Silverstein et al. (1967); 13. Guitton et al. (2005); 14. Chen et al. (2010); 15. Cazals et al. (1998); 16. Evans and Borerwe (1982); 17. Kumagai (1992); 18. Wei et al. (2010); 19. Basta et al. (2008); 20. Sun et al. (2009); 21. Ma et al. (2006); 22. Basta and Ernst (2004); 23. Jastreboff and Sasaki (1986); 24. Chen and Jastreboff (1995); 25. Lobarinas et al. (2006); 26. Norena et al. (2010); 27. Lu et al. (2011); 28. Lobarinas et al. (2006); 29. Paul et al. (2009); 30. Yang et al. (2007); 31. Eggermont and Kenmochi (1998); 32. Kenmochi and Eggermont (1997); 33. Zhang et al. (2011).

CN (vCN) or ventral MGB (vMGB) (Wallhausser-Franke, 1997; Wallhausser-Franke et al., 2003). The largest increases in c-fos expressing cells following salicylate (eight times the number of cells than control) were observed in AC, especially in primary AC (A1) and anterior auditory field (AAF) (Wallhausser-Franke et al., 2003). In contrast, the central nucleus of the IC (cIC) was virtually free of c-fos and only a moderate increase was observed in dorsomedial IC (dIC) (Wallhausser-Franke, 1997), which receives descending fibers from AC and does not belong to the ascending auditory pathway (Faye-Lund, 1985). Chronic dosing of salicylate in rats showed similar results for the CN and dIC, but differed in that increased c-fos was additionally observed in cIC (Wu et al., 2003). Interestingly, four times the number of cells expressing c-fos was observed in AC following systemic treatment of salicylate at a low dose (50 mg/kg), which is insufficient to induce behavioral evidence of tinnitus (Wallhausser-Franke et al., 2003). In the same study, a faint increase in c-fos expression was also observed in IC following the low, but not the high dose of salicylate. These results indicate that salicylate has effects on neural activity in the brain even at sub-tinnitus-inducing doses, indicating that the brain, and in particular AC, is highly sensitive to the presence of salicylate.

Paul and colleagues (2009) used a metabolic tracer, fluorine-18 deoxyglucose (FDG), and positron imaging tomography (PET) to image activity in the entire rat brain following a single dose of sodium salicylate (250 mg/kg i.p.). Metabolic activity was significantly increased in IC and AC; a small trend toward an increase was measured in the thalamus, but this did not reach statistical significance. The greatest increase in metabolic demands was observed in AC, followed by the IC, corroborating the results from immunocytochemistry experiments described above.

Holt and colleagues investigated the effects of chronic salicylate (3 consecutive days at 300 mg/kg i.p) in rats using manganese-enhanced MRI, a technique that assesses brain activity based on the uptake of manganese into active neurons (Holt et al., 2010). This technique, which has substantially higher spatial resolution than PET, measured significantly increased signal strength in dCN, but not in vCN, following chronic salicylate treatment, supporting the results of earlier *c-fos* studies. A significant increase in signal strength in cIC, dIC, and external nucleus of the IC (eIC) are consistent with earlier cytological studies after chronic salicylate dosing protocol (Wallhausser-Franke et al., 1996; Wu et al., 2003). Interestingly, this MRI study did not observe any significant changes in AC following salicylate treatment, whereas previous 2-DG studies with a similar dosing protocol had observed significant c-fos and metabolic activity in AC (Wallhausser-Franke et al., 1996; Paul et al., 2009).

Wallhäuser-Franke concluded: "If tinnitus is evoked by the effects of salicylate on the cochlea, increased c-fos immunoreactivity would be expected in auditory brainstem nuclei, especially since auditory stimulation readily evokes c-fos expression, for example in IC (see discussion in Wallhausser-Franke, 1997)." Following acoustic stimulation, the lemniscal auditory pathway structures (vCN, cIC, vMGB, and A1) all exhibit elevated c-fos expression (Carretta et al., 1999). As discussed in the previous section (see Section "Cochlear Effects"), if acute salicylate treatment does indeed increase spontaneous firing rates of AN fibers (Evans and Borerwe, 1982; Ruel et al., 2008) then 2-DG uptake and c-fos would be expected to be enhanced in the vCN, cIC, and vMGB. The apparent lack of c-fos within the lemniscal auditory structures following acute dosing of salicylate suggests that tinnitus-related hyperactivity originates within the brain and is related primarily to the AC and extralemniscal midbrain and brainstem structures (dMGB, dIC, and dCN). Results from immunocytochemistry studies are, therefore, more in line with the observations of reduced AN spontaneous firing rates recorded in gerbils following moderate systemic doses of salicylate sufficient to induce tinnitus (Muller et al., 2003).

While cytological studies support the hypothesis that central auditory structures play a critical role in tinnitus generation, it remains unclear if the hyperactivity in these auditory structures is the result of direct action of the drug on neural activity, the indirect result of dynamic adjustments of neural networks to decreased peripheral output, or a complex interaction between these peripheral and central effects. Furthermore, it should be noted that although this review is focused on alterations along the classical auditory pathway following salicylate, effects have been observed in other brain regions, such as limbic structures, and may play important roles in tinnitus (Wallhausser-Franke, 1997). In the following subsections, we will discuss evidence that salicylate does indeed directly modulate neurotransmission in the brain.

EFFECTS ON GABAergic NEUROTRANSMISSION

Salicylate has been shown to directly affect neurotransmitter systems in the brain. One important factor in salicylate-induced tinnitus is the drug's apparent direct actions on γ-aminobutyric acid (GABA) inhibitory neurotransmission in the brain.

Chronic treatment with salicylate in rats resulted in the increased expression of glutamic acid decarboxylase (GAD_{65}), the GABA synthesizing enzyme, in IC (Bauer et al., 2000). The increase in GAD was postulated to be compensatory for increased neural traffic. In the same study, a significant increase in $GABA_A$ receptor affinity in cIC, eIC, and dIC was measured. These changes may be the result of increased neural activity, direct effects of salicylate on GAD activity, or both. Indeed, changes in GAD concentration following salicylate treatment may be the result of direct inhibition of GAD enzymatic activity by salicylate (Gould et al., 1963; Gould and Smith, 1965); however, these effects were measured at relatively high concentrations *in vitro.*

Functional changes of GABAergic interneurons in the auditory system have also been observed. Salicylate applied to brain slices (1.4 mM) significantly decreased the frequency and amplitude of current-evoked and spontaneous-miniature inhibitory postsynaptic currents of AC layer 2/3 pyramidal cells (Wang et al., 2006). Furthermore, the same group later showed that salicylate selectively and reversibly silences current-evoked activity of fast-spiking inhibitory interneurons, but not of regular spiking inhibitory or excitatory pyramidal neurons within AC (Su et al., 2009). Such a decrease in GABAergic inhibition in AC by the direct action of salicylate has been proposed to permit hyperactivity within this region following acute treatment of salicylate observed in earlier cytological studies (see Section "Auditory Cortex").

Effects of salicylate on GABAergic neurotransmission have also been observed outside of the classic central auditory pathway. Similar to the results in A1 described above, both evoked and spontaneous inhibitory postsynaptic currents were decreased in excitatory neurons in the CA1 region of the hippocampus (Gong et al., 2008). Similar observations were made in the dorsal horn of rat spinal dorsal horn neurons (Xu et al., 2005). These results indicate that, at least *in vitro*, salicylate, at the concentrations used (generally 1.4 mM), exerts its greatest effects on highly active inhibitory neurons.

Taken together, both *in vitro* and *in vivo* experiments indicate that acute dosing of salicylate generally depresses GABAergic neurotransmission in the brain, whereas compensatory mechanisms, such as increased GAD expression, are initiated following chronic dosing protocols. Such modulation of GABAergic neurotransmission would be expected to significantly alter spontaneous and stimulus-driven neural activity. However, as discussed next, the results from some electrophysiology experiments corroborate the salicylate-induced disinhibition hypothesis, whereas other experiments indicate that salicylate has more complex modulation on neurotransmission in the brain.

ELECTROPHYSIOLOGY

The consequences of salicylate treatment on sound-evoked and spontaneous firing rates have been measured in many regions of the mammalian auditory brain *in vivo* and/or *in vitro* (summarized in **Figure 2**). In this section, we will review results from electrophysiology studies of salicylate's effects on brain regions along the auditory pathway and compare them to results from noise-exposures designed to induce tinnitus. Finding brain regions which exhibit similar alterations in neural activity following salicylate treatment or noise trauma will likely yield a framework for understanding phantom sound perception in general.

Cochlear nucleus

As detailed above (see Section "Identifying Key Brain Regions"), following acute systemic salicylate treatment, c-fos expression was increased in dCN, but not in vCN. This result can be taken as evidence that acute salicylate treatment primarily affects non-lemniscal auditory structures. Indeed, activity in vCN tends to follow AN activity, whereas activity in dCN is more heavily modulated by non-auditory brain regions (Koerber et al., 1966). To the best of our knowledge electrophysiological recordings in dCN following salicylate treatment have only been carried out in brain slice preparations. Salicylate was found to either increase (52.9%) or decrease (47.1%) spontaneous firing rates of a subpopulation (68%) of neurons in dCN (Basta et al., 2008). In a more recent patch clamp study, spontaneous and current-evoked firing rates of fusiform cells, but not cartwheel cells, in the dCN were selectively suppressed by salicylate (Wei et al., 2010). Furthermore, inhibitory postsynaptic currents recorded in fusiform cells of the dCN were significantly decreased by salicylate. These results indicated that suppressed firing rates in fusiform cells were most likely due to salicylate's direct effects on the intrinsic properties of this cell type and not the result of increased inhibition (Wei et al., 2010).

Significantly elevated spontaneous firing rates have been recorded from dCN fusiform cells in hamsters (Kaltenbach et al., 2004) and chinchillas (Brozoski et al., 2002) with behavioral evidence of tinnitus following exposure to loud tones. In subsequent studies by Brozoski and colleagues it was demonstrated that bilateral ablation of dCN in chinchillas with chronic tinnitus did not abolish tinnitus behavior in affected animals (Brozoski and Bauer, 2005); whereas ablation of dCN prior to noise trauma prevented the induction of tinnitus (Brozoski et al., 2012). While the dCN may play a role in the initial generation of tinnitus symptoms following intense sound exposure (Brozoski et al., 2012), the structure does not seem to be required to maintain the tinnitus percept (Brozoski and Bauer, 2005).

Inferior colliculus

Some of the earliest evidence that salicylate has direct effects on neural activity within the auditory brain was provided by electrophysiological recordings of altered neural activity in the IC following systemic delivery of salicylate. Following acute dosing in guinea pigs anesthetized with pentobarbital, spontaneous firing rates of a population of neurons in the eIC significantly increased (Jastreboff and Sasaki, 1986; Chen and Jastreboff, 1995), while the occurrence and duration of bursting type discharges in eIC increased for neurons sensitive to sound frequencies near the behaviorally assessed tinnitus pitch (Chen and Jastreboff, 1995). A mouse brain slice study observed similar frequency specific increases in spontaneous firing rates in cIC and eIC of neurons residing in anatomical regions receptive to sound frequencies at the animal's best hearing threshold (Basta and Ernst, 2004). Recordings from cIC of ketamine/xylazine anesthetized mice showed that acute salicylate treatment significantly decreased the occurrence of spontaneous bursting-type activity from single units as well as decreased the coefficient of variation for interspike intervals, indicating more regular spontaneous firing patterns (Ma et al., 2006). Furthermore, these changes were found to be greatest for single units with best frequencies below 27 kHz. Taken together, these electrophysiological results seem to corroborate observations of increased *c-fos* in eIC while the decreased spontaneous firing rates recorded *in vivo* agrees with the small decrease of *c-fos* observed in cIC following acute systemic treatment (Wallhausser-Franke, 1997).

Intravenous injection of lidocaine, a sodium channel blocker used to temporarily alleviate tinnitus in humans with chronic tinnitus (Perucca and Jackson, 1985; Reyes et al., 2002), reduced the salicylate-enhanced spontaneous firing rates of some guinea pig IC neurons for more than 30 minutes (Manabe et al., 1997). It is unclear from this study where in the IC these recordings were performed. We can speculate that since previous studies observed decreased spiking in cIC (Ma et al., 2006) and increased spiking in eIC (Chen and Jastreboff, 1995) that lidocaine may have been acting on neurons in eIC.

The amplitude of sound-evoked local field potentials (LFPs) recorded from the rat IC was unchanged following acute systemic salicylate injection; however, since the sound-evoked cochlear response (CAP) is decreased by salicylate treatment (see Section "Cochlear Effects"), the stable sound-evoked LFP amplitude of the IC indicates the neural signal was enhanced to a small degree in the brainstem (Sun et al., 2009). In the same study, application of sodium salicylate to the round window resulted in both decreased CAP amplitude and a correspondingly reduced sound-evoked LFP recorded from IC. These results provide further evidence that salicylate acts on the cochlea as well as directly on brain, most likely through the reduction of central inhibitory neurotransmission (see Section "Effects on GABAergic Neurotransmission").

Studies using the acute noise trauma model of tinnitus have observed increased spontaneous firing rates in the cIC near the exposure frequency after a week or more following noise exposure (Ma et al., 2006; Mulders and Robertson, 2009). Mulders and Robertson (2009) further demonstrated that inactivation, chemically, by cooling, or by complete ablation of the noise-exposed cochlea, reduced spontaneous firing rates of the contralateral cIC neurons compared to those of control animals. These results indicate that significantly enhanced spontaneous activity in cIC weeks after noise exposure still requires afferent input to exhibit these changes. While increased spontaneous activity weeks following noise trauma differs from acute salicylate treatment, where a decrease in c-fos was found in cIC (Wallhausser-Franke et al., 2003), chronic salicylate treatment similarly increased c-fos and 2-DG uptake in cIC (Wallhausser-Franke et al., 1996; Wu et al., 2003).

The role of the cIC in tinnitus may be different on short and long time scales. In acutely induced tinnitus from either noise trauma or salicylate, spontaneous firing rates in cIC do not increase immediately (salicylate or noise in mouse, Ma et al., 2006; noise in guinea pigs, Mulders and Robertson, 2009). In the case of noise trauma, spontaneous rates in the dCN and cIC increase starting 7 days or more after the exposure (Kaltenbach et al., 2004; Mulders and Robertson, 2009). Taken together, these results indicate that chronic, but not acute tinnitus may be associated with increased spontaneous firing in cIC.

One common feature between salicylate- and noise-induced tinnitus is the enhancement of the sound-evoked LFP recorded from the IC (Salvi et al., 1990; Mulders and Robertson, 2009; Sun et al., 2009). This enhanced response to sound may reflect a disinhibition in IC following manipulations that induce tinnitus. The precise location of this enhancement within the IC, (i.e., within cIC, dIC, or eIC), has yet to be determined.

Medial geniculate body

The only electrophysiological recordings of salicylate's effects on neural activity in MGB have been from extracellular recordings *in vitro* (Basta et al., 2008). In this study, the MGB (dorsal and ventral cells were analyzed together) exhibited the greatest proportion of neurons which had significantly altered spontaneous firing rates during salicylate application (dCN: 68.0%; MGB: 80.8%; AC: 71.4% of all recorded neurons); however, the direction of change in spontaneous firing rates of this MGB cell population were roughly equivalent (52.4% increase, 47.6% decrease).

We are unaware of any existing studies directly investigating the role of MGB in noise-induced tinnitus. Since MGB and the reticular nucleus of the thalamus play a critical role in gating auditory neural activity, these regions in concert with AC have been proposed to play a critical role in tinnitus perception (Llinas et al., 1999).

Auditory cortex

The effects of salicylate on spontaneous and sound-evoked neural activity within the auditory pathway have been most extensively studied in AC. The attention paid to this specific brain region may be warranted since several studies in animals have measured the largest changes in AC following acute systemic salicylate administration. Cytological studies indicate that metabolic activity in the core auditory cortex (A1 and AAF) was increased to the greatest extent over other auditory brain regions (Wallhausser-Franke et al., 2003, and see Section "Identifying Key Brain Regions"). The increased metabolic activity is presumed to reflect increased spontaneous neural activity; however, electrophysiology studies of AC do not seem to be in full agreement with this interpretation. In A1 and AAF, a small decrease in spontaneous firing rates has been measured following salicylate (Eggermont and Kenmochi, 1998; Yang et al., 2007; Lu et al., 2011), whereas a significant increase in secondary auditory cortex (A2) spontaneous firing rates was observed in anesthetized cats (Eggermont and Kenmochi, 1998). Since A1 and AAF receive projections primarily from the ascending lemniscal auditory pathway by way of vMGB (Huang and Winer, 2000), a small decrease observed in these regions may simply reflect the decreased cochlear output following salicylate treatment. In contrast, A2 is more heavily innervated by extralemniscal projections originating in dMGB (Huang and Winer, 2000). The increase in spontaneous neural activity in A2 may therefore indicate that the extralemniscal auditory structures play a more central role in salicylate-induced tinnitus. Furthermore, Eggermont and Kenmochi (1998) suggested that the presence of an incongruity in spontaneous firing rates across fields of AC may be an important feature distinguishing tinnitus-driven from acoustically driven sound perception.

The involvement of spontaneous activity in A1 during tinnitus induced by noise trauma has not been heavily investigated. Engineer et al. (2011) recorded sound-driven and spontaneous neural activity in A1 of rats 1 month following acute noise trauma. Rats with signs of tinnitus following noise exposure, assessed using the gap pre-pulse inhibition of the acoustic startle reflex paradigm, exhibited significantly increased spontaneous firing rates in A1; however, the reversal of signs of tinnitus using vagal-nerve stimulation paired with tones resulted in an additional increase in spontaneous firing rates. The authors conclude that increased spontaneous firing rates of neurons in A1 were not significantly correlated with evidence of tinnitus in rats.

In addition to simple spontaneous firing rates, other interesting changes in neural activity in AC have been observed following salicylate treatment. Ochi and Eggermont (1996) described changes in the temporal dynamics of spontaneous neural activity in A1 associated with salicylate treatment that may be more informative than simple statistics of population spontaneous firing rates. Salicylate was found to significantly increase the rebound to peak of the autocorrelation function, a mathematical tool used to look for repeating firing patterns of an individual neuron, indicating each spontaneous spike was followed by a prolonged interval before the next spike occurred. Furthermore, neurons in A1 were best modulated by click trains at slower presentation rates following salicylate. These changes in the temporal dynamics of A1 neural activity were hypothesized to be caused by increased afterhyperpolarization (AHP) resulting from enhanced activation of slow conducting Ca^{2+}-activated K^{+}-channels of cortical neurons (Ochi and Eggermont, 1996). The rationale for this hypothesis stems from studies of salicylate's action on peripheral nerve membranes at relatively high concentrations (20 mM, Neto et al., 1980) compared to those levels measured in cerebrospinal fluid following systemic treatment (1.4 mM, Jastreboff et al., 1986). In a more recent brain slice patch clamp study, a lower concentration of salicylate (1.4 mM) failed to significantly alter AHP amplitude in AC neurons (Su et al., 2009). Additional *in vivo* studies with pharmacological manipulations are required to better understand the basis for the altered temporal dynamics observed in A1.

Sound-evoked activity in AC is greatly altered by systemically administered or locally applied salicylate (Lobarinas et al., 2006; Sun et al., 2009; Norena et al., 2010; Lu et al., 2011). Since the sound-evoked CAP is decreased in the cochlea by either route of delivery, the enhanced AC response indicates a signal gain increase occurs within the brain (Sun et al., 2009). Sun et al. (2009) recorded sound-evoked LFPs from electrodes chronically implanted over AC in awake and anesthetized rats before and after salicylate treatment. In awake rats, the amplitude of sound-evoked AC response was significantly enhanced following systemic dose of salicylate (200 mg/kg i.p). Responses in AC were further enhanced in the same rats while under ketamine (NMDA receptor antagonist) anesthesia, whereas they were suppressed while under isoflurane ($GABA_A$ receptor agonist) anesthesia. In a subsequent study, application of salicylate (2 mM) to the brain surface over AC had similar effects on spontaneous (small decrease) and sound-evoked multiunit firing rates (significant increase) providing further evidence that these changes can be attributed to the direct effects of salicylate on the brain (Lu et al., 2011). Furthermore, co-application of the GABA transaminase inhibitor vigabatrin, which effectively increases the concentration of available GABA, or the $GABA_B$ receptor agonist baclofen to the brain surface reduced the salicylate-induced enhancement of sound-evoked multiunit firing rates (Lu et al., 2011).

Recently we showed that systemic salicylate treatment has significant and rapid effects on frequency receptive field tuning of neurons in the anesthetized rat A1 (Stolzberg et al., 2011). Following systemic administration of salicylate (250 or 300 mg/kg i.p.) the characteristic frequency, i.e., the sound frequency at which units were most sensitive, tended to shift toward 10–20 kHz (**Figure 3**), frequencies which coincide with the pitch of salicylate-induced tinnitus determined from previous behavioral studies. We hypothesized that this dramatic change in the frequency sensitivity of neurons in A1 may be the result of two coincident effects of salicylate. First, salicylate significantly altered the profile of OHC sensitivity with the greatest reduction at low (<10 kHz) and high (>20 kHz) sound frequencies (in rat, Stolzberg et al., 2011). Additionally, salicylate had greater effects on high frequencies resulting in a somewhat sloping high-frequency hearing loss beginning at 16 kHz. Second, a decrease in cortical inhibition (Wang et al., 2006; Su et al., 2009; Lu et al., 2011) may result in shifting of neuronal characteristic frequencies on a rapid timescale. The overrepresentation of frequency along the tonotopic gradient of A1 has been observed following acoustic trauma (Irvine et al., 2000; Eggermont and Komiya, 2000), various learning paradigms using acoustic stimuli (Edeline et al., 1993; Rutkowski and Weinberger, 2005), and in humans with chronic tinnitus (Wienbruch et al., 2006). It has been proposed that an overrepresentation of a frequency along the tonotopic gradient in A1 may reflect the relative behavioral importance of a sound to the organism (Rutkowski and Weinberger, 2005).

In humans, a magnetoencephalography study by Wienbruch et al. (2006) observed a flattening of the tonotopic gradient and an enhanced dipole response using 40-Hz auditory stimuli in A1

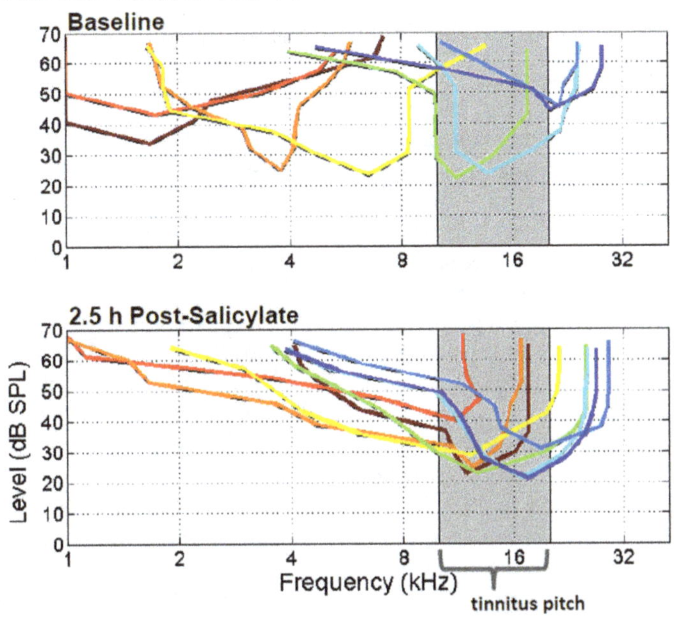

FIGURE 3 | Frequency tuning of eight simultaneously recorded extracellularly recorded multunits from primary auditory cortex before (top panel) and after systemic salicylate injection (bottom panel; 250 mg/kg i.p.). Following systemic salicylate treatment, the frequency tunings of tracked multiunits shifted maximal frequency sensitivities toward the 10–20 kHz frequency region, near the estimated tinnitus pitch. Please see Stolzberg et al., 2011 for population statistics. [From Stolzberg et al. (2011) with permission].

of tinnitus subjects compared with controls. Recently, Engineer et al. (2011) demonstrated that the pairing of vagal nerve stimulation with tones was able to retune the distorted tonotopic gradient in A1 of rats with evidence of noise-induced tinnitus. The retuning of A1 tonotopy using the vagal nerve stimulation protocol reduced the number of rats with evidence of tinnitus using the gap-prepulse inhibition of the acoustic startle reflex test. The authors also found that distortion of the tonotopic gradient and broadening of tuning curves in A1 was significantly correlated with the degree of gap detection impairment (interpreted as the presence of tinnitus); however, changes in spontaneous firing rates or synchronization were not found to be correlated with the presence of tinnitus (Engineer et al., 2011).

Tonotopic overrepresentation in A1 has been proposed to result from the unmasking of normally inhibited intracortical connections (Eggermont and Roberts, 2004). Furthermore, the overrepresentation of frequencies in A1 results in an enhanced sound-evoked field potential. It remains uncertain whether or not such an overrepresentation is responsible for the generation of tinnitus signal or if it reflects persistent spontaneous neural activation somewhere else along the auditory pathway.

DISCUSSION

The salicylate toxicity model differs from the noise trauma model of tinnitus in several respects; however, a few aspects shared by the two models may facilitate the identification of key brain regions and patterns of neural activity involved in tinnitus perception in general.

PERIPHERAL OR CENTRAL?

One critical aspect to understanding the origins of tinnitus is whether a persistent signal is generated in the ear or abnormal patterns of neural activity occur within the brain. In humans with persistent subjective tinnitus, neural activity closely linked to changes in tinnitus loudness have been observed in AC, medial geniculate and other sites within the central nervous system (Lockwood et al., 1998; Muhlnickel et al., 1998; Lockwood et al., 2001; Reyes et al., 2002). Since salicylate is delivered to the brain and cochlea simultaneously following systemic treatment (Jastreboff et al., 1986) it is difficult to make a clear dissociation between the drug's peripheral and central effects. One of the primary sources of confusion regarding the locus of salicylate's generation of tinnitus signal, and the utility of the drug as a model for more common manifestations of tinnitus (i.e., following noise trauma or presbycusis), stems from the use of very high concentrations of sodium salicylate in AN fiber recordings.

Systemic treatment with sodium salicylate at moderate doses capable of inducing tinnitus either does not affect or slightly decreases spontaneous firing rates of AN fibers (Kumagai, 1992; Muller et al., 2003); however, at very high concentrations, salicylate begins to induce effects in the inner ear resulting in increased AN spontaneous firing rates (Evans and Borerwe, 1982; Ruel et al., 2008). Since behavioral evidence of tinnitus can be induced at the moderate doses of salicylate (Myers and Bernstein, 1965; Lobarinas et al., 2006), effects observed at very high concentrations of the drug may be difficult to directly relate to tinnitus generation or perception. Evidence from cytological studies which used acute salicylate treatment at moderate doses indicate that brain regions associated with the ascending lemniscal auditory system show either a decrease or no change in markers related to neural activity (Wallhausser-Franke et al., 2003). Since acoustic stimulation activates the lemniscal auditory pathway (Carretta et al., 1999), whereas acute systemic salicylate treatment at a moderate dose does not (Wallhausser-Franke, 1997; Wallhausser-Franke et al., 2003), it is unlikely that salicylate concentrations sufficient to induce tinnitus increase AN spontaneous firing rates. With regards to spontaneous AN activity, the use of a moderate dose of salicylate seems to be in agreement with other manipulations which induce decreased cochlear sensitivity, such as noise trauma (Liberman and Kiang, 1978) or selective inner hair cell loss (Wang et al., 1997). Taken together, it is likely that an acute moderate dose of salicylate induces tinnitus by alteration of neural activity within the brain and not inherited from increased spontaneous AN activity. Following salicylate, changes in cochlear sensitivity may, however, play a role in determining the pitch of tinnitus (Stolzberg et al., 2011).

TIME COURSE OF SALICYLATE'S ACTIONS

Existing research on the central effects of salicylate seems to be approximately split equally between acute and chronic dosing protocols. As discussed throughout this review, it is critical to consider the time course of effects following systemic salicylate treatment. Immediately following acute systemic treatment with salicylate, the extralemniscal pathway rapidly becomes hyperactive whereas spontaneous firing rates within lemniscal auditory structures remain relatively stable. On the other hand, chronic systemic salicylate treatment increases spontaneous firing rates within the lemniscal pathway (Wallhausser-Franke et al., 1996; Wu et al., 2003). These differential effects of acute and chronic salicylate treatment regimens are important to keep in mind while seeking putative mechanisms of salicylate-induced tinnitus. Studying the effects of acute and chronic salicylate treatment may yield information about various aspects of the drug's actions in the cochlea and the brain. Since tinnitus occurs rapidly after systemic administration of salicylate, the results from acute salicylate treatment in animals are likely to be highly informative about which brain regions are involved in the tinnitus perception *per se*, whereas the results from studying chronic salicylate treatment may be more informative regarding compensatory biochemical and neural mechanisms which may be targets for tuning out the tinnitus. One example of a compensatory mechanism is enhanced prestin expression and increased DPOAE response following chronic salicylate treatment (Huang et al., 2005; Yang et al., 2009; Chen et al., 2010).

UTILITY OF SALICYLATE TOXICITY AS A MODEL FOR TINNITUS

Induction of tinnitus using salicylate has a few important advantages over other methods of induction such as noise trauma. First, salicylate acts rapidly to induce tinnitus in subjects and is metabolized within days in most species, providing the ability to monitor physiological changes before, during, and after tinnitus. Second, the drug's effects on GABAergic neurotransmission may model other conditions which similarly decrease GABAergic neurotransmission associated with tinnitus in humans such as aging (Caspary et al., 1995, 1999; Ling et al., 2005). Third, salicylate can be administered to humans whereas intense noise trauma is often unethical (however see Ortmann et al., 2011). A fourth advantage is that the locus of drug delivery can be controlled. This provides a means to dissociate the drug's effects on various brain regions *in vitro* and *in vivo*. Finally, with proper dosing, salicylate can reliably induce tinnitus behavior in animals (Jastreboff et al., 1988a,b; Lobarinas et al., 2006), whereas noise trauma is highly variable at inducing tinnitus behavior in animals (Kraus et al., 2010).

There are also some important inherent limitations of the salicylate model of tinnitus. One such limitation of systemic administration of salicylate is that the drug induces binaural hearing loss and the perception of tinnitus is binaural. Unilateral noise trauma provides the opportunity to study tinnitus-related changes ipsilateral or contralateral to the exposed ear within individual brains. The reliability of tinnitus induction by salicylate may be considered a limitation of the model. The variable success of noise trauma in inducing tinnitus permits experimenters to identify potential mechanisms of susceptibility to tinnitus.

The utility of the salicylate toxicity model of tinnitus may ultimately reside in which of the drug's effects are similar with those of noise induced tinnitus. On an acute time course, identifying brain regions and abnormal patterns of neural activity coincident between multiple methods of tinnitus induction will likely yield a greater understanding of tinnitus perception in general. The entrenchment of the tinnitus signal in neural circuits on the timescale of years (for example see Schlee et al., 2008), however, may not be an approachable aspect of subjective tinnitus to investigate using the salicylate model.

REMAINING QUESTIONS

Some important experimental questions remain for tinnitus researchers which may be best approached using the salicylate toxicity model:

- Why does acute salicylate administration increase neural activity in extralemniscal, but not lemniscal auditory structures?
- Does pre-ablation of the dCN prevent salicylate-induced tinnitus (see Section "Cochlear Nucleus").
- What determines the behaviorally identified pitch of salicylate-induced tinnitus? Is it determined solely by salicylate's effects in the cochlea? Or is it determined by alterations of tonotopic gradients within the auditory brain?
- What do the differential effects of acute and chronic dosing of salicylate tell us about neuroplasticity and the entrenchment of the tinnitus signal?

ACKNOWLEDGMENTS

The authors thank S. Hayes for her valuable feedback on the manuscript. Work supported in part by grants from NIH (R01DC009091, R01DC009219, R03DC011374-01, F31DC010931), Tinnitus Research Consortium and Tinnitus Research Initiative.

REFERENCES

Axelsson, A., and Sandh, A. (1985). Tinnitus in noise-induced hearing loss. *Br. J. Audiol.* 19, 271–276.

Basta, D., and Ernst, A. (2004). Effects of salicylate on spontaneous activity in inferior colliculus brain slices. *Neurosci. Res.* 50, 237–243.

Basta, D., Goetze, R., and Ernst, A. (2008). Effects of salicylate application on the spontaneous activity in brain slices of the mouse cochlear nucleus, medial geniculate body and primary auditory cortex. *Hear. Res.* 240, 42–51.

Bauer, C. A., Brozoski, T. J., Holder, T. M., and Caspary, D. M. (2000). Effects of chronic salicylate on GABAergic activity in rat inferior colliculus. *Hear. Res.* 147, 175–182.

Bokemeyer, C., Berger, C. C., Hartmann, J. T., Kollmannsberger, C., Schmoll, H. J., Kuczyk, M. A., and Kanz, L. (1998). Analysis of risk factors for cisplatin-induced ototoxicity in patients with testicular cancer. *Br. J. Cancer* 77, 1355–1362.

Brozoski, T. J., and Bauer, C. A. (2005). The effect of dorsal cochlear nucleus ablation on tinnitus in rats. *Hear. Res.* 206, 227–236.

Brozoski, T. J., Bauer, C. A., and Caspary, D. M. (2002). Elevated fusiform cell activity in the dorsal cochlear nucleus of chinchillas with psychophysical evidence of tinnitus. *J. Neurosci.* 22, 2383–2390.

Brozoski, T. J., Wisner, K. W., Sybert, L. T., and Bauer, C. A. (2012). Bilateral dorsal cochlear nucleus lesions prevent acoustic-trauma induced tinnitus in an animal model. *J. Assoc. Res. Otolaryngol.* 13, 55–66.

Carretta, D., Herve-Minvielle, A., Bajo, V. M., Villa, A. E., and Rouiller, E. M. (1999). c-Fos expression in the auditory pathways related to the significance of acoustic signals in rats performing a sensory-motor task. *Brain Res.* 841, 170–183.

Caspary, D. M., Holder, T. M., Hughes, L. F., Milbrandt, J. C., McKernan, R. M., and Naritoku, D. K. (1999). Age-related changes in GABA(A) receptor subunit composition and function in rat auditory system. *Neuroscience* 93, 307–312.

Caspary, D. M., Milbrandt, J. C., and Helfert, R. H. (1995). Central auditory aging: GABA changes in the inferior colliculus. *Exp. Gerontol.* 30, 349–360.

Cazals, Y. (2000). Auditory sensori-neural alterations induced by salicylate. *Prog. Neurobiol.* 62, 583–631.

Cazals, Y., Horner, K. C., and Huang, Z. W. (1998). Alterations in average spectrum of cochleoneural activity by long-term salicylate treatment in the guinea pig: a plausible index of tinnitus. *J. Neurophysiol.* 80, 2113–2120.

Chen, G. D., and Jastreboff, P. J. (1995). Salicylate-induced abnormal activity in the inferior colliculus of rats. *Hear. Res.* 82, 158–178.

Chen, G. D., Kermany, M. H., D'Elia, A., Ralli, M., Tanaka, C., Bielefeld, E. C., Ding, D., Henderson, D., and Salvi, R. (2010). Too much of a good thing: long-term treatment with salicylate strengthens outer hair cell function but impairs auditory neural activity. *Hear. Res.* 265, 63–69.

Day, R. O., Graham, G. G., Bieri, D., Brown, M., Cairns, D., Harris, G., Hounsell, J., Platt-Hepworth, S., Reeve, R., Sambrook, P. N., and Smith, J. (1989). Concentration-response relationships for salicylate-induced ototoxicity in normal volunteers. *Br. J. Clin. Pharmacol.* 28, 695–702.

Didier, A., Miller, J. M., and Nuttall, A. L. (1993). The vascular component of sodium salicylate ototoxicity in the guinea pig. *Hear. Res.* 69, 199–206.

Douek, E. E., Dodson, H. C., and Bannister, L. H. (1983). The effects of sodium salicylate on the cochlea of guinea pigs. *J. Laryngol. Otol.* 97, 793–799.

Durrant, J., Wang, J., Ding, D., and Salvi, R. (1998). Are inner or outer hair cells the source of summating potentials recorded from the round window? *J. Acoust. Soc. Am.* 104, 370–377.

Edeline, J. M., Pham, P., and Weinberger, N. M. (1993). Rapid development of learning-induced receptive field plasticity in the auditory cortex. *Behav. Neurosci.* 107, 539–551.

Eggermont, J. J., and Kenmochi, M. (1998). Salicylate and quinine selectively increase spontaneous firing rates in secondary auditory cortex. *Hear. Res.* 117, 149–160.

Eggermont, J. J., and Komiya, H. (2000). Moderate noise trauma in juvenile cats results in profound cortical topographic map changes in adulthood. *Hear. Res.* 142, 89–101.

Eggermont, J. J., and Roberts, L. E. (2004). The neuroscience of tinnitus. *Trends Neurosci.* 27, 676–682.

Engineer, N. D., Riley, J. R., Seale, J. D., Vrana, W. A., Shetake, J. A., Sudanagunta, S. P., Borland, M. S., and Kilgard, M. P. (2011). Reversing pathological neural activity using targeted plasticity. *Nature* 470, 101–104.

Evans, E. F., and Borerwe, T. A. (1982). Ototoxic effects of salicylates on the responses of single cochlear nerve fibres and on cochlear potentials. *Br. J. Audiol.* 16, 101–108.

Faye-Lund, H. (1985). The neocortical projection to the inferior colliculus in the albino rat. *Anat. Embryol.* 173, 53–70.

Fitzgerald, J. J., Robertson, D., and Johnstone, B. M. (1993). Effects of intra-cochlear perfusion of salicylates on cochlear microphonic and other auditory responses in the guinea pig. *Hear. Res.* 67, 147–156.

Gong, N., Zhang, M., Zhang, X. B., Chen, L., Sun, G. C., and Xu, T. L. (2008). The aspirin metabolite salicylate enhances neuronal excitation in rat hippocampal CA1 area through reducing GABAergic inhibition. *Neuropharmacology* 54, 454–463.

Gould, B. J., Huggins, A. K., and Smith, M. J. (1963). Effects of salicylate on glutamate dehydrogenase and glutamate decarboxylase. *Biochem. J.* 88, 346–349.

Gould, B. J., and Smith, M. J. (1965). Inhibition of rat brain glutamate decarboxylase activity by salicylate *in vitro*. *J. Pharm. Pharmacol.* 17, 15–18.

Graham, J. D., and Parker, W. A. (1948). The toxic manifestations of sodium salicylate therapy. *Q. J. Med.* 17, 153–163.

Guitton, M. J., Caston, J., Ruel, J., Johnson, R. M., Pujol, R., and Puel, J. L. (2003). Salicylate induces tinnitus through activation of cochlear NMDA receptors. *J. Neurosci.* 23, 3944–3952.

Guitton, M. J., Pujol, R., and Puel, J. L. (2005). m-Chlorophenylpiperazine exacerbates perception of salicylate-induced tinnitus in rats. *Eur. J. Neurosci.* 22, 2675–2678.

Halla, J. T., Atchison, S. L., and Hardin, J. G. (1991). Symptomatic salicylate ototoxicity: a useful indicator of serum salicylate concentration? *Ann. Rheum. Dis.* 50, 682–684.

Holt, A. G., Bissig, D., Mirza, N., Rajah, G., and Berkowitz, B. (2010). Evidence of key tinnitus-related brain regions documented by a unique combination of manganese-enhanced MRI and acoustic startle reflex testing. *PloS One* 5:e14260. doi: 10.1371/journal.pone.0014260

Huang, C. L., and Winer, J. A. (2000). Auditory thalamocortical projections in the cat: laminar and areal patterns of input. *J. Comp. Neurol.* 427, 302–331.

Huang, Z. W., Chen, P., Mei, L., Fan, Q. J., Xiao, B. K., and Wu, Z. Y. (2005). Differentially expressed gene profiles of cochlea in rats induced by acute and chronic sodium salicylate injection. *Zhonghua Er Bi Yan Hou Tou Jing Wai Ke Za Zhi* 40, 27–32.

Irvine, D. R., Rajan, R., and McDermott, H. J. (2000). Injury-induced reorganization in adult auditory cortex and its perceptual consequences. *Hear. Res.* 147, 188–199.

Janssen, T., Boege, P., Oestreicher, E., and Arnold, W. (2000). Tinnitus and 2f1–f2 distortion product otoacoustic emissions following salicylate overdose. *J. Acoust. Soc. Am.* 107, 1790–1792.

Jastreboff, P. J., Brennan, J. F., Coleman, J. K., and Sasaki, C. T. (1988a). Phantom auditory sensation in rats: an animal model for tinnitus. *Behav. Neurosci.* 102, 811–822.

Jastreboff, P. J., Brennan, J. F., and Sasaki, C. T. (1988b). An animal model for tinnitus. *Laryngoscope* 98, 280–286.

Jastreboff, P. J., Hansen, R., Sasaki, P. G., and Sasaki, C. T. (1986). Differential uptake of salicylate in serum, cerebrospinal fluid, and perilymph. *Arch. Otolaryngol. Head Neck Surg.* 112, 1050–1053.

Jastreboff, P. J., and Sasaki, C. T. (1986). Salicylate-induced changes in spontaneous activity of single units in the inferior colliculus of the guinea pig. *J. Acoust. Soc. Am.* 80, 1384–1391.

Kakehata, S., and Santos-Sacchi, J. (1996). Effects of salicylate and lanthanides on outer hair cell motility and associated gating charge. *J. Neurosci.* 16, 4881–4889.

Kaltenbach, J. A., Zacharek, M. A., Zhang, J., and Frederick, S. (2004). Activity in the dorsal cochlear nucleus of hamsters previously tested for tinnitus following intense tone exposure. *Neurosci. Lett.* 355, 121–125.

Kauer, J. S., Nemitz, J. W., and Sasaki, C. T. (1982). Tinnitus aurium: factor fancy. *Laryngoscope* 92, 1401–1407.

Kenmochi, M., and Eggermont, J. J. (1997). Salicylate and quinine affect the central nervous system. *Hear. Res.* 113, 110–116.

Kizawa, K., Kitahara, T., Horii, A., Maekawa, C., Kuramasu, T., Kawashima, T., Nishiike, S., Doi, K., and Inohara, H. (2010). Behavioral assessment and identification of a molecular marker in a salicylate-induced tinnitus in rats. *Neuroscience* 165, 1323–1332.

Koerber, K. C., Pfeiffer, R. R., Warr, W. B., and Kiang, N. Y. (1966). Spontaneous spike discharges from single units in the cochlear nucleus after destruction of the cochlea. *Exp. Neurol.* 16, 119–130.

Kraus, K. S., Mitra, S., Jimenez, Z., Hinduja, S., Ding, D., Jiang, H., Gray, L., Lobarinas, E., Sun, W., and Salvi, R. J. (2010). Noise trauma impairs neurogenesis in the rat hippocampus. *Neuroscience* 167, 1216–1226.

Kujawa, S. G., Fallon, M., and Bobbin, R. P. (1992). Intracochlear salicylate reduces low-intensity acoustic and cochlear microphonic distortion products. *Hear. Res.* 64, 73–80.

Kumagai, M. (1992). Effect of intravenous injection of aspirin on the cochlea. *Hokkaido Igaku Zasshi* 67, 216–233.

Liberman, M. C., and Kiang, N. Y. (1978). Acoustic trauma in cats. Cochlear pathology and auditory-nerve activity. *Acta Otolaryngol. Suppl.* 358, 1–63.

Ling, L. L., Hughes, L. F., and Caspary, D. M. (2005). Age-related loss of the GABA synthetic enzyme glutamic acid decarboxylase in rat primary auditory cortex. *Neuroscience* 132, 1103–1113.

Llinas, R. R., Ribary, U., Jeanmonod, D., Kronberg, E., and Mitra, P. P. (1999). Thalamocortical dysrhythmia: a neurological and neuropsychiatric syndrome characterized by magnetoencephalography. *Proc. Natl. Acad. Sci. U.S.A.* 96, 15222–15227.

Lobarinas, E., Yang, G., Sun, W., Ding, D., Mirza, N., Dalby-Brown, W., Hilczmayer, E., Fitzgerald, S., Zhang, L., and Salvi, R. (2006). Salicylate- and quinine-induced tinnitus and effects of memantine. *Acta Otolaryngol. Suppl.* 556, 13–19.

Lockwood, A. H., Salvi, R. J., Coad, M. L., Towsley, M. L., Wack, D. S., and Murphy, B. W. (1998). The functional neuroanatomy of tinnitus: evidence for limbic system links and neural plasticity. *Neurology* 50, 114–120.

Lockwood, A. H., Wack, D. S., Burkard, R. F., Coad, M. L., Reyes, S. A., Arnold, S. A., and Salvi, R. J. (2001). The functional anatomy of gaze-evoked tinnitus and sustained lateral gaze. *Neurology* 56, 472–480.

Lu, J., Lobarinas, E., Deng, A., Goodey, R., Stolzberg, D., Salvi, R. J., and Sun, W. (2011). GABAergic neural activity involved in salicylate-induced auditory cortex gain enhancement. *Neuroscience* 189, 187–198.

Ma, W. L., Hidaka, H., and May, B. J. (2006). Spontaneous activity in the inferior colliculus of CBA/J mice after manipulations that induce tinnitus. *Hear. Res.* 212, 9–21.

Manabe, Y., Yoshida, S., Saito, H., and Oka, H. (1997). Effects of lidocaine on salicylate-induced discharge of neurons in the inferior colliculus of the guinea pig. *Hear. Res.* 103, 192–198.

McFadden, D., Plattsmier, H., and Pasanen, E. (1984). Aspirin-induced hearing loss as a model of sensorineural hearing loss. *Hear. Res.* 16, 251–311.

McFadden, D., and Plattsmier, H. S. (1984). Aspirin abolishes spontaneous oto-acoustic emissions. *J. Acoust. Soc. Am.* 76, 443–448.

Miller, B., Sarantis, M., Traynelis, S. F., and Attwell, D. (1992). Potentiation of NMDA receptor currents by arachidonic acid. *Nature* 355, 722–725.

Mongan, E., Kelly, P., Nies, K., Porter, W. W., and Paulus, H. E. (1973). Tinnitus as an indication of therapeutic serum salicylate levels. *JAMA* 226, 142–145.

Muhlnickel, W., Elbert, T., Taub, E., and Flor, H. (1998). Reorganization of auditory cortex in tinnitus. *Proc. Natl. Acad. Sci. U.S.A.* 95, 10340–10343.

Mulders, W. H., and Robertson, D. (2009). Hyperactivity in the auditory midbrain after acoustic trauma: dependence on cochlear activity. *Neuroscience* 164, 733–746.

Muller, M., Klinke, R., Arnold, W., and Oestreicher, E. (2003). Auditory nerve fibre responses to salicylate revisited. *Hear. Res.* 183, 37–43.

Myers, E. N., and Bernstein, J. M. (1965). Salicylate ototoxicity; a clinical and experimental study. *Arch. Otolaryngol.* 82, 483–493.

Neto, M. S., Carvalho, A. C., and Callestini, E. A. (1980). Treatment of mandibular osteomyelitis in a pregnant syphilitic. Report of a clinical case. *Rev. Assoc. Paul. Cir. Dent. Reg. Aracatuba* 1, 7–13.

Norena, A., Micheyl, C., Chery-Croze, S., and Collet, L. (2002). Psychoacoustic characterization of the tinnitus spectrum: implications for the underlying mechanisms of tinnitus. *Audiol. Neurootol.* 7, 358–369.

Norena, A. J., Moffat, G., Blanc, J. L., Pezard, L., and Cazals, Y. (2010). Neural changes in the auditory cortex of awake guinea pigs after two tinnitus inducers: salicylate and acoustic trauma. *Neuroscience* 166, 1194–1209.

Ochi, K., and Eggermont, J. J. (1996). Effects of salicylate on neural activity in cat primary auditory cortex. *Hear. Res.* 95, 63–76.

Ochi, K., and Eggermont, J. J. (1997). Effects of quinine on neural activity in cat primary auditory cortex. *Hear. Res.* 105, 105–118.

Oliver, D., He, D. Z., Klocker, N., Ludwig, J., Schulte, U., Waldegger, S., Ruppersberg, J. P., Dallos, P., and Fakler, B. (2001). Intracellular anions as the voltage sensor of prestin, the outer hair cell motor protein. *Science* 292, 2340–2343.

Ortmann, M., Muller, N., Schlee, W., and Weisz, N. (2011). Rapid increases of gamma power in the auditory cortex following noise trauma in humans. *Eur. J. Neurosci.* 33, 568–575.

Paul, A. K., Lobarinas, E., Simmons, R., Wack, D., Luisi, J. C., Spernyak, J., Mazurchuk, R., Abdel-Nabi, H., and Salvi, R. (2009). Metabolic imaging of rat brain during pharmacologically-induced tinnitus. *Neuroimage* 44, 312–318.

Peng, B. G., Chen, S., and Lin, X. (2003). Aspirin selectively augmented *N*-methyl-D-aspartate types of glutamate responses in cultured spiral ganglion neurons of mice. *Neurosci. Lett.* 343, 21–24.

Perucca, E., and Jackson, P. (1985). A controlled study of the suppression of tinnitus by lidocaine infusion: (relationship of therapeutic effect with serum lidocaine levels). *J. Laryngol. Otol.* 99, 657–661.

Puel, J. L., Bobbin, R. P., and Fallon, M. (1990). Salicylate, mefenamate, meclofenamate, and quinine on cochlear potentials. *Otolaryngol. Head Neck Surg.* 102, 66–73.

Rachel, J. D., Kaltenbach, J. A., and Janisse, J. (2002). Increases in spontaneous neural activity in the hamster dorsal cochlear nucleus following cisplatin treatment: a possible basis for cisplatin-induced tinnitus. *Hear. Res.* 164, 206–214.

Ralli, M., Lobarinas, E., Fetoni, A. R., Stolzberg, D., Paludetti, G., and Salvi, R. (2010). Comparison of salicylate- and quinine-induced tinnitus in rats: development, time course, and evaluation of audiologic correlates. *Otol. Neurotol.* 31, 823–831.

Rauschka, H., Aboul-Enein, F., Bauer, J., Nobis, H., Lassmann, H., and Schmidbauer, M. (2007). Acute cerebral white matter damage in lethal salicylate intoxication. *Neurotoxicology* 28, 33–37.

Reyes, S. A., Salvi, R. J., Burkard, R. F., Coad, M. L., Wack, D. S., Galantowicz, P. J., and Lockwood, A. H. (2002). Brain imaging of the effects of lidocaine on tinnitus. *Hear. Res.* 171, 43–50.

Ruel, J., Chabbert, C., Nouvian, R., Bendris, R., Eybalin, M., Leger, C. L., Bourien, J., Mersel, M., and Puel, J. L. (2008). Salicylate enables cochlear arachidonic-acid-sensitive NMDA receptor responses. *J. Neurosci.* 28, 7313–7323.

Rutkowski, R. G., and Weinberger, N. M. (2005). Encoding of learned importance of sound by magnitude of representational area in primary auditory cortex. *Proc. Natl. Acad. Sci. U.S.A.* 102, 13664–13669.

Salvi, R. J., Saunders, S. S., Gratton, M. A., Arehole, S., and Powers, N. (1990). Enhanced evoked response amplitudes in the inferior colliculus of the chinchilla following acoustic trauma. *Hear. Res.* 50, 245–257.

Schlee, W., Weisz, N., Bertrand, O., Hartmann, T., and Elbert, T. (2008). Using auditory steady state responses to outline the functional connectivity in the tinnitus brain. *PloS One* 3:e3720. doi: 10.1371/journal.pone.0003720

Shargorodsky, J., Curhan, G. C., and Farwell, W. R. (2010). Prevalence and characteristics of tinnitus among US adults. *Am. J. Med.* 123, 711–718.

Shehata, W. E., Brownell, W. E., and Dieler, R. (1991). Effects of salicylate on shape, electromotility and membrane characteristics of isolated outer hair cells from guinea pig cochlea. *Acta Otolaryngol.* 111, 707–718.

Silverstein, H., Bernstein, J. M., and Davies, D. G. (1967). Salicylate ototoxicity. A biochemical and electrophysiological study. *Ann. Otol. Rhinol. Laryngol.* 76, 118–128.

Stolzberg, D., Chen, G. D., Allman, B. L., and Salvi, R. J. (2011). Salicylate-induced peripheral auditory changes and tonotopic reorganization of auditory cortex. *Neuroscience* 180, 157–164.

Su, Y. Y., Luo, B., Wang, H. T., and Chen, L. (2009). Differential effects of sodium salicylate on current-evoked firing of pyramidal neurons and fast-spiking interneurons in slices of rat auditory cortex. *Hear. Res.* 253, 60–66.

Sun, W., Lu, J., Stolzberg, D., Gray, L., Deng, A., Lobarinas, E., and Salvi, R. J. (2009). Salicylate increases the gain of the central auditory system. *Neuroscience* 159, 325–334.

Vane, S. J. (1998). Differential inhibition of cyclooxygenase isoforms: an explanation of the action of NSAIDs. *J. Clin. Rheumatol.* 4 (Suppl. 5), S3–S10.

Wallhausser-Franke, E. (1997). Salicylate evokes c-fos expression in the brain stem: implications for tinnitus. *Neuroreport* 8, 725–728.

Wallhausser-Franke, E., Braun, S., and Langner, G. (1996). Salicylate alters 2-DG uptake in the auditory system: a model for tinnitus? *Neuroreport* 7, 1585–1588.

Wallhausser-Franke, E., Mahlke, C., Oliva, R., Braun, S., Wenz, G., and Langner, G. (2003). Expression of c-fos in auditory and non-auditory brain regions of the gerbil after manipulations that induce tinnitus. *Exp. Brain Res.* 153, 649–654.

Walsh, B. T., Miller, J. B., Gacek, R. R., and Kiang, N. Y. S. (1972). Spontaneous activity in the eighth cranial nerve of the cat. *Int. J. Neurosci.* 3, 221–235.

Wang, H. T., Luo, B., Zhou, K. Q., Xu, T. L., and Chen, L. (2006). Sodium salicylate reduces inhibitory postsynaptic currents in neurons of rat auditory cortex. *Hear. Res.* 215, 77–83.

Wang, J., Powers, N. L., Hofstetter, P., Trautwein, P., Ding, D., and Salvi, R. (1997). Effects of selective inner hair cell loss on auditory nerve fiber threshold, tuning and spontaneous and driven discharge rate. *Hear. Res.* 107, 67–82.

Wei, L., Ding, D., Sun, W., Xu-Friedman, M. A., and Salvi, R. (2010). Effects of sodium salicylate on spontaneous and evoked spike rate in the dorsal cochlear nucleus. *Hear. Res.* 267, 54–60.

Weisz, N., Hartmann, T., Dohrmann, K., Schlee, W., and Norena, A. (2006). High-frequency tinnitus without hearing loss does not mean absence of deafferentation. *Hear. Res.* 222, 108–114.

Wienbruch, C., Paul, I., Weisz, N., Elbert, T., and Roberts, L. E. (2006). Frequency organization of the 40-Hz auditory steady-state response in normal hearing and in tinnitus. *Neuroimage* 33, 180–194.

Wier, C. C., Norton, S. J., and Kincaid, G. E. (1984). Spontaneous narrow-band oto-acoustic signals emitted by human ears: a replication. *J. Acoust. Soc. Am.* 76, 1248–1250.

Wier, C. C., Pasanen, E. G., and McFadden, D. (1988). Partial dissociation of spontaneous otoacoustic emissions and distortion products during aspirin use in humans. *J. Acoust. Soc. Am.* 84, 230–237.

Wilson, J. P. (1980). Evidence for a cochlear origin for acoustic re-emissions, threshold fine-structure and tonal tinnitus. *Hear. Res.* 2, 233–252.

Wu, J. L., Chiu, T. W., and Poon, P. W. (2003). Differential changes in Fos-immunoreactivity at the auditory brainstem after chronic injections of salicylate in rats. *Hear. Res.* 176, 80–93.

Xu, H., Gong, N., Chen, L., and Xu, T. L. (2005). Sodium salicylate reduces gamma aminobutyric acid-induced current in rat spinal dorsal horn neurons. *Neuroreport* 16, 813–816.

Yang, G., Lobarinas, E., Zhang, L., Turner, J., Stolzberg, D., Salvi, R., and Sun, W. (2007). Salicylate induced tinnitus: behavioral measures and neural activity in auditory cortex of awake rats. *Hear. Res.* 226, 244–253.

Yang, K., Huang, Z. W., Liu, Z. Q., Xiao, B. K., and Peng, J. H. (2009). Long-term administration of salicylate enhances prestin expression in rat cochlea. *Int. J. Audiol.* 48, 18–23.

Zhang, X., Yang, P., Cao, Y., Qin, L., and Sato, Y. (2011). Salicylate induced neural changes in the primary auditory cortex of awake cats. *Neuroscience* 172, 232–245.

Zheng, J., Shen, W., He, D. Z., Long, K. B., Madison, L. D., and Dallos, P. (2000). Prestin is the motor protein of cochlear outer hair cells. *Nature* 405, 149–155.

Zurek, P. M. (1981). Spontaneous narrowband acoustic signals emitted by human ears. *J. Acoust. Soc. Am.* 69, 514–523.

6

The auditory and non-auditory brain areas involved in tinnitus: An emergent property of multiple parallel overlapping subnetworks

Sven Vanneste * and Dirk De Ridder

Brai²n, TRI and Department of Neurosurgery, University Hospital Antwerp, Antwerp, Belgium

Tinnitus is the perception of a sound in the absence of an external sound source. It is characterized by sensory components such as the perceived loudness, the lateralization, the tinnitus type (pure tone, noise-like) and associated emotional components, such as distress and mood changes. Source localization of quantitative electroencephalography (qEEG) data demonstrate the involvement of auditory brain areas as well as several non-auditory brain areas such as the anterior cingulate cortex (dorsal and subgenual), auditory cortex (primary and secondary), dorsal lateral prefrontal cortex, insula, supplementary motor area, orbitofrontal cortex (including the inferior frontal gyrus), parahippocampus, posterior cingulate cortex and the precuneus, in different aspects of tinnitus. Explaining these non-auditory brain areas as constituents of separable subnetworks, each reflecting a specific aspect of the tinnitus percept increases the explanatory power of the non-auditory brain areas involvement in tinnitus. Thus, the unified percept of tinnitus can be considered an emergent property of multiple parallel dynamically changing and partially overlapping subnetworks, each with a specific spontaneous oscillatory pattern and functional connectivity signature.

Correspondence:
Sven Vanneste, Brai²n, TRI and Department of Neurosurgery, University Hospital Antwerp, Wilrijkstraat 10, 2650 Edegem, Belgium.
e-mail: sven.vanneste@ua.ac.be

Keywords: EEG, non-auditory brain areas, emergent property, multiple parallel overlapping subnetworks

INTRODUCTION

Consciousness is a crucial aspect of being human. One specific component of consciousness is the conscious perception of auditory stimuli. Hearing is a crucial sensory domain that helps to localize as well as recognize a sound source and is essential for communication. Our auditory function helps us to understand the world, maintain social contacts and to detect dangerous situations. In humans and other vertebrates, hearing is performed primarily by the auditory system. Vibrations are detected by the ear and translated into nerve impulses that are processed by the auditory cortex. Recent research has shown, however, that activity in the primary auditory cortex is necessary, but not sufficient condition for an auditory stimulus to gain access to consciousness (Boly et al., 2004). It has recently become clear that in order to perceive an auditory percept, hierarchically higher-order multimodal association areas are required (Boly et al., 2004; Laureys, 2005), similarly to what has been proposed in the visual (Dehaene et al., 2006) and somatosensory system (Laureys et al., 2002; Boly et al., 2005).

Understanding the brain mechanisms involved in the simplest forms of auditory conscious perception, such as noise and tones from the environment (i.e., externally generated) is a crucial start for gaining knowledge about auditory consciousness specifically and consciousness at large. However, a sound can also be internally generated. That is, perceiving a sound in the absence of an external sound source. This phenomenon is also known as tinnitus. In most cases this phantom sound resolves spontaneously within seconds or minutes. However, tinnitus persists in 5–10% of the population in western countries (Heller, 2003; Eggermont and Roberts, 2004), and interferes severely with the quality of life in 5–26% within this tinnitus population (Axelsson and Ringdahl, 1989; Heller, 2003). Moreover, the prevalence of chronic tinnitus increases with age, peaking at 14.3% in people between 60 and 69 years of age (Shargorodsky et al., 2010).

Phenomenologically, tinnitus can be perceived unilaterally or bilaterally and characterized as a pure tone, a narrow band noise or polyphonic. Tinnitus is usually evaluated both for its perceived loudness and annoyance or distress level. Yet, not everyone who experiences tinnitus becomes chronically distressed and measures of tinnitus loudness rarely correlate with experienced distress (Andersson and Westin, 2008). Distress can play an important part in the development of tinnitus, as distress might act as a potential trigger for sudden hearing loss and onset of tinnitus, but is not a necessity (Schmitt et al., 2000). Distress might unfavorably influence habituation via hyperarousal processes, but is not a requirement (Hallam, 1996). Tinnitus symptoms themselves can act as a stressor resulting in higher physiological arousal and psychological distress, but this is not always the case (Alpini and Cesarani, 2006).

In this review we try to map and disentangle the different brain areas generating an auditory phantom percept. We will only focus on simple auditory phantom percepts such as tones and noise and not on more complex sounds such as hearing voices or music. Although very common, tinnitus is not well understood. Clinical data indicate the involvement of peripheral auditory structures in tinnitus (Nicolas-Puel et al., 2002). This is suggested by the fact that tinnitus is often related to damage of the cochlea or the auditory nerve such as in presbyacusis, noise induced hearing loss, drug-related hearing loss, Meniere's disease, or other inner ear pathologies (Lockwood et al., 2002). Furthermore it has been demonstrated that psychoacoustic characteristics of tinnitus like pitch overlap with the frequency spectrum of an individual's hearing loss (Norena et al., 2002; Norena and Eggermont, 2003, 2006). In addition in animal models it was revealed that a peripheral mechanism involving the N-methyl-D-aspartate (NMDA) glutamatergic receptors in the cochlea can be generator of tinnitus (Guitton et al., 2003). On the other hand, an increasing amount of data shows the role played by activation and remodeling of various central cortical or subcortical structures to cause or to perpetuate tinnitus symptomatology (Muhlnickel et al., 1998; Eggermont and Roberts, 2004; Eggermont, 2005; Weisz et al., 2005). Investigating the neurophysiological differences in the characteristics of tinnitus perception could lead to a better understanding of pathological auditory neural activity. Therefore, we first discuss the different auditory and non-auditory brain areas involved in tinnitus and their potential function within the tinnitus network. Secondly, we try to combine these different brain areas involved in tinnitus in a multiple brain subnetworks.

THE AUDITORY AND NON-AUDITORY BRAIN AREAS INVOLVED IN TINNITUS

Based on previous quantitative electroencephalography (qEEG) research the following areas have been implicated in tinnitus: the auditory cortex, the subgenual and dorsal anterior cingulate cortex, the dorsolateral prefrontal cortex, the insula, the supplementary motor area, the orbitofrontal cortex (including the inferior frontal gyrus), the posterior cingulate cortex, the precuneus and the parahippocampus. **Table 1** and **Figure 1** give an overview of the different brain areas obtained based on qEEG research in tinnitus and their involvement in specific tinnitus characteristics.

THE AUDITORY CORTEX

Animal experiments have demonstrated that the degree of behavioral importance of an external sound is related to the representational expansion of its frequency in the primary auditory cortex (Rutkowski and Weinberger, 2005), and that the auditory cortex is involved in tinnitus (Engineer et al., 2011). But also in humans it was shown that the auditory cortex plays a role in tinnitus (van der Loo et al., 2009). In comparison to a control group both left and right-sided tinnitus patients had an increased gamma band activity in both the left and right primary and secondary auditory cortex (Vanneste et al., 2011a). This is the reason why primary and secondary auditory cortices are considered as important potential targets for the treatment of tinnitus (De Ridder et al., 2006a, 2007a,b). The rationale is that this phantom sound might be related to an increased neuronal activity within the auditory cortex secondary to the imbalance between excitatory and inhibitory mechanisms or an adjustment of auditory gain mechanisms (Norena, 2011). The difference could be triggered by altered auditory inputs which may support functional reorganization in synaptic connections. Neural hyperactivity has been found in subcortical structures (cochlear nuclei, inferior colliculi, medial geniculate bodies) and auditory cortical regions (primary and secondary auditory cortex) in animal models of tinnitus and hearing loss (Jastreboff and Sasaki, 1986; Jastreboff, 1990; Brozoski et al., 2002).

Based on MEG data, thalamocortical dysrhythmia has been proposed as a pathophysiological model for the development of gamma band activity related to the tinnitus percept (Llinás et al., 1999). According to this model tinnitus is caused by an abnormal, spontaneous, and constant gamma band activity (>30 Hz) generated as a consequence of hyperpolarization of specific thalamic nuclei, in casu the medial geniculate body. In normal circumstances auditory stimuli increase thalamocortical rhythms to gamma band activity (Joliot et al., 1994). In the deafferented state, however, oscillatory activity decreases from resting state alpha activity (8–12 Hz) to theta band activity (4–7 Hz) (Steriade, 2006). As a result, lateral inhibition is reduced inducing a surrounding gamma band activity known as the "edge effect" (Llinás et al., 1999, 2005). Lorenz et al. (Lorenz et al., 2009) reported an inverse relationship between alpha and gamma activity over subjects calculated for sources seeded in auditory regions. The inverse relationship was presented for tinnitus and control tinnitus group. Synchronized gamma band activity in the auditory cortex is proposed to bind auditory events into one coherent conscious auditory percept (Ribary et al., 1991; Tiitinen et al., 1993; Joliot et al., 1994; Llinas et al., 1994, 1998; Crone et al., 2001). In addition it was found that tinnitus perceived loudness is correlated to increased contralateral gamma band activity in the auditory cortex indicating that gamma band activity is important in tinnitus (van der Loo et al., 2009).

THE PARAHIPPOCAMPUS

The differences between uni- and bilateral tinnitus are reflected by high frequency EEG activity (i.e., beta and gamma) in the parahippocampus (Vanneste et al., 2011c). That is, unilateral tinnitus patients showed increased high frequency activity in the right parahippocampal area. This same brain area is also involved at an alpha rhythm in patients with a high distress and in non-coping with tinnitus. In addition, based on a region of interest analysis, whether tinnitus is perceived on the left side or right side tinnitus is dependent on gamma-band activity of the contralateral parahippocampal area (Vanneste et al., 2011c). In contrast to expectation, for the auditory cortex no differences were found between left-sided and right-sided tinnitus patients. In addition, narrow band noise tinnitus patients have increased activity in the parahippocampal area in comparison to pure tone tinnitus patients at the gamma frequency band (Vanneste et al., 2010a).

The involvement of the parahippocampus in tinnitus might be related to the constant updating of the tinnitus percept from memory thereby preventing habituation (De Ridder et al., 2006b). The posterior parahippocampal area is involved in auditory habituation as demonstrated by electrophysiological studies of auditory sensory gating both in animals (Bickford et al., 1993) and humans implanted with electrodes in the parahippocampus and hippocampus for epilepsy monitoring (Boutros et al., 2008). The hippocampal involvement in tinnitus pathophysiology is also demonstrated by histopathological findings of posterior hippocampus lesions in patients, who experience

Table 1 | Overview results based on resting-state EEG in tinnitus patients.

Brain region	BA	Function	Frequency band	Ref
Auditory cortex	BA21	Control group < Left and Right-sided tinnitus	gamma	Vanneste et al., 2011a
	BA22	Tinnitus with recent onset < Chronic tinnitus	gamma	Vanneste et al., 2011b
	BA40	Control group < Left and Right-sided tinnitus	gamma	Vanneste et al., 2011a
	BA41	Positive correlation with tinnitus intensity	gamma	van der Loo et al., 2009
Parahippocampus	BA36	Low distress < High distress	alpha1, alpha2	Vanneste et al., 2010b
	BA37	Coping with tinnitus < Non-coping	alpha1 alpha2	Vanneste et al., 2010b
	BA19	Left-sided tinnitus > Right-sided Tinnitus (right)	gamma	Vanneste et al., 2011a
		Left-sided tinnitus < Right-sided Tinnitus (left)	gamma	Vanneste et al., 2011a
		Control group < Left and Right-sided tinnitus	gamma	Vanneste et al., 2011a
		Pure tone < Narrow band noise tinnitus	gamma	Vanneste et al., 2010a
		Control group < Narrow band noise tinnitus	beta3, gamma	Vanneste et al., 2011c
		Unilateral tinnitus < Bilateral tinnitus		
Anterior cingulate cortex				
Dorsal	BA24	Tinnitus with recent onset < Chronic tinnitus	beta2, beta3	Vanneste et al., 2010b
	BA32	Control group < High distress	delta, theta	Vanneste et al., 2010b
		Control group > High distress	alpha, beta	Vanneste et al., 2010b
		Correlation with distress	alpha, beta	De Ridder et al., 2011b
Subgenual	BA25	Low distress < High distress	alpha1, alpha2	Vanneste et al., 2010b
		Coping with tinnitus < Non-coping	alpha1, alpha2	Vanneste et al., 2010b
		Correlation with TQ	alpha, beta	De Ridder et al., 2011b
DLPFC	BA9	Low distress coping > High distress coping	alpha1, alpha2	Vanneste et al., 2010b
	BA46			
Insula	BA13	Tinnitus with recent onset < Chronic tinnitus	beta3	Vanneste et al., 2011b
		Coping with tinnitus < Non-coping with tinnitus	alpha1, alpha2	Vanneste et al., 2010b
		Correlation with TQ and activity (left)	theta, alpha, gamma	van der Loo et al., 2011
		Correlation between TQ and activity (right)	delta, gamma	van der Loo et al., 2011
Supplementary motor area	BA6	Tinnitus with recent onset < Chronic tinnitus	theta	Vanneste et al., 2011b
	BA8	Low distress coping tinnitus > High distress coping	alpha1, alpha2	Vanneste et al., 2010b
		Unilateral tinnitus < Bilateral tinnitus	delta	Vanneste et al., 2011c
		Control group < Unilateral tinnitus	gamma	Vanneste et al., 2011c
		Control group < Bilateral tinnitus	gamma	Vanneste et al., 2011c
Orbitofrontal cortex	BA10	Pure tone > Narrow band noise tinnitus	delta	Vanneste et al., 2010a
(Inferior frontal gyrus)	BA11	Unilateral tinnitus > Bilateral tinnitus	delta	Vanneste et al., 2011c
	BA47	Control group < Bilateral tinnitus	beta3	Vanneste et al., 2011c
Posterior cingulate cortex	BA23	Low distress > High distress	alpha2	Vanneste et al., 2010b
		Pure tone < Narrow band noise tinnitus	beta3	Vanneste et al., 2010a
		Control group < Narrow band noise tinnitus	beta3	Vanneste et al., 2010a
		Control group Pure tone tinnitus	beta3, gamma	Vanneste et al., 2010a
Precuneus	BA7	Low distress > High distress	alpha2	Vanneste et al., 2010b
		Coping with tinnitus > Non-coping with tinnitus	alpha1, alpha2	Vanneste et al., 2010b
		Low distress coping tinnitus < High distress coping	alpha2	Vanneste et al., 2010b

DLPFC, dorsal lateral prefrontal cortex; Ref, reference.

tinnitus as a symptom of methyltin intoxications (Rey et al., 1984; Kreyberg et al., 1992). Furthermore, supraselective amytal injection in the anterior choroidal artery that supplies the amygdalohippocampal area is capable to suppress the pure tone component of tinnitus transiently by suppressing local activity (De Ridder et al., 2006b). The parahippocampal area together with the posterior cingulate cortex activity might be load dependent, as noise-like tinnitus constitutes multiple frequencies in contrast to pure tone tinnitus (Vanneste et al., 2010a). Hence, it has been proposed that a fundamental function of the (para)hippocampal structures is the establishment of auditory memory for tinnitus (Shulman, 1995).

THE DORSAL ANTERIOR CINGULATE CORTEX

A recent study, using source localization in EEG, revealed that distress in tinnitus patients is related to increased beta activity in the dorsal part of the anterior cingulate cortex and the amount of distress correlates with an alpha activity in several brain areas such as the amygdala, anterior cingulate cortex, insula, and parahippocampus (Vanneste et al., 2010b). A comparison

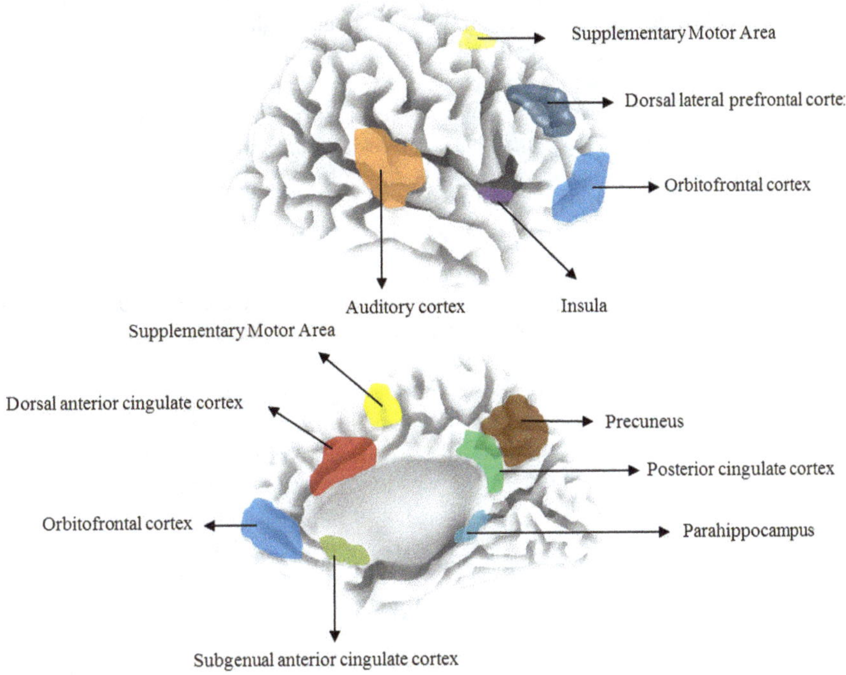

FIGURE 1 | Overview the different brain areas based on resting state EEG in tinnitus patients.

between recent onset and chronic tinnitus is related to differential activity and connectivity in a network comprising the auditory cortices, insula, dorsal anterior cingulate cortex and premotor cortex. Based on a blind source separation technique, tinnitus can be characterized by at least four independent components, two of which are posterior cingulate based, one based on the subgenual anterior cingulate and one based on the parahippocampus (De Ridder et al., 2011b). Only the subgenual component correlates with distress. When compared to a normative sample, group independent components analysis reveals that distress is characterized by two anterior cingulate based components. Spectral analysis of these components demonstrates that distress in tinnitus is related to alpha and beta changes in a network consisting of the subgenual anterior cingulate cortex extending to the pregenual and dorsal anterior cingulate cortex as well as the ventromedial prefrontal cortex/orbitofrontal cortex, insula, and parahippocampus. This network overlaps partially with brain areas implicated in distress in patients suffering from pain, functional somatic syndromes and, posttraumatic stress disorder, and might, therefore, represents an aspecific distress network. The dorsal part of the anterior cingulate cortex is one of the possible generators of frontal midline theta (Asada et al., 1999). Furthermore, it has been established that frontal midline theta oscillations are involved in attentional processes (Inanaga, 1998), and that both sympathetic and parasympathetic indices are increased during the appearance of frontal midline theta (Kubota et al., 2001). Whenever new information is presented, activity levels of the dorsal anterior cingulate cortex reflect the salience of the new information for predicting future outcomes (Critchley, 2005; Behrens et al., 2007), guiding optimal decision-making in an uncertain world (Kennerley et al., 2006). The human dorsal anterior cingulate cortex has developed a parallel specialization for motivational drive via a thalamocortical pathway relaying in the mediodorsal thalamus (Craig, 2002). Thus, the dorsal anterior cingulate might be involved in persisting attention to the tinnitus (Vanneste et al., 2010b; De Ridder et al., 2011b).

THE SUBGENUAL ANTERIOR CINGULATE CORTEX

The subgenual anterior cingulate cortex extending into nucleus accumbens-ventral tegmental area is involved in processing of aversive sounds (Zald and Pardo, 2002) and unpleasant music (Blood et al., 1999) as well as tinnitus (Muhlau et al., 2006). It has been implicated as the key component of social distress (Masten et al., 2009). This area in animals has been considered a visceromotor cortex, due to its connections with the parasympathetic nucleus tractus solitaries (Frysztak and Neafsey, 1994) and the sympathetic areas in the periaquaductal gray (Ongur and Price, 2000). Furthermore, it is functionally connected to the amygdala, insula, parahippocampus, orbitofrontal cortex, and ventrolateral prefrontal cortex and anticorrelated to the dorsal anterior cingulate cortex and precuneus. As such the subgenual anterior cingulate cortex could be important as an emotional component for tinnitus.

THE DORSOLATERAL PREFRONTAL CORTEX

Recently the dorsolateral prefrontal cortex has been associated with tinnitus-related distress (Vanneste et al., 2010b). It is known that the dorsal lateral prefrontal cortex has a bilateral facilitatory effect on auditory memory storage (Alain et al., 1998) and contains auditory memory cells (Bodner et al., 1996). The dorsal lateral prefrontal cortex also exerts early inhibitory modulation of input to primary auditory cortex in humans (Knight et al.,

1989) and has been found to be associated with auditory attention (Alain et al., 1998; Lewis et al., 2000; Voisin et al., 2006) resulting in top-down modulation of auditory processing (Mitchell et al., 2005). This was further confirmed by electrophysiological data indicating that tinnitus might occur as the result of a dysfunction in the top-down inhibitory processes (Norena et al., 1999). Interestingly, a recent study reported that coupling between dorsal anterior cingulate cortex and the right frontal lobe correlates negatively with tinnitus intrusiveness, which is defined by the authors as how bothersome and obtrusive the tinnitus is perceived (Schlee et al., 2008). However, in the above mentioned study it is not specified which part of the anterior cingulate cortex and prefrontal cortex is involved. Additionally, Jastreboff described the prefrontal cortex as a "candidate for the integration of sensory and emotional aspects of tinnitus" (Jastreboff, 1990). This is in accordance with the idea that the dorsal lateral prefrontal cortex in general could be considered as an area involved in the integration of emotion and cognition (Gray et al., 2002). Nevertheless, further research is needed to clarify the role of the dorsolateral prefrontal cortex in tinnitus.

INSULA

It was shown that the tinnitus questionnaire (TQ) scores are correlated to heart rate rariability markers, and related to neural activity in left and right anterior insula (van der Loo et al., 2011). It was shown that tinnitus distress is related to sympathetic activation, in part mediated via the right anterior insula. In addition the insula is activated in non-coping tinnitus at the alpha frequency band. The left insula is correlated with the TQ at theta, alpha, and gamma frequency band, while the right insula is correlated with delta and gamma frequency band.

The function of the dorsal anterior cingulate cortex and insula might be to integrate motivationally important information with appropriate bodily responses (Critchley et al., 2001) related to the survival needs of the body (Craig, 2003). In addition the insula together with the dorsal anterior cingulate cortex have also been referred to as the salience network (Seeley et al., 2007). This network has been implicated in bottom-up detection of salient events and coordinating appropriate responses (Medford and Critchley, 2010; Menon and Uddin, 2010). Activity in this network is correlated with improved sound detection thresholds, showing a role in the direction of attentional resources toward audition (Sadaghiani et al., 2009). The activation of the salience network suggests that the brain allocates an importance to auditory stimulus and might as such also signify importance to the internally generated tinnitus sound. Activation of the insula and dorsal anterior cingulate cortex during a phantom percept might be considered maladaptive. Imaging studies on the insula associated this area with subjective emotional and bodily awareness (Craig, 2003), as well as interoception (Craig, 2003). The anterior insula has been implicated in autonomic nervous system control (Oppenheimer et al., 1992; Oppenheimer, 1993; Critchley et al., 2004; Critchley, 2005) and might, therefore, be related to the autonomic components involved in distress (Critchley et al., 2000; Wang et al., 2005), induced by the phantom sound. Tinnitus distress is indeed correlated to sympathetic activation, in part mediated via the right anterior insula (van der Loo et al., 2011). Furthermore alpha activity in both the left and right anterior insula was also found for patients with severe tinnitus-related distress who can or cannot cope with these phantom sounds (Vanneste et al., 2010b). Although, the insula seems like an important brain area involved in tinnitus, further research is needed to elucidate what the exact role is of the insula in tinnitus.

THE SUPPLEMENTARY MOTOR AREA

For a sensory stimulus to be consciously perceived, activation of the early sensory areas is a prerequisite but not sufficient (Boly et al., 2005; Dehaene et al., 2006). The (visual) global workspace model suggests conscious perception of sensory events requires sensory cortex activation embedded in a cortical network, the global workspace, extending beyond the primary sensory regions including prefrontal, parietal, and cingulate cortices. Similarly, auditory stimuli need activation of the primary auditory cortex to be consciously perceived. However, this is not sufficient (Laureys et al., 2000; Boly et al., 2005). Studies performed on patients in vegetative state who do not have conscious auditory percepts reveal that auditory stimuli still activate the primary auditory cortex but that there is no functional connectivity to frontal areas in these patients. Primary auditory cortex activation might be only related to loudness coding (Jancke et al., 1998) and not the percept *per se*, similarly to what has been demonstrated at a single-cell level for somatosensory stimuli in the primary somatosensory cortex: stimulus intensity is encoded in the primary somatosensory cortex, while the conscious percept seems to be located in the frontal cortex, more precisely within the supplementary motor area (de Lafuente and Romo, 2005). In addition, Melloni et al., found that theta oscillations in the frontal regions including the supplementary motor area are essential for conscious perception during maintenance interval of visual stimuli (Melloni et al., 2007). Taking these findings together, it can be hypothesized that synchronized gamma activity in the auditory cortex is responsible for the tinnitus loudness (van der Loo et al., 2009), while synchronized theta activity in the supplementary motor area might be accountable for part of the conscious perception of the phantom sound, similar to the conscious perception for somatosensory stimuli.

THE ORBITOFRONTAL CORTEX (INCLUDING THE INFERIOR FRONTAL GYRUS)

Previous research has already shown that orbitofrontal cortex is important for emotional processing of sounds (Wheeler et al., 1993; Damasio, 1996; Dias et al., 1996; Blood et al., 1999). For example, it was revealed that patients with orbitofrontal cortex lesions had reduced self-evaluated perception of the unpleasantness of the acoustic probe stimulus (Angrilli et al., 2008). The orbitofrontal cortex has connections with other limbic areas important for processing of emotion (Beauregard, 2007). Female tinnitus patients have been found to be more emotionally responsive to tinnitus-related distress (Dineen et al., 1997). They also differ in physiological responses to negative emotional stimuli in comparison to males (Bradley et al., 2001; Gard and Kring, 2007). Koch et al. found that an interaction between negative emotion and working memory in females involved activation of the orbitofrontal cortex, suggesting that during the cognitive control of emotion, females mainly recruit the emotion-associated areas (Koch et al., 2007).

The orbitofrontal cortex together with the insula plays a key role in the top-down modulation of automatic or peripheral physiological responses to emotional experiences (Craig, 2003; Phillips et al., 2003; Critchley et al., 2004; Ohira et al., 2006). More synchronized connectivity between the orbitofrontal cortex and the insula is seen in tinnitus for females. It can, therefore, be hypothesized that the orbitofrontal cortex becomes recruited more often for female tinnitus patients in order to modulate the autonomic physiological responses evoked by tinnitus.

THE POSTERIOR CINGULATE CORTEX AND PRECUNEUS

qEEG data indicate that the posterior cingulate cortex is important in both pure tone and narrow band noise tinnitus (Vanneste et al., 2010a) as well as tinnitus-related distress (Vanneste et al., 2011c). In addition, the precuneus is active within the alpha frequency in patients who can cope with their tinnitus and have a low distress (Vanneste et al., 2011c). Together with the parahippocampal area, activation in the posterior cingulate cortex and precuneus has been associated with the brain's "default" network (Raichle et al., 2001). These regions deactivate when people engage in controlled processing and thought processes. According to this account, default activity is an inverse function of the task demand, where higher demands reduce activity in the default network because mental resources are used to perform a task (Gusnard et al., 2001; McKiernan et al., 2006). As the parahippocampal area as well as the posterior cingulate cortex and precuneus become more active, instead of becoming deactivated during the tinnitus perception, one can hypothesize the tinnitus generators might become integrated in the default mode in tinnitus patients. In addition, the precuneus area is a highly integrative structure, supposed to be involved in visuo-spatial imagery, episodic memory, self-consciousness, and the shifting of attention (Le et al., 1998). The precuneus is also involved in unpleasant music perception (Blood et al., 1999), auditory imagery (Yoo et al., 2001), and auditory memory retrieval (Buckner et al., 1996).

MULTIPLE PARALLEL DYNAMICALLY CHANGING AND PARTIALLY OVERLAPPING SUBNETWORKS

Taking the results in previous sections together the same brain areas occur in the different analyses for tinnitus that are related to different acoustic characteristics such as the tonal nature, lateralization, loudness level, tinnitus duration as well as for the affective components such as distress and mood changes. As such, tinnitus can be seen as the consequence of multiple brain subnetworks involved in the different aspects of tinnitus, both acoustic and affective. Thus, the unified percept of tinnitus, as perceived by the patient, e.g., a loud distressing left-sided pure tone tinnitus, might be considered as an emergent property of multiple parallel dynamically changing and partially overlapping subnetworks, each with a specific spontaneous oscillatory pattern signature. This interpretation casts doubts concerning the sole participation of only one critical circuit in phantom perception. Phantom percepts result from auditory deafferentation and reach awareness only when increased neuronal activity in the primary auditory cortex is connected to a larger network involving frontal and parietal areas (De Ridder et al., 2011a). It is possible that different brain subnetworks overlap and might all be involved in how a patient perceives his/her tinnitus.

CONCLUSION

Source localization of qEEG data demonstrate the involvement of auditory brain areas as well as several non-auditory brain areas such as the anterior cingulate cortex (dorsal and subgenual), auditory cortex (primary and secondary), dorsal lateral prefrontal cortex, insula, supplementary motor area, orbitofrontal cortex (including the inferior frontal gyrus), parahippocampus, posterior cingulate cortex and the precuneus, in different aspects of tinnitus. However, few conceptual explanations have been given for all these regions. Evaluating these areas as parts of separable subnetworks, each network representing a specific clinical aspect of tinnitus might help to explain their involvement in tinnitus. Thus, the unified percept of tinnitus can be considered an emergent property of multiple parallel dynamically changing and partially overlapping subnetworks, each with a specific spontaneous oscillatory pattern and functional connectivity signature.

REFERENCES

Alain, C., Woods, D. L., and Knight, R. T. (1998). A distributed cortical network for auditory sensory memory in humans. *Brain Res.* 812, 23–37.

Alpini, D., and Cesarani, A. (2006). Tinnitus as an alarm bell: stress reaction tinnitus model. *ORL J. Otorhinolaryngol. Relat. Spec.* 68, 31–36. discussion 36–37.

Andersson, G., and Westin, V. (2008). Understanding tinnitus distress: introducing the concepts of moderators and mediators. *Int. J. Audiol.* (Suppl. 2), S106–S111.

Angrilli, A., Bianchin, M., Radaelli, S., Bertagnoni, G., and Pertile, M. (2008). Reduced startle reflex and aversive noise perception in patients with orbitofrontal cortex lesions. *Neuropsychologia* 46, 1179–1184.

Asada, H., Fukuda, Y., Tsunoda, S., Yamaguchi, M., and Tonoike, M. (1999). Frontal midline theta rhythms reflect alternative activation of prefrontal cortex and anterior cingulate cortex in humans. *Neurosci. Lett.* 274, 29–32.

Axelsson, A., and Ringdahl, A. (1989). Tinnitus–a study of its prevalence and characteristics. *Br. J. Audiol.* 23, 53–62.

Beauregard, M. (2007). Mind does really matter: evidence from neuroimaging studies of emotional self-regulation, psychotherapy, and placebo effect. *Prog. Neurobiol.* 81, 218–236.

Behrens, T. E., Woolrich, M. W., Walton, M. E., and Rushworth, M. F. (2007). Learning the value of information in an uncertain world. *Nat. Neurosci.* 10, 1214–1221.

Bickford, P. C., Luntz-Leybman, V., and Freedman, R. (1993). Auditory sensory gating in the rat hippocampus: modulation by brainstem activity. *Brain Res.* 607, 33–38.

Blood, A. J., Zatorre, R. J., Bermudez, P., and Evans, A. C. (1999). Emotional responses to pleasant and unpleasant music correlate with activity in paralimbic brain regions. *Nat. Neurosci.* 2, 382–387.

Bodner, M., Kroger, J., and Fuster, J. M. (1996). Auditory memory cells in dorsolateral prefrontal cortex. *Neuroreport* 7, 1905–1908.

Boly, M., Faymonville, M. E., Peigneux, P., Lambermont, B., Damas, P., Del Fiore, G., Degueldre, C., Franck, G., Luxen, A., Lamy, M., Moonen, G., Maquet, P., and Laureys, S. (2004). Auditory processing in severely brain injured patients: differences between the minimally conscious state and the persistent vegetative state. *Arch. Neurol.* 61, 233–238.

Boly, M., Faymonville, M. E., Peigneux, P., Lambermont, B., Damas, F., Luxen, A., Lamy, M., Moonen, G., Maquet, P., and Laureys, S. (2005). Cerebral processing of auditory and noxious stimuli in severely brain injured patients: differences between VS and MCS. *Neuropsychol. Rehabil.* 15, 283–289.

Boutros, N. N., Mears, R., Pflieger, M. E., Moxon, K. A., Ludowig, E., and Rosburg, T. (2008). Sensory gating in the human hippocampal and rhinal regions: regional differences. *Hippocampus* 18, 310–316.

Bradley, M. M., Codispoti, M., Sabatinelli, D., and Lang, P. J. (2001). Emotion and motivation II: sex differences in picture processing. *Emotion* 1, 300–319.

Brozoski, T. J., Bauer, C. A., and Caspary, D. M. (2002). Elevated fusiform cell activity in the dorsal cochlear nucleus of chinchillas with psychophysical evidence of tinnitus. *J. Neurosci.* 22, 2383–2390.

Buckner, R. L., Raichle, M. E., Miezin, F. M., and Petersen, S. E. (1996). Functional anatomic studies of memory retrieval for auditory words and visual pictures. *J. Neurosci.* 16, 6219–6235.

Craig, A. D. (2002). How do you feel? Interoception: the sense of the physiological condition of the body. *Nat. Rev. Neurosci.* 3, 655–666.

Craig, A. D. (2003). Interoception: the sense of the physiological condition of the body. *Curr. Opin. Neurobiol.* 13, 500–505.

Critchley, H. D. (2005). Neural mechanisms of autonomic, affective, and cognitive integration. *J. Comp. Neurol.* 493, 154–166.

Critchley, H. D., Corfield, D. R., Chandler, M. P., Mathias, C. J., and Dolan, R. J. (2000). Cerebral correlates of autonomic cardiovascular arousal: a functional neuroimaging investigation in humans. *J. Physiol.* 523(Pt 1), 259–270.

Critchley, H. D., Mathias, C. J., and Dolan, R. J. (2001). Neural activity in the human brain relating to uncertainty and arousal during anticipation. *Neuron* 29, 537–545.

Critchley, H. D., Wiens, S., Rotshtein, P., Ohman, A., and Dolan, R. J. (2004). Neural systems supporting interoceptive awareness. *Nat. Neurosci.* 7, 189–195.

Crone, N. E., Boatman, D., Gordon, B., and Hao, L. (2001). Induced electrocorticographic gamma activity during auditory perception. Brazier Award-winning article, 2001. *Clin. Neurophysiol.* 112, 565–582.

Damasio, A. R. (1996). The somatic marker hypothesis and the possible functions of the prefrontal cortex. *Philos. Trans. R. Soc. Lond. B Biol. Sci.* 351, 1413–1420.

Dehaene, S., Changeux, J. P., Naccache, L., Sackur, J., and Sergent, C. (2006). Conscious, preconscious, and subliminal processing: a testable taxonomy. *Trends Cogn. Sci.* 10, 204–211.

de Lafuente, V., and Romo, R. (2005). Neuronal correlates of subjective sensory experience. *Nat. Neurosci.* 8, 1698–1703.

De Ridder, D., de Mulder, G., Verstraeten, E., Seidman, M., Elisevich, K., Sunaert, S., Kovacs, S., K. van der Kelen, van de Heyning, P., and Moller, A. (2007a). Auditory cortex stimulation for tinnitus. *Acta Neurochir. Suppl.* 97, 451–462.

De Ridder, D., de Mulder, G., Menovsky, T., Sunaert, S., and Kovacs, S. (2007b). Electrical stimulation of auditory and somatosensory cortices for treatment of tinnitus and pain. *Prog. Brain Res.* 166, 377–388.

De Ridder, D., de Mulder, G., Verstraeten, E., van der Kelen, K., Sunaert, S., Smits, M., Kovacs, S., Verlooy, J., van de Heyning, P., and Moller, A. R. (2006a). Primary and secondary auditory cortex stimulation for intractable tinnitus. *ORL J. Otorhinolaryngol. Relat. Spec.* 68, 48–54. discussion 54–55.

De Ridder, D., Fransen, H., Francois, O., Sunaert, S., Kovacs, S., and van de Heyning, P. (2006b). Amygdalohippocampal involvement in tinnitus and auditory memory. *Acta Otolaryngol. Suppl.* 556, 50–53.

De Ridder, D., Elgoyhen, A. B., Romo, R., and Langguth, B. (2011a). Phantom percepts: tinnitus and pain as persisting aversive memory networks. *Proc. Natl. Acad. Sci. U.S.A.* 108, 8075–8080.

De Ridder, D., Vanneste, S., and Congedo, M. (2011b). The distressed brain: a group blind source separation analysis on tinnitus. *PLoS One* 6:e24273. doi: 10.1371/journal.pone.0024273

Dias, R., Robbins, T. W., and Roberts, A. C. (1996). Dissociation in prefrontal cortex of affective and attentional shifts. *Nature* 380, 69–72.

Dineen, R., Doyle, J., and Bench, J. (1997). Audiological and psychological characteristics of a group of tinnitus sufferers, prior to tinnitus management training. *Br. J. Audiol.* 31, 27–38.

Eggermont, J. J. (2005). Tinnitus: neurobiological substrates. *Drug Discov. Today* 10, 1283–1290.

Eggermont, J. J., and Roberts, L. E. (2004). The neuroscience of tinnitus. *Trends Neurosci.* 27, 676–682.

Engineer, N. D., Riley, J. R., Seale, J. D., Vrana, W. A., Shetake, J. A., Sudanagunta, S. P., Borland, M. S., and Kilgard, M. P. (2011). Reversing pathological neural activity using targeted plasticity. *Nature* 470, 101–104.

Frysztak, R. J., and Neafsey, E. J. (1994). The effect of medial frontal cortex lesions on cardiovascular conditioned emotional responses in the rat. *Brain Res.* 643, 181–193.

Gard, M. G., and Kring, A. M. (2007). Sex differences in the time course of emotion. *Emotion* 7, 429–437.

Gray, J. R., Braver, T. S., and Raichle, M. E. (2002). Integration of emotion and cognition in the lateral prefrontal cortex. *Proc. Natl. Acad. Sci. U.S.A.* 99, 4115–4120.

Guitton, M. J., Caston, J., Ruel, J., Johnson, R. M., Pujol, R., and Puel, J. L. (2003). Salicylate induces tinnitus through activation of cochlear NMDA receptors. *J. Neurosci.* 23, 3944–3952.

Gusnard, D. A., Akbudak, E., Shulman, G. L., and Raichle, M. E. (2001). Medial prefrontal cortex and self-referential mental activity: relation to a default mode of brain function. *Proc. Natl. Acad. Sci. U.S.A.* 98, 4259–4264

Hallam, R. S. (1996). Correlates of sleep disturbance in chronic distressing tinnitus. *Scand. Audiol.* 25, 263–266.

Heller, A. J. (2003). Classification and epidemiology of tinnitus. *Otolaryngol. Clin. North Am.* 36, 239–248.

Inanaga, K. (1998). Frontal midline theta rhythm and mental activity. *Psychiatry Clin. Neurosci.* 52, 555–566.

Jancke, L., Shah, N. J., Posse, S., Grosse-Ryuken, M., and Muller-Gartner, H. W. (1998). Intensity coding of auditory stimuli: an fMRI study. *Neuropsychologia* 36, 875–883.

Jastreboff, P. J. (1990). Phantom auditory perception (tinnitus): mechanisms of generation and perception. *Neurosci. Res.* 8, 221–254.

Jastreboff, P. J., and Sasaki, C. T. (1986). Salicylate-induced changes in spontaneous activity of single units in the inferior colliculus of the guinea pig. *J. Acoust. Soc. Am.* 80, 1384–1391.

Joliot, M., Ribary, U., and Llinas, R. (1994). Human oscillatory brain activity near 40 Hz coexists with cognitive temporal binding. *Proc. Natl. Acad. Sci. U.S.A.* 91, 11748–11751.

Kennerley, S. W., Walton, M. E., Behrens, T. E., Buckley, M. J., and Rushworth, M. F. (2006). Optimal decision making and the anterior cingulate cortex. *Nat. Neurosci.* 9, 940–947.

Knight, R. T., Scabini, D., and Woods, D. L. (1989). Prefrontal cortex gating of auditory transmission in humans. *Brain Res.* 504, 338–342.

Koch, K., Pauly, K., Kellermann, T., Seiferth, N. Y., Reske, M., Backes, V., Stocker, T., Shah, N. J., Amunts, K., Kircher, T., Schneider, F., and Habel, U. (2007). Gender differences in the cognitive control of emotion: an fMRI study. *Neuropsychologia* 45, 2744–2754.

Kreyberg, S., Torvik, A., Bjorneboe, A., Wiik-Larsen, W., and Jacobsen, D. (1992). Trimethyltin poisoning: report of a case with postmortem examination. *Clin. Neuropathol.* 11, 256–259.

Kubota, Y., Sato, W., Toichi, M., Murai, T., Okada, T., Hayashi, A., and Sengoku, A. (2001). Frontal midline theta rhythm is correlated with cardiac autonomic activities during the performance of an attention demanding meditation procedure. *Brain Res. Cogn. Brain Res.* 11, 281–287.

Laureys, S. (2005). The neural correlate of (un)awareness: lessons from the vegetative state. *Trends Cogn. Sci.* 9, 556–559.

Laureys, S., Faymonville, M. E., Degueldre, C., Fiore, G. D., Damas, P., Lambermont, B., Janssens, N., Aerts, J., Franck, G., Luxen, A., Moonen, G., Lamy, M., and Maquet, P. (2000). Auditory processing in the vegetative state. *Brain* 123(Pt 8), 1589–1601.

Laureys, S., Faymonville, M. E., Peigneux, P., Damas, P., Lambermont, B., Del Fiore, G., Degueldre, C., Aerts, J., Luxen, A., Franck, G., Lamy, M., Moonen, G., and Maquet, P. (2002). Cortical processing of noxious somatosensory stimuli in the persistent vegetative state. *Neuroimage* 17, 732–741.

Le, T. H., Pardo, J. V., and Hu, X. (1998). 4 T-fMRI study of nonspatial shifting of selective attention: cerebellar and parietal contributions. *J. Neurophysiol.* 79, 1535–1548.

Lewis, J. W., Beauchamp, M. S., and deYoe, E. A. (2000). A comparison of visual and auditory motion processing in human cerebral cortex. *Cereb. Cortex* 10, 873–888.

Llinás, R., Urbano, F. J., Leznik, E., Ramirez, R. R., and van Marle, H. J. (2005). Rhythmic and dysrhythmic thalamocortical dynamics: GABA systems and the edge effect. *Trends Neurosci.* 28, 325–333.

Llinas, R., Ribary, U., Contreras, D., and Pedroarena, C. (1998). The neuronal basis for consciousness. *Philos. Trans. R. Soc. Lond. B Biol. Sci.* 353, 1841–1849.

Llinas, R., Ribary, U., Joliot, M., and Wang, X. (1994). "Content and context in temporal thalamocortical binding," in *Temporal Coding in the Brain*, eds G. Buzsaki, R. Llinasand, and W. Singer (Berlin: Springer-Verlag), 251–272.

Llinás, R. R., Ribary, U., Jeanmonod, D., Kronberg, E., and Mitra, P. P. (1999). Thalamocortical dysrhythmia: a neurological and neuropsychiatric syndrome characterized by magnetoencephalography. *Proc. Natl. Acad. Sci. U.S.A.* 96, 15222–15227.

Lockwood, A. H., Salvi, R. J., and Burkard, R. F. (2002). Tinnitus. *N. Engl. J. Med.* 347, 904–910.

Lorenz, I., Muller, N., Schlee, W., Hartmann, T., and Weisz, N. (2009). Loss of alpha power is related to increased gamma synchronization-A marker of reduced inhibition in tinnitus? *Neurosci. Lett.* 453, 225–228.

Masten, C. L., Eisenberger, N. I., Borofsky, L. A., Pfeifer, J. H., McNealy, K., Mazziotta, J. C., and Dapretto, M. (2009). Neural correlates of social exclusion during adolescence: understanding the distress of peer rejection. *Soc. Cogn. Affect. Neurosci.* 4, 143–157.

McKiernan, K. A., D'Angelo, B. R., Kaufman, J. N., and Binder, J. R. (2006). Interrupting the "stream of consciousness": an fMRI investigation. *Neuroimage* 29, 1185–1191.

Medford, N., and Critchley, H. D. (2010). Conjoint activity of anterior insular and anterior cingulate cortex: awareness and response. *Brain Struct. Funct.* 214, 535–549.

Menon, V., and Uddin, L. Q. (2010). Saliency, switching, attention and control: a network model of insula function. *Brain Struct. Funct.* 214, 655–667.

Melloni, L., Molina, C., Pena, M., Torres, D., Singer, W., and Rodriguez, E. (2007). Synchronization of neural activity across cortical areas correlates with conscious perception. *J. Neurosci.* 27, 2858–2865.

Mitchell, T. V., Morey, R. A., Inan, S., and Belger, A. (2005). Functional magnetic resonance imaging measure of automatic and controlled auditory processing. *Neuroreport* 16, 457–461.

Muhlau, M., Rauschecker, J. P., Oestreicher, E., Gaser, C., Rottinger, M., Wohlschlager, A. M., Simon, F., Etgen, T., Conrad, B., and Sander, D. (2006). Structural brain changes in tinnitus. *Cereb. Cortex* 16, 1283–1288.

Muhlnickel, W., Elbert, T., Taub, E., and Flor, H. (1998). Reorganization of auditory cortex in tinnitus. *Proc. Natl. Acad. Sci. U.S.A.* 95, 10340–10343.

Nicolas-Puel, C., Faulconbridge, R. L., Guitton, M., Puel, J. L., Mondain, M., and Uziel, A. (2002). Characteristics of tinnitus and etiology of associated hearing loss: a study of 123 patients. *Int. Tinnitus J.* 8, 37–44.

Norena, A., Cransac, H., and Chery-Croze, S. (1999). Towards an objectification by classification of tinnitus. *Clin. Neurophysiol.* 110, 666–675.

Norena, A., Micheyl, C., Chery-Croze, S., and Collet, L. (2002). Psychoacoustic characterization of the tinnitus spectrum: implications for the underlying mechanisms of tinnitus. *Audiol. Neurootol.* 7, 358–369.

Norena, A. J. (2011). An integrative model of tinnitus based on a central gain controlling neural sensitivity. *Neurosci. Biobehav. Rev.* 35, 1089–1109.

Norena, A. J., and Eggermont, J. J. (2003). Changes in spontaneous neural activity immediately after an acoustic trauma: implications for neural correlates of tinnitus. *Hear. Res.* 183, 137–153.

Norena, A. J., and Eggermont, J. J. (2006). Enriched acoustic environment after noise trauma abolishes neural signs of tinnitus. *Neuroreport* 17, 559–563.

Ohira, H., Nomura, M., Ichikawa, N., Isowa, T., Iidaka, T., Sato, A., Fukuyama, S., Nakajima, T., and Yamada, J. (2006). Association of neural and physiological responses during voluntary emotion suppression. *Neuroimage* 29, 721–733.

Ongur, D., and Price, J. L. (2000). The organization of networks within the orbital and medial prefrontal cortex of rats, monkeys and humans. *Cereb. Cortex* 10, 206–219.

Oppenheimer, S. (1993). The anatomy and physiology of cortical mechanisms of cardiac control. *Stroke* 24 (Suppl. 12), I3–I5.

Oppenheimer, S. M., Gelb, A., Girvin, J. P., and Hachinski, V. C. (1992). Cardiovascular effects of human insular cortex stimulation. *Neurology* 42, 1727–1732.

Phillips, M. L., Drevets, W. C., Rauch, S. L., and Lane, R. (2003). Neurobiology of emotion perception I: the neural basis of normal emotion perception. *Biol. Psychiatry* 54, 504–514.

Raichle, M. E., MacLeod, A. M., Snyder, A. Z., Powers, W. J., Gusnard, D. A., and Shulman, G. L. (2001). A default mode of brain function. *Proc. Natl. Acad. Sci. U.S.A.* 98, 676–682.

Rey, C., Reinecke, H. J., and Besser, R. (1984). Methyltin intoxication in six men; toxicologic and clinical aspects. *Vet. Hum. Toxicol.* 26, 121–122.

Ribary, U., Ioannides, A. A., Singh, K. D., Hasson, R., Bolton, J. P., Lado, F., Mogilner, A., and Llinas, R. (1991). Magnetic field tomography of coherent thalamocortical 40-Hz oscillations in humans. *Proc. Natl. Acad. Sci. U.S.A.* 88, 11037–11041.

Rutkowski, R. G., and Weinberger, N. M. (2005). Encoding of learned importance of sound by magnitude of representational area in primary auditory cortex. *Proc. Natl. Acad. Sci. U.S.A.* 102, 13664–13669.

Sadaghiani, S., Hesselmann, G., and Kleinschmidt, A. (2009). Distributed and antagonistic contributions of ongoing activity fluctuations to auditory stimulus detection. *J. Neurosci.* 29, 13410–13417.

Schlee, W., Weisz, N., Bertrand, O., Hartmann, T., and Elbert, T. (2008). Using auditory steady state responses to outline the functional connectivity in the tinnitus brain. *PLoS One* 3:e3720. doi: 10.1371/journal.pone.0003720

Schmitt, C., Patak, M., and Kroner-Herwig, B. (2000). Stress and the onset of sudden hearing loss and tinnitus. *Int. Tinnitus J.* 6, 41–49.

Seeley, W. W., Menon, V., Schatzberg, A. F., Keller, J., Glover, G. H., Kenna, H., Reiss, A. L., and Greicius, M. D. (2007). Dissociable intrinsic connectivity networks for salience processing and executive control. *J. Neurosci.* 27, 2349–2356.

Shargorodsky, J., Curhan, S. G., Curhan, G. C., and Eavey, R. (2010). Change in prevalence of hearing loss in US adolescents. *JAMA* 304, 772–778.

Shulman, A. (1995). A final common pathway for tinnitus – the medial temporal lobe system. *Int. Tinnitus J.* 1, 115–126.

Steriade, M. (2006). Grouping of brain rhythms in corticothalamic systems. *Neuroscience* 137, 1087–1106.

Tiitinen, H., Sinkkonen, J., Reinikainen, K., Alho, K., Lavikainen, J., and Naatanen, R. (1993). Selective attention enhances the auditory 40-Hz transient response in humans. *Nature* 364, 59–60.

van der Loo, E., Congedo, M., Vanneste, S., Van de Heyning, P., and De Ridder, D. (2011). Insular lateralization in tinnitus distress. *Auton. Neurosci.* 165, 191–194.

van der Loo, E., Gais, S., Congedo, M., Vanneste, S., Plazier, M., Menovsky, T., Van de Heyning, P., and De Ridder, D. (2009). Tinnitus intensity dependent gamma oscillations of the contralateral auditory cortex. *PLoS One* 4:e7396. doi: 10.1371/journal.pone.0007396

Vanneste, S., Plazier, M., van der Loo, E., Van de Heyning, P., and De Ridder, D. (2010a). The differences in brain activity between narrow band noise and pure tone tinnitus. *PLoS One* 5:e13618. doi: 10.1371/journal.pone.0013618

Vanneste, S., Plazier, M., der Loo, E., de Heyning, P. V., Congedo, M., and De Ridder, D. (2010b). The neural correlates of tinnitus-related distress. *Neuroimage* 52, 470–480.

Vanneste, S., Van de Heyning, P., and De Ridder, D. (2011a). Contralateral parahippocampal gamma-band activity determines noise-like tinnitus laterality: a region of interest analysis. *Neuroscience* 199, 481–490.

Vanneste, S., Van de Heyning, P., and De Ridder, D. (2011b). The neural network of phantom sound changes over time: a comparison between recent-onset and chronic tinnitus patients. *Eur. J. Neurosci.* 34, 718–731.

Vanneste, S., Plazier, M., van der Loo, E., Van de Heyning, P., and De Ridder, D. (2011c). The difference between uni- and bilateral auditory phantom percept. *Clin. Neurophysiol.* 122, 578–587.

Voisin, J., Bidet-Caulet, A., Bertrand, O., and Fonlupt, P. (2006). Listening in silence activates auditory areas: a functional magnetic resonance imaging study. *J. Neurosci.* 26, 273–278.

Wang, J., Rao, H., Wetmore, G. S., Furlan, P. M., Korczykowski, M., Dinges, D. F., and Detre, J. A. (2005). Perfusion functional MRI reveals cerebral blood flow pattern under psychological stress. *Proc. Natl. Acad. Sci. U.S.A.* 102, 17804–17809.

Weisz, N., Moratti, S., Meinzer, M., Dohrmann, K., and Elbert, T.

(2005). Tinnitus perception and distress is related to abnormal spontaneous brain activity as measured by magnetoencephalography. *PLoS Med.* 2:e153. doi: 10.1371/journal.pmed.0020153

Wheeler, R. E., Davidson, R. J., and Tomarken, A. J. (1993). Frontal brain asymmetry and emotional reactivity: a biological substrate of affective style. *Psychophysiology* 30, 82–89.

Yoo, S. S., Lee, C. U., and Choi, B. G. (2001). Human brain mapping of auditory imagery: event-related functional MRI study. *Neuroreport* 12, 3045–3049.

Zald, D. H., and Pardo, J. V. (2002). The neural correlates of aversive auditory stimulation. *Neuroimage* 16(3 Pt 1), 746–753.

7

Changes of oscillatory activity in pitch processing network and related tinnitus relief induced by acoustic CR neuromodulation

Ilya Adamchic[1] *, Christian Hauptmann[1] and Peter A. Tass[1,2]

[1] *Institute of Neuroscience and Medicine – Neuromodulation, Research Center Jülich, Jülich, Germany*

[2] *Department of Stereotactic and Functional Neurosurgery, University of Cologne, Cologne, Germany*

Correspondence:
Ilya Adamchic, Institute of Neuroscience and Medicine – Neuromodulation, Research Center Jülich, 52425 Jülich, Germany.
e-mail: i.adamchic@fz-juelich.de

Chronic subjective tinnitus is characterized by abnormal neuronal synchronization in the central auditory system. As shown in a controlled clinical trial, acoustic coordinated reset (CR) neuromodulation causes a significant relief of tinnitus symptoms along with a significant decrease of pathological oscillatory activity in a network comprising auditory and non-auditory brain areas, which is often accompanied with a significant tinnitus pitch change. Here we studied if the tinnitus pitch change correlates with a reduction of tinnitus loudness and/or annoyance as assessed by visual analog scale (VAS) scores. Furthermore, we studied if the changes of the pattern of brain synchrony in tinnitus patients induced by 12 weeks of CR therapy depend on whether or not the patients undergo a pronounced tinnitus pitch change. Therefore, we applied standardized low-resolution brain electromagnetic tomography (sLORETA) to EEG recordings from two groups of patients with a sustained CR-induced relief of tinnitus symptoms with and without tinnitus pitch change. We found that absolute changes of VAS loudness and VAS annoyance scores significantly correlate with the modulus, i.e., the absolute value, of the tinnitus pitch change. Moreover, as opposed to patients with small or no pitch change we found a significantly stronger decrease in gamma power in patients with pronounced tinnitus pitch change in right parietal cortex (Brodmann area, BA 40), right frontal cortex (BA 9, 46), left temporal cortex (BA 22, 42), and left frontal cortex (BA 4, 6), combined with a significantly stronger increase of alpha (10–12 Hz) activity in the right and left anterior cingulate cortex (ACC; BA 32, 24). In addition, we revealed a significantly lower functional connectivity in the gamma band between the right dorsolateral prefrontal cortex (BA 46) and the right ACC (BA 32) after 12 weeks of CR therapy in patients with pronounced pitch change. Our results indicate a substantial, CR-induced reduction of tinnitus-related auditory binding in a pitch processing network.

Keywords: tinnitus, coordinated reset neuromodulation, pitch, phantom perception, gamma band activity, electroencephalography

INTRODUCTION

Non-pulsatile subjective tinnitus is an auditory phantom phenomenon that is present in up to 15% of the population (Eggermont and Roberts, 2004). Tinnitus generation is considered to have a central basis, typically being initiated by damage to the peripheral hearing system (Eggermont and Roberts, 2004; Weisz et al., 2005, 2006). Cortical map reorganization is related to tinnitus (Robertson and Irvine, 1989; Muhlnickel et al., 1998; Lockwood et al., 2002; Moller, 2003; Yang et al., 2011). However, according to an MEG study, map reorganization cannot explain the emergence of tinnitus in a satisfactory manner (Weisz et al., 2006). Another important tinnitus-related phenomenon is the emergence of pathological neural synchrony (Ochi and Eggermont, 1997; Norena and Eggermont, 2003; Seki and Eggermont, 2003; Weisz et al., 2005, 2007; De Ridder et al., 2011b). In general, pathologically increased delta activity emerges in cortical regions deprived of afferent input (Steriade, 2006). In the context of tinnitus, pathologically enhanced neuronal synchronization was observed in the primary auditory cortex of animals following damage to the inner ear (Ochi and Eggermont, 1997; Norena and Eggermont, 2003; Seki and Eggermont, 2003) as well as in tinnitus patients (Llinas et al., 1999; Weisz et al., 2005, 2007; De Ridder et al., 2011b). Apart from a significant reduction of alpha band power (Weisz et al., 2005) abnormally strong synchrony was observed in tinnitus patients in the delta band (Weisz et al., 2005), theta band (De Ridder et al., 2011b), and gamma band (Weisz et al., 2007), e.g., in temporal areas. Several studies confirmed that pathological neural synchronization is related to the tinnitus percept (Dohrmann et al., 2007; Kahlbrock and Weisz, 2008; De Ridder et al., 2011b). However, a conscious perception of the tinnitus requires the involvement of larger networks of brain areas relevant to awareness and salience (De Ridder et al., 2011a).

Indeed, apart from auditory cortical areas also non-auditory areas such as amygdala, cingulate cortex, and parahippocampus are involved in the tinnitus generation, in particular, in patients with tinnitus distress (Rauschecker, 2005; Vanneste et al.,

2010; De Ridder et al., 2011a). Furthermore, an altered functional interaction between non-auditory and auditory areas with abnormal synchrony seems to be a hallmark of tinnitus distress (Schlee et al., 2009a).

To specifically counteract the electrophysiological correlate of tinnitus, i.e., the pathological neural synchrony, in a previous proof of concept study we have used a non-invasive desynchronizing stimulation technique, acoustic coordinated reset (CR) neuromodulation (Tass et al., 2012). CR neuromodulation has been developed computationally (Tass, 1999, 2003b) and is essentially based on fundamental dynamical self-organization principles (Tass, 2003a,b) as well as on the intimate relationship between neuronal dynamics and connectivity (Yuste and Bonhoeffer, 2004). As shown in theoretical and computational studies, CR neuromodulation causes a desynchronization (Tass, 2003b) which in turn shifts neural networks with spike timing-dependent plasticity (Gerstner et al., 1996; Markram, 1997) from a synchronized state with strong synaptic connectivity to a desynchronized state with weak connectivity (Tass and Majtanik, 2006; Hauptmann et al., 2007; Tass and Hauptmann, 2009). By doing so, the network unlearns pathological connectivity and pathological synchrony. Put otherwise, it undergoes an anti-kindling (Tass and Majtanik, 2006). CR neuromodulation has initially been developed for the application to electrical deep brain stimulation (DBS) in Parkinson's disease (Tass, 2003b). For this, brief electrical high-frequency pulse trains are sequentially delivered via different stimulation contacts of an implanted lead. In animal experiments acute desynchronizing effects (Neiman et al., 2007) as well as long-lasting desynchronizing after-effects (Tass et al., 2009) of electrical CR have been verified.

As shown computationally, due to the underlying biophysics and non-linear dynamics, CR neuromodulation can be applied invasively with electrical stimuli as well as non-invasively by means of sensory, e.g., auditory stimuli (Popovych and Tass, 2012; Tass and Popovych, 2012). Accordingly, in a proof of concept study the initially DBS-oriented CR concept was transformed into a non-invasive, acoustic treatment for subjective tonal tinnitus (Tass et al., 2012). Relying on the tonotopic organization of the central auditory system, the electrical brief high-frequency pulse trains were replaced by CR tones with different frequencies centered around the patient's individual tinnitus frequency. The CR approach aims at a desynchronization of a synchronized focus in the tonotopically organized auditory cortex located in an area corresponding to the dominant tinnitus frequency and the belonging tinnitus spectrum (Norena et al., 2002). To this end, we sequentially delivered CR tones, where the goal of each CR tone is to cause a phase reset or at least a soft phase reset (i.e., a phase reset achieved by an iterated administration of that CR tone (see Tass, 2002) of the pathological slow-wave oscillation in the delta frequency band in a neuronal sub-population tonotopically related to the frequency of the particular CR tone (Tass et al., 2012).

In a prospective, randomized, single blind, placebo-controlled proof of concept trial in 63 patients with chronic tonal tinnitus ("RESET study") CR treatment turned out to be safe and well-tolerated and resulted in a highly significant decrease of tinnitus loudness and symptoms as measured by VAS and tinnitus questionnaire (TQ) scores (Tass et al., 2012). Furthermore, as shown by means of EEG recordings, after 12 weeks of treatment with acoustic CR neuromodulation pathologically elevated delta and gamma activity were both decreased in a network of brain areas comprising primary and secondary auditory cortex as well as non-auditory, e.g., prefrontal areas (Tass et al., 2012). By the same token, the tinnitus-related reduction of alpha activity was reversed and alpha activity re-increased in auditory and prefrontal areas (Tass et al., 2012). In a relevant number of patients CR neuromodulation induced a tinnitus pitch change predominantly lowering tinnitus frequencies (Tass et al., 2012). Theoretical studies have predicted long-lasting (Tass and Majtanik, 2006) and cumulative (Hauptmann and Tass, 2009) desynchronizing effects of CR neuromodulation.

We here study if the tinnitus pitch change, observed in the RESET study, correlates with a reduction of tinnitus loudness and/or annoyance, and if the changes of the pattern of brain synchrony in tinnitus patients depends on whether or not the patients undergo a pronounced tinnitus pitch change. For this, we compare two groups of patients with very similar tinnitus relief, but significantly different tinnitus pitch change. According to previous studies different perceptual characteristics of tinnitus may be coded by an altered network activity of multiple parallel overlapping dynamic neural networks (De Ridder et al., 2011a). Also, it has been shown that different auditory modalities may be coded by different mechanisms and also by spatially separate neuronal networks: sound identification and sound localization were shown to depend on specialized and spatially distinct pathways (Clement et al., 1999; Alain et al., 2001; Banai et al., 2011). Clement et al. (1999) proposed that pitch and loudness are processed in separate modules of the auditory memory. Developmental trajectories of the abilities to detect auditory amplitude and frequency modulation were also shown to be distinct (Banai et al., 2011). Moreover, experiments in non-human primates indicate that an activation of primary sensory areas is not sufficient for the generation of the percept, and associative areas located in, e.g., frontal and parietal lobes are involved in sensory perception (Romo and Salinas, 2003; Lemus et al., 2009a,b). In summary, following current notions on parallel processing of different aspects of auditory information in general and in phantom perception in particular, we might expect differences in the change of brain synchrony in auditory, but also in non-auditory areas between our two patient groups, treated with acoustic CR neuromodulation and differing in the amount of their tinnitus pitch change.

The long-lasting and cumulative therapeutic (i.e., clinical) effects of acoustic CR neuromodulation along with its long-lasting desynchronizing effect on the pathological, tinnitus-related neuronal synchrony, both observed in our proof of concept study (Tass et al., 2012), are in accordance with these theoretical predictions. However, the CR-induced tinnitus pitch change was not predicted theoretically. In fact, the pitch change indicates CR-induced neuroplastic changes. We shall discuss possible mechanisms that may cause a CR-induced tinnitus pitch change below.

MATERIALS AND METHODS

PARTICIPANTS

The current work is based on existing data from patients who participated in a multicentric randomized, controlled clinical trial on Acoustic CR Neuromodulation in the Treatment of Chronic Tinnitus, performed in Germany between 2009 and 2010 ("RESET study[1]," Identifier: NCT00927121; Tass et al., 2012). For the present study patients were selected based on the following criteria: (i) EEG data had to be available for both baseline and the 12 weeks visit; (ii) clinical data, i.e., VAS loudness, VAS annoyance, and matched tinnitus pitch, had to be available for both base line and the 12 weeks visit. From the total population of 63 patients one patient dropped out of the study before the 12 weeks visit. For another patient there were no EEG data available, and in two patients matched tinnitus pitch could not be determined as tinnitus was absent at the 12 weeks visit. Thus 59 patients were selected for further analysis. All patients suffered from chronic subjective tonal tinnitus.

TREATMENT

Patients were stimulated for 12 weeks using a portable acoustic device and comfortable earphones (Tass et al., 2012). In the RESET study patients were randomly allocated to receive acoustic CR neuromodulation (group G1–G4) or placebo stimulation (G5): G1 ($n = 22$), G2 ($n = 12$), G3 ($n = 12$), G4 ($n = 12$), and G5 ($n = 5$). G1–G3 all received stimulation for 4–6 h every day. G4 and G5 all received stimulation for 1 h max every day. Stimulation signals were generated based on a specific formula reflecting the logarithmic tonotopic organization of the auditory cortex and on the matched tinnitus (frequency f_t) with an equal number of tones placed below and above the tinnitus frequency (except for placebo). Stimulation tones were perceived by patients as equally loud and just super-threshold. Four tones per cycle were played in random order with three stimulation cycles followed by two silent cycles. The four tones are based on a patient specific list of frequencies (see Tass et al., 2012): G1, G3, G4 (f_1 to f_4); G2 (G2, prior to each cycle four frequencies are chosen from f_1 to f_{12}, with the constraint that each cycle has to contain one frequency from each of the four groups f_1 to f_3, f_4 to f_6, f_7 to f_9, and f_{10} to f_{12}); G5 based on a modified tinnitus frequency [$f_p = 0.7071\, f_t/(2^n)$, f_p within 300–600 Hz]. The stimulation tones are equidistantly placed on a logarithmic scale within the interval [$0.5{\cdot}f_t$, $2{\cdot}f_t$] for G1–G4 and within [$0.5{\cdot}f_p$, $2{\cdot}f_p$] for G5. Cycle repetition rate was 1.5 Hz for G1, G2, G4, and G5 whereas in G3 the rate was harmonized to the patient's specific EEG data (Tass, 2003b; Tass et al., 2009; based on the highest peak in the delta frequency band). A readjustment of stimulation parameters was performed at each visit, provided the matched tinnitus frequency had changed. Visits took place after 1, 4, 8, 12, and 16 weeks. Data for this paper come from baseline and the 12 weeks visit as EEG recordings for all patients were performed at these visits. At each visit, tinnitus loudness and annoyance were assessed off-stimulation (at least 2.5 h after cessation of CR neuromodulation) and consecutively on-stimulation (15 min after turning on CR neuromodulation) using a VAS scale for loudness (VAS-L) and annoyance (VAS-A) ranging from 0 to 100. In this study we only use the off-stimulation VAS scores, because EEG recordings were performed off-stimulation. A pure tone matching procedure was used to determine the best matching tinnitus pitch (from 100 to 10,000 Hz). Patients were instructed to match the frequency of a pure tone to the perceived pitch of their tinnitus. During this procedure intensity and frequency of the matching tone were controlled by the patient. Tinnitus matching started either well below or well above the patient's tinnitus frequency. The patient had to adjust the matching tone to his/her tinnitus. Patients had to confirm a best matching pitch at least twice. The matching tone was repeatedly interrupted to facilitate the comparison between matching tone and tinnitus.

In general, the CR treatment was safe and well-tolerated and resulted in a highly significant decrease of tinnitus symptoms as measured by VAS and TQ scores (Tass et al., 2012): After 12 weeks of therapy a strong significant reduction (29.6–37.3 points) of VAS-L/VAS-A in G1 and G3 in the on-stimulation condition ($p \leq 0.01$ compared to baseline) was observed. This significant effect persisted in the off-stimulation condition for G1/G3 VAS-L/VAS-A (18.0–28.8 points $p < 0.004$). G2 (the noisy CR group) and G4 (stimulation time of 1 h/day) showed less pronounced reduction of tinnitus symptoms (for more details see Tass et al., 2012). In contrast, the placebo group G5 showed neither on- nor off-stimulation significant changes in VAS-L/VAS-A scores after 12 weeks. TQ scores were significantly reduced compared to baseline in G1–G4 with the strongest improvements in G1 and G3 (Tass et al., 2012). In contrast, there were no significant changes in TQ score in the placebo group G5.

DATA COLLECTION

Each patient underwent two recording sessions: on day 1 before start of treatment and after 12 weeks, minimum 2 h after stopping the last stimulation session. Subjects were instructed to retain from caffeinated beverages on the day of the recording to exclude caffeine induced changes of EEG activity. Patients were seated in upright position in a comfortable chair. EEG recordings were obtained in a dimly lit room in a Faraday cage. EEG data were collected from 128 surface electrodes using a HydroCel Geodesic Sensor Net. All electrodes were referenced to Cz. The EEG signals were amplified with the Net Amps 200 amplifier (Electrical Geodesics Inc, Eugene, USA), digitized at 1 kHz and analogous bandpass filtered from 0.1 to 400 Hz. Recordings were performed in the awake state during alternating 2 min intervals with eyes closed and eyes open. For all patients we selected the eyes closed data for further analysis, since they were less affected by artifacts. Photogrammetry was performed for all subjects using Geodesic Photogrammetry System, and the individual head shape was modeled for every subject in each EEG session. Offline the scalp EEG was re-referenced to an average reference. Signals were additionally digitally filtered with a 0.8–130 Hz digital filter. Each EEG recording was corrected for blink and eye movements in BESA using the surrogate model approach in BESA (Brain Electrical Source Analysis, MEGIS Software, 5.3 version; Scherg et al., 2002). Recordings were further analyzed in MATLAB (The Mathworks, Natick, MA, USA) using EEGLAB[2]. All EEG segments that contained large muscle or other artifacts were removed. The mean length of the recordings after artifact correction was 3 min 24 s $\pm$ 23 s.

[1]ClinicalTrials.gov

[2]http://sccn.ucsd.edu/eeglab

DATA ANALYSIS

Pearson correlation was performed between changes of VAS-L, VAS-A, matched tinnitus pitch (i.e., difference before and after CR treatment) and the corresponding modulus of the change of matched tinnitus pitch. We set out to investigate how spontaneous oscillatory brain activity changes in patients with pronounced tinnitus pitch change as opposed to patients with zero or minimal pitch change. Accordingly, to investigate differences in the changes of spontaneous oscillatory brain activity between patients with pronounced and with minimal/zero tinnitus pitch change, we created two groups of patients with a sustained relief of tinnitus symptoms as measured by VAS-L and VAS-A: (i) pitch change (PC) group, (ii) no tinnitus pitch change (NPC) or minimal tinnitus pitch change group. Sustained, clinically relevant relief of tinnitus symptoms, i.e., the minimal clinically important difference (MCID), was defined as ΔVAS ≤ -10 points ($n = 34$; Adamchic et al., submitted). This group of patients was divided into two equally large sub-populations based on the modulus of the individual pitch change ratio: Patients in the NPC group had a modulus of the pitch change ratio < 0.3, whereas patients in the PC group had pitch change ratio ≥ 0.3. Pitch change ratio was defined as (modified pitch at 12 weeks visit/initial pitch at baseline) $- 1$. Thus, 50% of patients were classified to the PC group and 50% to the NPC group. According to the significant positive correlation between VAS-L or VAS-A and the modulus of the change of the matched tinnitus pitch (see Results), the PC group had a greater VAS improvement (ΔVAS-L $= -29.4 \pm 10.8$, $n = 17$) compared to the NPC group (ΔVAS-L $= -25.1 \pm 18.9$, $n = 17$). To exclude the influence of different magnitudes of the reduction of tinnitus symptoms between the PC and NPC group on the further analysis, we excluded the patient with the greatest VAS-L improvement from PC and the patient with the smallest VAS-L improvement from NPC, in this way creating two groups (PC, $n = 16$ and NPC, $n = 16$) with a rather similar reduction of tinnitus symptoms, but significantly different matched pitch changes (**Table 1**).

None of the patients from the placebo group was classified to belong to PC. A current density analysis of the recorded electrical activity was performed in 3-D Talairach/MNI space using the sLORETA software package (Pascual-Marqui, 2002). sLORETA computed three-dimensional linear solutions for the EEG inverse problem with a three-shell spherical head model adapted to the Talairach human brain atlas digitized at the Brain Imaging Center of the Montreal Neurological Institute. sLORETA images represent the electrical activity of each voxel in terms of the amplitude of the computed current source density (CSD) in that voxel (μA/mm^2). LORETA has been validated using functional magnetic resonance imaging (fMRI) and positron emission tomography (PET; Pascual-Marqui et al., 1994; Vitacco et al., 2002; Mulert et al., 2004; Pizzagalli et al., 2004; Zumsteg et al., 2005). Also, it was shown that even deep structures with subcallosal cingulate and mesial hippocampal foci could be correctly identified by LORETA (Pizzagalli et al., 2004; Zumsteg et al., 2005). sLORETA is an advanced, further improved version of LORETA (Pascual-Marqui et al., 2002). The solution space used in this study was restricted to the gray matter voxels that belonged to cortical and hippocampal regions, comprising a total of 6430 voxels at a spatial resolution of 5 mm. The effects of the differential change of the matched tinnitus frequency on the spontaneous brain activity as assessed by sLORETA in the PC and the NPC group were revealed between the two groups with a voxel-by-voxel paired-groups comparison of the current density distribution applying t-statistical non-parametric mapping (SnPM; Robertson and Irvine, 1989). For this, a paired-groups design (A1–A2) = (B1–B2) was used, where A1 and A2 stand for the CSDs in the PC group (before vs. after CR therapy, respectively) and B1 and B2 stand for the CSDs in the NPC group (before vs. after CR therapy, respectively). In this way, we detected brain regions where oscillatory activity was specifically reduced or increased after 12 weeks of CR treatment in the PC group as opposed to the corresponding changes in the NPC group. The significance levels used were $p < 0.05$. sLORETA source localization was performed on the basis of fixed frequency bands: delta (1–3 Hz), theta (4–7 Hz), alpha1 (8–9 Hz), alpha2 (10–12 Hz), beta1 (13–18 Hz), beta2 (19–21 Hz), beta3 (22–30 Hz), and gamma (30–45 Hz). Put otherwise, previously we have shown that CR therapy induces significant power changes in different frequency bands and specific brain areas (Tass et al., 2012). We here study, how these changes depend on whether or not the tinnitus pitch changes strongly.

To study whether the CSD changes, that showed up as significant differences between PC and NPC groups in particular Brodmann areas (BAs), were correlated with tinnitus pitch changes or VAS changes, CSDs were extracted from spherical volumes of interest (radius 5 mm) centered on the voxels with maximal significance value in each of these BAs. These CSD values were used for a partial correlation analysis with data from matched tinnitus pitch, VAS-L and VAS-A in all 59 patients. By using partial correlations we measure the relationship of two variables with the effect of a control variable being removed. In our case we correlated changes of CSD extracted from spherical volumes of interest for a certain frequency band with pitch changes, controlling for VAS and vice versa, thus obtaining correlations specifically for pitch and VAS. Additionally, we assess functional connectivity as a pattern of statistical dependencies between separate brain regions. For this, we do not make any specific assumptions concerning the directional interactions between the brain regions under study. Measures of linear dependence (coherence-type) between two multivariate time series may be expressed as the sum of the lagged linear and instantaneous linear dependences (Pascual-Marqui, 2007b). However, any measure of instantaneous dependence is likely to be contaminated with a non-physiological contribution due to volume conduction (Pascual-Marqui, 2007b). Pascual-Marqui (2007a) introduced a technique that removes the instantaneous, non-physiological contribution resulting from volume

Table 1 | Clinical characteristics of NPC and PC groups, mean (SD).

	n	NPC	PC
VAS loudness	16	−26.9 (17.5)	−27.1 (10.3)
VAS annoyance	16	−25.7 (15.2)	−26.2 (12.1)
Tinnitus frequency change (Hz)	16	1197 (1002)	2438 (1190)
Tinnitus frequency ratio change	16	0.151 (0.084)	0.521 (0.177)

conduction. Accordingly, this measure of dependence can be applied to a large number of brain areas simultaneously. We calculated lagged linear connectivity (lagged coherence) for the same frequency bands as used for the sLORETA analysis. Calculations of lagged linear connectivity were performed using regions of interest (ROI), constructed for each hemisphere by defining all voxels located within a radius of 5 mm around designated seed points. Seed points were placed in the BAs that showed significant differences between PC and NPC and were defined as the voxel with the highest significance in a selected BA (see Results). In other words, we constrained our connectivity analysis to those brain areas which showed differential effects of CR therapy depending on whether or not tinnitus pitch changed strongly. Connectivity data were subjected to repeated-measures ANOVA (rmANOVA) with the within-group factor Time (1, base line; 2, after 12 weeks of acoustic CR neuromodulation) and between-group factor Group with two levels: PC and NPC. Where rmANOVA showed significant effects, *post hoc t*-tests were applied.

RESULTS

Baseline characteristics of the patient population are presented in **Table 2**.

No significant correlation was observed between changes in VAS-L or VAS-A and tinnitus pitch change ratio when all patients ($n = 59$) were included into the analysis (**Table 3**).

However, in patients with decreased tinnitus pitch the pitch change ratio positively correlated with both a decrease in VAS-L ($r = 0.37, p = 0.01; n = 46$) and VAS-A ($r = 0.48, p < 0.01; n = 46$; **Figure 1**).

A complementary trend was observed in patients with an increase in their tinnitus pitch (**Figure 1**). However, possibly due to the low number of patients ($n = 13$), the correlation between the increase of the tinnitus pitch and the VAS-L and VAS-A changes did not reach significance: correlation between the increase of the tinnitus pitch change ratio and VAS changes were $r = -0.37$, $p = 0.11$ for VAS-L and $r = -0.25$, $p = 0.42$ for VAS-A. One patient (an "outlier") had a much greater tinnitus pitch change ratio, i.e., = 1.49 than all other patients. However inclusion of this patient into the analysis set did not dramatically affect the results (**Figure 1**). Based on these findings, the modulus of the tinnitus pitch change was used for further analysis. A reduction of the tinnitus symptoms negatively correlated with the modulus of the tinnitus pitch change (**Figure 2**; **Table 3**). In general, we found a high correlation between the CR-induced changes in ΔVAS-L and ΔVAS-A, i.e., $r = 0.92$ (baseline to 12 weeks, $p < 0.01$).

Standardized low resolution brain electromagnetic tomography revealed regions were oscillatory activity was specifically reduced or increased after 12 weeks of treatment in the PC group as compared to the changes in the NPC group. A significantly different effect on the power of the oscillatory activity after 12 weeks of CR therapy between the two groups was observed in the gamma band in PC compared to NPC in the following areas: left parietal cortex (BA 40), right frontal cortex (BA 9, 46), left frontal cortex (BA 4, 6), and left temporal cortex (BA 22, 42; **Figure 3**). In these brain areas gamma band power decreased significantly more strongly in the PC group.

In addition, we found a differential effect of the CR therapy on the power of the oscillatory activity in the alpha2 band: The power of alpha2 increased significantly more strongly in the PC as compared to the NPC group in the right anterior cingulate cortex (ACC; BA 32, 24). No significant results were found for any other frequency bands. BAs containing significant voxels are listed in **Table 4**.

The modulus of the tinnitus pitch change ratio correlated negatively (controlling for VAS-L, i.e., statistically ruling out the influence of VAS-L) with the CSD changes in the gamma band in the left temporal cortex $r = -0.31, p = 0.02$ (volumes of interest

Table 2 | Patient's characteristics at baseline ($n = 59$).

Sex	Female	18 (31%)
	Male	41 (69%)
Age, years (SD)		48.8 (11.0)
Tinnitus duration, years (SD)		6.5 (6.4)
VAS-L (SD)		63.6 (20.0)
VAS-A (SD)		61.5 (20.6)
Tinnitus side	Right	8 (13.6%)
	Left	19 (32.2%)
	Both sides	32 (54.2%)

Table 3 | Correlation (p value) between change in VAS-L, VAS-A, and tinnitus pitch change ratio.

	n	Tinnitus pitch change ratio (*p*)	Modulus of tinnitus pitch change ratio (*p*)
VAS-L	59	0.10 (0.43)	−0.34 (<0.01)
VAS-A	59	0.19 (0.16)	−0.32 (<0.01)

Table 4 | Locations (Talairach coordinates) of maximal t-values in each BA containing significant voxels revealed by comparing oscillatory power changes between groups (PC and NPC) by means of sLORETA.

Side	BA	ROI center		
		x	*y*	*z*
Left	4	−41	−20	51
Left	6	−43	−8	62
Right	9	53	14	32
Left	22	−58	−45	16
Right	24	6	37	11
Left	24	−4	38	10
Right	32	4	36	16
Left	32	−7	37	14
Left	40	−59	−43	20
Left	42	−60	−33	15
Right	46	46	27	19

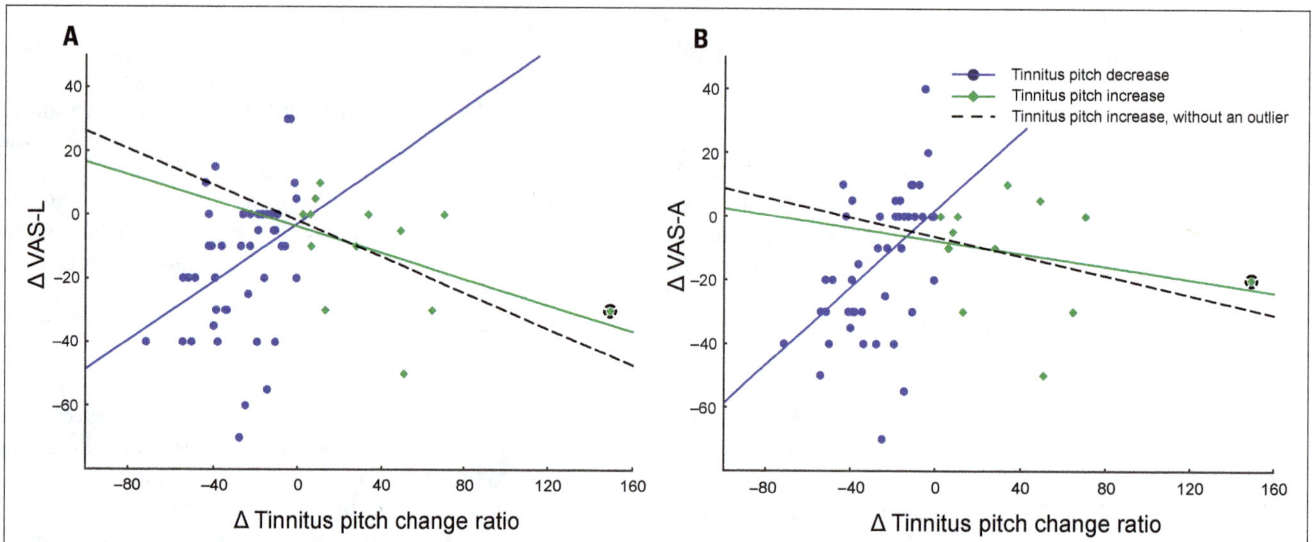

FIGURE 1 | Changes in VAS-L **(A)** and VAS-A **(B)** as a function of a tinnitus pitch change ratio. Patients are divided into two groups: (1) tinnitus pitch decrease (blue, $n = 46$); (2) tinnitus pitch increase (green, $n = 13$ or red dashed line after removal of an outlier, $n = 12$). An outlier patient is marked by the red circle.

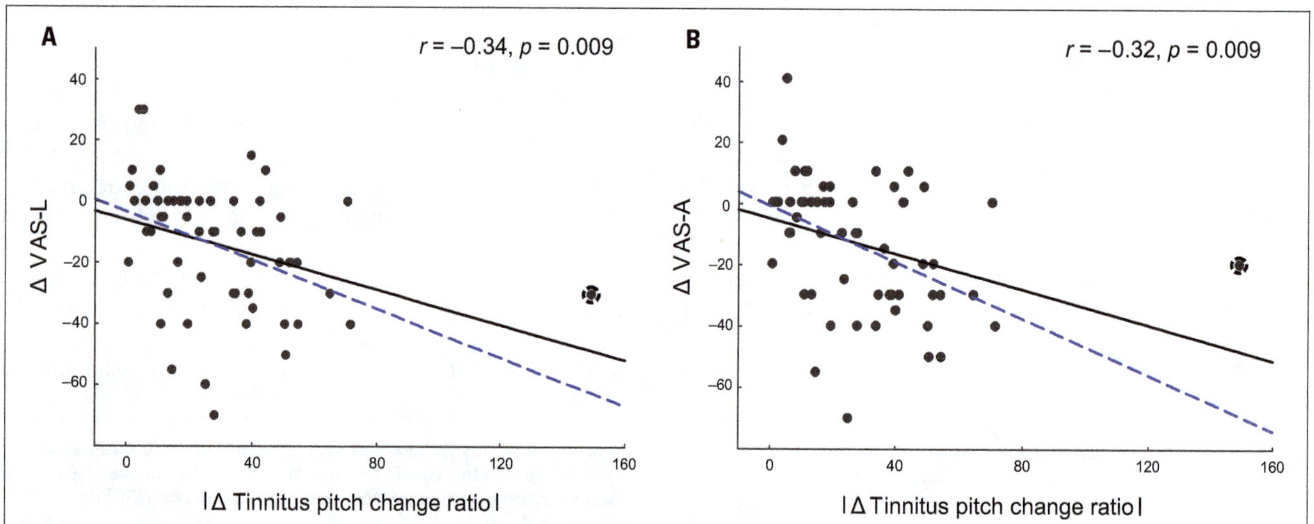

FIGURE 2 | Changes in VAS-L **(A)** and VAS-A **(B)** as a function of the modulus tinnitus pitch change ratio with all patients included ($n = 59$, solid red line) or with the outlier (marked by the red circle) excluded from the analysis ($n = 58$, dashed blue line).

center *x* −58, *y* −45, *z* 16; BA 22). Changes in the VAS-A negatively correlated with changes in CSD (controlling for the modulus of the tinnitus pitch change ratio, i.e., statistically ruling out the influence of the modulus of the tinnitus pitch change ratio) in the alpha2 band in the right frontal cortex $r = -0.33$, $p = 0.01$ (volumes of interest center *x* 6, *y* 37, *z* 11; BA 24; **Figure 4**). The correlation between modulus of the pitch change ratio and CSD gamma power remained significant ($r = -0.29$, $p = 0.03$, $n = 58$) also after removing the outlier from the complete ($n = 59$) dataset.

No further significant correlations between clinical data and CSD were found for other regions and bands.

Repeated-measures ANOVA of functional connectivity values between BAs containing significant voxels revealed a significant interaction of Group (PC vs. NPC, $F = 5.3$, $p = 0.03$) for the right BA 32 – BA 46 connectivity. Subsequent *post hoc t*-tests showed a significantly lower linear connectivity at the end of 12 weeks than at the baseline ($p = 0.007$). Comparison between NPC and PC at the 12 weeks visit revealed significantly lower functional connectivity in the gamma band between the right dorsolateral prefrontal cortex (DLPFC; BA 46) and the right ACC (BA 32) in the PC group ($p = 0.008$; **Figure 5**). Accordingly no significant differences in functional connectivity were found between PC and NPC at baseline ($p > 0.05$).

DISCUSSION

To our knowledge, this is the first study in a group of tinnitus patients that reveals an association of therapy-induced changes

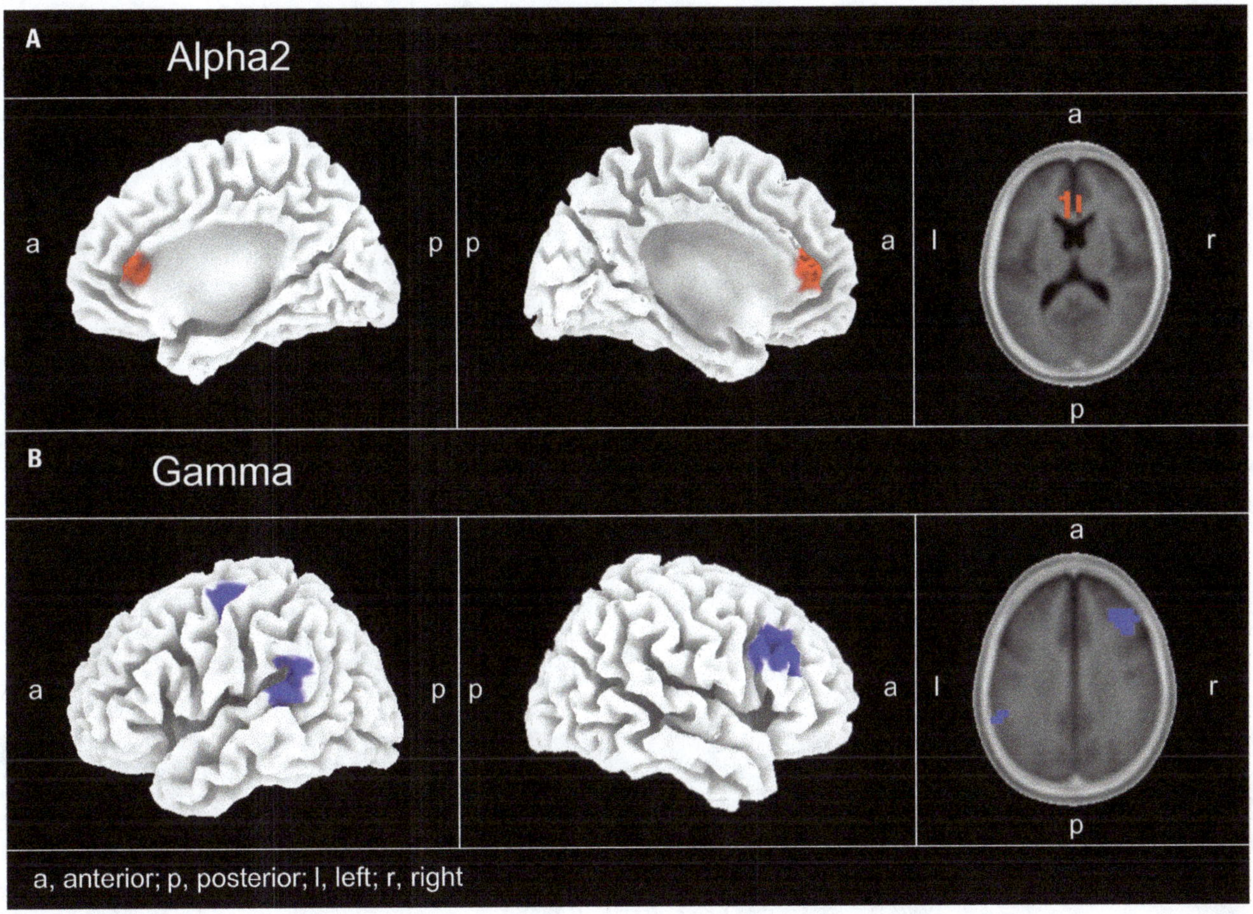

FIGURE 3 | EEG source localization (sLORETA) power maps for the PC–NPC paired-groups comparison. (A) Alpha2 (10–12 Hz) increased (color-coded red) in the right and left anterior cingulate cortex (BA 24, 32). **(B)** Gamma band power decreased (color-coded blue) with pitch change in the left parietal (BA 40), left temporal (BA 22, 42), right frontal (BA 9, 46), and left frontal (BA 4, 6) cortex.

in tinnitus pitch to both a reduction of tinnitus symptoms and changes in oscillatory brain activity.

Notably, we observe a significant correlation between long-lasting CR therapy-induced changes of tinnitus pitch and changes of tinnitus loudness and annoyance. These findings are in agreement with a study conducted by Baguley et al. (2005) who showed that intravenous infusion of lidocaine in tinnitus patients leads to a short-term reduction of tinnitus loudness and annoyance paralleled by a tinnitus pitch reduction of roughly similar size. In that study, the measurement of pitch change, however, was performed with VAS and no analysis of an interdependence between changes in tinnitus loudness or annoyance and tinnitus pitch was performed. Another, substantial difference to our study is that changes of pitch as well as reduction in VAS-L and VAS-A disappeared 20 min after lidocaine injection, whereas VAS and matched tinnitus pitch measurements in our study were performed minimally 2.5 h after cessation of the acoustic CR neuromodulation.

In another study, investigating the treatment of tinnitus with chronic electrical neurostimulation of the vestibulocochlear nerve, the transformation of the tinnitus spectrum *per se* was perceived by patients as pleasant (Bartels et al., 2007). The significant correlation between changes in tinnitus loudness, tinnitus annoyance and changes in tinnitus pitch, obtained in our study, demonstrates the relation of the perceived CR therapy-induced tinnitus pitch change to the change of tinnitus symptoms.

Significant group differences in oscillatory brain activity are a reduction in gamma power over the left superior temporal gyrus, the left supramarginal gyrus and the left premotor cortex and the right DLPFC and an accompanying enhancement in alpha2 power in frontal lobe in patients with tinnitus pitch change. Human functional imaging studies indicate that supramarginal gyrus (left > right) is a part of a distributed and dynamic brain network that subserves pitch memory (Gaab et al., 2003). The area with reduced gamma activity in the left temporal lobe also roughly overlaps with the planum temporale (PT), a large region, located in the superior temporal plane posterior to Heschl's gyrus (Westbury et al., 1999). PT was proposed to be a computational interface segregating incoming sound patterns that are then used for comparison with the previously stored patterns (Griffiths and Warren, 2002). The association of a CSD change in this area with changes in tinnitus pitch suggests that changes in the left superior temporal region might be more associated with changes in processing

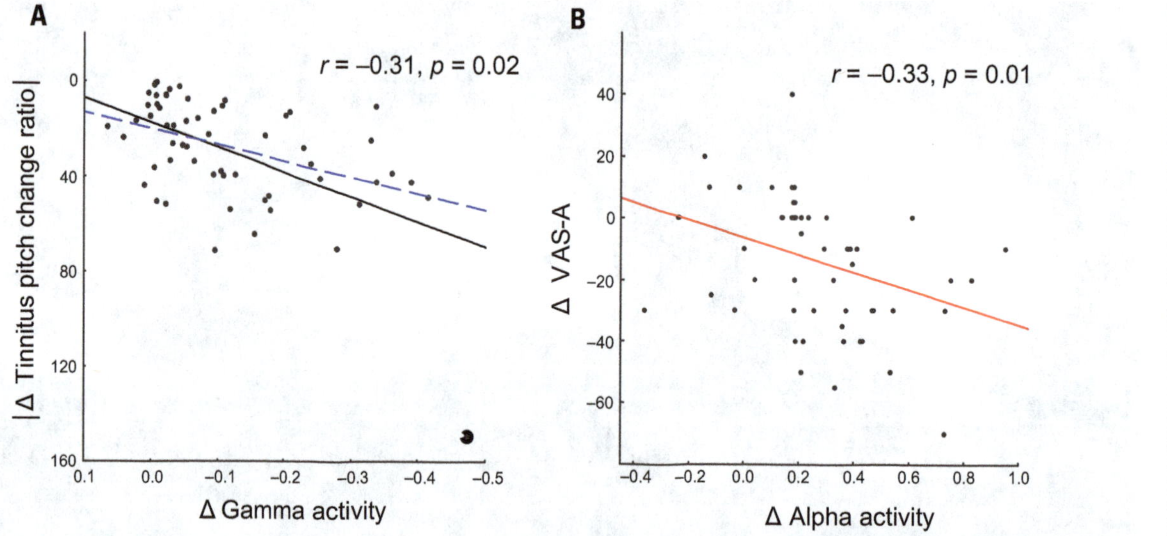

FIGURE 4 | Significant negative partial correlation between relative change of CSD gamma power and modulus of tinnitus pitch change ratio (A) with all patients included ($r = -0.31$, $p = 0.02$, solid red line) or with the outlier excluded ($r = -0.29$, $p = 0.03$, dashed blue line). The outlier patient is marked by the red circle. A significant negative correlation ($r = -0.33$, $p = 0.01$, $n = 59$) between relative change of anterior cingulate CSD alpha power and difference in VAS-A **(B)**.

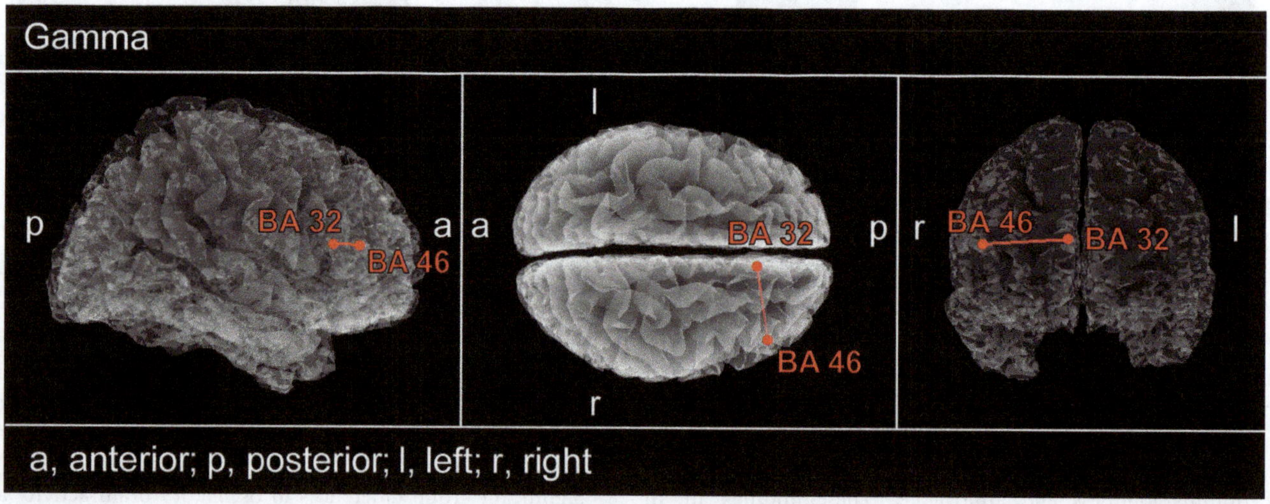

FIGURE 5 | Connectivity contrast analysis between PC and NPC patients. rmANOVA analysis was applied to those brain areas which showed differential effects of CR therapy depending on whether or not tinnitus pitch changed strongly (see **Figure 3**). Decreased gamma lagged linear connectivity can be seen in PC patients between right ACC (BA 32) and DLPFC (BA 46).

of tinnitus pitch *per se*. This region might not be the locus of conscious perception of pitch change, but instead a relay-station necessary for processing and gating pitch related information to higher-order cortical areas involved in the tinnitus aversive network.

Another region with lower gamma in the PC group roughly corresponds to the DLPFC. The right DLPFC was proposed to be a part of the tinnitus network related to the affective components of tinnitus (Schlee et al., 2009a,b; Vanneste et al., 2010; Langguth et al., 2011). It is also a part of a fronto-parietal network proposed to perform the retrieval and comparison of incoming auditory information (Arnott et al., 2005). Frontal regions were also shown to play a role in the maintenance of tonal patterns and auditory working memory, e.g., experimental evidence even suggests that the prefrontal cortex has cells related to auditory memory (Bodner et al., 1996; Chao and Knight, 1996; Celsis et al., 1999). Thus the prefrontal cortex could be one of the higher-order centers in the tinnitus aversive network that integrates sensory (e.g., tinnitus pitch) aspects of tinnitus possibly coming from PT with other modalities (Jastreboff, 1990; Mirz et al., 2000). An increase in alpha2 oscillatory brain activity in the PC group was found in a region corresponding to ACC. This is in line with data reported by Vanneste and De Ridder (2011) where the stimulation of DLPFC in tinnitus patients resulted in an increase of alpha activity in ACC. Moreover in our study CSD changes in the anterior cingulate area negatively correlated with changes in tinnitus annoyance. These results correspond to data obtained from patients suffering with pain where a correlation between changes in ACC activity and pain perception was observed (Davis et al., 1997).

Furthermore, we found a decreased connectivity in the gamma band between DLPFC and ACC regions in patients with tinnitus pitch change. The DLPFC has anatomical connections to the ACC permitting functional connectivity between these two areas (Pandya et al., 1981; Petrides and Pandya, 1999). In particular, gamma band oscillations appear to be crucial for the binding of information originating from different sources into coherent percept (Singer and Gray, 1995; Schulte et al., 2002; Herrmann et al., 2010). This finding is in line with previous data showing a modulation of activity in the ACC as a result of rTMS or transcranial direct current stimulation of the prefrontal cortex over the DLPFC (Paus et al., 2001; Vanneste and De Ridder, 2011). Remarkably decreased functional connectivity in the gamma band was also found between the right DLPFC and ACC after transcranial direct current stimulation of DLPFC (Vanneste and De Ridder, 2011). Premotor cortex was proposed to have hidden sensory function, however it's relation to tinnitus is not yet clear (de Lafuente and Romo, 2002).

In summary, our study revealed changes in a distributed brain network which involved the left superior temporal and supramarginal gyrus, dorsolateral prefrontal region, and the ACC. CSD in the gamma band positively correlated with the modulus of the tinnitus pitch change in the region of the superior temporal gyrus (BA 22) indicating that this region may be related to processing and gating tinnitus pitch related information to higher-order cortical hubs of the tinnitus network. The ACC, in turn, could be more associated with affective tinnitus distress, being one of the higher-order centers in tinnitus network.

What mechanism may turn a greater tinnitus pitch change into a greater change of tinnitus annoyance and loudness? Different auditory modalities were proposed to be coded by different mechanisms and spatially separate brain networks (Clement et al., 1999; Alain et al., 2001; Banai et al., 2011). Thus, one can assume that different perceptual characteristics of tinnitus (e.g., pitch and loudness) could also be coded by spatially and functionally parallel and overlapping brain networks. This notion would be in line with the notion that tinnitus arises as the result of altered activity in multiple parallel overlapping dynamic brain networks (De Ridder et al., 2011b). Thus, tinnitus characteristic pitch associated with a negative emotional context related to tinnitus, can lead to the formation of a strong, aversive memory trace of this particular sound in a separate brain network specific for pitch processing and memory. This may at the same time be paralleled by increased synchronized neural activity, indicating its more intensive involvement, in the brain network subserving perceptual modality, i.e., pitch related to negative emotions. According to the binding theory (Singer and Gray, 1995; Schulte et al., 2002; Herrmann et al., 2010) different features of an object have to be combined into a coherent percept to be consciously perceived. Oscillatory neural activity in the gamma band have been proposed to be a representation of this binding process (Singer and Gray, 1995; Schulte et al., 2002; Herrmann et al., 2010). From the standpoint of auditory binding, the sLORETA results obtained in our study can be interpreted to reflect a substantial, CR-induced reduction of a tinnitus-related auditory binding process. Moreover persistent tinnitus would support this aversive emotional association and hinders its decline (De Ridder et al., 2011a). In this network superior temporal gyrus and/or PT could play the role of a tinnitus pitch processing and gating center and constitute a distinctive part of a pitch aversive network. After having been processed by this pitch hub, the information might enter a non-specific network comprising DLPFC for sensory information integration and ACC for associative and emotional processing. A change in tinnitus pitch might break the synchrony in one part of the tinnitus network of brain areas that otherwise supports aversive emotional associations and prevents from a decline of the memory of the tinnitus. In the absence of a reinforcement these aversive associations may gradually diminish and, finally, fade away. A destruction of such aversive emotional associations may, in turn, contribute to the reduction in chronic tinnitus distress.

As shown here, the amount of tinnitus pitch change determines in which way the amount of pathological (gamma) and physiological (alpha) synchrony in a network of tinnitus-related brain areas together with the interactions between different hubs within that network change. However, the question of the underlying physiological mechanism of the CR-induced tinnitus pitch change still remains open. Given the tonotopic organization of the primary auditory cortex, a CR-induced tinnitus pitch change may likely correspond to a spatial shift of the synchronized, tinnitus-related synchronous focus within the primary auditory cortex. Based on the dynamical mechanisms of action of CR neuromodulation (Tass, 2003a,b; Tass and Majtanik, 2006; Hauptmann et al., 2007; Tass and Hauptmann, 2009) asymmetries of both the stimulation and the network subjected to stimulation might cause such an effect. For instance, in an elegant modeling study on the emergence of the Zwicker tone (Zwicker, 1964; Franosch et al., 2003), an auditory after-effect, the impact of a spatial gradient of the lateral inhibition in the auditory cortex on the neuronal dynamics in the central auditory cortex has been explored. It was shown that a gradient of the lateral inhibition has significant impact on the neuronal dynamics and, in particular, that a noise reduction mechanism together with a dominantly unilateral inhibition is able to explain the emergence of the Zwicker tone. A gradient of the lateral inhibition combined with a spatially equidistant delivery of acoustic stimuli might explain a spatial shift of a synchronous focus in the primary auditory cortex. By the same token, in case of a spatially well-balanced lateral inhibition asymmetries of the arrangement of the CR tones (with respect to the patient's individual tonotopic organization of the primary auditory cortex) might also cause a spatial shift of the synchronous focus in the primary auditory cortex. This issue will be in the focus of forthcoming theoretical and experimental studies.

Our results support the idea that tinnitus might be a consequence of altered activity in multiple parallel and overlapping dynamic networks. In this network elementary sensory dimensions may be represented by segregated mechanisms and networks that probably involve cortical areas encoding sensory features of the stimulus as well as prefrontal and cingulate regions necessary for perception.

Additional studies are required to further deepen our understanding of the involvement of pitch processing networks in the pathophysiology of tinnitus. Such studies will further elaborate which brain areas are critically involved in pitch processing in auditory phantom perception and how these areas interact with or depend on areas required for the percept to reach consciousness.

REFERENCES

Alain, C., Arnott, S. R., Hevenor, S., Graham, S., and Grady, C. L. (2001). "What" and "where" in the human auditory system. *Proc. Natl. Acad. Sci. U.S.A.* 98, 12301–12306.

Arnott, S. R., Grady, C. L., Hevenor, S. J., Graham, S., and Alain, C. (2005). The functional organization of auditory working memory as revealed by fMRI. *J. Cogn. Neurosci.* 17, 819–831.

Baguley, D. M., Jones, S., Wilkins, I., Axon, P. R., and Moffat, D. A. (2005). The inhibitory effect of intravenous lidocaine infusion on tinnitus after translabyrinthine removal of vestibular schwannoma: a double-blind, placebo-controlled, crossover study. *Otol. Neurotol.* 26, 169–176.

Banai, K., Sabin, A. T., and Wright, B. A. (2011). Separable developmental trajectories for the abilities to detect auditory amplitude and frequency modulation. *Hear. Res.* 280, 219–227.

Bartels, H., Staal, M. J., Holm, A. F., Mooij, J. J., and Albers, F. W. (2007). Long-term evaluation of treatment of chronic, therapeutically refractory tinnitus by neurostimulation. *Stereotact. Funct. Neurosurg.* 85, 150–157.

Bodner, M., Kroger, J., and Fuster, J. M. (1996). Auditory memory cells in dorsolateral prefrontal cortex. *Neuroreport* 7, 1905–1908.

Celsis, P., Boulanouar, K., Doyon, B., Ranjeva, J. P., Berry, I., Nespoulous, J. L., and Chollet, F. (1999). Differential fMRI responses in the left posterior superior temporal gyrus and left supramarginal gyrus to habituation and change detection in syllables and tones. *Neuroimage* 9, 135–144.

Chao, L. L., and Knight, R. T. (1996). Prefrontal and posterior cortical activation during auditory working memory. *Brain Res. Cogn. Brain Res.* 4, 27–37.

Clement, S., Demany, L., and Semal, C. (1999). Memory for pitch versus memory for loudness. *J. Acoust. Soc. Am.* 106, 2805–2811.

Davis, K. D., Taylor, S. J., Crawley, A. P., Wood, M. L., and Mikulis, D. J. (1997). Functional MRI of pain- and attention-related activations in the human cingulate cortex. *J. Neurophysiol.* 77, 3370–3380.

de Lafuente, V., and Romo, R. (2002). A hidden sensory function for motor cortex. *Neuron* 36, 785–786.

De Ridder, D., Elgoyhen, A. B., Romo, R., and Langguth, B. (2011a). Phantom percepts: tinnitus and pain as persisting aversive memory networks. *Proc. Natl. Acad. Sci. U.S.A.* 108, 8075–8080.

De Ridder, D., Van Der Loo, E., Vanneste, S., Gais, S., Plazier, M., Kovacs, S., Sunaert, S., Menovsky, T., and Van De Heyning, P. (2011b). Theta-gamma dysrhythmia and auditory phantom perception. *J. Neurosurg.* 114, 912–921.

Dohrmann, K., Weisz, N., Schlee, W., Hartmann, T., and Elbert, T. (2007). Neurofeedback for treating tinnitus. *Prog. Brain Res.* 166, 473–554.

Eggermont, J. J., and Roberts, L. E. (2004). The neuroscience of tinnitus. *Trends Neurosci.* 27, 676–682.

Franosch, J. M., Kempter, R., Fastl, H., and Van Hemmen, J. L. (2003). Zwicker tone illusion and noise reduction in the auditory system. *Phys. Rev. Lett.* 90, 178103.

Gaab, N., Gaser, C., Zaehle, T., Jancke, L., and Schlaug, G. (2003). Functional anatomy of pitch memory – an fMRI study with sparse temporal sampling. *Neuroimage* 19, 1417–1426.

Gerstner, W., Kempter, R., Van Hemmen, J. L., and Wagner, H. (1996). A neuronal learning rule for sub-millisecond temporal coding. *Nature* 383, 76–81.

Griffiths, T. D., and Warren, J. D. (2002). The planum temporale as a computational hub. *Trends Neurosci.* 25, 348–353.

Hauptmann, C., Popovych, O., and Tass, P. A. (2007). Desynchronizing the abnormally synchronized neural activity in the subthalamic nucleus: a modeling study. *Expert Rev. Med. Devices* 4, 633–650.

Hauptmann, C., and Tass, P. A. (2009). Cumulative and after-effects of short and weak coordinated reset stimulation: a modeling study. *J. Neural Eng.* 6, 016004.

Herrmann, C. S., Frund, I., and Lenz, D. (2010). Human gamma-band activity: a review on cognitive and behavioral correlates and network models. *Neurosci. Biobehav. Rev.* 34, 981–992.

Jastreboff, P. J. (1990). Phantom auditory perception (tinnitus): mechanisms of generation and perception. *Neurosci. Res.* 8, 221–254.

Kahlbrock, N., and Weisz, N. (2008). Transient reduction of tinnitus intensity is marked by concomitant reductions of delta band power. *BMC Biol.* 6, 4. doi: 10.1186/1741-7007-6-4

Langguth, B., Landgrebe, M., Kleinjung, T., Sand, G. P., and Hajak, G. (2011). Tinnitus and depression. *World J. Biol. Psychiatry* 12, 489–500.

Lemus, L., Hernandez, A., and Romo, R. (2009a). Neural codes for perceptual discrimination of acoustic flutter in the primate auditory cortex. *Proc. Natl. Acad. Sci. U.S.A.* 106, 9471–9476.

Lemus, L., Hernandez, A., and Romo, R. (2009b). Neural encoding of auditory discrimination in ventral premotor cortex. *Proc. Natl. Acad. Sci. U.S.A.* 106, 14640–14645.

Llinas, R. R., Ribary, U., Jeanmonod, D., Kronberg, E., and Mitra, P. P. (1999). Thalamocortical dysrhythmia: a neurological and neuropsychiatric syndrome characterized by magnetoencephalography. *Proc. Natl. Acad. Sci. U.S.A.* 96, 15222–15227.

Lockwood, A. H., Salvi, R. J., and Burkard, R. F. (2002). Current concepts: tinnitus. *N. Eng. J. Med.* 347, 904–910.

Markram, H. (1997). Regulation of synaptic efficacy by coincidence of postsynaptic APs and EPSPs. *Science* 275, 213–215.

Mirz, F., Gjedde, A., Ishizu, K., and Pedersen, C. B. (2000). Cortical networks subserving the perception of tinnitus – a PET study. *Acta Otolaryngol. Suppl.* 543, 241–243.

Moller, A. R. (2003). Pathophysiology of tinnitus. *Otolaryngol. Clin. North Am.* 36, 249–266, v–vi.

Muhlnickel, W., Elbert, T., Taub, E., and Flor, H. (1998). Reorganization of auditory cortex in tinnitus. *Proc. Natl. Acad. Sci. U.S.A.* 95, 10340–10343.

Mulert, C., Jager, L., Schmitt, R., Bussfeld, P., Pogarell, O., Moller, H. J., Juckel, G., and Hegerl, U. (2004). Integration of fMRI and simultaneous EEG: towards a comprehensive understanding of localization and time-course of brain activity in target detection. *Neuroimage* 22, 83–94.

Neiman, A. B., Russell, D. F., Yakusheva, T. A., Dilullo, A., and Tass, P. A. (2007). Response clustering in transient stochastic synchronization and desynchronization of coupled neuronal bursters. *Phys. Rev. E Stat. Nonlin. Soft Matter Phys.* 76, 021908.

Norena, A., Micheyl, C., Chery-Croze, S., and Collet, L. (2002). Psychoacoustic characterization of the tinnitus spectrum: implications for the underlying mechanisms of tinnitus. *Audiol. Neurootol.* 7, 358–369.

Norena, A. J., and Eggermont, J. J. (2003). Changes in spontaneous neural activity immediately after an acoustic trauma: implications for neural correlates of tinnitus. *Hear. Res.* 183, 137–153.

Ochi, K., and Eggermont, J. J. (1997). Effects of quinine on neural activity in cat primary auditory cortex. *Hear. Res.* 105, 105–118.

Pandya, D. N., Van Hoesen, G. W., and Mesulam, M. M. (1981). Efferent connections of the cingulate gyrus in the rhesus monkey. *Exp. Brain Res.* 42, 319–330.

Pascual-Marqui, R. D. (2002). Standardized low-resolution brain electromagnetic tomography (sLORETA): technical details. *Methods Find. Exp. Clin. Pharmacol.* 24(Suppl. D), 5–12.

Pascual-Marqui, R. D. (2007a). Discrete, 3D distributed, linear imaging methods of electric neuronal activity. Part 1: exact, zero error localization. arXiv:0710.3341 [math-ph], http://arxiv.org/pdf/0710.3341

Pascual-Marqui, R. D. (2007b). Instantaneous and lagged measurements of linear and nonlinear dependence between groups of multivariate time series: frequency decomposition. arXiv:0711.1455 [stat.ME], http://arxiv.org/abs/0711.1455

Pascual-Marqui, R. D., Esslen, M., Kochi, K., and Lehmann, D. (2002). Functional imaging with low-resolution brain electromagnetic tomography (LORETA): a review. *Methods Find. Exp. Clin. Pharmacol.* 24(Suppl. C), 91–95.

Pascual-Marqui, R. D., Michel, C. M., and Lehmann, D. (1994). Low resolution electromagnetic tomography:

a new method for localizing electrical activity in the brain. *Int. J. Psychophysiol.* 18, 49–65.

Paus, T., Castro-Alamancos, M. A., and Petrides, M. (2001). Corticocortical connectivity of the human mid-dorsolateral frontal cortex and its modulation by repetitive transcranial magnetic stimulation. *Eur. J. Neurosci.* 14, 1405–1411.

Petrides, M., and Pandya, D. N. (1999). Dorsolateral prefrontal cortex: comparative cytoarchitectonic analysis in the human and the macaque brain and corticocortical connection patterns. *Eur. J. Neurosci.* 11, 1011–1036.

Pizzagalli, D. A., Oakes, T. R., Fox, A. S., Chung, M. K., Larson, C. L., Abercrombie, H. C., Schaefer, S. M., Benca, R. M., and Davidson, R. J. (2004). Functional but not structural subgenual prefrontal cortex abnormalities in melancholia. *Mol. Psychiatry* 9, 325, 393–405.

Popovych, O. V., and Tass, P. A. (2012). Desynchronizing electrical and sensory coordinated reset neuromodulation. *Front. Hum. Neurosci.* 6:58. doi: 10.3389/fnhum.2012.00058

Rauschecker, J. P. (2005). Neural encoding and retrieval of sound sequences. *Ann. N. Y. Acad. Sci.* 1060, 125–135.

Robertson, D., and Irvine, D. R. (1989). Plasticity of frequency organization in auditory cortex of guinea pigs with partial unilateral deafness. *J. Comp. Neurol.* 282, 456–471.

Romo, R., and Salinas, E. (2003). Flutter discrimination: neural codes, perception, memory and decision making. *Nat. Rev. Neurosci.* 4, 203–218.

Scherg, M., Ille, N., Bornfleth, H., and Berg, P. (2002). Advanced tools for digital EEG review: virtual source montages, whole-head mapping, correlation, and phase analysis. *J. Clin. Neurophysiol.* 19, 91–112.

Schlee, W., Hartmann, T., Langguth, B., and Weisz, N. (2009a). Abnormal resting-state cortical coupling in chronic tinnitus. *BMC Neurosci.* 10, 11. doi: 10.1186/1471-2202-10-11

Schlee, W., Mueller, N., Hartmann, T., Keil, J., Lorenz, I., and Weisz, N. (2009b). Mapping cortical hubs in tinnitus. *BMC Biol.* 7, 80. doi: 10.1186/1741-7007-7-80

Schulte, M., Knief, A., Seither-Preisler, A., and Pantev, C. (2002). Different modes of pitch perception and learning-induced neuronal plasticity of the human auditory cortex. *Neural Plast.* 9, 161–175.

Seki, S., and Eggermont, J. J. (2003). Changes in spontaneous firing rate and neural synchrony in cat primary auditory cortex after localized tone-induced hearing loss. *Hear. Res.* 180, 28–38.

Singer, W., and Gray, C. M. (1995). Visual feature integration and the temporal correlation hypothesis. *Annu. Rev. Neurosci.* 18, 555–586.

Steriade, M. (2006). Grouping of brain rhythms in corticothalamic systems. *Neuroscience* 137, 1087–1106.

Tass, P., Silchenko, A., Hauptmann, C., Barnikol, U., and Speckmann, E. J. (2009). Long-lasting desynchronization in rat hippocampal slice induced by coordinated reset stimulation. *Phys. Rev. E Stat. Nonlin. Soft Matter Phys.* 80, 011902.

Tass, P. A. (1999). *Phase Resetting in Medicine and Biology: Stochastic Modelling and Data Analysis.* Berlin: Springer Verlag.

Tass, P. A. (2002). Desynchronization of brain rhythms with soft phase-resetting techniques. *Biol. Cybern.* 87, 102–115.

Tass, P. A. (2003a). Desynchronization by means of a coordinated reset of neural sub-populations – a novel technique for demand-controlled deep brain stimulation. *Prog. Theor. Phys. Suppl.* 150, 281–296.

Tass, P. A. (2003b). A model of desynchronizing deep brain stimulation with a demand-controlled coordinated reset of neural subpopulations. *Biol. Cybern.* 89, 81–88.

Tass, P. A., Adamchic, I., Freund, H.-J., Von Stackelberg, T., and Hauptmann, C. (2012). Counteracting tinnitus by acoustic coordinated reset neuromodulation. *Restor. Neurol. Neurosci.* 30, 137–159.

Tass, P. A., and Hauptmann, C. (2009). Anti-kindling achieved by stimulation targeting slow synaptic dynamics. *Restor. Neurol. Neurosci.* 27, 589–609.

Tass, P. A., and Majtanik, M. (2006). Long-term anti-kindling effects of desynchronizing brain stimulation: a theoretical study. *Biol. Cybern.* 94, 58–66.

Tass, P. A., and Popovych, O. P. (2012). Unlearning tinnitus-related cerebral synchrony with acoustic coordinated reset stimulation – theoretical concept and modelling. *Biol. Cybern.* 106, 27–36.

Vanneste, S., and De Ridder, D. (2011). Bifrontal transcranial direct current stimulation modulates tinnitus intensity and tinnitus-distress-related brain activity. *Eur. J. Neurosci.* 34, 605–614.

Vanneste, S., Plazier, M., Der Loo, E., De Heyning, P. V., Congedo, M., and De Ridder, D. (2010). The neural correlates of tinnitus-related distress. *Neuroimage* 52, 470–480.

Vitacco, D., Brandeis, D., Pascual-Marqui, R., and Martin, E. (2002). Correspondence of event-related potential tomography and functional magnetic resonance imaging during language processing. *Hum. Brain Mapp.* 17, 4–12.

Weisz, N., Hartmann, T., Dohrmann, K., Schlee, W., and Norena, A. (2006). High-frequency tinnitus without hearing loss does not mean absence of deafferentation. *Hear. Res.* 222, 108–114.

Weisz, N., Moratti, S., Meinzer, M., Dohrmann, K., and Elbert, T. (2005). Tinnitus perception and distress is related to abnormal spontaneous brain activity as measured by magnetoencephalography. *PLoS Med.* 2, e153. doi: 10.1371/journal.pmed.0020153

Weisz, N., Muller, S., Schlee, W., Dohrmann, K., Hartmann, T., and Elbert, T. (2007). The neural code of auditory phantom perception. *J. Neurosci.* 27, 1479–1484.

Westbury, C. F., Zatorre, R. J., and Evans, A. C. (1999). Quantifying variability in the planum temporale: a probability map. *Cereb. Cortex* 9, 392–405.

Yang, S., Weiner, B. D., Zhang, L. S., Cho, S. J., and Bao, S. (2011). Homeostatic plasticity drives tinnitus perception in an animal model. *Proc. Natl. Acad. Sci. U.S.A.* 108, 14974–14979.

Yuste, R., and Bonhoeffer, T. (2004). Genesis of dendritic spines: insights from ultrastructural and imaging studies. *Nat. Rev. Neurosci.* 5, 24–34.

Zumsteg, D., Wennberg, R. A., Treyer, V., Buck, A., and Wieser, H. G. (2005). H2(15)O or 13NH3 PET and electromagnetic tomography (LORETA) during partial status epilepticus. *Neurology* 65, 1657–1660.

Zwicker, E. (1964). "Negative afterimage" in hearing. *J. Acoust. Soc. Am.* 36, 2413.

8

Gamma-aminobutyric acid and glutamic acid levels in the auditory pathway of rats with chronic tinnitus: A direct determination using high resolution point-resolved proton magnetic resonance spectroscopy (^{1}H-MRS)

Thomas Brozoski[1]*, Boris Odintsov[2] and Carol Bauer[1]

[1] *Division of Otolaryngology, Southern Illinois University School of Medicine, Springfield, IL, USA*
[2] *Biomedical Imaging Center, Beckman Institute for Advanced Science and Technology, University of Illinois, Urbana Champaign, Urbana, IL, USA*

***Correspondence:**
Thomas Brozoski, Division of Otolaryngology, Southern Illinois University School of Medicine, 801 N. Rutledge Street, Rm 3205, PO Box 19629, Springfield, IL, USA.
e-mail: tbrozoski@siumed.edu

Damage to the auditory system following high-level sound exposure reduces afferent input. Homeostatic mechanisms appear to compensate for the loss. Overcompensation may produce the sensation of sound without an objective physical correlate, i.e., tinnitus. Several potential compensatory neural processes have been identified, such as increased spontaneous activity. The cellular mechanisms enabling such compensatory processes may involve down-regulation of inhibitory neurotransmission mediated by γ-amino butyric acid (GABA), and/or up-regulation of excitatory neurotransmission, mediated by glutamic acid (Glu). Because central processing systems are integrated and well-regulated, compensatory changes in one system may produce reactive changes in others. Some or all may be relevant to tinnitus. To examine the roles of GABA and Glu in tinnitus, high resolution point-resolved proton magnetic resonance spectroscopy (^{1}H-MRS) was used to quantify their levels in the dorsal cochlear nucleus (DCN), inferior colliculus (IC), medial geniculate body (MGB), and primary auditory cortex (A1) of rats. Chronic tinnitus was produced by a single high-level unilateral exposure to noise, and was measured using a psychophysical procedure sensitive to tinnitus. Decreased GABA levels were evident only in the MGB, with the greatest decrease, relative to unexposed controls, obtained in the contralateral MGB. Small GABA increases may have been present bilaterally in A1 and in the contralateral DCN. Although Glu levels showed considerable variation, Glu was moderately and bilaterally elevated both in the DCN and in A1. In the MGB Glu was increased ipsilaterally but decreased contralaterally. These bidirectional and region-specific alterations in GABA and Glu may reflect large-scale changes in inhibitory and excitatory equilibrium accompanying chronic tinnitus. The present results also suggest that targeting both neurotransmitter systems may be optimal in developing more effective therapeutics.

Keywords: tinnitus animal model, ^{1}H-MRS, GABA, glutamate, dorsal cochlear nucleus, inferior colliculus, medial geniculate, primary auditory cortex

INTRODUCTION

Chronic tinnitus affects a large number of people, with perhaps 3–5 percent of the tinnitus population significantly disturbed by their condition. Exposure to damaging high-level sound is likely the leading cause of tinnitus in young people (Muhr and Rosenhall, 2011) and the second leading cause in older adults (Nondahl et al., 2002). Damage to the peripheral auditory system, in the long-term, reduces afferent input to the central auditory system and appears to stimulate compensatory central changes. The compensation, or perhaps overcompensation, may produce the sensation of sound where none exists, i.e., tinnitus. The neural correlates of tinnitus identified in animal studies are summarized in **Table 1**. Cellular mechanisms responsible for these changes have been hypothesized to include a down-regulation of inhibitory neurotransmission, such as that mediated by the neurotransmitter γ-amino butyric acid (GABA) and/or an up-regulation of excitatory neurotransmission, such as that mediated by the excitatory neurotransmitter glutamate (Glu). Can alterations in the concentration of these compounds be directly detected in the brains of animals with objectively confirmed evidence of tinnitus?

Over the past decade animal models have contributed significantly to the neuroscience of tinnitus (Roberts et al., 2010). While diverse, all animal models assume that the sensation of tinnitus results from relatively primitive alterations in central auditory processing. In animals, tinnitus is induced by manipulations, such as high-level sound exposure, that commonly produce tinnitus in humans. The presence of tinnitus can be revealed by appropriately designed psychophysical procedures (Brozoski and Bauer, 2008). In the present experiment, the brains of rats with

Table 1 | Candidate compensatory mechanisms potentially responsible for compensatory "restoration" of central function following sensory organ damage.

Increased spontaneous neural activity.
Increased synchronous activity across parallel afferents.
Increased regularity of action potentials within individual neurons.
High-frequency discharge clustered into bursts of action potentials.
Over-representation of "lost" frequency bands in tonotopic organization.

psychophysical evidence of sound-induced chronic tinnitus were imaged, and point-resolved proton magnetic resonance spectra (^{1}H-MRS) were obtained from tissue volumes localized to areas in the auditory pathway that have been identified in one or more studies as potentially involved in mediating tinnitus. Analyzed areas included the dorsal cochlear nucleus (DCN), the inferior colliculus (IC), the medial geniculate body (MGB) or auditory thalamus, and primary auditory cortex (A1).

Recent technical improvements have enabled the acquisition of well-resolved spectra from small tissue volumes. Point-resolved spectroscopy (PRESS) can be used to optimize signal strength from small volumes, while ultra-short echo times can be used to reduce signal multiplets thereby improving peak dispersion and the resolution of complex spectra such as those obtained from brain tissue. Insertion of asymmetric variable power RF pulses into the probe sequence can be used to reduce the otherwise intrusive water peak that obscures signals above 3 ppm (Mlynarik et al., 2008). Separation of spectral lines and extraction of weak signals can be further enhanced by using very high-level magnetic fields and additionally through the use of a tunable pickup coil (Odintsov, 2011).

In the present investigation spectra were obtained from brain volumes of interest (VOI). The brain spectra were calibrated against spectra obtained from glass phantoms, filled with known concentrations of GABA and Glu, and comparable in size to the VOI. GABA and Glu were selected for analysis because they are, respectively, the major inhibitory and excitatory neurotransmitters in the auditory pathway; their concentrations are at detectible levels in small brain volumes, and they have been identified as potentially playing a significant role in tinnitus.

MATERIALS AND METHODS

SUBJECTS

Twenty adult male Long–Evans rats (Harlan, Indianapolis, IN), 90 days old at the start of the experiment, were individually housed and maintained at 25°C with a 12/12 h reversed light/dark schedule. Ten months prior to spectroscopy 16 of the animals participated in a study examining the effect of supplementary dietary taurine on tinnitus. The experimental protocol was approved by the Laboratory Animal Care and Use Committee of Southern Illinois University School of Medicine and the University of Illinois at Urbana Champaign.

TINNITUS INDUCTION

Half of the animals ($n = 10$) were unilaterally exposed once to band limited noise for 1 h. These subjects will be referred to as "exposed." The remaining animals ($n = 10$) were treated identically, but unexposed. They will be referred to as "unexposed." Sound exposure parameters were identical to those reported previously to produce tinnitus in rats (Bauer and Brozoski, 2001; Brozoski et al., 2012). All subjects, exposed and unexposed, were anesthetized to an areflexive state, using either an isoflurane/O2 mixture (Aerrane, Baxter Healthcare Corp., Deerfield, IL, USA), or a ketamine/xylazine mixture (24.6 and 3 mg/kg, respectively; ketamine, Ketaset, Fort Dodge Animal Health, Fort Dodge, IA; xylazine, Anased, Lloyd Laboratories, Shenandoah, IA). For the exposed animals, peak level was 116 dB (SPL) centered at 16 kHz, with the noise band falling to ambient level at 8 kHz and 24 kHz. The sound was delivered monaurally using a speaker driver (FT17H, Fostex, Tokyo, Japan) in a custom enclosure funneling the sound to a flexible tube that fit snugly into the auditory canal. Sound levels were calibrated using a Brüel and Kjaer (Norcross, GA, USA) Pulse sound measurement system (Pulse 13 software), equipped with a 3560C high-frequency module, and a 4138 pressure-field microphone (Brüel and Kjaer) coupled to the transducer using rubber tubing with the internal dimensions of an adult rat external auditory canal. All sound levels reported in the present experiment are unweighted pressure levels re 20 μPa.

HEARING LEVELS

Hearing thresholds were determined immediately before and after exposure (for exposed rats) using auditory brainstem-evoked potentials (ABR). They were also obtained at the conclusion of tinnitus testing. ABR measurements were obtained using either a TDT System 3 Real Time Signal Processing System running BioSig32 and SigGen (Tucker Davis Technologies, Alachua, FL, USA), or an IHS Smart EP System, running IHS High Frequency Software (v. 2.33) and using IHS high frequency transducers (HFT9911–20–0035, Intelligent Hearing Systems, Miami, FL). Evoked responses were differentially recorded from a subcutaneous vertex needle electrode referenced to an electrode at the occiput. Evoked responses for 10 msec epochs following stimulus onset were amplified × 100,000, bandpass filtered (100–3000 Hz), and averaged for 512 repetitions of each frequency-intensity level combination. Digitized records of the evoked responses (40 μsec resolution) were exported to Excel (Microsoft, Redmond, WA, USA) for analysis and threshold determination. Hearing thresholds for each ear were defined by the lowest stimulus level that produced statistically distinct and visually distinct evoked waveforms, defined as the maximum peak-to-peak deflection within the 10 msec window following stimulus onset. Custom applications written for Excel were used for analysis.

TINNITUS ASSESSMENT

Tinnitus was measured after sound exposure, using a behavioral assay shown to be sensitive to tinnitus in rats, and described in detail elsewhere (Bauer and Brozoski, 2001; Brozoski et al., 2012). Briefly, an operant conditioned-suppression procedure was used to determine the animal's perception of test tones and silent periods embedded in an ambient of low level (60 dB, SPL) broad-band noise (BBN). The key feature of the procedure was that animals were required to discriminate between the presence and absence of sound when tested with a variety of sounds varying in composition, frequency, and level. While the features of tinnitus in rats (and humans) cannot be directly known, it is certain that tinnitus cannot sound like silence. The animals were tested daily in commercial operant test chambers (Lafayette Instruments, Mod. 80001, Lafayette, IN, USA) equipped with lid-mounted speakers. Speaker-off periods (i.e., silence) had a special significance because lever pressing for food during the silent periods led to a foot shock at the end of that period. The behavior of interest was lever pressing during randomly presented test sounds (1 min duration) that substituted for some of the speaker-off presentations (also 1 min duration). Assessment sessions consisted of 10 randomly inserted, non-contiguous, presentations. Two of the 10 were always silent (i.e., speaker-off) periods. The remaining eight presentations were of a randomly selected tone or noise, with different levels in each presentation. Lever pressing was quantified using a relative rate measure, the suppression ratio (R). R was determined as a running measure for successive 1 min segments of each session using the formula $R = B/(A + B)$, where A was the number of lever presses in the preceding 1 min segment and B the number of lever presses in the current 1 min segment. R can vary between 0 and 1. A value of 0 is attained when lever pressing in the current minute is 0, a value of 0.5 when lever pressing in the current minute is equal to that of the previous minute and a value of 1 when lever pressing in the previous minute is zero. R provided a running index of behavior, in 1 min segments, and enabled a quantitative comparison between subjects as well as unbiased compilation of group data. R is a useful index of perceptual performance in that it is very sensitive to short-term behavioral effects, such as those produced by sensory events, but it is very insensitive to gradual behavioral effects, such as those produced by changes in motivational status, for example, satiation. In the context of the present procedure, it was expected that exposed rats with tinnitus would have lower R values than unexposed rats, when tested with stimuli that resembled their tinnitus. All test sessions were 60 min in duration. Further details of the psychophysical procedure appear in an open-source document (Brozoski et al., 2012).

Exposed and unexposed rats were treated identically and tested in parallel. Individual animal and group discrimination functions were derived from the final 3–5 sessions of each test series, where performance variability was minimal. Test stimuli were BBN, and 8, 10, 16, 20, 24, and 32 kHz tones. Each stimulus was tested across a range of levels from low to high audibility. Evidence of tinnitus was determined by the divergence of group discrimination functions. For subjects with tinnitus, test stimuli that resembled their tinnitus served as a signal for response (lever press) suppression. In contrast, for unexposed subjects without tinnitus, the signal for suppression was silence. Test stimuli with sensory features resembling tinnitus, therefore, produced greater suppression (i.e., fewer lever presses) in subjects with tinnitus. Previous research (Bauer and Brozoski, 2001) has shown that Long–Evans adult rats, unilaterally exposed to high-level band-limited noise centered at 16 kHz, show evidence of tinnitus in a range between 10 and 30 kHz.

SPECTROSCOPY: PREPARATION

Prior to spectroscopy, each animal in its home cage, was placed in a double-wall sound insulated booth for 20 h without food but with freely available water. The objective was to equate the baseline acoustic environment for all subjects, and to reduce the acoustic ambient to a low-level. The sound floor in this environment across the audible frequency range for rats was less than 10 dB (SPL). Ten minutes prior to spectroscopy, animals were pretreated i.p. with 10 mg/kg 3-mercaptopropionic acid (product M5801, Sigma-Aldrich, St. Louis, MO) to arrest post-mortem GABA inflation (van der Heyden and Korf, 1978). Immediately before acquisition, animals were given a lethal dose of anesthetic (Euthasol, Virbac, Ft. Worth, TX), decapitated, the mandible removed, and excess muscle tissue dissected away from the skull. The head was placed in a polyethylene holder along with a 1 mm diameter glass capillary filled with CuSO4 (3 mM). The image phantom of the capillary indexed the left hemisphere, making VOI laterality unambiguous.

SPECTROSCOPY: CALIBRATION

Prior to spectrum acquisition, glass vessels 2 mm in diameter were prepared with either 10 mM of GABA or 10 mM of Glu dissolved in sterile normal saline. Initial attempts to include one or more calibration vessels along with the brain during spectrographic data acquisition distorted the field, making shimming impossible. Therefore, calibration spectra were obtained either before or after acquisition of brain spectra. Initial calibrations were done with GABA and Glu in combination with compounds, such as creatine, that were expected to produce unwanted spectral lines potentially obscuring those of GABA and Glu. Spectrograms of the mixtures were used to identify GABA and Glu peaks, from among their multiplets, that provided the clearest separation from background. Calibration and peak selection were further refined using arrays of phantoms distributed in the field of view as shown in **Figure 1**. Taking into account all calibration results, GABA levels were determined using the peak at 2.18 ppm and Glu using the peak at 3.68 ppm (**Figure 2**).

SPECTROSCOPY: DATA ACQUISITION

At the conclusion of behavioral testing, the rats were individually imaged and volume-localized ^{1}H-MRS spectra were determined. Spectra were obtained using a vertical bore Varian Unity/Inova 600 mHz NMR spectrometer with a 14.1 T magnet. To reduce the displacement error of microvolume localized ^{1}H-MRS, caused by large chemical shifts in the strong magnetic field, a hybrid short-pulse sequence, obtained from R. Gruetter (Mlynarik et al., 2008), was used. The pulse sequence was optimized for signal acquisition in the spectral band containing the neurochemicals of interest, i.e., GABA and Glu. Signals were further optimized using a tunable pickup coil (Odintsov, 2011).

For each animal, an initial MRI brain scan was used to locate the VOI for ^{1}H-MRS. Contiguous transverse (i.e., coronal) slices, 0.5 mm thick (26 μm planar resolution), were obtained, extending 13 mm caudally from Bregma (26 slices total). VOI for ^{1}H-MRS were determined within the auditory pathway as indicated in **Table 2**. The VOI for each auditory region was kept constant and its placement was made as standard as possible using image

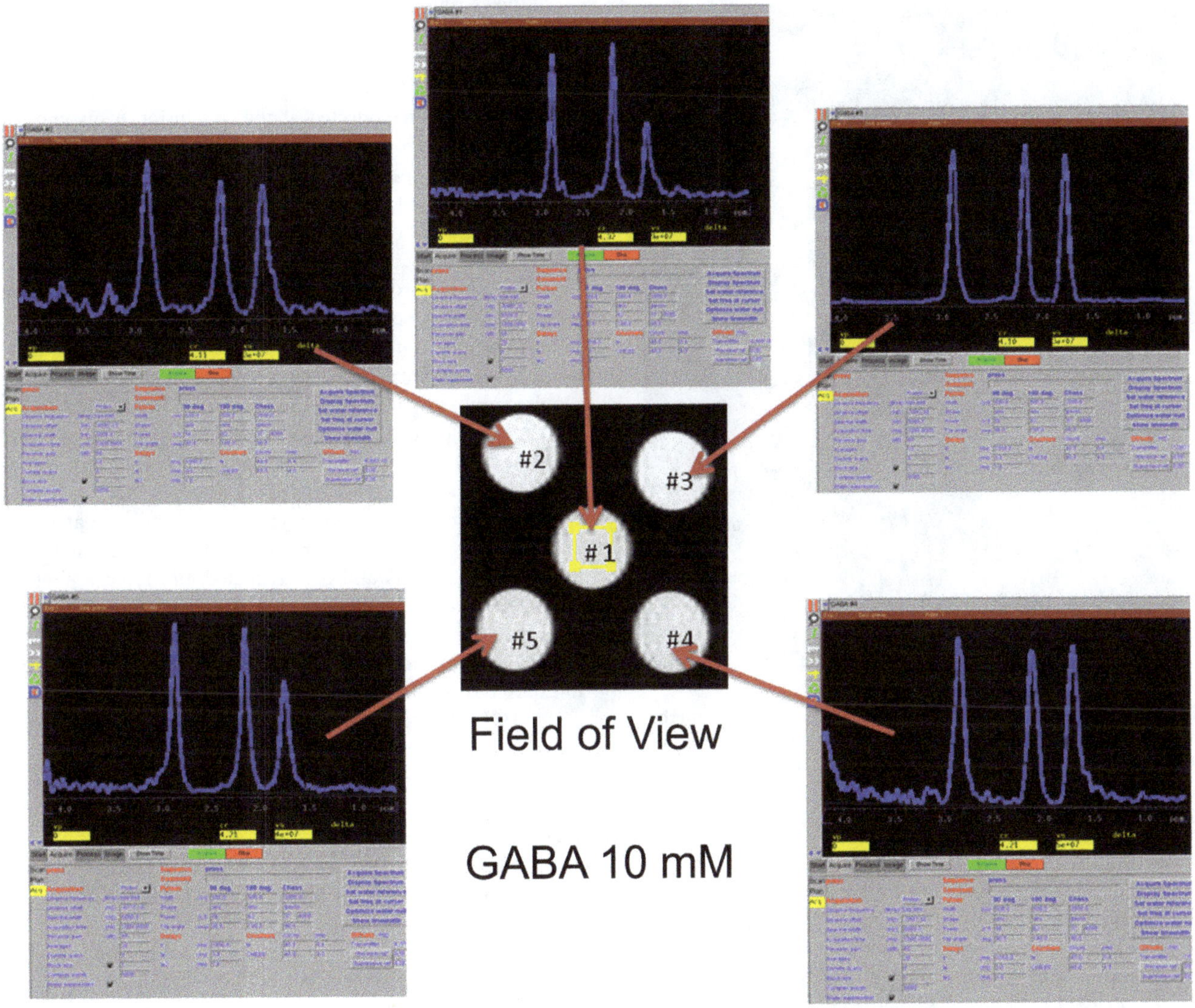

FIGURE 1 | Calibration of GABA spectra using an array of phantoms, each containing 10 mM GABA in sterile normal saline, distributed across the imaging field of view. Using multiple phantoms arrayed throughout the field of view illustrates optimized field shimming and selection of the least-variant spectral peak, from among the multiplets at each location, used to quantify the compound of interest (in this example, GABA).

reference points. ^{1}H-MRS spectra were obtained bilaterally in the order indicated in **Table 2**, with acquisition parameters optimized for each VOI. When shimming, the water peak for all spectra was held constant at 4.7 ppm, and its line width minimized (typically 30–45 Hz). Three hundred scan repetitions were adequate to resolve all spectra, with the exception of the DCN (**Table 2**).

SPECTROSCOPY: DATA ANALYSIS

Spectra, as TIFF images, were imported into Image J (ver. 1.44p, http://imagej.nih.gov/ij). Peaks in closest approximation to the calibration peaks for GABA and Glu, were outlined, and the area under each curve (AUC) for each was determined. AUCs were expressed in spectrum baseline (i.e., curve lower bound) units in order to correct for image gain. AUC values were copied to an Excel (2007, Microsoft, Redmond, WA) spreadsheet for analysis. The AUC of each neurochemical was converted to concentration level (mM), taking into account VOI volume, calibration vessel volume, known calibration concentration, and calibration AUC, as indicated in Equation 1.

$$\text{VOI est conc} = [(\text{VOI AUC}/\text{calib AUC}) \times (\text{calib conc})] \times (\text{calib vol}/\text{VOI vol}) \quad (1)$$

Pair-wise comparisons were made between exposed and unexposed VOI. Reported significance levels were derived from independent *t*-tests.

RESULTS

EVIDENCE OF TINNITUS

Significant tinnitus was evident in the exposed rats approximately four months after exposure. The protocol in the present experiment (exposure before psychophysical training and testing),

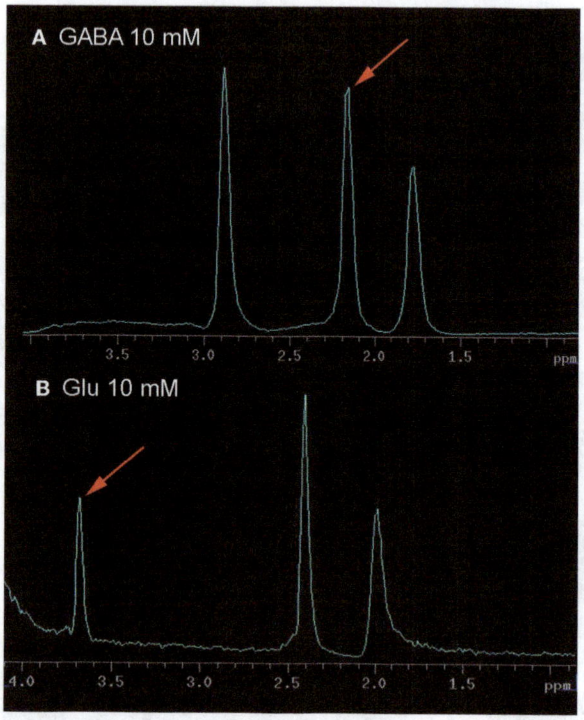

FIGURE 2 | Calibration spectra of GABA and Glu, obtained using the same scanning parameters (see Methods for details) used to capture VOI spectra. The peak, from among the multiplets, used to quantify GABA and Glu is shown by the pointer.

reveals tinnitus as a downshift in discrimination functions. This happens because the sensory correlate of speaker-off periods, i.e., tinnitus in exposed animals, is the conditioned stimulus for response suppression. Therefore, stimuli resembling the speaker-off sensation suppress responding. Frequency-specific suppression was evident in both individual (**Figure 3**) as well as group data (**Figure 4**), between 16 and 24 kHz. Individual subjects showed some variation in the frequency range of their suppression, from rather narrow (**Figure 3A**) to broad (**Figure 3B**). This may reflect the tonality of their tinnitus. In addition, some individuals showed evidence of tinnitus plus hyperacusis. Nevertheless, all of the exposed rats showed some evidence of tinnitus.

GABA AND Glu LEVELS

^{1}H-MRS data were collected at the conclusion of psychophysical testing. Data from six exposed and five unexposed rats were included in the spectral analysis. Data from seven initial rats were used to adjust and optimize experimental parameters and were not included in the final analysis. Data from two rats were discarded when pituitary tumors were detected. Mean age at the time of spectroscopy was 19.8 and 17.8 months, respectively, for the exposed and unexposed animals. The mean interval between exposure and spectroscopy was 16.2 months. Acquisition of spectra from one animal, along with attendant field shimming, required approximately 7 h to complete. One session was run per day. Spectra for the four auditory areas of interest, DCN, IC, MGB, and A1, are summarized in **Figures 5–8**. Each figure depicts selection of the VOI in the top panel, a representative individual spectrum from that VOI in the center panel, and estimated GABA and Glu average levels for exposed and control animals in the bottom panel. GABA and Glu estimated mM levels are reported separately for each hemisphere, ipsilateral, and contralateral, with respect to sound exposure. Decreased GABA concentration was evident only in the MGB, with the greatest decrease, relative to unexposed controls, obtained in the contralateral MGB (**Figure 7**; $p = 0.033$). GABA levels in the exposed MGB were 0.38 mM (±0.18) contralateral and 1.62 mM (±0.64) ipsilateral, as compared to unexposed levels of 2.77 mM (±1.04) contralateral and 2.57 mM (±1.39) ipsilateral. Error (±) is the standard error of the mean. Therefore, a GABA decrease, and potential loss of GABA-mediated inhibition, was most evident in the auditory thalamus in the direct pathway from the exposed ear, i.e., the contralateral MGB. Small GABA increases may have been present bilaterally in A1 (**Figure 8**) and in the contralateral DCN (**Figure 5**) however, these differences were not statistically significant.

Glu level variation, both within and between treatment groups, was higher than GABA variation. Despite the variation, Glu was significantly ($p = 0.039$) elevated in the exposed ipsilateral DCN, 18.77 mM (±9.76) while unexposed was 12.36 mM (±2.32). Contralateral DCN Glu levels were not significantly different in exposed and unexposed rats. The contralateral

Table 2 | ^{1}H-MRS acquisition parameters.

Area of interest	Hemisphere	Volume (mm) of analysis *x, y, z* dimension	Approximate on-center caudal distance from Bregma	Spectrum acquisition		
				Number of repetitions	Duration (min)	Measurement sequence
Dorsal cochlear nucleus (DCN)	Right (ipsilat)	1.5, 2, 1.5	−10.5	2900	74	5
	Left (contra)	1.5, 2, 1.5	−10.5	2900	74	8
Inferior colliculus (IC)	Right (ipsilat)	2, 2, 2	−7.5	300	7	1
	Left (contra)	2, 2, 2	−7.5	300	7	2
Medial geniculate body (MGB)	Right (ipsilat)	1.5, 2, 2	−5	300	7	6
	Left (contra)	1.5, 2, 2	−5	300	7	7
Primary auditory cortex (A1)	Right (ipsilat)	1.5, 2, 3	−3.5	300	7	3
	Left (contra)	1.5, 2, 3	−3.5	300	7	4

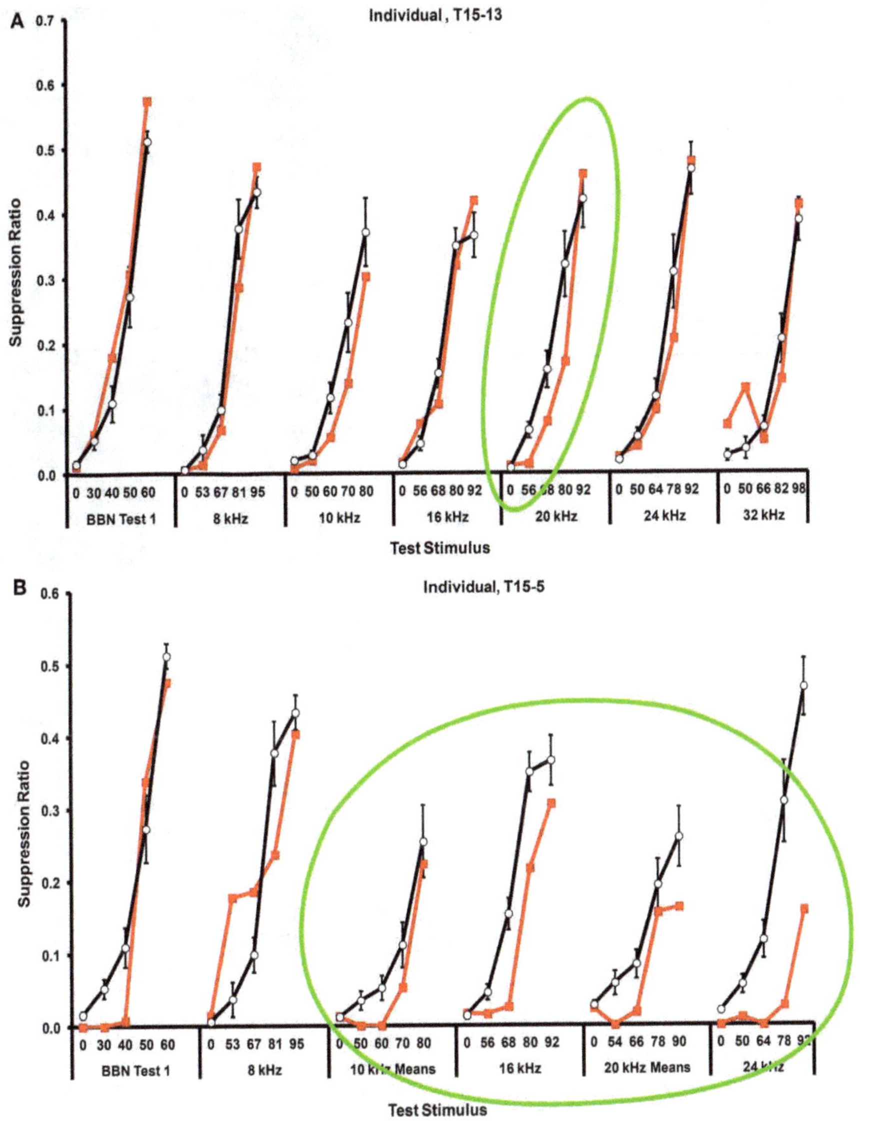

FIGURE 3 | Examples of tinnitus in individual rats. (A) A rat with focal narrow-band tinnitus in the vicinity of 20 kHz, and **(B)** A rat with rather broad-band tinnitus localized between 10 and 24 kHz. Error bars show the standard error of the mean of the unexposed group. Relative rate of lever pressing, as indicated by the suppression ratio (see Text), is shown on the *y*-axis, and test stimulus across stimulus levels (dB, SPL) is shown on the *x*-axis.

exposed level was 6.52 mM (±5.00) while unexposed was 3.08 mM (±2.09) (**Figure 5**). Exposed ipsilateral and contralateral Glu levels were elevated in A1 with respect to unexposed controls, but not significantly so (**Figure 8**; $p = 0.082$, ipsilateral; $p = 0.145$, contralateral). However, significance was negatively impacted by high variation in spectra obtained from A1. Field shimming was difficult for A1, and this suggested that the measurement variation may have been a consequence of field anisotropy near the periphery, rather than intrinsic tissue factors. A1 exposed ipsilateral Glu was 3.12 mM (±1.64) while unexposed was 1.32 mM (±0.54). Exposed contralateral A1 Glu was 2.60 mM (±1.55) while unexposed was 0.81 mM (±0.59).

In the MGB Glu was significantly decreased contralaterally (1.24, ± 0.67 vs. 4.55, ± 1.13; $p = 0.029$) and non-signficantly increased ipsilaterally (4.36, ± 1.91 vs. 2.59, ± 1.11; $p = 0.448$). In summary, these results suggest enhanced Glu-mediated excitation in the DCN, and potentially in A1, although variation in cortical levels obscured significance. In the IC, exposed vs. unexposed differences in both GABA and Glu were small (**Figure 6**).

HEARING THRESHOLDS

The sound exposure used to produce tinnitus was unilateral. This was done to preserve free-field hearing thresholds, a requirement for psychophysical testing. Immediately after exposure (peak sound level at 116 dB, SPL), exposed ear hearing thresholds, as indicated by ABR, were elevated approximately 60 dB at 20 kHz (**Figure 9**, top panel). Thresholds for unexposed ears were not affected by the exposure. At the conclusion of psychophysical

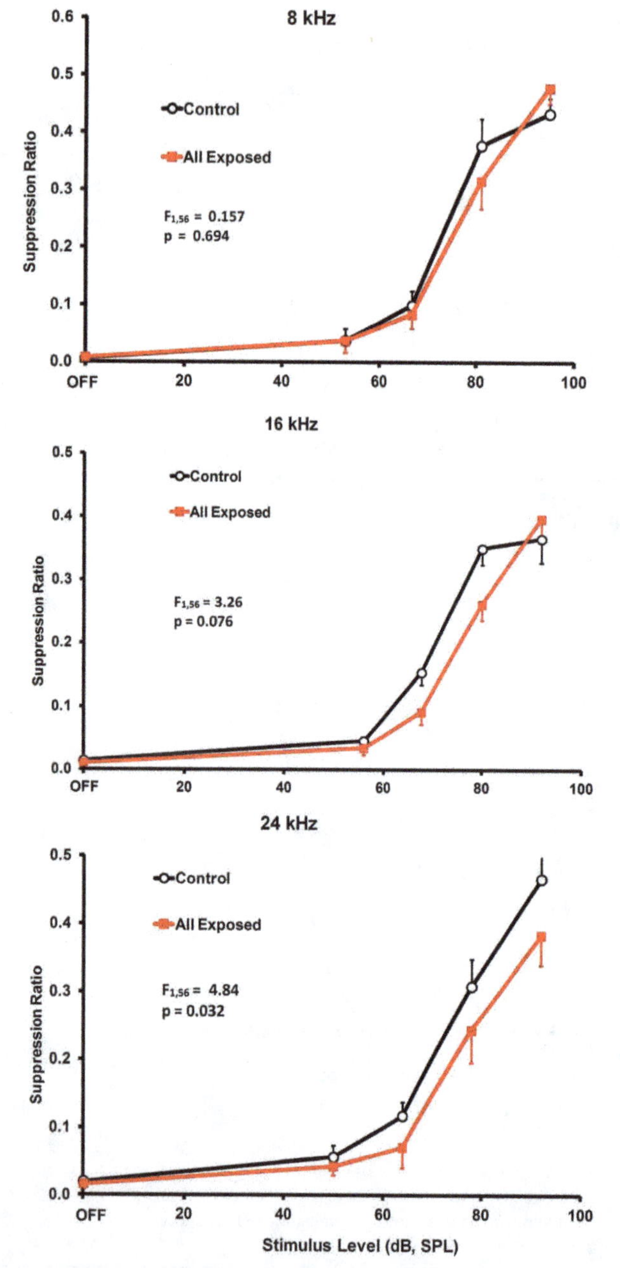

FIGURE 4 | Frequency-specific group evidence of tinnitus. The statistics in each panel represent a comparison of exposed and unexposed groups for stimulus levels above the OFF setting. As in **Figure 3**, relative lever pressing is shown on the *y*-axis and test stimulus across levels is shown on the *x*-axis. Error bars show the standard error of the mean.

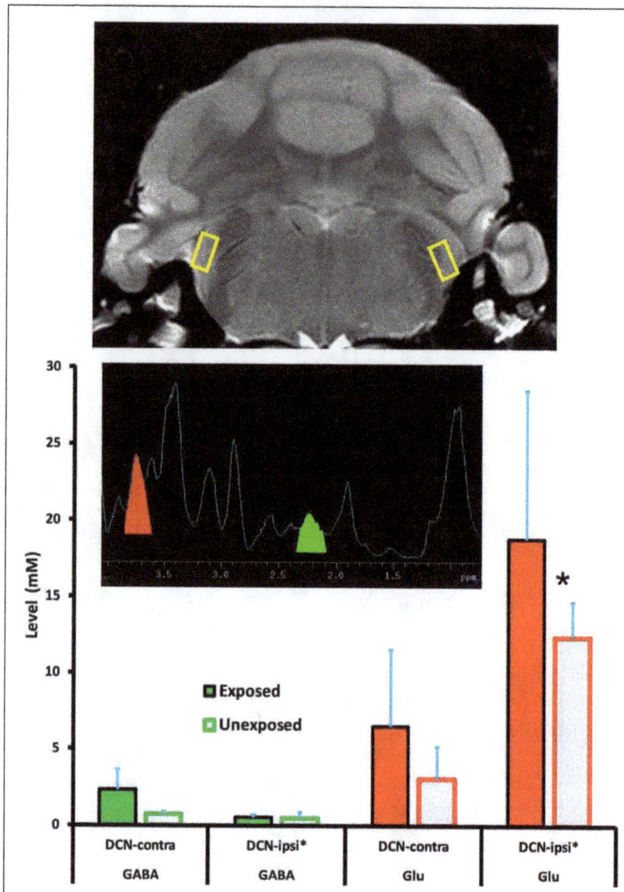

FIGURE 5 | GABA and Glu levels (mM/ml) in the dorsal cochlear nucleus (DCN) of exposed and unexposed rats. Top panel: size and location of the VOI; Mid panel: a typical individual ^{1}H-MRS; Lower panel: group average GABA and Glu levels. Error bars show the standard error of the mean. Asterisk next to the axis label indicates the direct pathway with respect to the trauma-exposed ear. Asterisk next to the data bar indicates statistical significance ($p \leq 0.05$).

testing, and prior to MRS data collection, ABR thresholds for exposed ears returned to normal levels (**Figure 9**, bottom panel). Recovery of threshold sensitivity is typical for this level of exposure (Bauer and Brozoski, 2001) in Long Evans rats.

DISCUSSION

VOLUME LEVEL VS. NEUROTRANSMITTER LEVEL

The present results indicated that there was a GABA decrease in the MGB and Glu increase in both the DCN and A1, accompanying chronic tinnitus in a rat model. This would support the hypothesis that region-specific loss of inhibition and increased excitatory neurotransmission, underpins chronic acoustically induced tinnitus. However, support of the neurotransmitter hypothesis must be tempered when taking into account limitations of the current method. Neurochemical concentrations were determined *ex vivo* using point-resolved ^{1}H-MRS and a 14.1 T magnet. Spectra were effectively resolved from volumes down to 4.5 mm^3 (i.e., the DCN volume). But the reported levels reflect concentrations of the compounds of interest throughout the tissue volume from which spectra were obtained. Using an MRI scan of each brain, care was taken to place the measurement volume entirely within each area of interest. Within each VOI, however, ^{1}H-MRS cannot distinguish concentrations in specific sub-VOI compartments, for example, within neurotransmitter vesicles. In addition to their role as neurotransmitters, GABA and Glu also participate in general metabolic functions, for example as components of the tricarboxylic acid cycle GABA shunt. A further complexity is that GABA is derived from Glu by enzymatic decarboxylation. Therefore, the concentration

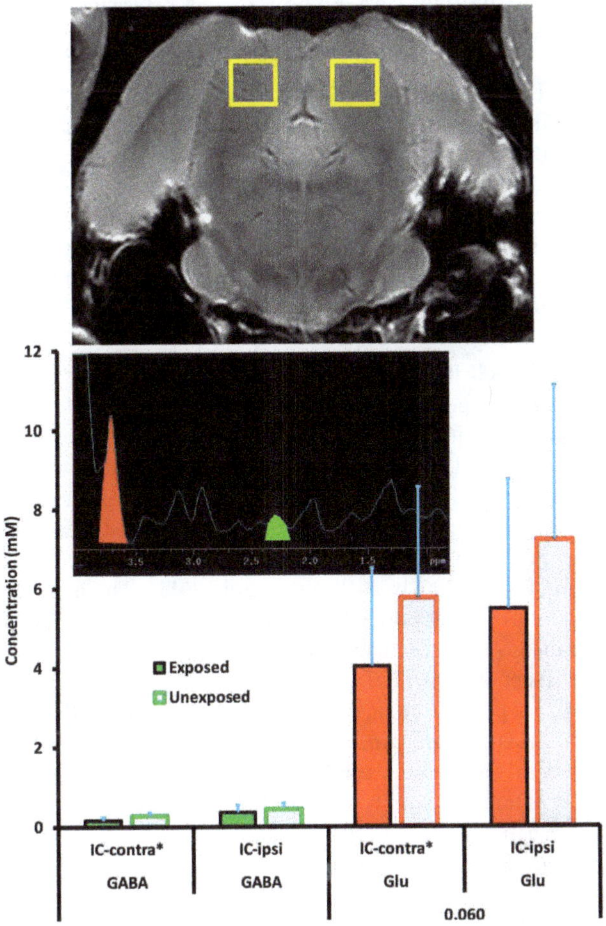

FIGURE 6 | GABA and Glu levels (mM/ml) in the inferior colliculus (IC) of exposed and unexposed rats. No significant differences were obtained between exposed and unexposed animals in the IC. Graphic parameters as in **Figure 5**.

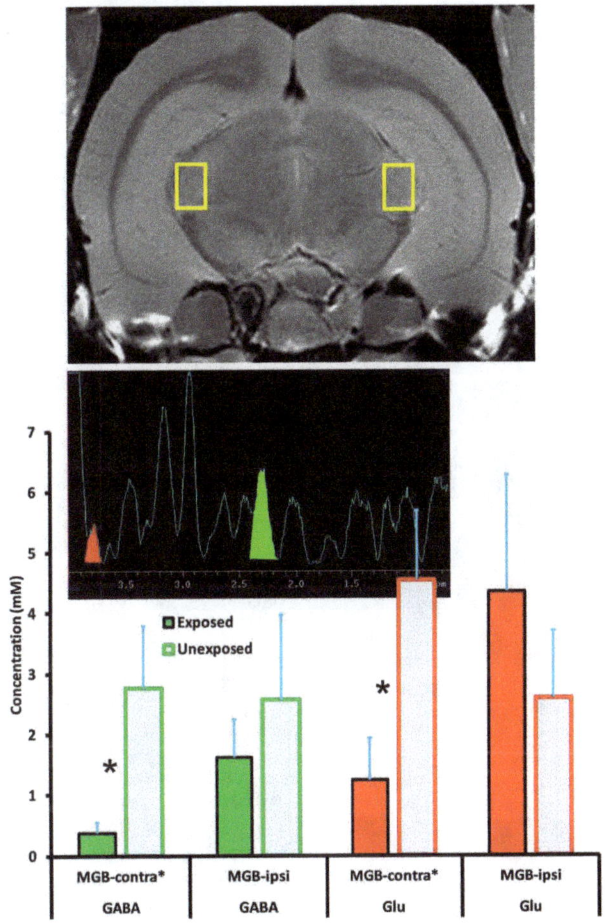

FIGURE 7 | GABA and Glu levels (mM/ml) in the medial geniculate body (MGB) of exposed and unexposed rats. GABA and Glu concentrations were significantly lower in the contralateral MGB of exposed animals. Graphic parameters as in **Figure 5**.

levels reported in the present research cannot be construed as neurotransmitter levels. However, in the present experiment comparisons were made between exposed and unexposed rats, treated identically except for one high-level sound exposure. On average the sound exposure occurred 16 months prior to spectroscopy. It is unlikely that general metabolic consequences of the exposure would linger to influence the results. A reasonable interpretation would be that between-treatment-group variation in GABA and Glu levels reflects functional changes heavily dependent upon neurotransmitter variation (Stagg et al., 2011b).

REPORTED LEVELS, CALIBRATION, AND COMPARISON TO OTHER ESTIMATES

The GABA and Glu levels reported in the present study were concentrations determined in reference to external calibration standards (see Methods). In contrast, many ^{1}H-MRS studies report relative levels with respect to an internal standard, which is another signal within the spectrum, such as that of N-acetyl aspartate (Stagg et al., 2011a), or water (Puts et al., 2011). When using an internal standard it must be assumed that the standard compound remains constant in concentration across conditions and VOI. The advantage of using an internal standard is that variation in local measurement conditions, for example shimming parameters, does not affect the reported values. The primary disadvantage of using an internal standard is that concentration of the standard compound might not be constant across individuals and conditions, thus affecting the reported ratios. A second disadvantage is that only relative level ratios can be reported, actual concentration levels remain unknown. When using an external standard, as in the present research, physical concentration levels are known and internal standard variation is irrelevant. However, when using an external standard, accuracy is dependent upon the calibration method. The external method described in the present study attempted to establish both realistic and stable calibration conditions (**Figures 1** and **2**). Calibration spectra were determined from phantoms similar in volume to the VOI and filled with realistic concentrations of GABA and Glu. Calibration spectra were also determined proximate in time to the brain spectra. Unfortunately attempts to simultaneously calibrate by including phantoms along with the brain at the time of data acquisition

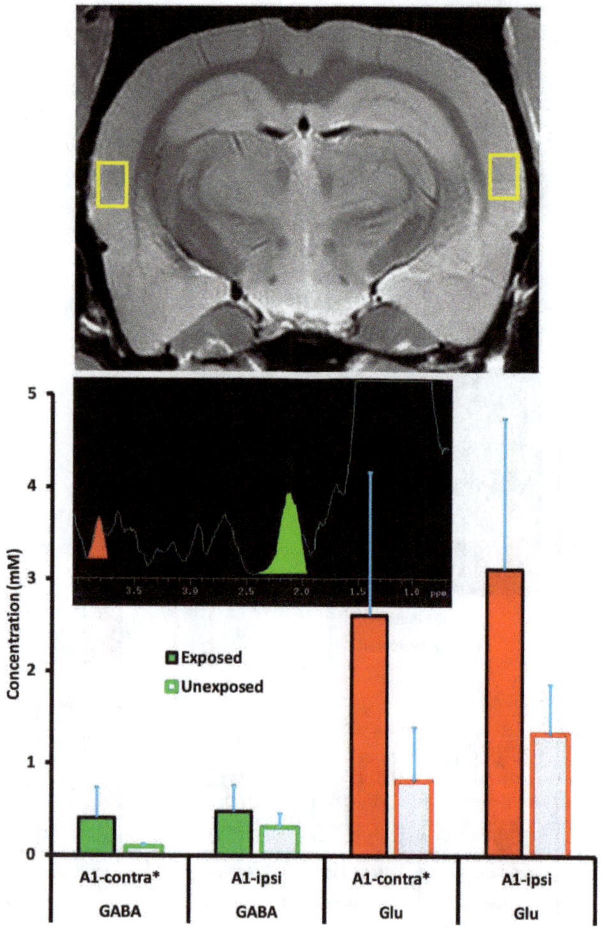

FIGURE 8 | GABA and Glu levels (mM/ml) in primary auditory cortex (A1) of exposed and unexposed rats. Although differences between exposed and unexposed animals were not statistically significant, significance levels may have been masked by measurement variability stemming from field anisotropy rather that neurochemical variability. Graphic parameters as in **Figure 5**.

were not fruitful. Calibration phantoms included along with the brain produced field distortions that made shimming impossible. Also, placing phantoms alongside the brain put the phantoms in the field periphery where locally poor isotropy yielded calibration spectra of low quality.

Glu levels reported in the present study varied between 0.81 and 18.77 mM, while GABA levels varied between 0.09 and 2.77 mM, depending upon the VOI. These *ex vivo* levels are comparable to levels reported by others using similar ^{1}H-MRS methods. Mlynarik et al. (Mlynarik et al., 2008) reported whole rat brain Glu levels of 10.3 (±8%) and GABA levels of 1.5 (±13%) mM/kg. In comparison to contemporary studies using traditional quantitative analytic methods, Glu levels reported in the present study were within range while GABA levels were somewhat higher. For example a recent report by (Zhu et al., 2011) using current-generation high performance liquid chromatography and whole brain homogenates, reported adult rat brain GABA levels of about 0.5 (±25%) mM/mg and Glu levels of 10 (±10%) mM/mg. The GABA discrepancy between the present study and that of (Zhu et al., 2011) may derive from differences between the methods, liquid chromatography depending upon solvent extraction from whole brain homogenates, and ^{1}H-MRS depending on spectra derived from *in situ* tissue in the auditory pathway. It may also be that in the present study there was some GABA inflation, despite the use of 3-mercaptopropionic acid to arrest post-mortem elevation. A GABA inflation error, if present, should have affected exposed and unexposed rats equally since GABA (and Glu) levels were determined using the same procedural sequence for all animals (**Table 2**).

GABA DECREASE IN THE MGB

It has been hypothesized that a loss of inhibition in the central auditory pathway underpins chronic tinnitus (Holt et al., 2010; Wang et al., 2011; Brozoski et al., 2012). Indirect evidence supporting the hypothesis comes from pharmacological studies where systemically administered GABA agonists have been shown to decrease or eliminate behavioral evidence of tinnitus (Brozoski et al., 2007b, 2010; Yang et al., 2011). The hypothesis is also indirectly supported by studies showing increased levels of spontaneous neural activity in animals with evidence of tinnitus (Brozoski et al., 2002; Kaltenbach and Godfrey, 2008; Middleton et al., 2011). The role of the MGB, i.e., the auditory thalamus, in tinnitus is currently not well defined. Recent imaging evidence suggests that altered thalamic circuits may gate abnormal brainstem spontaneous activity to the cortex and limbic structures in tinnitus patients (Rauschecker et al., 2010). The MGB is an obligatory relay for ascending auditory information. Loss of inhibition in the MGB could increase the impact of spontaneous brainstem activity on higher processes, and induce the perception of sound in the absence of peripheral stimulation. Understanding the function of GABA in the MGB is currently evolving. The density of post-synaptic GABA-A receptors is quite low (Halonen et al., 2009). However, GABA-A receptors containing a δ subunit in substitution for the more common γ subunit, have a high density in the MGB compared to other forebrain areas (Halonen et al., 2009; Richardson et al., 2011). δ-subunit-containing GABA-A receptors appear to be primarily extra-synaptic and are responsible for mediating tonic inhibition (Richardson et al., 2011). This suggests that ambient extracellular GABA is important for regulating the general balance of inhibition/excitation in the MGB. Tinnitus may be mediated by loss of inhibitory volume transmission in the MGB mediated by down-regulation of extracellular GABA. Although the density of GABAergic interneurons in the rat MGB is apparently very low (Winer and Larue, 1996), glia have been shown to be a significant source of GABA in other brain areas (Olah et al., 2009). The loss of MGB GABA reported in the present experiment may reflect decreased extracellular-levels as well as lowered levels in glia. The net decrease in inhibition would increase rostral excitation.

Llinas et al. (2005) present a cortico-thalamic network model to account for tinnitus and other neuro-psychiatric disorders. In their model, cortical pyramidal cell feedback to the auditory thalamus, both indirectly, via the thalamic reticular nucleus, and directly, enables low-frequency thalmo-cortical oscillation. In this model, loss of afferent inhibitory input to the thalamus

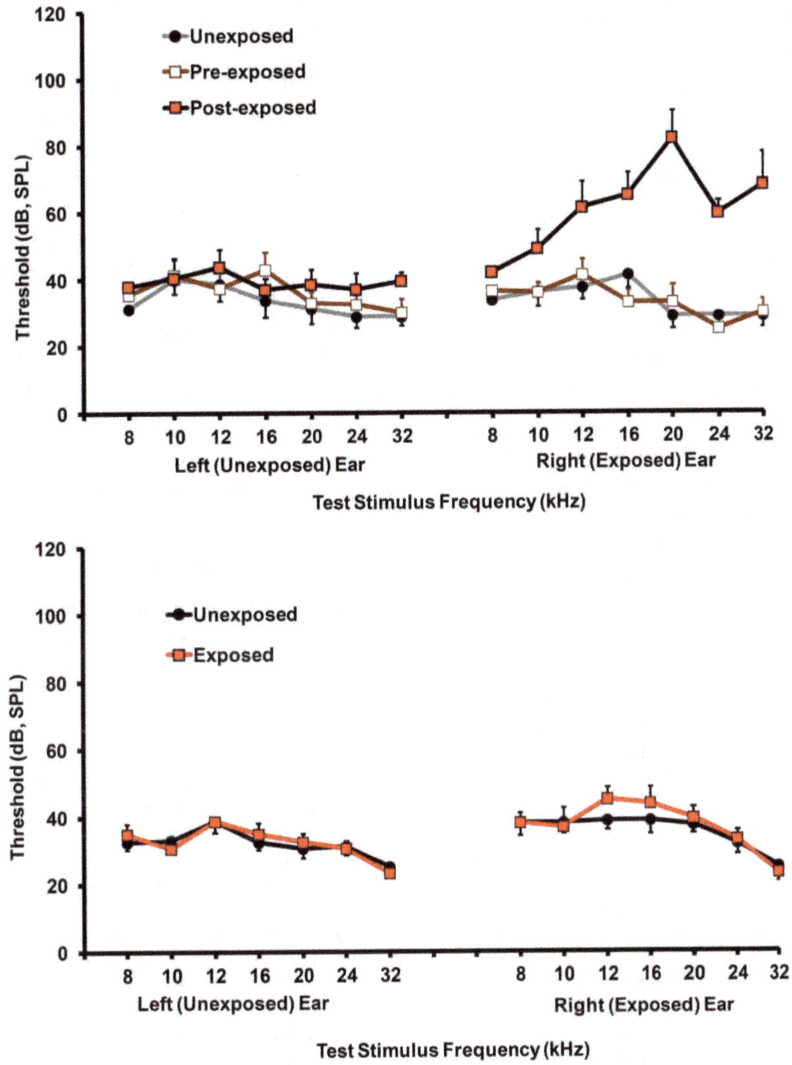

FIGURE 9 | Auditory brainstem response thresholds for exposed and unexposed rats. Top panel: thresholds before and immediately after acoustic exposure. Significant threshold elevation was evident only in the exposed ear. Bottom panel: thresholds prior to spectroscopy show normal levels in both groups. Error bars show the standard error of the mean.

is hypothesized to lead to "edge effect" enhancement of low-frequency (8 Hz) oscillation, the result being the sensation of tinnitus. Interestingly the model also predicts increased low-frequency oscillation, and presumably, associated tinnitus, in the presence of "protracted hyperpolarization of thalamic cells" (Llinas et al., 2005). Therefore, in the Llinas model, elevated GABA intrinsic to the MGB would be expected to produce chronic tinnitus. The present results, however, show just the opposite, with MGB GABA decreased in rats with tinnitus. Further research with cellular-level resolution will be required to answer more detailed questions concerning the role of GABA in specific circuits.

Glu INCREASE IN DCN

In addition to lowered MGB GABA levels, the present research also showed moderately elevated Glu levels in the DCN. Increased spontaneous neural activity in the DCN is associated with tinnitus in rodent models (Brozoski et al., 2002; Kaltenbach et al., 2004), while altered tonotopic organization of the auditory cortex has also been associated with tinnitus in rats (Yang et al., 2011). In fact there may be widespread increases in central gain functions following sensory loss, such as that produced by traumatic high-level sound exposure (Norena, 2011). Adaptive alterations in brain function are primarily mediated by plastic glutamatergic synapses via long-term potentiation (LTP) and long-term depression (LTD) (Zhuo, 2009; Lovinger, 2010; Kullmann and Lamsa, 2011). While LTP and LTD, as characterized *in vitro*, have durations of only an hour or so, it is clear that the same processes are involved in chronic changes that have been reported in adult rat A1 in the context of specific pharmacological and acoustic exposures (Hogsden et al., 2011). Increased Glu levels in the DCN and A1 found in the present study, in rats with chronic tinnitus, may well reflect very long-term increases in excitatory neurotransmission. Both LTP and LTD have been identified in DCN local networks (Tzounopoulos et al., 2007). Furthermore, Glu associated alterations of cochlear nucleus function have been identified following cochlear damage (Zeng et al., 2009).

NULL EFFECT IN THE INFERIOR COLLICULUS (IC)

Given considerable evidence that the IC is involved in chronic tinnitus in animals (Brozoski et al., 2007a; Holt et al., 2010) and humans (Gu et al., 2010), it was somewhat surprising that neither GABA nor Glu levels in the IC were different in exposed versus unexposed animals (**Figure 6**). One explanation may be that average neural activity level was only slightly elevated in the IC of exposed animals. While significantly involved in tinnitus, the neural correlate in the IC may involve alterations in patterns of neural activity, such as infrequent bursts of high-frequency spikes and decreased inter-spike interval variance (Bauer et al., 2008), rather than gross level increases. As such, volume GABA and Glu alterations may not be evident. It also might be noted that studies reporting loss of IC GABA receptors after cochlear damage, also report permanent threshold elevations (Dong et al., 2010). In the present study hearing thresholds were essentially normal at the time of tinnitus testing and spectroscopy (**Figure 9**, bottom panel).

IMPLICATIONS FOR TINNITUS THERAPY

There is no generally effective therapeutic intervention for tinnitus in current clinical application. In contrast, in animal models of tinnitus, several GABA agonists have been found to effectively attenuate or eliminate evidence of tinnitus (Brozoski et al., 2007b, 2010; Yang et al., 2011). Interestingly, while peripheral blockade of cochlear glutamatergic NMDA receptors has been shown to attenuate acoustic-trauma-induced tinnitus in a rat model (Guitton and Dudai, 2007), administration of the systemic NMDA antagonist ketamine, was not effective (Yang et al., 2011). Clinically, neither GABA agonists, for example the many available benzodiazepine derivatives, nor NMDA antagonists, have been shown to be effective in well-controlled trials. The present research suggests that a combined approach, targeting both decreased GABA function and elevated Glu function, may be more fruitful.

ACKNOWLEDGMENTS

Supported by the National Institute on Deafness and Other Communication Disorders, #1R01DC009669–01.

REFERENCES

Bauer, C. A., and Brozoski, T. J. (2001). Assessing tinnitus and prospective tinnitus therapeutics using a psychophysical animal model. *J. Assoc. Res. Otolaryngol.* 2, 54–64.

Bauer, C. A., Turner, J. G., Caspary, D. M., Myers, K. S., and Brozoski, T. J. (2008). Tinnitus and inferior colliculus activity in chinchillas related to three distinct patterns of cochlear trauma. *J. Neurosci. Res.* 86, 2564–2578.

Brozoski, T. J., and Bauer, C. A. (2008). Learning about tinnitus from an animal model. *Semin. Hear.* 29, 242–258.

Brozoski, T. J., Bauer, C. A., and Caspary, D. M. (2002). Elevated fusiform cell activity in the dorsal cochlear nucleus of chinchillas with psychophysical evidence of tinnitus. *J. Neurosci.* 22, 2383–2390.

Brozoski, T. J., Caspary, D. M., Bauer, C. A., and Richardson, B. D. (2010). The effect of supplemental dietary taurine on tinnitus and auditory discrimination in an animal model. *Hear. Res.* 270, 71–80.

Brozoski, T. J., Ciobanu, L., and Bauer, C. A. (2007a). Central neural activity in rats with tinnitus evaluated with manganese-enhanced magnetic resonance imaging (MEMRI). *Hear. Res.* 228, 168–179.

Brozoski, T. J., Spires, T. J., and Bauer, C. A. (2007b). Vigabatrin, a GABA transaminase inhibitor, reversibly eliminates tinnitus in an animal model. *J. Assoc. Res. Otolaryngol.* 8, 105–118.

Brozoski, T. J., Wisner, K. W., Sybert, L. T., and Bauer, C. A. (2012). Bilateral dorsal cochlear nucleus lesions prevent acoustic-trauma induced tinnitus in an animal model. *J. Assoc. Res. Otolaryngol.* 13, 55–66.

Dong, S., Rodger, J., Mulders, W. H., and Robertson, D. (2010). Tonotopic changes in GABA receptor expression in guinea pig inferior colliculus after partial unilateral hearing loss. *Brain Res.* 1342, 24–32.

Gu, J. W., Halpin, C. F., Nam, E. C., Levine, R. A., and Melcher, J. R. (2010). Tinnitus, diminished sound-level tolerance, and elevated auditory activity in humans with clinically normal hearing sensitivity. *J. Neurophysiol.* 104, 3361–3370.

Guitton, M. J., and Dudai, Y. (2007). Blockade of cochlear NMDA receptors prevents long-term tinnitus during a brief consolidation window after acoustic trauma. *Neural Plast.* 2007, 80904.

Halonen, L. M., Sinkkonen, S. T., Chandra, D., Homanics, G. E., and Korpi, E. R. (2009). Brain regional distribution of GABA(A) receptors exhibiting atypical GABA agonism: roles of receptor subunits. *Neurochem. Int.* 55, 389–396.

Hogsden, J. L., Rosen, L. G., and Dringenberg, H. C. (2011). Pharmacological and deprivation-induced reinstatement of juvenile-like long-term potentiation in the primary auditory cortex of adult rats. *Neuroscience* 186, 208–219.

Holt, A. G., Bissig, D., Mirza, N., Rajah, G., and Berkowitz, B. (2010). Evidence of key tinnitus-related brain regions documented by a unique combination of manganese-enhanced MRI and acoustic startle reflex testing. *PLoS One* 5, e14260. doi: 10.1371/journal.pone.0014260

Kaltenbach, J. A., and Godfrey, D. A. (2008). Dorsal cochlear nucleus hyperactivity and tinnitus: are they related? *Am. J. Audiol.* 17, S148–S161.

Kaltenbach, J. A., Zacharek, M. A., Zhang, J., and Frederick, S. (2004). Activity in the dorsal cochlear nucleus of hamsters previously tested for tinnitus following intense tone exposure. *Neurosci. Lett.* 355, 121–125.

Kullmann, D. M., and Lamsa, K. P. (2011). LTP and LTD in cortical GABAergic interneurons: emerging rules and roles. *Neuropharmacology* 60, 712–719.

Llinas, R., Urbano, F. J., Leznik, E., Ramirez, R. R., and van Marle, H. J. (2005). Rhythmic and dysrhythmic thalamocortical dynamics: GABA systems and the edge effect. *Trends Neurosci.* 28, 325–333.

Lovinger, D. M. (2010). Neurotransmitter roles in synaptic modulation, plasticity and learning in the dorsal striatum. *Neuropharmacology* 58, 951–961.

Middleton, J. W., Kiritani, T., Pedersen, C., Turner, J. G., Shepherd, G. M., and Tzounopoulos, T. (2011). Mice with behavioral evidence of tinnitus exhibit dorsal cochlear nucleus hyperactivity because of decreased GABAergic inhibition. *Proc. Natl. Acad. Sci. U.S.A.* 108, 7601–7606.

Mlynarik, V., Cudalbu, C., Xin, L., and Gruetter, R. (2008). 1H NMR spectroscopy of rat brain *in vivo* at 14.1Tesla: improvements in quantification of the neurochemical profile. *J. Magn. Reson.* 194, 163–168.

Muhr, P., and Rosenhall, U. (2011). The influence of military service on auditory health and the efficacy of a Hearing Conservation Program. *Noise Health* 13, 320–327.

Nondahl, D. M., Cruickshanks, K. J., Wiley, T. L., Klein, R., Klein, B. E., and Tweed, T. S. (2002). Prevalence and 5-year incidence of tinnitus among older adults: the epidemiology of hearing loss study. *J. Am. Acad. Audiol.* 13, 323–331.

Norena, A. J. (2011). An integrative model of tinnitus based on a central gain controlling neural sensitivity. *Neurosci. Biobehav. Rev.* 35, 1089–1109.

Odintsov, B. (2011). *Tunable Radio-Frequency Coil.* USA patent application 61081954. November 1, 2011.

Olah, S., Fule, M., Komlosi, G., Varga, C., Baldi, R., Barzo, P., and Tamas, G. (2009). Regulation of cortical microcircuits by unitary GABA-mediated volume transmission. *Nature* 461, 1278–1281.

Puts, N. A., Edden, R. A., Evans, C. J., Mcglone, F., and Mcgonigle, D.

J. (2011). Regionally specific human GABA concentration correlates with tactile discrimination thresholds. *J. Neurosci.* 31, 16556–16560.

Rauschecker, J. P., Leaver, A. M., and Muhlau, M. (2010). Tuning out the noise: limbic-auditory interactions in tinnitus. *Neuron* 66, 819–826.

Richardson, B. D., Ling, L. L., Uteshev, V. V., and Caspary, D. M. (2011). Extrasynaptic GABA(A) receptors and tonic inhibition in rat auditory thalamus. *PLoS One* 6, e16508. doi: 10.1371/journal.pone.0016508

Roberts, L. E., Eggermont, J. J., Caspary, D. M., Shore, S. E., Melcher, J. R., and Kaltenbach, J. A. (2010). Ringing ears: the neuroscience of tinnitus. *J. Neurosci.* 30, 14972–14979.

Stagg, C. J., Bachtiar, V., and Johansen-Berg, H. (2011a). The role of GABA in human motor learning. *Curr. Biol.* 21, 480–484.

Stagg, C. J., Bachtiar, V., and Johansen-Berg, H. (2011b). What are we measuring with GABA magnetic resonance spectroscopy? *Commun. Integr. Biol.* 4, 573–575.

Tzounopoulos, T., Rubio, M. E., Keen, J. E., and Trussell, L. O. (2007). Coactivation of pre- and postsynaptic signaling mechanisms determines cell-specific spike-timing-dependent plasticity. *Neuron* 54, 291–301.

van der Heyden, J. A., and Korf, J. (1978). Regional levels of GABA in the brain: rapid semiautomated assay and prevention of postmortem increase by 3-mercapto-propionic acid. *J. Neurochem.* 31, 197–203.

Wang, H., Brozoski, T. J., and Caspary, D. M. (2011). Inhibitory neurotransmission in animal models of tinnitus: maladaptive plasticity. *Hear. Res.* 279, 111–117.

Winer, J. A., and Larue, D. T. (1996). Evolution of GABAergic circuitry in the mammalian medial geniculate body. *Proc. Natl. Acad. Sci. U.S.A.* 93, 3083–3087.

Yang, S., Weiner, B. D., Zhang, L. S., Cho, S. J., and Bao, S. (2011). Homeostatic plasticity drives tinnitus perception in an animal model. *Proc. Natl. Acad. Sci. U.S.A.* 108, 14974–14979.

Zeng, C., Nannapaneni, N., Zhou, J., Hughes, L. F., and Shore, S. (2009). Cochlear damage changes the distribution of vesicular glutamate transporters associated with auditory and nonauditory inputs to the cochlear nucleus. *J. Neurosci.* 29, 4210–4217.

Zhu, K. Y., Fu, Q., Leung, K. W., Wong, Z. C., Choi, R. C., and Tsim, K. W. (2011). The establishment of a sensitive method in determining different neurotransmitters simultaneously in rat brains by using liquid chromatography-electrospray tandem mass spectrometry. *J. Chromatogr. B Analyt. Technol. Biomed. Life Sci.* 879, 737–742.

Zhuo, M. (2009). Plasticity of NMDA receptor NR2B subunit in memory and chronic pain. *Mol. Brain* 2, 4.

9

Neuroimaging and neuromodulation: Complementary approaches for identifying the neuronal correlates of tinnitus

Berthold Langguth[1,2]*, Martin Schecklmann[1,2], Astrid Lehner[1,2], Michael Landgrebe[1,2], Timm Benjamin Poeppl[1,2], Peter Michal Kreuzer[1,2], Winfried Schlee[3], Nathan Weisz[4], Sven Vanneste[5] and Dirk De Ridder[5]

[1] *Department of Psychiatry and Psychotherapy, University of Regensburg, Regensburg, Germany*
[2] *Tinnitus Center, University of Regensburg, Regensburg, Germany*
[3] *OBOB Laboratory, Department of Psychology, University of Konstanz, Konstanz, Germany and University of Trento, Trento, Italy*
[4] *Clinical and Biological Psychology, Institute of Psychology and Education, University of Ulm, Ulm, Germany*
[5] *TRI, BRAI²N and Department of Neurosurgery, University Hospital Antwerp, Antwerp, Belgium*

****Correspondence:***
Berthold Langguth, Department of Psychiatry and Psychosomatics, Bezirksklinikum, University of Regensburg, Universitaetsstr. 84, 93053 Regensburg, Germany.
e-mail: berthold.langguth@medbo.de

An inherent limitation of functional imaging studies is their correlational approach. More information about critical contributions of specific brain regions can be gained by focal transient perturbation of neural activity in specific regions with non-invasive focal brain stimulation methods. Functional imaging studies have revealed that tinnitus is related to alterations in neuronal activity of central auditory pathways. Modulation of neuronal activity in auditory cortical areas by repetitive transcranial magnetic stimulation (rTMS) can reduce tinnitus loudness and, if applied repeatedly, exerts therapeutic effects, confirming the relevance of auditory cortex activation for tinnitus generation and persistence. Measurements of oscillatory brain activity before and after rTMS demonstrate that the same stimulation protocol has different effects on brain activity in different patients, presumably related to interindividual differences in baseline activity in the clinically heterogeneous study cohort. In addition to alterations in auditory pathways, imaging techniques also indicate the involvement of non-auditory brain areas, such as the fronto-parietal "awareness" network and the non-tinnitus-specific distress network consisting of the anterior cingulate cortex, anterior insula, and amygdale. Involvement of the hippocampus and the parahippocampal region putatively reflects the relevance of memory mechanisms in the persistence of the phantom percept and the associated distress. Preliminary studies targeting the dorsolateral prefrontal cortex, the dorsal anterior cingulate cortex, and the parietal cortex with rTMS and with transcranial direct current stimulation confirm the relevance of the mentioned non-auditory networks. Available data indicate the important value added by brain stimulation as a complementary approach to neuroimaging for identifying the neuronal correlates of the various clinical aspects of tinnitus.

Keywords: chronic tinnitus, neuromodulation, neuroimaging, neuronal correlates, brain stimulation

INTRODUCTION

Tinnitus is a common and distressing symptom that is characterized by the perceived sensation of sound in the absence of an external stimulus, most commonly known as the perception of "ringing in the ears"). Moreover it has been generally recognized that tinnitus is clinically heterogeneous, with respect to its etiology, its perceptual characteristics and its accompanying symptoms. Neuroimaging studies have increasingly contributed to a better understanding of the neuronal correlates of the different forms of tinnitus. In detail they demonstrated involvement of both auditory pathways and non-auditory brain areas, such as dorsolateral prefrontal cortex, orbitofrontal cortex, anterior cingulate, subgenual cingulate, posterior cingulate, parietal cortex, amygdala, hippocampus, parahippocampus, and cerebellum (for review see Lanting et al., 2009). In a recent working model these areas were suggested to be implicated in attentional, emotional, cognitive, and memory aspects related to tinnitus (De Ridder et al., 2011a). However an inherent limitation of functional imaging studies is its correlational approach. In other words, functional imaging can only reveal alterations of neuronal activity that are related to tinnitus, but cannot distinguish, which alterations are of causal relevance and which may just represent epiphenomena. More information about critical contributions of specific brain regions can be gained by transient perturbation of neural activity in these regions. This can be done by investigating the behavioral effects of focal brain stimulation methods. Brain stimulation techniques can be non-invasive, e.g., transcranial magnetic stimulation (TMS) or transcranial direct current stimulation (tDCS) or invasive, e.g., epidural or deep brain electrical stimulation.

Notably the still incomplete understanding of the mechanisms by which brain stimulation methods exert their behavioral effects limits their informative value for mapping brain function

(Borchers et al., 2011). TMS for example represents a multimodal stimulation approach involving stimulation of somatosensory afferents and auditory stimulation in addition to cortical stimulation, all of which may be relevant for the observed behavioral effect (Schecklmann et al., 2011b; Vanneste et al., 2011b; Zunhammer et al., 2011). However, with these limitations in mind brain stimulation techniques still represent useful tools for complementing neuroimaging techniques in the study of brain function by testing hypotheses of causal relationships between the behavioral effects and imaging results. In detail, performing neuroimaging before and after brain stimulation can directly reveal, which changes of brain activity are related to subjective perceptual changes. Here we will review how neuroimaging and brain stimulation studies have complemented each other in the identification of neuronal correlates of tinnitus.

BRAIN STIMULATION TECHNIQUES

TRANSCRANIAL MAGNETIC STIMULATION

Transcranial magnetic stimulation is an experimental tool for stimulating neuronal cell assemblies via brief magnetic pulses delivered by a coil placed on the scalp (Barker et al., 1985). A short lasting, high intensity current pulse through an insulated stimulating coil induces a magnetic field perpendicular to the coil which penetrates the scalp with little attenuation inducing an electrical current in the brain area under the coil, which in turn induces depolarization of nerve cells. Magnetic coils with a variety of shapes are available. Figure-eight-shaped coils are preferentially used, since they produce a more focal magnetic field than round coils. Their maximal current is delivered at the intersection of the two round components (Hallett, 2000). Due to the strong decline of the magnetic field with increasing distance from the coil, the direct stimulation is limited to superficial cortical areas. However, stimulation effects propagate transsynaptically to functionally connected remote areas and thus modulate brain network activity (Siebner et al., 2003; May et al., 2007). More recently newer coils have been developed that might be able to penetrate deeper into the brain, such as the H-coil (Rosenberg et al., 2011) or double cone coil (Hayward et al., 2007).

Whereas single magnetic pulses do not seem to have longer lasting effects on the brain, the application of multiple pulses, called repetitive TMS (rTMS), can induce changes in neuronal excitability that outlast the duration of the stimulation (Hallett, 2000). These effects resemble those seen in animal experiments where repeated electrical stimulation has been shown to produce changes in the effectiveness of synapses in the same circuits (Hoffman and Cavus, 2002). These changes include the phenomena of long term potentiation (LTP) and long term depression (LTD), which have been shown to be important for learning and memory processes (Wang et al., 1996). rTMS can also be used to transiently disturb ongoing neural activity in the stimulated cortical area, thus creating a transient functional lesion. Such an approach can help to identify whether a given brain area is critically involved in a specific behavioral task. However in the interpretation of the effects it has to be considered that effects of rTMS are not limited to the directly stimulated brain regions, but can also induce changes in remote functionally connected brain areas. Moreover it has to be taken into consideration that rTMS always represents a multimodal stimulation approach involving not only cortical stimulation, but also the stimulation of somatosensory afferents (Vanneste et al., 2011b; Zunhammer et al., 2011) by the stimulation of scalp neurons and auditory stimulation (Schecklmann et al., 2011b) by its acoustic artifact, all of which may be relevant for the observed behavioral effect.

TRANSCRANIAL DIRECT CURRENT STIMULATION

Transcranial Direct Current stimulation is another non-invasive procedure for cortical stimulation. For tDCS a relatively weak constant direct current (between 0.5 and 2 mA) is transiently applied via scalp electrodes. The current flows from the anode to the cathode (George and ston-Jones, 2010), and about 50% of the current is shunted through the skin and subcutaneous tissues, whereas 50% goes through the brain (Dymond et al., 1975). Depending on the polarity of the stimulation, tDCS can increase or decrease cortical excitability in the brain regions under the electrode (Nitsche and Paulus, 2000). Anodal tDCS typically has an excitatory effect on the local cerebral cortex by depolarizing neurons, while the opposite is the case under the cathode, where hyperpolarization occurs. This effect of tDCS typically outlasts the stimulation by an hour or longer after a single treatment session of about 20–30 min (Nitsche and Paulus, 2000, 2001)

EPIDURAL STIMULATION

Epidural stimulation via implanted electrodes is an invasive neuromodulation technique used to permanently modulate activity of the cerebral cortex, which is in contrast to non-invasive techniques that usually yield a transient modulation. Electrodes can be placed anywhere on the cortex, e.g., motor cortex (Nguyen et al., 1997), somatosensory cortex (De Ridder et al., 2007b), auditory cortex (De Ridder et al., 2007a), or dorsolateral prefrontal cortex (De Ridder et al., 2011d). The target is usually retrieved by functional imaging such as fMRI (De Ridder et al., 2004) or PET scan, but can also be done using a combination of intraoperative electrophysiological measures (ERP; Pirotte et al., 2005) and functional imaging data (MRI; Pirotte et al., 2008). Attempts have been made to use non-invasive TMS prognostically showing moderate (De Ridder et al., 2011c) to good results (Lefaucheur et al., 2011).

DEEP BRAIN STIMULATION

Deep brain stimulation (DBS) uses the same technique as epidural stimulation to modulate electrical activity in the deeper brain structures. It has been shown that DBS alters neurotransmitter release and electrical activity locally, and also exerts a certain network effect (Kringelbach et al., 2007). For localization purposes Cartesian coordinates derived from brain atlases are used to integrate in stereotactic frames. This permits to accurately positioning a wire electrode in the elected neurostimulation target. Recordings from the inserted electrode can be performed for confirming the localization of the electrode at the intended target.

THE INVOLVEMENT OF CENTRAL AUDITORY PATHWAYS IN TINNITUS

Traditionally, tinnitus was considered to be a disorder that was primarily confined to the ear. However, the observation that tinnitus persists in general after transsection of the auditory nerve clearly indicates its central nervous system origin (House and Brackmann, 1981). Both animal models of tinnitus and neuroimaging research in patients suffering from tinnitus have provided important insight into the neuronal mechanisms involved in the pathophysiology of tinnitus. Based on animal studies, three mechanisms have been proposed to underlie tinnitus: (1) changes in the firing rates of spontaneous neural activity in the central auditory system, (2) changes in the temporal pattern of neural activity (synchrony), and (3) reorganization of tonotopic maps (Eggermont and Roberts, 2004).

The first functional neuroimaging studies of tinnitus have been focused on the auditory system either by analyzing steady-state neural activity in the auditory cortex (Arnold et al., 1996) or by investigating sound-evoked responses (Lockwood et al., 1998; Melcher et al., 2000). All studies with $[^{15}O]$-H_2O PET have consistently provided evidence for tinnitus-related elevated blood flow in auditory structures. Measurements of regional glucose uptake (FDG-PET), which is a marker for steady-state neuronal activity, found an asymmetric activation of the auditory cortex with an increase predominantly on the left side and independent of tinnitus perceived laterality (Arnold et al., 1996; Langguth et al., 2006a). In several (Melcher et al., 2000; Smits et al., 2007; Lanting et al., 2008) but not all (Melcher et al., 2009) studies investigating individuals with unilateral tinnitus, altered activation patterns were observed in the auditory pathway contralateral to where the tinnitus was perceived.

Alterations of neuronal activity in central auditory pathways have also been investigated by electroencephalography (EEG) and magnetoencephalography (MEG). In people with chronic tinnitus MEG (Llinas et al., 1999; Weisz et al., 2005b, 2007) and EEG (van der Loo et al., 2009; Moazami-Goudarzi et al., 2010) resting state measurements revealed relatively consistent a reduction of alpha activity (8–12 Hz), and an increase in both slow wave activity (delta and theta 1–6 Hz) and gamma activity (>30 Hz) in the temporal cortex.

Alterations of neuronal activity in auditory pathways of tinnitus patients have also been documented by using auditory evoked potentials, where both increases (Santos and Matas, 2010) and decreases (Attias et al., 1993, 1996) of amplitudes have been found. The increases were observed in patients without hearing loss (i.e., <25 dB; Santos and Matas, 2010), whereas the decreases in patients with hearing loss (Attias et al., 1993). Significantly increased N1–P2 amplitudes were found at higher stimulus intensities for the tinnitus ear in comparison to the non-tinnitus ear in patients with unilateral tinnitus (Norena et al., 1999).

It is assumed that the observed alterations of neural activity in the auditory pathways arise as a consequence of altered sensory input, namely auditory deprivation in most cases (Norena et al., 2002; Norena and Eggermont, 2005), but can also be due to altered somatosensory input (Roberts et al., 2010). Several lines of evidence indicate that the mentioned adaptive processes are mainly driven by mechanisms of homeostatic plasticity which alter the balance between excitatory and inhibitory function of the auditory system at several levels in order to compensate for the reduced input (Schaette and Kempter, 2006; Norena, 2011; Schaette and McAlpine, 2011; Yang et al., 2011).

Even if neuroimaging findings largely contributed to a more detailed understanding of tinnitus, important knowledge gaps still remain. Thus it is not clear to which extent the observed findings are really related to tinnitus ("state") or whether they reflect a predisposition for developing tinnitus ("trait").

Moreover, the alterations of neuronal structure and function in tinnitus patients may represent the neuronal correlates of tinnitus, but they may also represent compensatory mechanisms for auditory deprivation and be unrelated to tinnitus or even beneficial for attenuating tinnitus. Answering these questions is challenging due to (1) the lack of longitudinal studies in humans with neuroimaging measurements before and after tinnitus onset, (2) the limited reliability of behavioral assessment of tinnitus in animals, and (3) the limited sensitivity for assessing auditory dysfunction in humans. Many cross-sectional imaging studies which compared tinnitus patients and controls, did not control for hearing loss. Thus it remains unclear whether the observed changes are related to tinnitus or to hearing loss. But even when the studies controlled for hearing loss, this was done based on the audiogram which provides only limited information about the integrity of the cochlea (Schaette and McAlpine, 2011).

Thus, the modulation of neuronal activity in the auditory pathways of tinnitus patients by means of focal brain stimulation represents an elegant way to further address the question whether alterations in the auditory pathway depict a trait or a state factor

MODULATION OF AUDITORY CORTEX ACTIVITY

Transcranial magnetic stimulation

As mentioned before, tinnitus is related to altered activity of central auditory areas. If the perception of tinnitus can be influenced by rTMS over auditory cortical areas and given that rTMS reliably changes auditory cortex activity, this would provide support for a causal relationship between abnormal neural activity in these areas and tinnitus perception. Many studies have investigated the effects of both single sessions and repeated sessions of rTMS over temporal or temporoparietal brain areas.

Single sessions of rTMS for transient tinnitus suppression. Within the last years 11 studies involving over 300 patients have been published, in which single sessions of rTMS over temporal or temporoparietal areas have been applied (see **Table 1**). These studies differed with respect to the applied stimulation protocols, the exact stimulation areas, the method for coil localization, the chosen control condition, and the used assessment instruments. Nevertheless almost all studies reported a transient tinnitus reduction in a subgroup of tinnitus patients (for detailed results see **Table 1**). This indicates the relevance of the stimulated area for tinnitus perception in those patients. Only few studies have compared different stimulation protocols.

In one study different brain areas were stimulated with high-frequency rTMS (10 Hz). Best tinnitus suppression was found for stimulation of the left temporoparietal cortex resulting in a transient reduction of tinnitus in 57% of the participants (Plewnia et al., 2003).

In one study rTMS at frequencies between 1 and 20 Hz was applied over the auditory cortex contralateral to the site of tinnitus

Table 1 | Effects of single sessions of rTMS over auditory brain areas.

Authors	*N*	Stimulation site	Coil positioning	Frequency	Intensity	Pulses/session	Control condition	Results
Plewnia et al. (2003)	14	Various scalp positions	10–20 EEG system	10 Hz	120% MT	30	Stimulation of non-auditory cortical areas	In eight patients (58%) tinnitus suppression after left temporal/temporoparietal stimulation
De Ridder et al. (2005)	114	Auditory cortex contralateral to tinnitus site	Anatomical landmarks	1, 5, 10, 20 Hz	90% MT	200	Coil angulation	In 60 patients (53%) good or partial tinnitus suppression after active rTMS, in 33% suppression after sham rTMS
Fregni et al. (2006)	7	Left temporoparietal areas	10–20 EEG system	10 Hz	120% MT	30	Sham coil and active stimulation of mesial parietal cortex	In three patients (42%) tinnitus suppression after left temporoparietal stimulation, no effect for both control rTMS conditions
Folmer et al. (2006)	15	Left and right temporal cortex	10–20 EEG system	10 Hz,	100% MT	150	Sham coil	In six patients (40%) tinnitus suppression after active rTMS, in four of the patients after contralateral rTMS in two patient after ipsilat. TMS; in two patients suppression after sham rTMS
Londero et al. (2006)	13	contralateral auditory cortex	fMRI-guided neuronavigation	1, 10 Hz	120% MT	30	Stimulation over non-auditory cortical areas	Eight patients were stimulated over the auditory cortex with 1 Hz; in five of them (62.5%) tinnitus suppression; no suppression after 1 Hz rTMS of non-auditory targets; no suppression after 10 Hz, in two patients suppression after stimulation of a control position
Plewnia et al. (2007a)	8	Area of maximum tinnitus-related PET activation (temporoparietal cortex)	neuronavigational system, based on H_2O PET with and without Lidocaine	1 Hz	120% MT	300, 900, 1800	control position (occipital cortex)	In six patients (75%) tinnitus reduction after active rTMS, better suppression with more pulses
De Ridder et al. (2007a,b)	46	Auditory cortex contralateral to tinnitus site	Anatomical landmarks	5, 10, 20 Hz tonic; 5, 10, 20 Hz burst	90% MT	200	Coil angulation	Fourteen placebo-negative patients were analyzed: In those with narrow band/white noise tinnitus burst TMS was more effective in tinnitus suppression as compared to tonic TMS, whereas for pure tone tinnitus no difference was found between burst and tonic.
Poreisz et al. (2009)	20	Inferior temporal cortex	10–20 EEG electrode system, T3	continuous theta burst, intermittent theta burst, immediate theta burst	80% MT	600	No placebo condition	Significant tinnitus reduction only for continuous theta burst immediately after stimulation

Meeus et al. (2009)	50	Auditory cortex contralateral to tinnitus site	Anatomical landmarks	1, 5, 10, 20 Hz tonic; 5, 10, 20 Hz burst	50% maximal stimulator output (independently of individual MT)	200	Coil angulation	No difference between tonic and burst rTMS in pure tone tinnitus (about 50% average suppression in unilateral and 30% in bilateral tinnitus). For bilateral narrow band tinnitus superiority of burst stimulation compared to tonic stimulation; better effects in patients with lower MT
Lorenz et al. (2010)	10	Left auditory cortex	10–20 EEG electrode system	1 Hz, individual alpha, continuous theta burst, intermittent theta burst, sham	110% MT for 1 Hz, individual alpha and sham; 80% MT for the theta burst protocols	1000 for 1 Hz, individual alpha and sham; 600 for the theta burst protocols	Coil angulation	Significant tinnitus reduction for 1 Hz rTMS and continuous theta burst
Minami et al. (2011)	16	Left auditory cortex	Anatomical landmarks	1 Hz	110% MT	1200	Open study	significant reduction in the VAS (loudness and annoyance) immediately after rTMS

MT, Motor threshold.

perception. The best transient tinnitus suppression was achieved by using higher stimulation frequencies for tinnitus of recent onset and lower frequencies for tinnitus of longer duration. Patients who had their tinnitus for a shorter duration experienced the best results (De Ridder et al., 2005). One study (Londero et al., 2006) demonstrated reliable tinnitus suppression in only 1 out of 13 subjects after a single session of 10 Hz rTMS, whereas 5 out of 8 reported tinnitus suppression after 1 Hz rTMS. Dose-dependent effects were observed in one study, where single sessions of low-frequency (1 Hz) rTMS were applied to areas of altered blood flow during lidocaine injection (Plewnia et al., 2007a). With longer lasting stimulation sessions a longer lasting tinnitus reduction was observed.

Repetitive TMS can be applied in tonic and burst mode. Bursts of three stimuli at a frequency of 50 Hz (interval of 20 ms between each stimulus), applied every 200 ms (5 Hz, Theta burst) have been shown to induce more pronounced and longer lasting effects on the human motor cortex than tonic stimulation (Huang et al., 2005). Single sessions of continuous theta burst stimulation (three pulses at 50 Hz, repeated at 200 ms intervals for up to 600 pulses for 40 s) over the temporal cortex in tinnitus patients did only result in short lasting reduction of tinnitus loudness, comparable to effects achieved with single sessions of tonic stimulation, whereas other theta burst protocols had no effect at all (Poreisz et al., 2009; Lorenz et al., 2010). In two other studies single sessions of burst stimulation were compared with tonic stimulation (De Ridder et al., 2007c,d). Burst stimulation had similar effects as tonic stimulation in patients with pure tone tinnitus but was superior in patients with noise-like tinnitus. It was hypothesized that pure tone tinnitus may be due to increased neuronal activity in the classical (lemniscal) tonotopically organized auditory pathways, which mainly fire tonically, whereas noise-like tinnitus may be the result of increased activity in the non-classical (extralemniscal) non- (or less) tonotopically organized auditory pathways, characterized by burst firing (Hu et al., 1994; De Ridder et al., 2010).

Even if single studies indicate some relationship between specific tinnitus characteristics, stimulation parameters, and behavioral effects, available data are by far not sufficient to draw firm conclusions about such relationships. An unspecific effect by the acoustic artifact can be largely excluded since practically all studies controlled for this confounding factor, e.g., by using a sham coil that produces the same sound like the real coil. In contrast the involvement of peripheral stimulation of somatosensory afferents cannot be entirely excluded. Comparison of rTMS effects and effects of transcutaneous electrical stimulation (TENS) at the neck in the same patient group demonstrate a relationship between response to these two interventions which might serve as a hint for either the involvement of unspecific effects or for the involvement of peripheral somatosensory nerve structures in the mediation of the rTMS effect. However, these peripheral or unspecific effects do not explain the entire rTMS effect (Vanneste et al., 2011b).

In summary the available data provide evidence that interference with temporal or temporoparietal cortex by single sessions of rTMS have a transient effect on the tinnitus percept in about half of the stimulated patients.

Repeated sessions of rTMS. In 21 studies with a total of over 600 participants the effects of repeated sessions of rTMS over temporal or temporoparietal areas have been investigated (**Table 2**). Among these studies 10 randomized placebo-controlled trials with 234 participants are counted. Most rTMS treatment studies applied low-frequency rTMS in long trains of 1200–2000 pulses repeatedly over 5–10 days. Repeated sessions of rTMS were first investigated in a placebo-controlled cross-over study with 14 participants. The site of maximum activation in the auditory cortex was determined by [^{18}F]deoxyglucose (FDG) PET and a neuronavigational system was used for exact placement of the TMS coil over this area (Kleinjung et al., 2005). After active treatment the participants experienced a significant decrease in their tinnitus reflected by the score of the tinnitus questionnaire, whereas sham treatment showed no effect. Treatment effects were still detectable 6 months after treatment. Another study concerned the effects of 2 weeks of rTMS applied over the cortical area where lidocaine-induced activity change was largest as determined by [^{15}O]H_2O PET (Plewnia et al., 2007b). This approach also resulted in moderate but significant effects after active stimulation. Placing the coil over the left temporal area according to the 10–20 EEG coordinate systems (Langguth et al., 2006b) also resulted in a significant reduction of tinnitus severity after 10 sessions of 1 Hz rTMS. Beneficial effects of low-frequency rTMS have been confirmed by many (Rossi et al., 2007; Smith et al., 2007; Khedr et al., 2008, 2010; Anders et al., 2010; Marcondes et al., 2010; Chung et al., 2011; Mennemeier et al., 2011) but not by all controlled studies (Piccirillo et al., 2011). Unspecific effects can largely be excluded since all mentioned studies controlled for the acoustic artifact by using a sham condition and in two recent studies the control condition even involved additional electrical superficial nerve stimulation (Rossi et al., 2007; Mennemeier et al., 2011). The degree of improvement and the duration of treatment effects varied across the studies. This may be due to differences in study design, outcome variables, stimulation parameters, selection criteria of the participants, and the stimulation target. In this context it should be mentioned that the exact cortical region in which temporal rTMS exerts clinical effects in tinnitus patients is still a matter of debate (Langguth et al., 2010). It has been argued that the primary auditory cortex is difficult to reach by TMS since it is located far from the brain surface in the Sylvian fissure in lateromedial direction. Furthermore, following the tonotopic organization of the primary auditory cortex the representation of low frequencies is located more lateral whereas the representation of high frequencies resides more medial. Thus one would expect better outcomes in patients with low-frequent tinnitus since the related abnormalities in the auditory cortex are expected to be more lateral and should therefore be better reached by rTMS. However such a relationship could not be demonstrated (Frank et al., 2010). It has been proposed that rTMS might exert direct effects on the superficial secondary auditory cortex which then further propagate to the primary auditory cortex, analogously to what has been described for electrical stimulation of the secondary auditory cortex in tinnitus (De Ridder et al., 2004).

In summary most studies investigating rTMS over temporal or temporoparietal cortical areas found a statistically significant reduction of tinnitus complaints. However, the available data do not provide a hint for superiority of specific stimulation paradigms or stimulation targets. Since most studies assessed treatment effects only by questionnaires which do not differentiate between changes in tinnitus loudness and tinnitus annoyance it is also not clear whether rTMS reduces primarily tinnitus loudness, tinnitus annoyance, or both.

Neuronal correlates of rTMS effects on tinnitus. The above mentioned studies which assessed the behavioral effect of rTMS over auditory brain areas on tinnitus perception could demonstrate that interfering with neuronal activity in these areas results in a reduction in tinnitus perception. However, they do not provide information about which neuronal changes are related to these perceptual changes. Such information can be obtained by performing neuroimaging studies before and after brain stimulation. The observed changes of neuronal activity can be related to the behavioral changes and differentiate (1) between state and trait related changes and (2) between neuronal alterations in tinnitus patients that are really causally relevant for tinnitus, unrelated to tinnitus, or even represent a beneficial compensatory mechanism.

Moreover the identification of neuronal mechanisms of rTMS induced tinnitus reduction is essential for developing optimization strategies for rTMS treatment (Kleinjung and Langguth, 2009). Unfortunately the number of studies investigating neuronal correlates of rTMS treatment is still relatively limited.

In one study voxel based morphometry and auditory evoked potentials were used to investigate the effects of TMS over the auditory cortex in healthy controls. An increase in the N2–P2 amplitude was found after active rTMS and transient structural alterations in the temporal cortex and in the thalamus (May et al., 2007). No comparison with behavioral effects can be made, since the study was performed in healthy controls, in which no behavioral changes were observed. Nevertheless the results indicate that structural changes are not automatically a trait marker, but could also serve as a state marker, since they can be induced by 1 week of rTMS. The observed changes in the thalamus and the stimulated cortical area were interpreted as a hint for an influence of rTMS on thalamocortical processing. This interpretation has been further supported by electrophysiologic studies both in healthy controls (Eichhammer et al., 2007) and in tinnitus patients (Langguth et al., 2008) before and after stimulation. By investigating motor cortex excitability it has been shown that the cortical silent period, a marker for inhibitory thalamic function, increased after stimulation (Eichhammer et al., 2007) and that this increase was related to improvement of tinnitus (Langguth et al., 2008).

One study used single photon emission computed tomography (SPECT) for exploring neuronal changes induced by five sessions of left temporoparietal low-frequency (1 Hz) rTMS (Marcondes et al., 2010). Comparison of SPECT data before and 2 weeks after active rTMS revealed no change in the directly stimulated area, but reduction of neuronal activity in both the left and the right temporal lobe and increased activity in the right uncus and the right cingulate gyrus. In contrast, sham rTMS resulted in increased activity in the left temporal lobe, the cingulated gyrus bilaterally, and in the right insula.

In a recent study FDG-PET scans were performed before and after five sessions of active and sham rTMS (Mennemeier

Table 2 | Effects of repeated sessions of rTMS in tinnitus patients.

Authors	*N*	Stimulation site	Coil positioning	Frequency	Intensity	sessions	Pulses / session	Design	Control condition	Results
Kleinjung et al. (2005)	14	Area of maximum PET activation in the temporal cortex, (12 left, 2 right)	Neuronavigational system, based on FDG-PET	1 Hz,	110% MT	5	2000	Sham-controlled, cross-over	Sham coil	Significant reduction of tinnitus after active rTMS as compared to sham rTMS; lasting tinnitus reduction (6 months)
Langguth et al. (2006a)	28	Left auditory cortex	10–20 EEG system	1 Hz	110% MT	10	2000	open	No control condition	Significant reduction of tinnitus until end of follow-up (3 months)
Plewnia et al. (2007a)	6	Area of maximum tinnitus-related PET activation (temporoparietal cortex; three left, three right)	Neuronavigational system, based on H_2O PET with and without Lidocaine	1 Hz	120% MT	10	1800	Sham-controlled, cross-over	Occipital cortex	Significant reduction of tinnitus after active rTMS, as compared to the control condition; no lasting effects
Kleinjung et al. (2007)	45	Left auditory cortex	Neuronavigational system, based on structural MRI	1 Hz	110% MT	10	2000	open	No control condition	Significant tinnitus reduction after rTMS, lasting up during follow-up period (3 months) responders were characterized by shorter tinnitus duration and less hearing impairment
Rossi et al. (2007)	16	Left secondary auditory cortex	Eight patients: neuronavigational system Eight patients: according to 10–20 EEG system, halfway between T3 and C3/T5	1 Hz	120% MT	5	1200	Sham-controlled, cross-over	Coil angulation + electrical stimulation of facial nerve	Significant reduction of tinnitus after active rTMS, as compared to the control condition, no lasting effects
Smith et al. (2007)	4	Area of maximal PET activation in the temporal cortex, neuronavigational system	Neuronavigational system, based on FDG-PET	1 Hz	110% MT	5	1800	Sham-controlled, cross-over	Coil angulation	Modest response to active treatment in three patients (75%)
Khedr et al. (2008, 2009)	66	Left temporoparietal cortex	10–20 EEG system	1, 10, 25 Hz	100% MT	10	1500	Sham-controlled, parallel group design	Occipital cortex	Significant reduction of tinnitus after all three active rTMS conditions, as compared to the control condition; tinnitus reduction lasting during follow-up period (4 and 12 months)

(Continued)

Table 2 | Continued

Authors	N	Stimulation site	Coil positioning	Frequency	Intensity	sessions	Pulses / session	Design	Control condition	Results
Langguth et al. (2008)	32	Left auditory cortex	Neuronavigational system, based on structural MRI	1, 6 + 1 Hz	110% MT (90% MT for 6 Hz rTMS)	10	2000	Two active treatment conditions, parallel group design	No sham control condition	Significant improvement for both stimulation conditions, no difference between conditions, no lasting effects
Lee et al. (2008)	8	Left temporoparietal cortex	10–20 EEG system	0.5 Hz	100% MT	5	600	Open study	No control condition	No significant reduction of tinnitus
Kleinjung et al. (2008)	32	Left auditory cortex; left dorsolateral prefrontal cortex	Neuronavigational system, based on structural MRI	1, 20 (DLPFC) + 1 Hz	110% MT	10	2000	Two active treatment conditions, parallel group design	No sham control condition	Directly after stimulation significant improvement for both stimulation conditions, at 3 months follow-up significantly better results for the combined frontal and temporal stimulation
Kleinjung et al. (2009)	32	Left auditory cortex	Neuronavigational system, based on structural MRI	1 Hz, 1 Hz + Levodopa	110% MT	10	2000	Two active treatment conditions, parallel group design	No sham control condition	Significant improvement for both stimulation conditions, no difference between conditions, no lasting effects
Marcondes et al. (2010)	19	Left temporoparietal cortex	10–20 EEG system	1 Hz,	110% MT	5	1020	Randomized sham controlled, parallel group design	Sham coil	Significant improvement after active rTMS but not after sham rTMS, beneficial treatment effects still detectable at 6 months follow-up
Khedr et al. (2010)	62	Temporoparietal cortex	10–20 EEG system	1, 25 Hz				Randomization between 1 and 25 Hz and between ipsil- and contralateral stimulation	No sham control condition	Significant improvement for the whole group. Stimulation contralateral to perceived tinnitus significantly more efficient than ipsilateral stimulation; No significant difference between 1 and 25 Hz
Anders et al. (2010)	52	Left temporal cortex	10–20 EEG system	1 Hz	110% MT	10	1500	Randomized sham controlled, parallel group design	Coil angulation	Significant reduction in TQ and THI scores in the active treated group compared to the sham group in the follow-up period (2–26 weeks)

Frank et al. (2010)	194	Left temporal cortex	10–20 EEG system or neuronavigated	1 Hz	110% MT	10	2000	Retrospective analysis	No control condition	Reduction of the TQ score for the whole group; better effects in patients with left-sided or bilateral tinnitus
Mennemeier et al. (2011)	21	Temporal or temporoparietal cortex	Neuronavigated based on FDG PET findings	1 Hz	110% MT	5	1800	Randomized sham-controlled cross-over trial	Sham coil with electrical stimulation	Visual analog scale ratings of tinnitus loudness decreased after active, but not sham treatment; 43% of patients had at least 33% loudness reduction; tinnitus reduction was not reflected by reduction of PET activation in the stimulated brain area
Piccirillo et al. (2011)	14	Temporoparietal cortex	10–20 EEG system or neuronavigated	1 Hz	110% MT	10	2000	Double-blind randomized sham-controlled cross-over trial	Sham coil system	THI score reductions after both sham and active rTMS; no difference between groups
Kleinjung et al. (2011)	18	Left temporal cortex	10–20 EEG system or neuronavigated	1 Hz + bupropion	110% MT	10	2000	Comparison with historical control group	No control condition	TQ score reduction for the whole group, no enhancing effect of bupropion
Chung et al. (2011)	22	Left temporal cortex	Neuronavigated	Continuous theta burst	80% MT	10	900 (300 bursts)	Randomized sham controlled, parallel group design	Sham coil system	Significant reductions of TQ and THI scores in the actively treated group compared to sham treatment, reduction of tinnitus loudness match after active rTMS
Kreuzer et al. (2011)	56	Left temporal cortex; right dorsolateral prefrontal cortex	10–20 EEG system	1 Hz	110% MT	10	2000	Two active treatment conditions, parallel group design	No sham control condition	TQ reduction in both groups immediately after stimulation, in the combined stimulated group tendency toward higher efficacy

MT, Motor threshold.

et al., 2011). The site most consistently associated with a positive response was the secondary auditory cortex either hemisphere. Whereas PET activity decreased significantly beneath the stimulating coil following active treatment, similar changes occurred at control sites and after sham stimulation. Moreover no relationship between the treatment related change of metabolic activation of the auditory cortex and clinical effects could be detected, indicating that FDG-PET does not represent a sensitive method for identifying the neuronal correlates of rTMS induced tinnitus reduction and probably also not useful for defining the stimulation target (Mennemeier et al., 2011).

Another recent study used MEG to record auditory evoked potentials of three different tones before and after five different stimulation protocols in patients with tinnitus (1 Hz, stimulation at the individual alpha frequency, continuous theta burst, intermittent theta burst, sham; Lorenz et al., 2010). An important finding was that the effect of the different protocols varied from patient to patient. On average, the 1-Hz protocol revealed the most pronounced tinnitus reduction, but in individual patients other protocols turned out to be more efficient. The most consistent electrophysiological finding was a significant reduction of the auditory steady-state response (aSSR) after rTMS, indicating significant changes of neuronal activity in the directly stimulated auditory cortex ipsilateral to the coil placement. The reduction of the aSSR also correlated significantly with the perceived reduction of tinnitus loudness. Interestingly a similar relationship has been observed in a study where tinnitus reduction was achieved by a specific auditory stimulation (Okamoto et al., 2010). Importantly, the reduction of the aSSR was not related to the TMS intervention, but to the reduction of tinnitus induced by TMS.

The rTMS effect on the N1 depended on the frequency of the tone for which the auditory evoked response was assessed with inverse effects for low and high-frequency tones. Different explanations may account for this frequency-specific effect. First the cortical representations of the tested high-, middle-, and low-frequency tones have different localizations in the auditory cortex and may as such be reached by TMS differently. A second explanation may relate to the dependency of rTMS effects on the activity of the stimulated cortical area. Animal models of tinnitus have demonstrated differential effects of noise trauma induced tinnitus on auditory cortex excitability. Excitability in the deafferentiated area is characterized by reduced inhibitory function, whereas the normal hearing region exhibits increased inhibitory and excitatory transmission (Yang et al., 2011). Thus the differential effects of rTMS on the N1 of the different tones may reflect differential TMS effects due to differences in the excitability state of different areas in the auditory cortex of tinnitus patients.

Resting state measurements before and after the different rTMS protocols revealed a correlation between tinnitus reduction and reduction of gamma activity and increase in alpha activity (Müller et al., submitted). Similar like for the aSSR measurements these effects were only observed when rTMS resulted in a reduction of tinnitus loudness.

Thus in summary there are only few studies that assessed TMS effects over the auditory cortex on both behavioral and neuronal level. Available data suggest, that rTMS modulates thalamocortical activity and that the neuronal effects are rather related to the behavioral effects of rTMS than to the rTMS protocol itself. Thus the same rTMS protocol can have different effects on the neuronal activity of a stimulated patient. However if rTMS is able to induce specific effects on neuronal activity, this is accompanied by a reduction in tinnitus loudness.

Transcranial direct current stimulation

Based on findings of increased neuronal activity in the auditory cortex of tinnitus patients tDCS over the left temporoparietal cortex has been investigated by two studies involving relatively small sample sizes ($N = 7$, Fregni et al., 2004 and $N = 20$, Garin et al., 2011). In both studies single sessions of anodal tDCS applied over the left temporoparietal area and with the cathode placed contralateral over the supraorbital area resulted in a transient reduction of tinnitus, whereas no effect was found from a single session of cathodal tDCS applied over the left temporoparietal area. These findings are remarkable since anodal tDCS is assumed to increase cortical excitability. In some patients these effects lasted for several days (Garin et al., 2011). No studies with repeated applications of tDCS over auditory brain areas have been performed and there are also no data available that provide information about neuronal effects of temporal tDCS in tinnitus patients.

Stimulation of the auditory cortex with implanted electrodes

Neuronal activity in the auditory cortex can be also modified by direct electrical stimulation via implanted electrodes. In contrast to rTMS which can only be applied for a limited amount of time electrical stimulation via implanted electrodes can be performed permanently.

Clinical effects of stimulation of the auditory cortex with implanted electrodes. The largest sample derives from the TRI Tinnitus Clinic in Antwerp, Belgium, where 43 patients with severe treatment resistant tinnitus were implanted with a cortical electrode overlying the secondary auditory cortex (De Ridder et al., 2011c). Patients were only eligible to implantation when TMS over the auditory cortex resulted in a placebo-controlled suppression of the tinnitus on two separate occasions. Although all patients reacted to TMS, one out of three patients did not respond to the cortical stimulation after implantation. Among the responders to cortical stimulation there was an average decrease in the perceived tinnitus loudness of 51.3%. There was a significant but weak positive correlation ($r = 0.34, p < 0.05$) between the amount of the suppression effect from the preceding test TMS and cortical stimulation after implantation (De Ridder et al., 2011c).

With respect to epidural stimulation protocols, it has been observed that burst stimulation (five stimuli of 1 ms pulse width, 1 ms interpulse interval delivered at 500 Hz, 40 times a second) is more efficient than tonic stimulation. With tonic stimulation only one in three patients responded to stimulation. With burst stimulation half of the non-responding patients did benefit, resulting in a total response rate of two out of three patients. Burst stimulation was specifically superior to tonic stimulation for suppressing noise-like tinnitus (De Ridder et al., 2011c). Furthermore, treatment effects depended on tinnitus type. Pure tone tinnitus can be suppressed better than narrow band noise or the combination of pure tone and narrow band noise, and unilateral tinnitus better than bilateral tinnitus. This approach has been replicated by other centers. A French study obtained long-lasting 65% tinnitus reduction in a woman using a fMRI based extradural auditory cortex implant (Litre et al., 2009, 2010). Another study of eight patients using a similar technique but different hardware found no permanent tinnitus suppression (Friedland et al., 2007). In six out of the eight patients, temporary effects on tinnitus perception were observed. However, tinnitus distress decreased slowly over time, even without suppression of tinnitus intensity. This may be related to the fact that an electrode with only two contacts was used which limits the way the electrodes can be programmed. The finding of decreased tinnitus distress with unchanged tinnitus intensity could possibly be explained by disruption of phase synchronization between the "general distress network" and the tinnitus-related activity in the auditory cortex (De Ridder et al., 2008). Since the reduction of tinnitus distress in that study (Friedland et al., 2007) occurred slowly during the follow-up period, which was not anymore sham controlled non-specific effects cannot be ruled as well. Intracortical microstimulation in the auditory cortex of animals not only disrupts local ongoing activity but also affects long-range connections in a larger network (Deliano et al., 2009), which is similar to findings in humans using TMS of the auditory cortex (Langguth et al., 2008; May et al., 2007).

In four patients an intradural electrode on the primary auditory cortex was inserted in the Sylvian fissure, stimulating gray matter of the primary auditory cortex (De Ridder et al., 2004, 2006a). In two patients the purpose was to obtain stabilization of tinnitus suppression, because the stimulus parameters had to be reprogrammed every 2–3 days. In both patients the intradural positioning resulted in a stabilized suppression of their tinnitus. However, in the two patients who did not respond at all to epidural stimulation the intradural extracerebral stimulation was not beneficial either.

Also wire electrodes have been inserted in the primary auditory cortex, with comparable results (De Ridder et al., 2007a; Seidman et al., 2008).

Neuronal effects of stimulation of the auditory cortex with implanted electrodes. MEG during electrical stimulation of the auditory cortex revealed that the electrical stimulation increased spectral correlation across low and high gamma band activity and between alpha and beta activity, whereas delta/theta activity decreased, suggesting that auditory cortex stimulation affects thalamocortical dysrhythmia (Ramirez et al., 2009). This has been confirmed by recordings from electrodes overlying the secondary auditory cortex. Maximal tinnitus suppression was obtained by current delivery exactly at the BOLD spot, identified by tinnitus-matched sound presentation during fMRI. Recordings from this electrode revealed increased gamma and theta activity in contrast to the other electrode poles. These spectral changes normalize when stimulation induces tinnitus suppression, both on electrode and source localized EEG recordings (De Ridder et al., 2011b). Furthermore, only at the BOLD area autocorrelations showed theta–gamma coupling. These findings are in line with the hypothesis that changes in the theta- and gamma-frequency band may be causally related to a conscious auditory phantom percept as proposed by the model of thalamocortical dysrhythmia (Llinas et al., 1999; De Ridder et al., 2011b). Thus in summary EEG, MEG, and recordings from the implanted electrode support the notion that electrical stimulation reduces tinnitus perception by interfering with the abnormal thalamocortical dysrhythmia embedded in a larger tinnitus network.

Electrical stimulation of the auditory cortex has also been investigated in animal experiments where it significantly suppressed behavioral evidence of noise induced tinnitus and enhanced hearing detection (Zhang et al., 2011). In contrast auditory cortex stimulation did not induce behavioral changes in animals that did not manifest any behavioral evidence of tinnitus following the same noise exposure. These results have been interpreted in the sense that electrical stimulation of the auditory cortex may involve restoration of abnormal central auditory processing (Zhang et al., 2011).

THE RELEVANCE OF NON-AUDITORY BRAIN AREAS FOR TINNITUS

It is assumed that the activation in the auditory system is necessary but not sufficient for causing an auditory percept. Activation in the auditory system only becomes conscious if it is synchronously connected to larger co-activated "awareness" and "salience" brain networks consisting of the inferior parietal cortex, the dorsolateral prefrontal cortex, the anterior cingulated cortex (ACC), anterior insula, and the posterior cingulate cortex (PCC). Thus analogous to the global workspace model elaborated for the visual system (Dehaene et al., 2006; Baars and Franklin, 2007) and recently extended to the auditory system (Bekinschtein et al., 2009; Pegado et al., 2010), the function of the primary sensory cortices may be mainly to generate an appropriate neural discriminatory representation of the sensory input, but tinnitus only becomes conscious when activity in the auditory cortex becomes functionally connected to a network of higher order brain areas (De Ridder et al., 2011a; see **Figure 1**). This is in line with the neuroimaging literature that demonstrates involvement of both auditory and non-auditory areas in tinnitus (for an overview see **Table 3**; Adjamian et al., 2009; Lanting et al., 2009). Tinnitus-related neural networks overlap with brain regions involved in attention (Doesburg et al., 2012) to and processing of normal sounds, and in auditory memory (Schulze et al., 2011), including the primary and secondary auditory cortex, the anterior cingulate, the dorsolateral prefrontal, and the parietal cortex. Tinnitus-related brain activity also overlaps with brain areas activated by aversive sound stimulation (Mirz et al., 2000), those related to the reward and emotional system, such as nucleus accumbens, insula, and amygdala and to the hippocampal area related to memory (Langguth et al., 2011).

Tinnitus distress may then be reflected by a simultaneously co-activated distress network consisting of the anterior cingulate cortex, anterior insula, and amygdale (De Ridder et al., 2006b, 2011; Schlee et al., 2008; Vanneste et al., 2010b). This distress network is non-specific and is similarly activated in chronic pain or somatoform disorders (Landgrebe et al., 2008). An oversensitivity of this network as consequence of sensory discrimination impairment has been proposed as an additional factor in the pathogenesis of tinnitus (Landgrebe et al., 2009a).

Memory mechanisms may play a role in the persistence of the awareness of the phantom percept as well as in the reinforcement of the associated distress. Hippocampal involvement has been documented in animal models of tinnitus (Goble et al., 2009; Kraus et al., 2010) as well as by neuroimaging (Landgrebe et al., 2009b; Vanneste et al., 2011d). Accordingly, invasive supraselective amytal injection in the anterior choroidal artery, supplying the amygdalo-hippocampal area, resulted in transient reduction of the pure tone component of the contralateral tinnitus loudness (De Ridder et al., 2006b). There is an important mutual interaction between the different involved networks which may be relevant for the maintenance of tinnitus even after disappearance of the initial trigger. As an example, it has been proposed that tinnitus may be the result of a deficient sensory attentional gating mechanism originating in the subgenual cingulate cortex/nucleus accumbens area and acting on the reticular thalamic nucleus thereby modulating thalamocortical processing in the auditory system (Rauschecker et al., 2010).

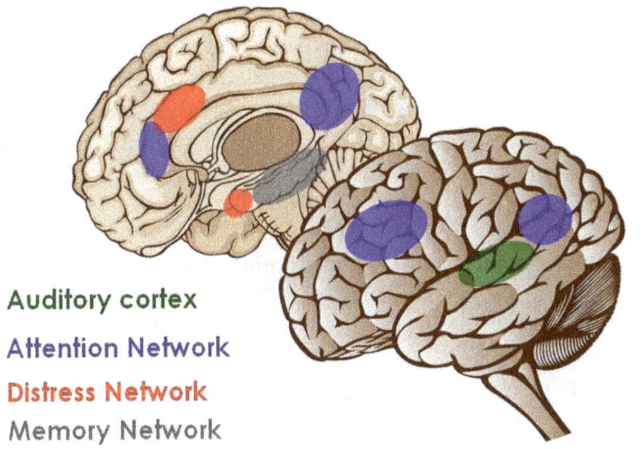

FIGURE 1 | Brain networks involved in tinnitus. Auditory deafferentation causes neuroplastic changes resulting in increased activation of the primary auditory cortex (green). Awareness of the stimulus arises when this activity is connected to a larger co-activated awareness or perceptual network. This perceptual network involves anterior and posterior cingulate cortex, precuneus, parietal cortex, and frontal cortex (blue). As a consequence of a constant learning process, the phantom percept becomes associated to distress, which is reflected by a non-specific distress network consisting of the anterior cingulate cortex, anterior insula, and amygdala (red). The persistence of the phantom percept is due to memory mechanisms involving the parahippocampal area, amygdala, and hippocampus (gray; modified from De Ridder et al., 2011a).

Pilot data suggest that the generators involved in tinnitus of recent onset seem to change over time with increased activity in several brain areas [auditory cortex, supplementary motor area, and dorsal anterior cingulate cortex (dACC) plus insula], associated with changes in connectivity between the different auditory and non-auditory brain structures. This is so both for EEG recordings (Vanneste et al., 2011e) and MEG recordings (Schlee et al., 2009). The MEG study looking at phase-locked connectivity in the tinnitus network found that in patients with a tinnitus history of less than 4 years, the left temporal cortex is predominant in the gamma band network, whereas this network is more widely distributed, including more frontal and parietal regions, in patients with tinnitus duration of more than 4 years (Schlee et al., 2009). The EEG study demonstrates a decrease of overall connectivity with increasing tinnitus duration (Vanneste et al., 2011e). An exception to this general connectivity decrease is an increase in gamma-band connectivity between the left primary and secondary auditory cortex and the left insula, and also between the auditory cortices and the right dorsolateral prefrontal cortex. These networks are both connected to the left parahippocampal area (Vanneste et al., 2011e). Thus both studies find that acute and chronic tinnitus are related to differential activity and connectivity in a network comprising the auditory cortices, insula, dACC, and premotor cortex. A recent FDG-PET study confirmed that the

Table 3 | Functional imaging studies in individuals with tinnitus: synopsis of results.

Area	Individuals with tinnitus compared to controls		Individuals with tinnitus: changes in tinnitus, induced by		
	Steady-state metabolism	Effects of sound stimulation	Somatosensory modulation	Gaze	Lidocaine
Primary auditory cortex	↑[1,2,3]	↑[4,6,17] **A**[12,13]	↕[4]		
Secondary auditory cortex		**A**[12,13]			
Auditory assoc. cortex			↕[4]	↕[5]	↕[6,7,9,10]
Thalamus		**A**[13]	↕[4]		
Inferior colliculus		↑[14,15] ↓[11] **A**[13]			
Auditory brainstem			↕[16]	↕[8]	
Limbic system		↑[4, 18]			↕[7,10]
Frontal lobe					↕[6,7]

↑, *increased asymmetry of FDG uptake.*
↓, *increased response to sound: reduced response to sound.*
↕, *increased and reduced rCBF corresponding to increased and reduced tinnitus.*
A, *abnormal assymetry.*
Studies: FDG-PET: [1]Arnold et al. (1996), [2]Wang et al. (2001), [3]Langguth et al. (2006a); H_2O-PET: [4]Lockwood et al. (1998), [5]Giraud et al. (1999), [6]Mirz et al. (1999), [7]Mirz et al. (2000), [8]Lockwood et al. (2001), [9]Reyes et al. (2002), [10]Plewnia et al. (2007a); fMRI: [11]Melcher et al. (2000), [12]Kovacs et al. (2006), [13]Smits et al. (2007), [14]Lanting et al. (2008), [15]Melcher et al. (2009), [16]Lanting et al. (2010), [17]Gu et al. (2010), [18]Leaver et al. (2011).

relative contribution of the different brain networks depends on tinnitus characteristics such as tinnitus distress or tinnitus duration (Schecklmann et al., 2011a). Thus, in summary the functional neuroimaging literature converges in the finding that tinnitus is related to functional and structural alterations in auditory and non-auditory brain areas involving an architecture of interacting and separable tinnitus-related subnetworks (De Ridder et al., 2011a; see **Figure 1**).

MODULATION OF NON-AUDITORY BRAIN AREAS

Findings of the involvement of non-auditory areas in tinnitus are limited by the correlational approach of neuroimaging which cannot inform about the real relevance of the observed alterations. Hypotheses about a causal relation can be tested by interfering with the activity in the various identified brain areas and investigating changes in tinnitus perception or annoyance. Compared to the stimulation of auditory areas much less data are available.

Effects of rTMS of non-auditory brain areas

The effects of rTMS over the dorsolateral prefrontal cortex (DLPFC), the dorsal anterior cingulated cortex (dACC), the ventrolateral prefrontal cortex (VLPFC), and the intraparietal sulcus (IPS) have been investigated. Results are summarized in **Table 4** (single sessions) and **Table 5** (repeated sessions). All mentioned studies only investigated behavioral effects of stimulation. Thus there is no information available about the neuronal changes underlying the reported behavioral changes in tinnitus patients.

Single sessions of rTMS over the dorsolateral prefrontal cortex (DLPFC). As mentioned, activity in the auditory cortex has to be linked to other "global workspace" areas such as the dorsolateral prefrontal cortex (DLPFC) in order to gain access to consciousness. The DLPFC seems to play a specific role in auditory processing. The DLPFC has a bilateral facilitatory effect on auditory memory storage and contains auditory memory cells (Bodner et al., 1996). The DLPFC also exerts early inhibitory modulation of input to primary auditory cortex in humans (Knight et al., 1989) and has been found to be associated with auditory attention (Alain et al., 1998; Voisin et al., 2006) resulting in top-down modulation of auditory processing (Mitchell et al., 2005). In order to test the involvement of the DLPFC in tinnitus it has been investigated whether rTMS of the DLPFC results in tinnitus suppression. In this study in 62 patients 1 Hz rTMS (200 pulses) over the right DLPFC resulted in a significant reduction of tinnitus loudness as compared to sham stimulation (Vanneste et al., unpublished data; **Table 4**). These data enlarge the knowledge from imaging studies by indicating the critical involvement of the right DLPFC in the pathophysiology of a subgroup of tinnitus patients.

Repeated sessions of rTMS with combined stimulation over the DLPFC and the temporal cortex. There is no published study reporting results from repeated sessions of rTMS of the DLPFC alone. However both high-frequency left rTMS and low-frequency right rTMS over the DLPFC have been combined with low-frequency rTMS over the left temporal cortex (**Table 5**). It has also been shown that left DLPFC stimulation followed by auditory cortex TMS results in better tinnitus suppression after 3 months than isolated auditory cortex stimulation (Kleinjung et al., 2008). These results could be confirmed in a large controlled trial (Langguth et al., submitted) and in a retrospective analysis of 47 patients who were treated with the combined protocol as compared to 188 patients who were stimulated only over the left temporal cortex only (Burger et al., 2011). In a recent study left temporal stimulation combined with low-frequency rTMS over the right DLPFC showed also a trend toward more pronounced effects as compared to temporal stimulation alone (Kreuzer et al., 2011).

Table 4 | Effects of single sessions of rTMS over non-auditory brain areas.

Authors	*N*	Stimulation site	Coil positioning	Frequency	Intensity	Pulses/ session	Control condition	Results
Vanneste (submitted)	62	Right DLPFC	10–20 EEG system	11 Hz	90% MT	200	Coil angulation	Significant VAS reduction/10% reduction for group, 35% for responders. 56% of patients respond
Vanneste et al. (2011c)	78	Bifrontal targeting dACC	Anatomical landmarks: 1.5 cm anterior to 1/3 of the distance from the nasion- inion	1, 3, 5, 10, 20 Hz	50% machine output	200	Coil angulation	52 placebo-negative (21 non-responders, 31 responders): 1&3 Hz significantly better than sham, 5Hz equal to sham, 10&20 Hz worse than sham.
Vanneste (submitted)	60	Left VLPFC	Anatomical landmarks	1 and 10 Hz	90% MT	200	Coil angulation	Only 10 Hz better than sham. 35 placebo negative. 22% improvement for group, 37% for responders.
Vanneste (submitted)	64 (40 + 24)	Bilateral IPS (40 patients) Left IPS (24 patients)	Anatomical landmarks	1, 5, 10 Hz	50% of maximal stimulator output	200	Coil angulation	Only 5 &10 Hz significant for bilateral IPS: 9% improvement. Only 10 Hz significant for left IPS: 10% improvement

Table 5 | Effects of repeated sessions of rTMS over non-auditory brain areas.

Authors	N	Stimulation site	Coil positioning	Frequency	Intensity	sessions	Pulses/ session	Design	Control condition	Results
Kleinjung et al. (2008)	32	Left auditory cortex; left dorsolateral prefrontal cortex	neuron avigational system, based on structural MRI	1 Hz, 20 Hz (DLPFC) + 1 Hz	110%MT	10	2000	Two active treatment conditions, parallel group design	No sham control condition	Directly after stimulation significant improvement for both stimulation conditions, at 3 months follow-up significantly better results for the combined frontal and temporal stimulation
Kreuzer et al., 2011	56	Left temporal cortex; right dorsolateral prefrontal cortex	10–20 EEg system	1 Hz	110%MT	10	2000	Two active treatment conditions, parallel group design	No sham control condition	TQ reduction in both groups immediately after stimulation, in the combined stimulated group tendency toward higher efficacy

rTMS of the dorsal anterior cingulated cortex with the double cone coil. Resting state EEG and MEG recordings in tinnitus patients have shown that the dorsal part of the anterior cingulate cortex is involved both in chronification of tinnitus (Schlee et al., 2009; Vanneste et al., 2011d) as well as in tinnitus-related distress (Weisz et al., 2005a; Vanneste et al., 2010b; De Ridder et al., 2011). The use of a double cone coil permits to modulate the activity in the dorsal part of the anterior cingulate cortex as demonstrated by a PET study (Hayward et al., 2007). In a study on 78 tinnitus patients it was shown that 1 and 3 Hz of DCC frontal TMS can improve both tinnitus intensity and tinnitus distress, 5 Hz is equal to sham and 20 Hz is significantly worse than sham (Vanneste et al., 2011c; **Table 4**). Of 78 tinnitus patients, 52 had no response to sham stimulation. Of these 52 sham negative participants, 31 patients were TMS responders. For this latter group the mean reduction of the VAS score for tinnitus intensity was 34.38%, for tinnitus-related distress 26%. These findings confirm the relevance of the dACC for tinnitus intensity and distress in a substantial part of the investigated population.

TMS of the ventrolateral prefrontal cortex. It has recently been proposed that tinnitus may be a compensatory mechanism related to incongruity emerging from a discrepancy between an expected sound and the perceived sound that is distorted due to cochlear impairment (De Ridder et al., 2011a). Visual incongruity is known to involve the ventrolateral prefrontal cortex, the anterior cingulate cortex, the supplementary motor area, and the inferior parietal area (Michelon et al., 2003). Thus a study was initiated in 60 patients targeting the left VLPFC for tinnitus suppression at 1 and 10 Hz (Vanneste et al., submitted; **Table 4**). 1 Hz TMS was no better than sham, but 10 Hz had a significant effect on tinnitus. Among those participants who did not respond to sham 10 Hz over the VLPFC suppressed tinnitus perception in average by 21.9 and by 36.7% when only responders were analyzed. Of interest is the frequency dependent effect for stimulation of the left VLPFC, which is contrary to the DLPFC where only 1 Hz revealed a reduction of tinnitus perception.

rTMS of the parietal cortex. The extremely emotional context of disabling tinnitus often leads to a higher level of selective attention directed toward the tinnitus. As such, tinnitus is a continuously distracting auditory event. Auditory attention activates the intra-partietal sulcus (IPS), and modulating the IPS with 10 Hz TMS creates the ability to ignore salient distractors (Mevorach et al., 2010). Thus it is expected that modulating the IPS may interfere with the perception of tinnitus. The effect of TMS on tinnitus has recently been evaluated using a double cone coil overlying the left IPS in 24 individuals (study 1) and in 40 individuals with the double cone coil symmetrically overlying both IPS areas (study 2; Vanneste et al., submitted; **Table 4**). In study 1 patients reported a significant transient reduction of the tinnitus percept after 10 Hz stimulation in comparison to pre-treatment, sham, and 1 Hz stimulation, respectively, with a suppression effect of 11.36%. No significant effect was obtained for 1 Hz stimulation with the coil tilted toward the left IPS. In study 2 patients revealed a significant suppression effect on 1, 5, and 10 Hz in comparison to pre-treatment. However, only stimulation at 5 and 10 Hz had a significant difference in comparison to sham with a suppression effect of respectively 8.78 and 9.50%. These data suggest that the IPS is involved in tinnitus perception and that 10 Hz TMS using the double cone coil overlying the IPS can modulate tinnitus, predominantly via the left IPS.

Effects of tDCS of non-auditory brain areas

Several studies have used tDCS to interfere with tinnitus by modulation of activity in the dorsolateral prefrontal cortex (DLPFC; Vanneste et al., 2010a; Faber et al., 2011; Vanneste and De Ridder, 2011; Frank et al., 2012). In a large study involving 448 individuals with non-pulsatile tinnitus, it was shown that a single session of tDCS with the anode over the right DLPFC and the cathode over the left DLPFC could cause tinnitus suppression in 29.9% of the participants (Vanneste et al., 2010a). In contrast the opposite stimulation procedure with the cathode over the right DLPFC and the anode over the left DLPFC had no effects in a sample of 30 patients (Vanneste et al., 2010a). Six repeated bifrontal tDCS sessions within 3 weeks with the cathode over the left DLPFC and the anode over the right DLPFC reduced tinnitus loudness, unpleasantness, and discomfort especially in female tinnitus patients (Frank et al., 2012). In a double-blind, placebo-controlled cross-over study 15 subjects with tinnitus were randomly assigned to active and sham anodal tDCS over left ($N = 8$) or right DLPFC ($N = 7$) for six sessions in a counterbalanced order, with the cathode electrode placed on the contralateral DLPFC. Both active conditions, irrespective of the anodal position decreased tinnitus annoyance but not tinnitus intensity. Furthermore, anodal stimulation of the left DLPFC had a significant effect on depression, whereas anodal stimulation of the right DLPFC reduced symptoms of anxiety (Faber et al., 2011).

In conclusion, these preliminary studies indicate that both anodal stimulation of the left auditory cortex and bifrontal tDCS with the cathode left and the anode right can have beneficial effects on tinnitus in some individuals. The interindividual variability of treatment effects is high in all studies, suggesting that there may be pathophysiologically distinct forms of tinnitus that respond particularly well to different tDCS protocols (Vanneste et al., 2011c).

In order to unravel the mechanism by which tDCS suppresses tinnitus EEG measurements were performed before and after single sessions of bifrontal tDCS in 12 patients who responded to tDCS. Reduction of tinnitus intensity and tinnitus-related distress was related to modulation of neuronal activity in pregenual anterior cingulate cortex, parahippocampal area, and right primary auditory cortex regions (Vanneste et al., 2011a). These findings are comparable to those obtained in healthy controls after a similar tDCS intervention (anode positioned over the left DLPFC and the cathode over the right supraorbital region), that revealed a tDCS induced modulation of regional electrical activity in the left subgenual prefrontal cortex, the anterior cingulate cortex and the left parahippocampus (Keeser et al., 2011b) and significant changes of regional brain connectivity both for the default mode network and the fronto-parietal network (Keeser et al., 2011a).

Effects of direct electric stimulation of non-auditory brain areas

In a few tinnitus patients also implanted electrodes have been used to stimulate non-auditory brain areas. In one patient with intractable tinnitus electrodes have been implanted over the DLPFC (De Ridder et al., 2011d). Knowledge about the effects of DBS derives from patients who received DBS for movement disorders and suffered from comorbid tinnitus.

Effects of epidural electrodes over the DLPFC. In a patient intractable to conservative medical management and TMS of the auditory cortex, a neuronavigation-based auditory fMRI-guided frontal cortex TMS session was performed in a placebo-controlled way, yielding 50% tinnitus suppression. Based on the same concept of epidural auditory cortex stimulation and motor cortex stimulation, this TMS result was used as a predictive indication to implant two extradural electrodes (De Ridder et al., 2011d). The exact localization was determined by the fMRI–BOLD response in the DLPFC during presentation of a sound that was matched to the individual tinnitus sound. Postoperatively the tinnitus immediately improved by 66.67% and has progressively continued to improve for more than 1 year. The initial VAS of 8/10 has decreased after 1 year to 2/10. This suggests that in selected patients focal extradural electrical stimulation of the dorsolateral prefrontal cortex at the area of tinnitus-matched sound elected BOLD activation is capable of suppressing contralateral tinnitus partially.

Effects of deep brain stimulation. Whereas rTMS, tDCS, and epidural stimulation exert their effects primarily in superficial brain regions, DBS can modulate brain activity very focally in deeper brain regions. To our knowledge there are no published reports of patients who received DBS for the treatment of tinnitus. However, results are available from patients who received DBS in the ventralis intermedius nucleus of the thalamus (Shi et al., 2009) or in the caudate nucleus (Cheung and Larson, 2010) for movement disorders who also reported having tinnitus.

In one study, seven patients implanted with DBS systems for movement disorders who also reported having tinnitus were interviewed and asked about their tinnitus conditions. Three of the seven patients reported reduced tinnitus loudness when DBS was turned on. Of the four patients tested in a specialized tinnitus clinic, results indicated that DBS of the ventralis intermedius nucleus of the thalamus caused decreases in tinnitus loudness in two patients with relatively prolonged residual inhibition (Shi et al., 2009).

The caudate is routinely traversed during DBS implantation of the subthalamic nucleus and ventral intermediate nucleus in awake patients for treatment of Parkinson's disease and essential tremor, respectively. In six tinnitus patients who underwent DBS for movement disorders. the effect of DBS in the locus of caudate neurons (area LC) was evaluated with respect to the patients' tinnitus (Cheung and Larson, 2010). In five subjects tinnitus loudness in both ears was suppressed to an intensity level 2/10 or less. In one subject, where the DBS lead was outside the area LC, tinnitus was not modulated. Hearing thresholds were unchanged by area LC stimulation.

These results suggest that DBS of non-auditory thalamus and caudate structures may provide tinnitus relief for some patients. The mechanisms involved in tinnitus suppression by DBS are yet unknown, but it has been suggested that stimulation of area LC of the caudate nucleus may modulate auditory gating function (Larson and Cheung, 2012).

CONCLUSION

Imaging studies demonstrate that tinnitus is related to structural and functional alterations in multiple brain structures including auditory cortex, thalamus, dorsal, and subgenual anterior and posterior cingulated cortex, ventromedial prefrontal, and dorsolateral prefrontal cortex, parietal cortex, precuneus, insula, amygdale, hippocampus, and parahippocampus. The findings from imaging studies are complemented by brain stimulation studies that demonstrate reduction of tinnitus loudness and/or distress after stimulation of temporal, temporoparietal, parietal, dorsolateral and ventromedial prefrontal cortex, and ACC.

It has been suggested that different aspects of tinnitus such as perceptual aspects (loudness, tone-, or noise-like, laterality), attention, salience, distress, mood, memory, and duration are reflected by the involvement of specific networks (De Ridder et al., 2011a), a claim which is currently only partly supported by empirical evidence from imaging or brain stimulation studies. This may also be due to methodological difficulties related to (1) reliable assessment of the different aspects of tinnitus, (2) the need for large samples in order to differentiate the neuronal correlate of specific aspects, (3) the limited resolution and sensitivity of the currently used imaging techniques, and (4) incomplete understanding of the mechanisms of action of the various brain stimulation techniques.

In spite of these constraints the available data demonstrate that focal modulation of neuronal activity by brain stimulation techniques provides a useful complementary approach to neuroimaging, which is limited by its strictly correlational character. Important added value can be obtained by investigating the effects of focal modulation of the different areas showing up in functional imaging studies of tinnitus. Assessment of neuronal changes related to tinnitus reduction or worsening can reveal important information about which neuronal changes are directly related to tinnitus and which reflect predisposition, compensatory changes, or epiphenomena. Thus, correlations between brain activity and/or connectivity and tinnitus can tentatively be turned into causal relationships. This can be performed for tinnitus as a unified percept, or for specific aspects of tinnitus (e.g., distress, depression, loudness,...) if well controlled for other aspects. This will ultimately lead to a better understanding of which areas or subnetworks are critically involved in the generation of each aspect of tinnitus and ultimately in tinnitus as a unified percept. The pathophysiological neural correlates could subsequently provide important information for improving brain stimulation techniques as a treatment strategy.

REFERENCES

Adjamian, P., Sereda, M., and Hall, D. A. (2009). The mechanisms of tinnitus: perspectives from human functional neuroimaging. *Hear. Res.* 253, 15–31.

Alain, C., Woods, D. L., and Knight, R. T. (1998). A distributed cortical network for auditory sensory memory in humans. *Brain Res.* 812, 23–37.

Anders, M., Dvorakova, J., Rathova, L., Havrankova, P., Pelcova, P., Vaneckova, M., Jech, R., Holcat, M., Seidl, Z., and Raboch, J. (2010). Efficacy of repetitive transcranial magnetic stimulation for the treatment of refractory chronic tinnitus: a randomized, placebo controlled study. *Neuro Endocrinol. Lett.* 31, 238–249.

Arnold, W., Bartenstein, P., Oestreicher, E., Romer, W., and Schwaiger, M. (1996). Focal metabolic activation in the predominant left auditory cortex in patients suffering from tinnitus: a PET study with [18F]deoxyglucose. *ORL J. Otorhinolaryngol. Relat. Spec.* 58, 195–199.

Attias, J., Furman, V., Shemesh, Z., and Bresloff, I. (1996). Impaired brain processing in noise-induced tinnitus patients as measured by auditory and visual event-related potentials. *Ear Hear.* 17, 327–333.

Attias, J., Urbach, D., Gold, S., and Shemesh, Z. (1993). Auditory event related potentials in chronic tinnitus patients with noise induced hearing loss. *Hear. Res.* 71, 106–113.

Baars, B. J., and Franklin, S. (2007). An architectural model of conscious and unconscious brain functions: global workspace theory and IDA. *Neural Netw.* 20, 955–961.

Barker, A. T., Jalinous, R., and Freeston, I. L. (1985). Non-invasive magnetic stimulation of human motor cortex. *Lancet* 1, 1106–1107.

Bekinschtein, T. A., Dehaene, S., Rohaut, B., Tadel, F., Cohen, L., and Naccache, L. (2009). Neural signature of the conscious processing of auditory regularities. *Proc. Natl. Acad. Sci. U.S.A.* 106, 1672–1677.

Bodner, M., Kroger, J., and Fuster, J. M. (1996). Auditory memory cells in dorsolateral prefrontal cortex. *Neuroreport* 7, 1905–1908.

Borchers, S., Himmelbach, M., Logothetis, N., and Karnath, H. O. (2011). Direct electrical stimulation of human cortex – the gold standard for mapping brain functions? *Nat. Rev. Neurosci.* 3, 63–70.

Burger, J., Frank, E., Kreuzer, P., Kleinjung, T., Vielsmeier, V., Landgrebe, M., Hajak, G., and Langguth, B. (2011). Transcranial magnetic stimulation for the treatment of tinnitus: 4-year follow-up in treatment responders-a retrospective analysis. *Brain Stimul.* 4, 222–227.

Cheung, S. W., and Larson, P. S. (2010). Tinnitus modulation by deep brain stimulation in locus of caudate neurons (area LC). *Neuroscience* 169, 1768–1778.

Chung, H. K., Tsai, C. H., Lin, Y. C., Chen, J. M., Tsou, Y. A., Wang, C. Y., Lin, C. D., Jeng, F. C., Chung, J. G., and Tsai, M. H. (2011). Effectiveness of theta-burst repetitive transcranial magnetic stimulation for treating chronic tinnitus. *Audiol. Neurootol.* 17, 112–120.

De Ridder, D., De Mulder, G., Verstraeten, E., Seidman, M., Elisevich, K., Sunaert, S., Kovacs, S., Van der Kelen, K., Van de Heyning, P., and Moller, A. (2007a). Auditory cortex stimulation for tinnitus. *Acta Neurochir. Suppl.* 97, 451–462.

De Ridder, D., De Mulder, G., Verstraeten, E., Sunaert, S., and Moller, A. (2007b). Somatosensory cortex stimulation for deafferentation pain. *Acta Neurochir. Suppl.* 97, 67–74.

De Ridder, D., van der Loo, E., Van der Kelen, K., Menovsky, T., Van de Heyning, P., and Moller, A. (2007c). Do tonic and burst TMS modulate the lemniscal and extralemniscal system differentially? *Int. J. Med. Sci.* 4, 242–246.

De Ridder, D., van der Loo, E., Van der Kelen, K., Menovsky, T., Van de Heyning, P., and Moller, A. (2007d). Theta, alpha and beta burst transcranial magnetic stimulation: brain modulation in tinnitus. *Int. J. Med. Sci.* 4, 237–241.

De Ridder, D., De Mulder, G., Verstraeten, E., Van der Kelen, K., Sunaert, S., Smits, M., Kovacs, S., Verlooy, J., Van de Heyning, P., and Moller, A. R. (2006a). Primary and secondary auditory cortex stimulation for intractable tinnitus. *ORL J. Otorhinolaryngol. Relat. Spec.* 68, 48–54.

De Ridder, D., Fransen, H., Francois, O., Sunaert, S., Kovacs, S., and Van de Heyning, P. (2006b). Amygdalohippocampal involvement in tinnitus and auditory memory. *Acta Otolaryngol. Suppl.* 556, 50–53.

De Ridder, D., De Mulder, G., Walsh, V., Muggleton, N., Sunaert, S., and Moller, A. (2004). Magnetic and electrical stimulation of the auditory cortex for intractable tinnitus. Case report. *J. Neurosurg.* 100, 560–564.

De Ridder, D., Elgoyhen, A. B., Romo, R., and Langguth, B. (2011a). Phantom percepts: tinnitus and pain as persisting aversive memory networks. *Proc. Natl. Acad. Sci. U.S.A.* 108, 8075–8080.

De Ridder, D., van der Loo, E., Vanneste, S., Gais, S., Plazier, M., Kovacs, S., Sunaert, S., Menovsky, T., and Van de Heyning, P. (2011b). Theta-gamma dysrhythmia and auditory phantom perception. *J. Neurosurg.* 114, 912–921.

De Ridder, D., Vanneste, S., Kovacs, S., Sunaert, S., Menovsky, T., Van de Heyning, P., and Moller, A. (2011c). Transcranial magnetic stimulation and extradural electrodes implanted on secondary auditory cortex for tinnitus suppression. *J. Neurosurg.* 114, 903–911.

De Ridder, D., Vanneste, S., Plazier, M., Menovsky, T., Van de, H. P., Kovacs, S., and Sunaert, S. (2011d). Dorsolateral prefrontal cortex transcranial magnetic stimulation and electrode implant for intractable tinnitus. *World Neurosurg.* PMID: 22120273. [Epub ahead of print].

De Ridder, D., Menovsky, T., and Van de Heyning, P. (2008). Auditory cortex stimulation for tinnitus suppression. *Otol. Neurotol.* 29, 574–575.

De Ridder, D., Vanneste, S., and Congedo, M. (2011). The distressed brain: a group blind source separation analysis on tinnitus. *PLoS ONE* 6, e24273. doi:10.1371/journal.pone.0024273

De Ridder, D., Vanneste, S., van der Loo, E., Plazier, M., Menovsky, T., and Van de Heyning, P. (2010). Burst stimulation of the auditory cortex: a new form of neurostimulation for noise-like tinnitus suppression. *J. Neurosurg.* 112, 1289–1294.

De Ridder, D., Verstraeten, E., Van der, K. K., De Mulder, G., Sunaert, S., Verlooy, J., Van de, H. P., and Moller, A. (2005). Transcranial magnetic stimulation for tinnitus: influence of tinnitus duration on stimulation parameter choice and maximal tinnitus suppression. *Otol. Neurotol.* 26, 616–619.

Dehaene, S., Changeux, J. P., Naccache, L., Sackur, J., and Sergent, C. (2006). Conscious, preconscious, and subliminal processing: a testable taxonomy. *Trends Cogn. Sci. (Regul. Ed.)* 10, 204–211.

Deliano, M., Scheich, H., and Ohl, F. W. (2009). Auditory cortical activity after intracortical microstimulation and its role for sensory processing and learning. *J. Neurosci.* 29, 15898–15909.

Doesburg, S. M., Green, J. J., McDonald, J. J., and Ward, L. M. (2012). Theta modulation of inter-regional gamma synchronization during auditory attention control. *Brain Res.* 1431, 77–85.

Dymond, A. M., Coger, R. W., and Serafetinides, E. A. (1975). Intracerebral current levels in man during electrosleep therapy. *Biol. Psychiatry* 10, 101–104.

Eggermont, J. J., and Roberts, L. E. (2004). The neuroscience of tinnitus. *Trends Neurosci.* 27, 676–682.

Eichhammer, P., Kleinjung, T., Landgrebe, M., Hajak, G., and Langguth, B. (2007). TMS for treatment of chronic tinnitus: neurobiological effects. *Prog. Brain Res.* 166, 369–375.

Faber, M., Vanneste, S., Fregni, F., and De, R. D. (2011). Top down prefrontal affective modulation of tinnitus with multiple sessions of tDCS of dorsolateral prefrontal cortex. *Brain Stimul.* doi: 10.1016/j.brs.2011.09.003. [Epub ahead of print].

Folmer, R. L., Carroll, J. R., Rahim, A., Shi, Y., and Hal Martin, W. (2006). Effects of repetitive transcranial magnetic stimulation (rTMS) on chronic tinnitus. *Acta Otolaryngol. Suppl.* 556, 96–101.

Frank, E., Schecklmann, M., Landgrebe, M., Burger, J., Kreuzer, P., Poeppl, T. B., Kleinjung, T., Hajak, G., and Langguth, B. (2012). Treatment of chronic tinnitus with repeated sessions of prefrontal transcranial direct current stimulation: outcomes from an open-label pilot study. *J. Neurol.* 259, 327–333.

Frank, G., Kleinjung, T., Landgrebe, M., Vielsmeier, V., Steffenhagen, C., Burger, J., Frank, E., Vollberg, G., Hajak, G., and Langguth, B. (2010). Left temporal low-frequency rTMS for the treatment of tinnitus: clinical predictors of treatment outcome – a retrospective study. *Eur. J. Neurol.* 17, 951–956.

Fregni, F., Santos, C. M., Myczkowski, M. L., Rigolino, R., Gallucci-Neto, J., Barbosa, E. R., Valente, K. D., Pascual-Leone, A., and Marcolin, M. A. (2004). Repetitive transcranial magnetic stimulation is as effective as fluoxetine in the treatment of depression in patients with Parkinson's disease. *J. Neurol. Neurosurg. Psychiatr.* 75, 1171–1174.

Fregni, F., Marcondes, R., Boggio, P. S., Marcolin, M. A., Rigonatti, S. P., Sanchez, T. G., Nitsche, M. A., and Pascual-Leone, A. (2006). Transient tinnitus suppression induced by repetitive transcranial magnetic stimulation and transcranial direct current stimulation. *Eur. J. Neurol.* 13, 996–1001.

Friedland, D. R., Gaggl, W., Runge-Samuelson, C., Ulmer, J. L., and Kopell, B. H. (2007). Feasibility of auditory cortical stimulation for the treatment of tinnitus. *Otol. Neurotol.* 28, 1005–1012.

Garin, P., Gilain, C., Van Damme, J. P., de, F. K., Jamart, J., Ossemann, M., and Vandermeeren, Y. (2011). Short- and long-lasting tinnitus relief induced by transcranial direct current stimulation. *J. Neurol.* 258, 1940–1948.

George, M. S., and ston-Jones, G. (2010). Noninvasive techniques for probing neurocircuitry and treating illness: vagus nerve stimulation (VNS), transcranial magnetic stimulation (TMS) and transcranial direct current stimulation (tDCS). *Neuropsychopharmacology* 35, 301–316.

Giraud, A. L., Chéry-Croze, S., Fischer, G., Fischer, C., Vighetto, A., Grégoire, M. C., Lavenne, F., and Collet, L. (1999). A selective imaging of tinnitus. *Neuroreport* 10, 1–5.

Goble, T. J., Moller, A. R., and Thompson, L. T. (2009). Acute high-intensity sound exposure alters responses of place cells in hippocampus. *Hear. Res.* 253, 52–59.

Gu, J. W., Halpin, C. F., Nam, E. C., Levine, R. A., and Melcher, J. R. (2010). Tinnitus, diminished sound-level tolerance, and elevated auditory activity in humans with clinically normal hearing sensitivity. *J. Neurophysiol.* 104, 3361–3370.

Hallett, M. (2000). Transcranial magnetic stimulation and the human brain. *Nature* 406, 147–150.

Hayward, G., Mehta, M. A., Harmer, C., Spinks, T. J., Grasby, P. M., and Goodwin, G. M. (2007). Exploring the physiological effects of double-cone coil TMS over the medial frontal cortex on the anterior cingulate cortex: an H2(15)O PET study. *Eur. J. Neurosci.* 25, 2224–2233.

Hoffman, R. E., and Cavus, I. (2002). Slow transcranial magnetic stimulation, long-term depotentiation, and brain hyperexcitability disorders. *Am. J. Psychiatry* 159, 1093–1102.

House, J. W., and Brackmann, D. E. (1981). Tinnitus: surgical treatment. *Ciba Found. Symp.* 85, 204–216.

Hu, B., Senatorov, V., and Mooney, D. (1994). Lemniscal and non-lemniscal synaptic transmission in rat auditory thalamus. *J. Physiol. (Lond.)* 479(Pt 2), 217–231.

Huang, Y. Z., Edwards, M. J., Rounis, E., Bhatia, K. P., and Rothwell, J. C. (2005). Theta burst stimulation of the human motor cortex. *Neuron* 45, 201–206.

Keeser, D., Meindl, T., Bor, J., Palm, U., Pogarell, O., Mulert, C., Brunelin, J., Moller, H. J., Reiser, M., and Padberg, F. (2011a). Prefrontal transcranial direct current stimulation changes connectivity of resting-state networks during fMRI. *J. Neurosci.* 31, 15284–15293.

Keeser, D., Padberg, F., Reisinger, E., Pogarell, O., Kirsch, V., Palm, U., Karch, S., Moller, H. J., Nitsche, M. A., and Mulert, C. (2011b). Prefrontal direct current stimulation modulates resting EEG and event-related potentials in healthy subjects: a standardized low resolution tomography (sLORETA) study. *Neuroimage* 55, 644–657.

Khedr, E. M., bo-Elfetoh, N., Rothwell, J. C., El-Atar, A., Sayed, E., and Khalifa, H. (2010). Contralateral versus ipsilateral rTMS of temporoparietal cortex for the treatment of chronic unilateral tinnitus: comparative study. *Eur. J. Neurol.* 17, 976–983.

Khedr, E. M., Rothwell, J. C., Ahmed, M. A., and El-Atar, A. (2008). Effect of daily repetitive transcranial magnetic stimulation for treatment of tinnitus: comparison of different stimulus frequencies. *J. Neurol. Neurosurg. Psychiatr.* 79, 212–215.

Khedr, E. M., Rothwell, J. C., El-Atar, A. (2009). One-year follow up of patients with chronic tinnitus treated with left temporoparietal rTMS. *Eur. J. Neurol.* 16, 404–408.

Kleinjung, T., Eichhammer, P., Landgrebe, M., Sand, P., Hajak, G., Steffens, T., Strutz, J., and Langguth, B. (2008). Combined temporal and prefrontal transcranial magnetic stimulation for tinnitus treatment: a pilot study. *Otolaryngol. Head Neck Surg.* 138, 497–501.

Kleinjung, T., Eichhammer, P., Langguth, B., Jacob, P., Marienhagen, J., Hajak, G., Wolf, S. R., and Strutz, J. (2005). Long-term effects of repetitive transcranial magnetic stimulation (rTMS) in patients with chronic tinnitus. *Otolaryngol. Head Neck Surg.* 132, 566–569.

Kleinjung, T., Steffens, T., Landgrebe, M., Vielsmeier, V., Frank, E., Burger, J., Strutz, J., Hajak, G., and Langguth, B. (2011). Repetitive transcranial magnetic stimulation for tinnitus treatment: no enhancement by the dopamine and noradrenaline reuptake inhibitor bupropion. *Brain Stimul.* 4, 65–70.

Kleinjung, T., Steffens, T., Landgrebe, M., Vielsmeier, V., Frank, E., Hajak, G., Strutz, J., and Langguth, B. (2009). Levodopa does not enhance the effect of low-frequency repetitive transcranial magnetic stimulation in tinnitus treatment. *Otolaryngol. Head Neck Surg.* 140, 92–95.

Kleinjung, T., and Langguth, B. (2009). Strategies for enhancement of transcranial magnetic stimulation effects in tinnitus patients. *Int. Tinnitus J.* 15, 154–160.

Kleinjung, T., Steffens, T., Sand, P., Murthum, T., Hajak, G., Strutz, J., Langguth, B., and Eichhammer, P. (2007). Which tinnitus patients benefit from transcranial magnetic stimulation? *Otolaryngol. Head Neck Surg.* 137, 589–595.

Knight, R. T., Scabini, D., and Woods, D. L. (1989). Prefrontal cortex gating of auditory transmission in humans. *Brain Res.* 504, 338–342.

Kovacs, S., Peeters, R., Smits, M., De Ridder, D., Van Hecke, P., and Sunaert, S. (2006). Activation of cortical and subcortical auditory structures at 3 T by means of a functional magnetic resonance imaging paradigm suitable for clinical use. *Invest. Radiol.* 41, 87–96.

Kraus, K. S., Mitra, S., Jimenez, Z., Hinduja, S., Ding, D., Jiang, H., Gray, L., Lobarinas, E., Sun, W., and Salvi, R. J. (2010). Noise trauma impairs neurogenesis in the rat hippocampus. *Neuroscience* 167, 1216–1226.

Kreuzer, P. M., Landgrebe, M., Schecklmann, M., Poeppl, T. B., Vielsmeier, V., Hajak, G., Kleinjung, T., and Langguth, B. (2011). Can temporal repetitive transcranial magnetic stimulation be enhanced by targeting affective components of tinnitus with frontal rTMS? A randomized controlled pilot trial. *Front. Syst. Neurosci.* 5:88. doi:10.3389/fnsys.2011.00088

Kringelbach, M. L., Jenkinson, N., Owen, S. L., and Aziz, T. Z. (2007). Translational principles of deep brain stimulation. *Nat. Rev. Neurosci.* 8, 623–635.

Landgrebe, M., Barta, W., Rosengarth, K., Frick, U., Hauser, S., Langguth, B., Rutschmann, R., Greenlee, M. W., Hajak, G., and Eichhammer, P. (2008). Neuronal correlates of symptom formation in functional somatic syndromes: a fMRI study. *Neuroimage* 41, 1336–1344.

Landgrebe, M., Frick, U., Hauser, S., Hajak, G., and Langguth, B. (2009a). Association of tinnitus and electromagnetic hypersensitivity: hints for a shared pathophysiology? *PLoS*

ONE 4, e5026. doi:10.1371/journal.pone.0005026

Landgrebe, M., Langguth, B., Rosengarth, K., Braun, S., Koch, A., Kleinjung, T., May, A., De Ridder, D., and Hajak, G. (2009b). Structural brain changes in tinnitus: grey matter decrease in auditory and non-auditory brain areas. *Neuroimage* 46, 213–218.

Langguth, B., Eichhammer, P., Kreutzer, A., Maenner, P., Marienhagen, J., Kleinjung, T., Sand, P., and Hajak, G. (2006a). The impact of auditory cortex activity on characterizing and treating patients with chronic tinnitus – first results from a PET study. *Acta Otolaryngol. Suppl.* 556, 84–88.

Langguth, B., Zowe, M., Landgrebe, M., Sand, P., Kleinjung, T., Binder, H., Hajak, G., and Eichhammer, P. (2006b). Transcranial magnetic stimulation for the treatment of tinnitus: a new coil positioning method and first results. *Brain Topogr.* 18, 241–247.

Langguth, B., Kleinjung, T., Landgrebe, M., De Ridder, D., and Hajak, G. (2010). rTMS for the treatment of tinnitus: the role of neuronavigation for coil positioning. *Neurophysiol. Clin.* 40, 45–58.

Langguth, B., Kleinjung, T., Frank, E., Landgrebe, M., Sand, P., Dvorakova, J., Frick, U., Eichhammer, P., Hajak, G. (2008). High-frequency priming stimulation does not enhance the effect of low-frequency rTMS in the treatment of tinnitus. *Exp. Brain Res.* 184, 587–591.

Langguth, B., Landgrebe, M., Kleinjung, T., Sand, G. P., and Hajak, G. (2011). Tinnitus and depression. *World J. Biol. Psychiatry* 12, 489–500.

Lanting, C. P., De, K. E., Bartels, H., and Van, D. P. (2008). Functional imaging of unilateral tinnitus using fMRI. *Acta Otolaryngol.* 128, 415–421.

Lanting, C. P., de Kleine, E., Eppinga, R. N., and van Dijk, P. (2010). Neural correlates of human somatosensory integration in tinnitus. *Hear. Res.* 267, 78–88.

Lanting, C. P., De Kleine, E., and Van Dijk, P. (2009). Neural activity underlying tinnitus generation: results from PET and fMRI. *Hear. Res.* 255, 1–13.

Larson, P. S., and Cheung, S. W. (2012). Deep brain stimulation in area LC controllably triggers auditory phantom percepts. *Neurosurgery* 70, 398–405.

Leaver, A. M., Renier, L., Chevillet, M. A., Morgan, S., Kim, H. J., and Rauschecker, J. P. (2011). Dysregulation of limbic and auditory networks in tinnitus. *Neuron* 69, 33–43.

Lee, S. L., Abraham, M., Cacace, A. T., and Silver, S. M. (2008). Repetitive transcranial magnetic stimulation in veterans with debilitating tinnitus: a pilot study. *Otolaryngol. Head Neck Surg.* 138, 398–399.

Lefaucheur, J. P., Menard-Lefaucheur, I., Goujon, C., Keravel, Y., and Nguyen, J. P. (2011). Predictive value of rTMS in the identification of responders to epidural motor cortex stimulation therapy for pain. *J. Pain.* 12, 1102–1111.

Litre, C. F., Giersky, F., Theret, E., Leveque, M., Peruzzi, P., and Rousseaux, P. (2010). Feasibility of auditory cortical stimulation for the treatment of tinnitus. Three case reports. *Neurochirurgie* 56, 303–308.

Litre, C. F., Theret, E., Tran, H., Leveque, M., Portefaix, C., Gierski, F., Emeriau, S., and Peruzzi, P. (2009). Surgical treatment by electrical stimulation of the auditory cortex for intractable tinnitus. *Brain Stimul.* 2, 132–137.

Llinas, R. R., Ribary, U., Jeanmonod, D., Kronberg, E., and Mitra, P. P. (1999). Thalamocortical dysrhythmia: a neurological and neuropsychiatric syndrome characterized by magnetoencephalography. *Proc. Natl. Acad. Sci. U.S.A.* 96, 15222–15227.

Lockwood, A. H., Salvi, R. J., Coad, M. L., Towsley, M. L., Wack, D. S., and Murphy, B. W. (1998). The functional neuroanatomy of tinnitus: evidence for limbic system links and neural plasticity. *Neurology* 50, 114–120.

Lockwood, A. H., Wack, D. S., Burkard, R. F., Coad, M. L., Reyes, S. A., Arnold, S. A., and Salvi, R. J. (2001). The functional anatomy of gaze-evoked tinnitus and sustained lateral gaze. *Neurology* 56, 472–480.

Londero, A., Lefaucheur, J. P., Malinvaud, D., Brugieres, P., Peignard, P., Nguyen, J. P., Avan, P., and Bonfils, P. (2006). Magnetic stimulation of the auditory cortex for disabling tinnitus: preliminary results. *Presse Med.* 35, 200–206.

Lorenz, I., Muller, N., Schlee, W., Langguth, B., and Weisz, N. (2010). Short-term effects of single repetitive TMS sessions on auditory evoked activity in patients with chronic tinnitus. *J. Neurophysiol.* 104, 1497–1505.

Marcondes, R. A., Sanchez, T. G., Kii, M. A., Ono, C. R., Buchpiguel, C. A., Langguth, B., and Marcolin, M. A. (2010). Repetitive transcranial magnetic stimulation improve tinnitus in normal hearing patients: a double-blind controlled, clinical and neuroimaging outcome study. *Eur. J. Neurol.* 17, 38–44.

May, A., Hajak, G., Ganssbauer, S., Steffens, T., Langguth, B., Kleinjung, T., and Eichhammer, P. (2007). Structural brain alterations following 5 days of intervention: dynamic aspects of neuroplasticity. *Cereb. Cortex* 17, 205–210.

Meeus, O., Blaivie, C., Ost, J., De Ridder, D., and Van de Heyning, P. (2009). Influence of tonic and burst transcranial magnetic stimulation characteristics on acute inhibition of subjective tinnitus. *Otol. Neurotol.* 30, 697–703.

Melcher, J. R., Levine, R. A., Bergevin, C., and Norris, B. (2009). The auditory midbrain of people with tinnitus: abnormal sound-evoked activity revisited. *Hear. Res.* 257, 63–74.

Melcher, J. R., Sigalovsky, I. S., Guinan, J. J. Jr., and Levine, R. A. (2000). Lateralized tinnitus studied with functional magnetic resonance imaging: abnormal inferior colliculus activation. *J. Neurophysiol.* 83, 1058–1072.

Mennemeier, M., Chelette, K. C., Allen, S., Bartel, T. B., Triggs, W., Kimbrell, T., Crew, J., Munn, T., Brown, G. J., and Dornhoffer, J. (2011). Variable changes in PET activity before and after rTMS treatment for tinnitus. *Laryngoscope* 121, 815–822.

Mevorach, C., Hodsoll, J., Allen, H., Shalev, L., and Humphreys, G. (2010). Ignoring the elephant in the room: a neural circuit to downregulate salience. *J. Neurosci.* 30, 6072–6079.

Michelon, P., Snyder, A. Z., Buckner, R. L., McAvoy, M., and Zacks, J. M. (2003). Neural correlates of incongruous visual information. An event-related fMRI study. *Neuroimage* 19, 1612–1626.

Minami, S. B., Shinden, S., Okamoto, Y., Watada, Y., Watabe, T., Oishi, N., Kanzaki, S., Saito, H., Inoue, Y., and Ogawa, K. (2011). Repetitive transcranial magnetic stimulation (rTMS) for treatment of chronic tinnitus. *Auris Nasus Larynx* 38, 301–306.

Mirz, F., Gjedde, A., Sodkilde-Jrgensen, H., and Pedersen, C. B. (2000). Functional brain imaging of tinnitus-like perception induced by aversive auditory stimuli. *Neuroreport* 11, 633–637.

Mirz, F., Pedersen, B., Ishizu, K., Johannsen, P., Ovesen, T., Stødkilde-Jørgensen, H., and Gjedde, A. (1999). Positron emission tomography of cortical centers of tinnitus. *Hear. Res.* 134, 133–144.

Mitchell, T. V., Morey, R. A., Inan, S., and Belger, A. (2005). Functional magnetic resonance imaging measure of automatic and controlled auditory processing. *Neuroreport* 16, 457–461.

Moazami-Goudarzi, M., Michels, L., Weisz, N., and Jeanmonod, D. (2010). Temporo-insular enhancement of EEG low and high frequencies in patients with chronic tinnitus. QEEG study of chronic tinnitus patients. *BMC Neurosci.* 11, 40. doi:10.1186/1471-2202-11-40

Nguyen, J. P., Keravel, Y., Feve, A., Uchiyama, T., Cesaro, P., Le, G. C., and Pollin, B. (1997). Treatment of deafferentation pain by chronic stimulation of the motor cortex: report of a series of 20 cases. *Acta Neurochir. Suppl.* 68, 54–60.

Nitsche, M. A., and Paulus, W. (2000). Excitability changes induced in the human motor cortex by weak transcranial direct current stimulation. *J. Physiol. (Lond.)* 527(Pt 3), 633–639.

Nitsche, M. A., and Paulus, W. (2001). Sustained excitability elevations induced by transcranial DC motor cortex stimulation in humans 3. *Neurology* 57, 1899–1901.

Norena, A., Cransac, H., and Chery-Croze, S. (1999). Towards an objectification by classification of tinnitus. *Clin. Neurophysiol.* 110, 666–675.

Norena, A., Micheyl, C., Chery-Croze, S., and Collet, L. (2002). Psychoacoustic characterization of the tinnitus spectrum: implications for the underlying mechanisms of tinnitus. *Audiol. Neurootol.* 7, 358–369.

Norena, A. J. (2011). An integrative model of tinnitus based on a central gain controlling neural sensitivity. *Neurosci. Biobehav. Rev.* 35, 1089–1109.

Norena, A. J., and Eggermont, J. J. (2005). Enriched acoustic environment after noise trauma reduces hearing loss and prevents cortical map reorganization. *J. Neurosci.* 25, 699–705.

Okamoto, H., Stracke, H., Stoll, W., and Pantev, C. (2010). Listening to tailor-made notched music reduces tinnitus loudness and tinnitus-related auditory cortex activity. *Proc. Natl. Acad. Sci. U.S.A.* 107, 1207–1210.

Pegado, F., Bekinschtein, T., Chausson, N., Dehaene, S., Cohen, L., and Naccache, L. (2010). Probing the lifetimes of auditory novelty detection processes. *Neuropsychologia* 48, 3145–3154.

Piccirillo, J. F., Garcia, K. S., Nicklaus, J., Pierce, K., Burton, H., Vlassenko, A. G., Mintun, M., Duddy, D., Kallogjeri, D., and Spitznagel, E. L. Jr. (2011). Low-frequency repetitive transcranial magnetic stimulation to the temporoparietal junction for tinnitus. *Arch. Otolaryngol. Head Neck Surg.* 137, 221–228.

Pirotte, B., Neugroschl, C., Metens, T., Wikler, D., Denolin, V., Voordecker, P., Joffroy, A., Massager, N., Brotchi, J., Levivier, M., and Baleriaux, D. (2005). Comparison of functional MR imaging guidance to electrical cortical mapping for targeting selective motor cortex areas in neuropathic pain: a study based on intraoperative stereotactic navigation. *AJNR Am. J. Neuroradiol.* 26, 2256–2266.

Pirotte, B., Voordecker, P., Neugroschl, C., Baleriaux, D., Wikler, D., Metens, T., Denolin, V., Joffroy, A., Massager, N., Brotchi, J., and Levivier, M. (2008). Combination of functional magnetic resonance imaging-guided neuronavigation and intraoperative cortical brain mapping improves targeting of motor cortex stimulation in neuropathic pain. *Neurosurgery* 62(6 Suppl. 3), 941–956.

Plewnia, C., Bartels, M., and Gerloff, C. (2003). Transient suppression of tinnitus by transcranial magnetic stimulation. *Ann. Neurol.* 53, 263–266.

Plewnia, C., Reimold, M., Najib, A., Brehm, B., Reischl, G., Plontke, S. K., and Gerloff, C. (2007a). Dose-dependent attenuation of auditory phantom perception (tinnitus) by PET-guided repetitive transcranial magnetic stimulation. *Hum. Brain Mapp.* 28, 238–246.

Plewnia, C., Reimold, M., Najib, A., Reischl, G., Plontke, S. K., and Gerloff, C. (2007b). Moderate therapeutic efficacy of positron emission tomography-navigated repetitive transcranial magnetic stimulation for chronic tinnitus: a randomised, controlled pilot study. *J. Neurol. Neurosurg. Psychiatr.* 78, 152–156.

Poreisz, C., Paulus, W., Moser, T., and Lang, N. (2009). Does a single session of theta-burst transcranial magnetic stimulation of inferior temporal cortex affect tinnitus perception? *BMC Neurosci.* 10, 54.doi:10.1186/1471-2202-10-54

Ramirez, R. R., Kopell, B. H., Butson, C. R., Gaggl, W., Friedland, D. R., and Baillet, S. (2009). Neuromagnetic source imaging of abnormal spontaneous activity in tinnitus patient modulated by electrical cortical stimulation. *Conf. Proc. IEEE Eng. Med. Biol. Soc.* 2009, 1940–1944.

Rauschecker, J. P., Leaver, A. M., and Muhlau, M. (2010). Tuning out the noise: limbic-auditory interactions in tinnitus. *Neuron* 66, 819–826.

Reyes, S. A., Salvi, R. J., Burkard, R. F., Coad, M. L., Wack, D. S., Galantowicz, P. J., and Lockwood, A. H. (2002). Brain imaging of the effects of lidocaine on tinnitus. *Hear. Res.* 171, 43–50.

Roberts, L. E., Eggermont, J. J., Caspary, D. M., Shore, S. E., Melcher, J. R., and Kaltenbach, J. A. (2010). Ringing ears: the neuroscience of tinnitus. *J. Neurosci.* 30, 14972–14979.

Rosenberg, O., Roth, Y., Kotler, M., Zangen, A., and Dannon, P. (2011). Deep transcranial magnetic stimulation for the treatment of auditory hallucinations: a preliminary open-label study. *Ann. Gen. Psychiatry* 10, 3.

Rossi, S., De, C. A., Ulivelli, M., Bartalini, S., Falzarano, V., Filippone, G., and Passero, S. (2007). Effects of repetitive transcranial magnetic stimulation on chronic tinnitus: a randomised, crossover, double blind, placebo controlled study. *J. Neurol. Neurosurg. Psychiatr.* 78, 857–863.

Santos, F. V., and Matas, C. G. (2010). Late auditory evoked potentials in individuals with tinnitus. *Braz. J. Otorhinolaryngol.* 76, 263–270.

Schaette, R., and Kempter, R. (2006). Development of tinnitus-related neuronal hyperactivity through homeostatic plasticity after hearing loss: a computational model. *Eur. J. Neurosci.* 23, 3124–3138.

Schaette, R., and McAlpine, D. (2011). Tinnitus with a normal audiogram: physiological evidence for hidden hearing loss and computational model. *J. Neurosci.* 31, 13452–13457.

Schecklmann, M., Landgrebe, M., Poeppl, T. B., Kreuzer, P., Manner, P., Marienhagen, J., Wack, D. S., Kleinjung, T., Hajak, G., and Langguth, B. (2011a). Neural correlates of tinnitus duration and distress: a positron emission tomography study. *Hum. Brain Mapp.* doi: 10.1002/hbm.21426. [Epub ahead of print].

Schecklmann, M., Volberg, G., Frank, G., Hadersdorfer, J., Steffens, T., Weisz, N., Landgrebe, M., Hajak, G., Greenlee, M., Classen, J., and Langguth, B. (2011b). Paired associative stimulation of the auditory system: a proof-of-principle study. *PLoS ONE* 6, e27088. doi:10.1371/journal.pone.0027088

Schlee, W., Dohrmann, K., Hartmann, T., Lorenz, N., Mülller, N., Elbert, T., and Weisz, N. (2008). Assessment and modification of the tinnitus-related cortical network. *Semin. Hear.* 29, 270–287.

Schlee, W., Hartmann, T., Langguth, B., and Weisz, N. (2009). Abnormal resting-state cortical coupling in chronic tinnitus. *BMC Neurosci.* 10, 11. doi:10.1186/1471-2202-10-11

Schulze, K., Zysset, S., Mueller, K., Friederici, A. D., and Koelsch, S. (2011). Neuroarchitecture of verbal and tonal working memory in nonmusicians and musicians. *Hum. Brain Mapp.* 32, 771–783.

Seidman, M. D., De, R. D., Elisevich, K., Bowyer, S. M., Darrat, I., Dria, J., Stach, B., Jiang, Q., Tepley, N., Ewing, J., Seidman, M., and Zhang, J. (2008). Direct electrical stimulation of Heschl's gyrus for tinnitus treatment. *Laryngoscope* 118, 491–500.

Shi, Y., Burchiel, K. J., Anderson, V. C., and Martin, W. H. (2009). Deep brain stimulation effects in patients with tinnitus. *Otolaryngol. Head Neck Surg.* 141, 285–287.

Siebner, H. R., Filipovic, S. R., Rowe, J. B., Cordivari, C., Gerschlager, W., Rothwell, J. C., Frackowiak, R. S., and Bhatia, K. P. (2003). Patients with focal arm dystonia have increased sensitivity to slow-frequency repetitive TMS of the dorsal premotor cortex. *Brain.*

Smith, J. A., Mennemeier, M., Bartel, T., Chelette, K. C., Kimbrell, T., Triggs, W., and Dornhoffer, J. L. (2007). Repetitive transcranial magnetic stimulation for tinnitus: a pilot study. *Laryngoscope* 117, 529–534.

Smits, M., Kovacs, S., De, R. D., Peeters, R. R., Van, H. P., and Sunaert, S. (2007). Lateralization of functional magnetic resonance imaging (fMRI) activation in the auditory pathway of patients with lateralized tinnitus. *Neuroradiology* 49, 669–679.

van der Loo, E., Gais, S., Congedo, M., Vanneste, S., Plazier, M., Menovsky, T., Van de Heyning, P., and De Ridder, D. (2009). Tinnitus intensity dependent gamma oscillations of the contralateral auditory cortex. *PLoS ONE* 4, e7396. doi:10.1371/journal.pone.0007396

Vanneste, S., and De Ridder, D. (2011). Bifrontal transcranial direct current stimulation modulates tinnitus intensity and tinnitus-distress-related brain activity. *Eur. J. Neurosci.* 34, 605–614.

Vanneste, S., Focquaert, F., Van de Heyning, P., and De Ridder, D. (2011a). Different resting state brain activity and functional connectivity in patients who respond and not respond to bifrontal tDCS for tinnitus suppression. *Exp. Brain Res.* 210, 217–227.

Vanneste, S., Langguth, B., and De Ridder, D. (2011b). Do tDCS and TMS influence tinnitus transiently via a direct cortical and indirect somatosensory modulating effect? A combined TMS-tDCS and TENS study. *Brain Stimul.* 4, 242–252.

Vanneste, S., Plazier, M., Van de Heyning, P., and De Ridder, D. (2011c). Repetitive transcranial magnetic stimulation frequency dependent tinnitus improvement by double cone coil prefrontal stimulation. *J. Neurol. Neurosurg. Psychiatr.* 82, 1160–1164.

Vanneste, S., Van de Heyning, P., and De Ridder, D. (2011d). Contralateral parahippocampal gamma-band activity determines noise-like tinnitus laterality: a region of interest analysis. *Neuroscience* 199, 481–490.

Vanneste, S., Van de Heyning, P., and De Ridder, D. (2011e). The neural network of phantom sound changes over time: a comparison between recent-onset and chronic tinnitus patients. *Eur. J. Neurosci.* 34, 718–731.

Vanneste, S., Plazier, M., Ost, J., van der Loo, E., Van de Heyning, P., and De Ridder, D. (2010a). Bilateral dorsolateral prefrontal cortex modulation for tinnitus by transcranial direct current stimulation: a preliminary clinical study. *Exp. Brain Res.* 202, 779–785.

Vanneste, S., Plazier, M., van der Loo, E., Van de Heyning, P., Congedo, M., and De Ridder, D. (2010b). The neural correlates of tinnitus-related distress. *Neuroimage* 52, 470–480.

Voisin, J., Bidet-Caulet, A., Bertrand, O., and Fonlupt, P. (2006). Listening in silence activates auditory areas: a functional magnetic resonance imaging study. *J. Neurosci.* 26, 273–278.

Wang, H., Tian, J., Yin, D., Jiang, S., Yang, W., Han, D., Yao, S., and Shao, M. (2001). Regional glucose metabolic increases in left auditory cortex in tinnitus patients: a preliminary study with positron emission tomography. *Chin. Med. J. (Engl)* 114, 848–851.

Wang, H., Wang, X., and Scheich, H. (1996). LTD and LTP induced by transcranial magnetic stimulation in auditory cortex. *Neuroreport* 7, 521–525.

Weisz, N., Dohrmann, K., and Elbert, T. (2007). The relevance of spontaneous activity for the coding of the tinnitus sensation. *Prog. Brain Res.* 166, 61–70.

Weisz, N., Moratti, S., Meinzer, M., Dohrmann, K., and Elbert, T. (2005a). Tinnitus perception and distress is related to abnormal spontaneous brain activity as measured by magnetoencephalography. *PLoS Med.* 2, e153. doi:10.1371/journal.pmed.0020153

Weisz, N., Wienbruch, C., Dohrmann, K., and Elbert, T. (2005b). Neuromagnetic indicators of auditory cortical reorganization of tinnitus. *Brain* 128(Pt 11), 2722–2731.

Yang, S., Weiner, B. D., Zhang, L. S., Cho, S. J., and Bao, S. (2011). Homeostatic plasticity drives tinnitus perception in an animal model. *Proc. Natl. Acad. Sci. U.S.A.* 108, 14974–14979.

Zhang, J., Zhang, Y., and Zhang, X. (2011). Auditory cortex electrical stimulation suppresses tinnitus in rats. *J. Assoc. Res. Otolaryngol.* 12, 185–201.

Zunhammer, M., Busch, V., Griesbach, F., Landgrebe, M., Hajak, G., and Langguth, B. (2011). rTMS over the cerebellum modulates temperature detection and pain thresholds through peripheral mechanisms. *Brain Stimul.* 4, 210–217.

10

Tinnitus suppression by electric stimulation of the auditory nerve

Janice E. Chang[1]* and Fan-Gang Zeng[1,2]*

[1] *Department of Anatomy and Neurobiology, University of California Irvine, Irvine, CA, USA*
[2] *Department of Otolaryngology – Head and Neck Surgery, University of California Irvine, Orange, CA, USA*

Correspondence:
Janice E. Chang and Fan-Gang Zeng, Department of Anatomy and Neurobiology, Hearing and Speech Lab, University of California, Irvine, 110 Medical Science E, Irvine, CA 92697, USA.
e-mail: janicec@uci.edu, fzeng@uci.edu

Electric stimulation of the auditory nerve via a cochlear implant (CI) has been observed to suppress tinnitus, but parameters of an effective electric stimulus remain unexplored. Here we used CI research processors to systematically vary pulse rate, electrode place, and current amplitude of electric stimuli, and measure their effects on tinnitus loudness and stimulus loudness as a function of stimulus duration. Thirteen tinnitus subjects who used CIs were tested, with nine (70%) being "Responders" who achieved greater than 30% tinnitus loudness reduction in response to at least one stimulation condition and the remaining four (30%) being "Non-Responders" who had less than 30% tinnitus loudness reduction in response to any stimulus condition tested. Despite large individual variability, several interesting observations were made between stimulation parameters, tinnitus characteristics, and tinnitus suppression. If a subject's tinnitus was suppressed by one stimulus, then it was more likely to be suppressed by another stimulus. If the tinnitus contained a "pulsating" component, then it would be more likely suppressed by a given combination of stimulus parameters than tinnitus without these components. There was also a disassociation between the subjects' clinical speech processor and our research processor in terms of their effectiveness in tinnitus suppression. Finally, an interesting dichotomy was observed between loudness adaptation to electric stimuli and their effects on tinnitus loudness, with the Responders exhibiting higher degrees of loudness adaptation than the Non-Responders. Although the mechanisms underlying these observations remain to be resolved, their clinical implications are clear. When using a CI to manage tinnitus, the clinical processor that is optimized for speech perception needs to be customized for optimal tinnitus suppression.

Keywords: tinnitus, cochlear implant, loudness adaptation, electric stimulation

INTRODUCTION

Tinnitus is an auditory disorder known as "ringing of the ears or head" which affects 50 million Americans and an estimated 600 million worldwide, according to the American Tinnitus Association (ATA; www.ata.org). Its severity can range from being temporary and unobtrusive to debilitating and life-impairing. Tinnitus has steadily increased by 18% per year since 2001 in soldiers returning from the Global War on Terror, and is currently the number one cause of service-connected disability (ATA, 2011). Although management treatments and therapies are available, there currently exists no cure (Goodey, 2007).

While neural mechanisms causing tinnitus and hearing loss are not identical, the incidence of tinnitus is highly correlated with, and believed to be related to hearing loss (Axelsson and Ringdahl, 1989). A study by the National Study of Hearing showed that hearing impairment is the dominant factor in predicting the occurrence of prolonged spontaneous tinnitus (Coles et al., 1988; Tyler, 2000). Although not all individuals experiencing tinnitus have hearing loss, those who have a hearing loss experience an 83% higher risk of developing tinnitus over those who do not have a hearing loss (Nondahl et al., 2002). Interestingly, when these individuals are fit with hearing aids, approximately half of hearing aid users with tinnitus report that their amplification also provides either partial or total relief from their tinnitus (Surr et al., 1985).

Individuals with more severe hearing loss may receive a cochlear implant (CI) to help restore hearing (Zeng, 2004). While most individuals who have tinnitus are not profoundly deaf (Tyler, 2000), a reported 66–86% of CI users indeed experience tinnitus (Tyler and Kelsay, 1990; Hazell et al., 1995; Miyamoto et al., 1997; Quaranta et al., 2004; Bovo et al., 2010). Evidence of cochlear electrical stimulation has been noted to benefit tinnitus, and CIs have been suggested as a potential therapeutic since they became commercially available in the early 1980s (House and Brackmann, 1981). In recent years, the benefit of CI on tinnitus has been widely reported in many studies. Efficacy rates range from 34 to 93% (Tyler and Kelsay, 1990; Miyamoto et al., 1997; Pan et al., 2009; Bovo et al., 2010). On the other hand, a smaller percentage of 16.7–41.5% of CI users reports no effect of the CI on their tinnitus (Tyler and Kelsay, 1990; Miyamoto et al., 1997; Bovo et al., 2010).

Significantly, most studies investigating CI effects on tinnitus have used standard multichannel CIs using speech processors optimized for speech. Observational questionnaires comparing pre- and post-implantation tinnitus have found reduction in tinnitus intensity or loudness (Ito and Sakakihara, 1994; Miyamoto et al., 1997; Ruckenstein et al., 2001), decreased annoyance, and general reports that "the majority of patients thought that their CI was helpful in tinnitus suppression" (Souliere et al., 1992). Changes in tinnitus pitch and timber following implantation have also been noted (Souliere et al., 1992; Miyamoto et al., 1997). These effects have been attributed to surgical insertion of the intra-cochlear electrode (Baguley and Atlas, 2007) as well as plastic changes in the auditory system brought about by CI use (Quaranta et al., 2004; Baguley and Atlas, 2007). Of note, current candidacy requirements for CI implantation are strictly based on hearing capabilities, as measured by severe-to-profound sensorineural hearing loss that is not substantially improved by hearing aids, and speech recognition test scores in the United States, Canada, and the United Kingdom (UK Cochlear Implant Study Group, 2004; Balkany et al., 2007; Amoodi et al., 2012). Because clinical processors used in CIs are designed to improve speech perception (Wilson et al., 1991; Zeng et al., 2008), their effects on tinnitus are usually considered to be secondary.

There is limited literature on optimizing electric stimulation for tinnitus suppression. Rubinstein et al. (1999) used high-rate stimulation to produce a pattern of spontaneous-like firing similar to that seen in the healthy auditory nerve, which is thought to represent the auditory "code for silence." He tested the effectiveness of high-rate stimulation [4800 pulses per second (pps)] in three Cochlear CI users with tinnitus and found that one subject showed level-dependent tinnitus suppression with complete adaptation to the electric stimulus, one subject showed tinnitus suppression only in the presence of a stimulus percept, and one subject reported no change in tinnitus at her maximal comfort level of stimulation (Rubinstein et al., 2003). On the other hand, Dauman et al. (1993) explored low-rate bipolar stimulation in two Cochlear CI patients, finding that 125 pps stimuli was the most effective in that it required the lowest amount of current to achieve suppression, and that the effectiveness of stimulation could vary by place. A parametric study exploring various combinations of stimuli parameters also found low-rate stimuli effective at completely suppressing tinnitus in a single Advanced Bionics HiRes CI user (Zeng et al., 2011). In this study we sought to corroborate these findings in a larger subject size using various CI devices. The goal of the present study is twofold: (1) to use flexible research processors to systematically vary electric stimulation parameters and measure their effects on tinnitus suppression, and (2) to identify relationships between tinnitus characteristics and electric stimulation to tinnitus suppression.

MATERIALS AND METHODS

SUBJECTS

Subjects who had chronic tinnitus and a CI were screened for the study. Prior to enrollment, subjects completed an online tinnitus survey, including a questionnaire about their hearing loss and tinnitus, the Beck Depression Inventory (BDI), Beck Anxiety Inventory, Tinnitus Handicap Index, and Tinnitus Severity Index. They also provided audiological records, which included their speech recognition scores as assessed by the standardized Hearing in Noise Test (HINT; Nilsson et al., 1994). Subjects who had not been evaluated by a physician for their tinnitus, had a treatable type of tinnitus, or were on medications or other treatments for their tinnitus were excluded from the study. All subjects perceived their tinnitus for a minimum of six months.

Thirteen CI users with chronic tinnitus, 11 female and two male of average age 60.8 ± 13.6 years (mean ± SD) participated in the study (**Table 1**). Etiology of hearing loss varied, and all subjects had severe to profound hearing loss in the non-implanted ear except for S11, who had sudden sensorineural hearing loss in one ear and normal hearing in the other. Average duration of hearing loss was 27.9 ± 11.7 years and subjects had an average

Table 1 | Patient demographics.

	Gender	Age	Hearing loss		Cochlear implant (CI)		
			Etiology	Duration (years)	CI use (years)	CI side	HINT sentence (% correct)
S1	F	59	Otosclerosis	26	1	L	76
S2	F	67	Genetic	34	6	R	100
S3	F	74	Sensorineural	28	9	L	97
S4	F	77	Autoimmune	21	4	L	75
S5	F	50	Autoimmune	31	13	Both	96 (L) 63 (R)
S6	F	61	Meniere's	29	2	L	96
S7	F	72	Idiopathic	15	9	Both	n.a. (L) 87 (R)
S8	F	59	Sensorineural	43	8	L	44
S9	M	86	Noise-induced	39	3	R	8
S10	F	43	Radiation-induced	14	1	L	76
S11	M	50	Idiopathic	5	4	R	70
S12	F	45	Congenital rubella	45	6	L	0
S13	F	47	Genetic	33	1	R	100

n.a. = not available.

CI use of 5.15 ± 3.8 years with at least one year of experience. Six subjects used Cochlear devices, four used Advanced Bionics, and three used Med-El. These CI users had sentence recognition ranged from 0 to 100%, and covered the full range from poor to good performers (Nilsson et al., 1994; Friesen et al., 2001).

TINNITUS CHARACTERISTICS

Patient tinnitus characteristics are shown in **Table 2.** Prior to testing, patients were asked if "their tinnitus has improved since cochlear implantation." Seven (54%) patients reported "Yes" or "sometimes," while five subjects (38%) reported "No" and one subject was unsure. All patients had experienced tinnitus for a minimum of one year, ranging from 1 to 49 years with an average of 20.5 ± 15.3 years. Tinnitus Handicap Inventory (THI) scores showed 38% of subjects (5 of 13) with moderate handicap, 31% (4 of 13) with mild handicap, and 31% (4 of 13) with slight or no tinnitus handicap. Ninety-two percent (12 of 13) of patients had minimal depression (the lowest grade possible) based on the BDI, and one subject experienced mild depression.

Average baseline loudness rating (LR) of their tinnitus was 4.4 ± 1.9 on a numeric scale from 0–10 (**Table 3**). Subjects reported a variety of different sounds descriptive of their tinnitus. The most common sound perceived was humming (85%, 11 subjects), followed by ringing and roaring (both 77%, 10 subjects each), then buzzing and the "inside of a seashell" (both 69%, nine subjects each). Two subjects reported hearing music alongside their tinnitus.

STIMULI AND PROCEDURE

All stimuli were delivered to the subject's CI using a research processor, controlled by a customizable research interface connected to a computer. Use of the customizable research interfaces allowed fixed pulse trains to be continuously delivered to only a single electrode at a given stimulation rate, place, or level, as distinct from commercial speech processors. Stimuli were fixed, charge-balanced, biphasic anodic-first pulse trains, delivered with a given stimulation rate (low: 100 or 200 pps and high: 5000 pps), stimulation place (apical, middle, or basal electrode) and stimulation level (corresponding to soft, medium, and loud) for a total combination of 18 stimuli conditions. Stimulated electrodes were selected as the apical- and basal-most electrodes, as well as the electrode in the middle of the array. Apical, middle, and basal electrodes were selected, respectively as electrodes 22, 11, and 1 for Cochlear devices; 1, 8, 16 for Advanced Bionics; and 1, 6, and 12 for Med-El (see **Figure 1**). Loudness levels were determined via subject feedback, using a LR numeric scale from 0 to 10 (0 = no sound, 10 = very uncomfortable) as a guide. On this scale, LR 3 corresponded to "soft," LR 5 to "medium," and LR 7 to "loud but comfortable."

- For Cochlear users, electric stimuli were delivered through a programmable SPEAR3 Speech Processor (Hearworks, Pty, Melbourne, Australia) and controlled via the Woomera software (Cochlear Ltd., Sydney, Australia); source code was written in Motorola DSP563xx assembly language. Subjects adjusted the volume to the appropriate loudness using a dial on the speech processor.
- For Advanced Bionics users, electric stimuli were delivered via a research interface provided by Advanced Bionics Corporation and controlled via the BionicEar Data Collection System software (Advanced Bionics LLC; Sylmar, CA, USA).
- For Med-El users, electric stimuli were delivered via the Diagnostic Interface Box connected to the CIS-PRO + processor and controlled using the CI.Studio+ 2.0 software (Med-El Corporation, Innsbruck, Austria). The clinical mapping software was used to turn off all but one electrode, which was set at the appropriate stimulation rate. A steady state sound was then delivered directly through the processor via an audio input cable to activate that given electrode.

Table 2 | Patient tinnitus characteristics.

	CI benefit (self-report)	Duration (years)	Tinnitus Handicap Inventory (THI)		Beck Depression Inventory	
			THI	THI score	BDI	BDI score
S1[a]	No	1	20	Mild (Grade 2)	1	Minimal
S2	Sometimes	14	18	Mild (Grade 2)	5	Minimal
S3[b]	Sometimes	Unsure	6	Slight or None (Grade 1)	10	Minimal
S4	Sometimes	21	22	Mild (Grade 2)	6	Minimal
S5[b]	No	32	40	Moderate (Grade 3)	8	Minimal
S6[b]	No	20	40	Moderate (Grade 3)	9	Minimal
S7	Yes	14	14	Slight or None (Grade 1)	4	Minimal
S8[b]	Yes	44	14	Slight or None (Grade 1)	2	Minimal
S9	Sometimes	49	22	Mild (Grade 2)	13	Minimal
S10	Unsure	12	0	Slight or None (Grade 1)	0	Minimal
S11	No	5	52	Moderate (Grade 3)	15	Mild
S12	No	5	52	Moderate (Grade 3)	4	Minimal
S13	Sometimes	29	48	Moderate (Grade 3)	6	Minimal

[a] *Onset of tinnitus after implantation.*

[b] *Experienced bilateral tinnitus, with distinct sounds reported by ear.*

Table 3 | Tinnitus characteristics.

	Baseline loudness	Buzz	Hum	Ring	Blow	Hiss	Roar	Whistling	Pulsating	Constant high pitches	Constant low pitches	Running water	Inside of a seashell	Sizzle	Other
S1	4.0										X				X
S2	3.2	X	X	X		X	X	X	X			X	X	X	X[a]
S3	1.0 (L) 5.0 (R)	X	X	X		X	X	X		X	X		X	X	
S4	6.7	X	X	X	X		X	X		X	X		X		X[a]
S5	8.3 (L) 7.3 (R)	X	X	X			X			X	X		X		X
S6	4.5 (L) 4.9 (R)	X	X	X			X		X				X		X
S7	2.4	X	X			X							X		
S8	1.6 (L) 4.0 (R)		X		X	X	X	X	X	X	X		X		
S9	3.6	X	X	X			X			X		X			
S10	3.4			X											X
S11	5.2	X	X	X		X	X	X	X	X	X	X	X	X	X
S12	3.9		X	X			X				X	X			
S13	6.0	X	X	X		X	X		X	X		X	X		X
#	4.4 ± 1.9	9	11	10	2	6	10	5	5	7	7	5	9	3	8
%		69	85	77	15	46	77	38	38	54	54	38	69	23	62

[a] *S2 and S4 reported hearing music.*

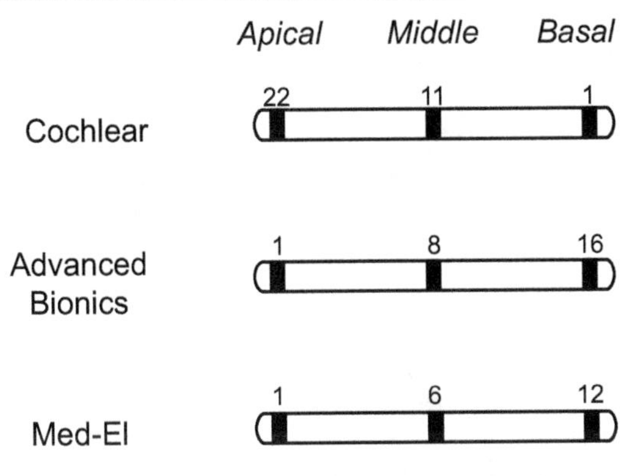

FIGURE 1 | Electrode stimulation site by condition and CI manufacturer. Diagrammatic representations of electrode arrays are presented by CI manufacturer, with the stimulated electrode number listed above the appropriate electrode (shaded in black) for apical (left), middle (center), and basal (right) stimulation conditions.

Prior to each trial, baseline tinnitus was assessed as the LR of the tinnitus prior to delivery of the test stimulus. Fixed, unmodulated pulse trains were then delivered to a single electrode at a fixed stimulation level for 6 min. LRs of the tinnitus and the electric stimuli were each reported by the subject every 30 s for the duration of the stimuli. Tinnitus was allowed to return to baseline prior to the next testing condition. S10 had a dead region in the basal region of her cochlea secondary to radiation for a cerebellar tumor (Moore et al., 2000); S3, S6, S7, and S9 did not complete testing conditions. Testing conditions were presented in a randomized order. Due to thorough evaluation of stimulation conditions and time required between trials, total testing time could span two full days for each subject.

All patients gave informed, written consent and protocols were approved by the Institutional Review Board at the University of California Irvine.

ANALYSIS

LRs for tinnitus and electric stimuli were reported as loudness adaptation percentages, calculated as such:

$$\text{Loudness adaptation percentage} = \frac{L_t - L_0}{L_0} \times 100,$$

where L_t is LR at time t and L_0 is the initial LR at time $t = 0$. A value of -100% means that the tinnitus or sound is inaudible ($L_t = 0$), while 0% means that the tinnitus or sound is unchanged from the baseline ($L_t = L_0$). The adaptation data were fitted using the following equation:

$$y(t) = s(1 - e^{-t/\tau}),$$

where s represents the plateaued adaptation percentage, calculated as the average of the final five loudness estimates in terms of percentage of the original loudness at the onset of stimulation. τ represents the time constant at which the loudness percept adapted. For cases where no adaptation occurred, both s (plateaued adaptation percentage) and τ (time constant) were set to 0.

Subjects were also classified based on their responses to the tested stimuli. Tinnitus suppression outcome were based on a 30% cutoff; a tinnitus suppression of 30% or more was considered "successful" while suppression of less than 30% was considered as "no suppression." Thus, subjects tested in this paradigm fit into one of two categories: "Responder" subjects, whose tinnitus adapted to at least one condition by 30% or more, or "Non-Responder" subjects, whose tinnitus remained uninfluenced by electric stimulation.

Statistical analyses were performed for all subjects. Data were analyzed using Generalized Estimating Equations to control for repeated measures, using a linear scale response outcome of the minimum tinnitus adaptation percentage, or plateaued adaptation and time constant of the curve-fit variables for adaptation of the electric stimulus (SPSS/PASW Statistics 18; Somers, NY, USA).

Another Generalized Estimating Equations model using binary logistic regression was used to evaluate effects of stimulation parameters on tinnitus suppression outcome of greater or less than −30%. All regression models were built using rate, place and level as main effects; two-way interactions were consequently assessed. The statistical significance of each regression coefficient was determined using Wald Chi-square analyses, and the model was reduced by backward elimination. Variables of clinical interest were evaluated in the final model, and post-hoc analyses were performed based on pairwise contrasts.

RESULTS

TINNITUS SUPPRESSION

Figure 2 shows representative data from three subjects (S1, S2, and S5) at a high rate (5000 pps) and an apical electrode, with the loudness of the electric stimuli at soft, medium and loud levels represented in columns. Subjects S1 and S2 (in the first two rows) show loudness adaptation of both the tinnitus (filled circles) and the electric stimuli (open triangles). Note in the first panel S1 particularly—-both the tinnitus and electric stimulus adapted from a soft level (LR: 3) to a barely audible sensation (LR: 1) for a total adaptation of −66.7%. Subject S2 also showed loudness adaptation to both her tinnitus and the electric stimuli, with her tinnitus percept adapting completely to −100% (LR: 0) in the medium and loud conditions. Subject S5 is a bilateral user who showed no loudness adaptation to the tinnitus in either ear (right ear: filled circles; left ear: X's) or the electric stimuli (open triangles).

Figure 3 shows the spread of suppression across tinnitus subjects, with each circle representing a single trial condition. Of 227 trials tested, 37% (83 of 227) were successful conditions that elicited a tinnitus suppression of 30% or more, represented by the dotted line in **Figure 3**. Of these, 49% (41/83) of the successful conditions yielded complete tinnitus suppression, where the

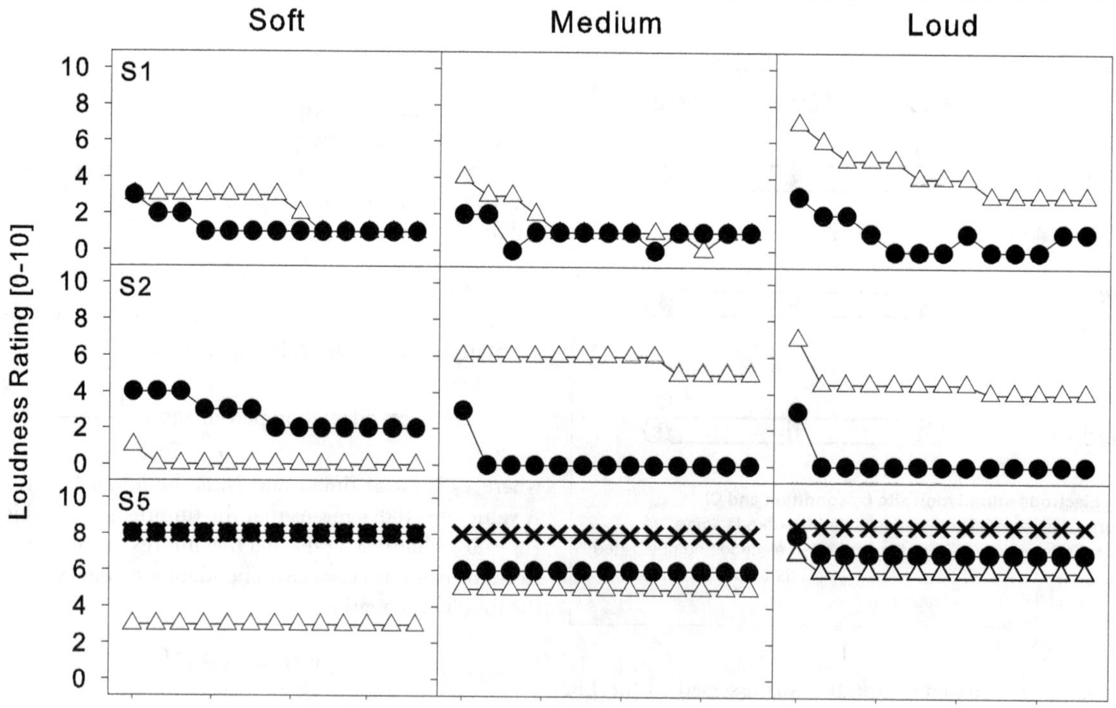

FIGURE 2 | Representative data from three subjects at a high rate (5000 pps), apical electrode. Plots show tinnitus and electric stimulus loudness percepts across time at three different loudness levels for three representative subjects. Loudness levels are shown in columns; subjects S1, S2, and S5 are displayed in rows. For S1 and S2, plots show LRs (scale: 0–10) of tinnitus (filled circles) and electric stimuli (open triangles). S5 is a user who reported bilateral tinnitus; tinnitus from her right ear (filled circles) is shown alongside tinnitus from her left ear (filled X's), and electric stimuli (open triangles).

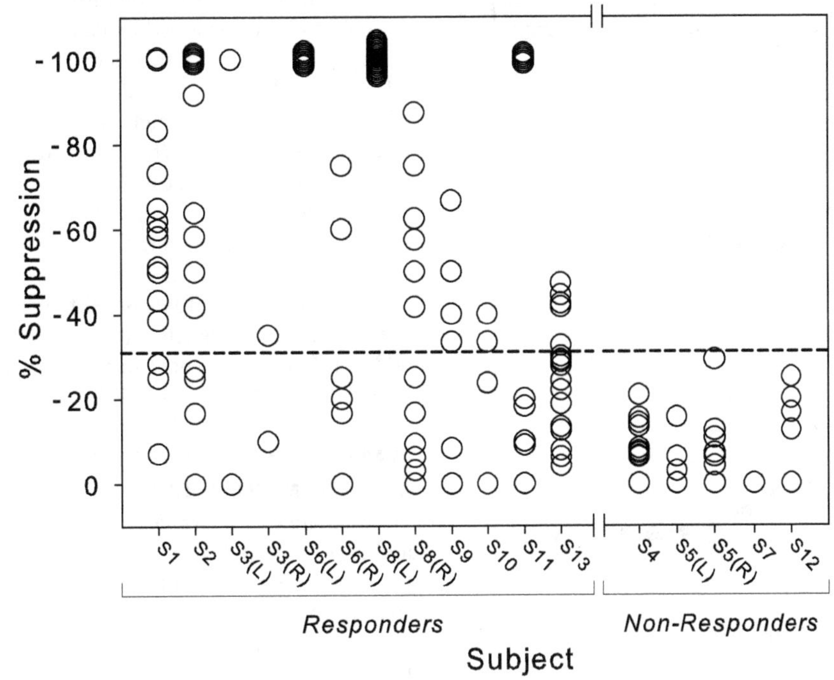

FIGURE 3 | Spread of suppression, by subject. The spread of variability in tinnitus suppression percentage across all conditions is shown for each subject. Subjects are listed across the *x*-axis and grouped as Responders (left) or Non-Responders (right). Each open circle represents the maximal tinnitus suppression for a given condition. Bilateral tinnitus percepts for subjects S3, S5, S6, and S8 are listed by ear. Symbols at −100% suppression (complete adaptation) were shifted by up to 5% for visualization purposes. A dotted line is shown at −30% suppression to indicate the cutoff for successful suppression.

tinnitus percept dropped to be completely imperceptible (LR: 0). Sixty-nine percent (9 of 13) of subjects responded to at least one condition tested: S1, S2, S3, S6, S8, S9, S10, S11, and S13. For subjects with bilateral tinnitus, ears responded uniformly: both ears responded to stimuli for S3, S6, and S8; neither ear responded for S5.

The large individual variability produced no significant effect of stimulation rate, place of stimulation, or loudness level of the electric stimulus on tinnitus suppression outcome. However, subjects who responded to one stimulus were much more likely to respond a second stimuli ($\chi^2 = 93.5$, $df = 1$, $p < 0.001$, likelihood ratio Chi-square test). Subjects who responded to at least one stimuli responded to a minimum of 27% of conditions tested (S9) and up to 78% conditions tested (S1) for an average of 50% of successful conditions.

Figure 4 shows the percentage of successful suppression conditions based on the total number of conditions tested, with low rate stimuli represented as open bars and high rate stimuli as filled bars. A binary logistic regression model found a significant effect of loudness level on tinnitus suppression ($p = 0.049$, Wald Chi-square analysis), along with a significant rate-level interaction ($p = 0.030$). Only loud sounds were significantly more effective than soft sounds ($p = 0.027$). The significant rate-level interaction showed additionally that, for high rate sounds, medium sounds were more effective than soft sounds ($p = 0.043$) and loud sounds ($p = 0.008$). No other significant effects or interactions were found.

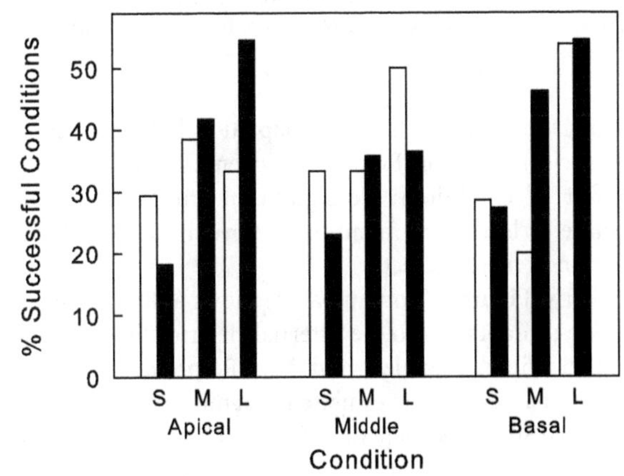

FIGURE 4 | Percentage of successful suppression conditions, by condition. Percentage of successful conditions (achieving tinnitus suppression of −30% or greater) of conditions tested are reported by stimulus condition. Open bars denote low rate stimuli; filled bars denote high rate stimuli. Electrodes for an apical, middle and basal place are grouped in clusters, and loudness levels are shown for each electrode (S = soft; M = medium; L = loud).

RESPONDER VERSUS NON-RESPONDER SUBJECTS

We sought to evaluate adaptation differences to external sounds (electric stimulus) as compared to internal ones (tinnitus) under the same stimulation conditions. **Figure 5** (top panel) shows

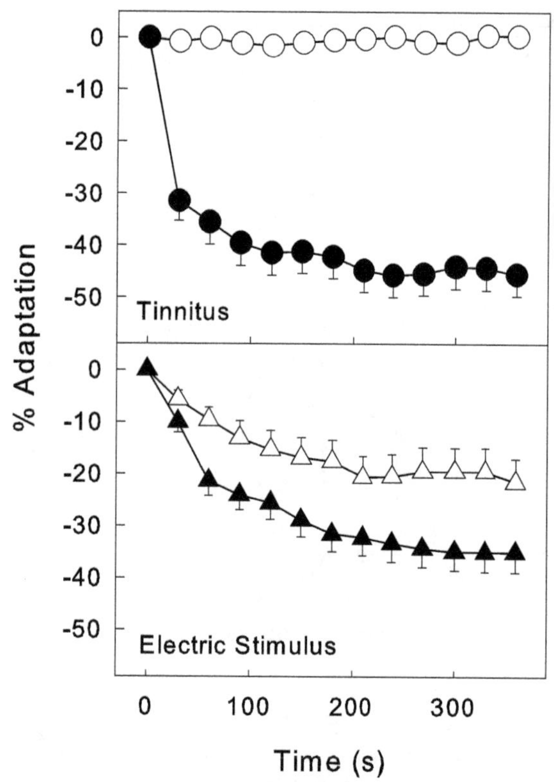

FIGURE 5 | Adaptation of tinnitus and electric stimuli, Responders versus Non-Responders. Tinnitus adaptation is shown across time in the top panel, averaged across Responder (filled circles) and Non-Responder subjects (open circles). Electric stimuli adaptation is shown across time in the bottom panel, averaged across Responder (filled triangles) and Non-Responder subjects (open triangles). Error bars indicate SEM.

a distinctive pattern of tinnitus adaptation between Responder (filled circles) and Non-Responder (open circles) subjects averaged over all conditions. No significant effects of stimulation rate, place or level were found on the overall degree of tinnitus adaptation in these subjects.

Similarly, **Figure 5** (bottom panel) shows a distinctive pattern of loudness adaptation to the external electric stimulus between Responder (filled triangles) and Non-Responder (open triangles) subjects. Responders exhibited a significantly greater degree of plateaued stimulus adaptation (−29%) than Non-Responders (−22%), but a similar rate of loudness adaptation $\tau = 0.03$ (Responders) versus $\tau = 0.02$ (Non-Responders). Effects of loudness adaptation were significant at $T(225) = 1.686$, $p = 0.030$. The similar patterns between Responders and Non-Responders suggest that mechanisms of tinnitus adaptation may be related to loudness adaptation to external stimuli.

DISCUSSION

COMPARISON TO PREVIOUS STUDIES

Our findings are in line with published results reporting effectiveness of electrical stimulation of the auditory nerve via a CI to suppress tinnitus. In our study, a fixed pulse train delivered to a single electrode of the CI effectively suppressed tinnitus for 69% of our subjects, while published efficacy rates of the CI range from 46 to 93% (reviewed by Pan et al., 2009). Two recent studies reported 80–95% of their subjects to respond positively to the CI (van de Heyning et al., 2008; Arndt et al., 2011). While our efficacy rates are not as high, our study populations are also different. These two studies focus on individuals with incapacitating unilateral tinnitus and deafness, implanted primarily for their tinnitus, while our subjects are individuals with bilateral hearing loss treated by cochlear implantation who have coincident tinnitus. By nature of our study design and patient selection, our subjects are also those whose tinnitus was resistant to complete suppression by the CI (hence seeking relief in our study). Furthermore, we found additional tinnitus benefit in four subjects who did not initially report tinnitus benefit with their own speech processor.

CHARACTERIZING DIFFERENCES BETWEEN RESPONDER AND NON-RESPONDER SUBJECTS

We evaluated demographics, hearing loss, and tinnitus profiles, and past medical histories of the two groups of subjects to identify any characteristic differences of the two groups. However, no significant differences were found between the Responder and Non-Responder groups with regard to gender, age, duration of hearing loss, duration of CI use, CI ear implant, CI device type (manufacturer), tinnitus duration, tinnitus severity (TSI), tinnitus handicap (THI), anxiety levels (BAI), or depression status (BDI). No differences were found in patient self-report of if their CI was beneficial to their tinnitus or not. No significant differences were found in general health status between the two groups either, based on self-reported past medical history of: endolymphatic shunt, vestibular neurectomy, chronic upper respiratory infection, noise exposure, sudden hearing loss, vertigo, Meniere's disease, chronic ear infections, abnormal bone growth, otorrhea, balance problems, hypertension, hypothyroidism, anemia, head tumor, autoimmune disorder(s), genetic disorder, heavy smoking, excessive caffeine use, chronic pain, insomnia, anxiety, depression, allergies, sinus congestion, or chronic infection. Interestingly, all four subjects with reported previous history of motor vehicle collision (MVC; S3, S8, S11, and S13) were Responders while none of the four Non-Responders reported having been involved in a MVC [$T(8) = 2.530$, $p = 0.035$].

Lastly, only one of the tinnitus sound component qualities was seen more highly associated with Responder subjects: Responders were significantly more likely than Non-Responders to have pulsatile-type tinnitus, $T(8) = 3.162$, $p = 0.013$. No significant differences were noted for individuals with tinnitus components of: buzzing, humming, ringing, blowing, hissing, roaring, whistling, constant high pitches, constant low pitches, water-like, seashell sounds, sizzling, or any other reported sounds. Furthermore, no differences were seen between the groups either in baseline levels of tinnitus, or in the overall standard deviation (or variability) of baseline tinnitus for each subject.

EFFECTIVENESS OF SOUND STIMULI BY TINNITUS QUALITY

We also ran an analysis comparing effectiveness of each of the eighteen stimuli by the sound components of tinnitus (**Table 4**). No stimuli were significantly more or less effective for tinnitus with buzzing, humming, blowing, constant high pitches, constant low pitches, water-like, seashell sounds, or any "other" reported sound components. However, for several sounds, particular stimuli were found to be significantly more effective for subjects reporting that given tinnitus sound component, than for subjects who did not report that sound. For example, individuals reporting tinnitus with a "roaring" component achieved a significantly greater amount of tinnitus suppression with a low rate, soft stimuli to an apical electrode as compared to subjects without a roaring tinnitus component, $T(14.140) = 2.853, p = 0.013$; T-values are reported in **Table 4**. Ringing was the only sound that was predictive of negative predictability; namely, individuals with ringing tinnitus were *less likely to respond* to high rate stimuli of a soft-loudness level to either middle or basal electrodes. Tinnitus with a pulsatile component was easily suppressed with any of the six loud sound conditions except to an apical electrode with a low stimulation rate.

TINNITUS AND ELECTRIC STIMULUS ADAPTATION: INSIGHTS INTO UNDERLYING MECHANISMS

Loudness adaptation to externally presented electric stimuli in these subjects, as compared to simultaneous tinnitus adaptation, may also be insightful to mechanisms of tinnitus production. Despite a large variability in tinnitus response between subjects, a significant level-dependence was observed for tinnitus adaptation, with loud sounds achieving more tinnitus adaptation than soft sounds. While this may be partially attributed to a masking effect of electric stimuli on the tinnitus percept (Vernon, 2000; Vernon and Meikle, 2000), simple masking may not fully explain the observed results.

First, a large variability in tinnitus suppression results may indicate a heterogeneous population of tinnitus subjects. Where a final common pathway has been implicated for the perception of tinnitus (Shulman et al., 2009), evidence of tinnitus-related activity has been observed from the peripheral auditory system, through the brainstem and up to the cortex (Muhlnickel et al., 1998; Eggermont and Roberts, 2004; Roberts et al., 2010; Kaltenbach, 2011). Variability in both tinnitus characteristics described and responses to the stimuli tested here may indicate tinnitus manifesting from different sources.

Next, patterns of adaptation to electric stimuli are different from those to tinnitus adaptation. Loudness adaptation to electric stimuli showed significant effects of stimulation rate ($p = 0.011$), stimulation place ($p = 0.000$), and stimulation level ($p = 0.020$) (similar results were found in Tang et al., 2006), while tinnitus suppression is unaffected by these same parameters. This suggests that neural mechanisms underlying loudness adaptation to electric stimuli are likely distinct from those underlying tinnitus adaptation.

Despite these differences, electric stimuli are able to elicit tinnitus suppression in a subset of this heterogeneous group of tinnitus subjects. Responder individuals who experienced tinnitus suppression here also exhibited a higher degree of adaptation to the electric stimuli, while Non-Responders achieved a lesser degree of adaptation to both their tinnitus and the electric stimulation percepts. This result supports the auditory gain hypothesis, in which increased central gain in response to reduced input from the periphery results in tinnitus (Salvi et al., 2000; Norena, 2011). If physiological mechanisms underlying loudness growth are mediated by cochlear and central non-linearities (Zeng and Shannon, 1994; Moore, 2004) and loudness adaptation may be mediated by a central feedback loop dependent on peripheral nerve activity (Tang et al., 2006), then our observation here of increased stimulus adaptation in Responder individuals may indicate that their tinnitus is such that the external stimulus, applied at the auditory periphery, can induce adaptation to the tinnitus as well. Accordingly, Non-Responders who exhibit less adaptation to both the stimulus and their tinnitus may have tinnitus which originates more centrally within the auditory system, making their tinnitus less susceptible to adaptation via peripheral stimulation.

CLINICAL IMPLICATIONS

We also compared an individual's tinnitus suppression outcome using our testing paradigm to their self-reported answer to the question "Has your tinnitus improved since cochlear implantation?" In **Table 5**, we see the patient's self-reported answer as "Helpful" or "Not Helpful" in rows, with any actual, validated effectiveness using the sounds in our study reported in columns as "Effective" or "Not Effective." Nearly half (6 of 13 subjects; 46.2%) of the subjects inaccurately predicted actual effectiveness with our testing paradigm. Of these, two subjects predicted that their CI was helpful towards their tinnitus while not actually finding any effective sounds, while four subjects reported no benefit of their CI, but found relief with our testing stimuli.

Table 4 | Effectiveness of sound stimuli by tinnitus quality.

LOW RATE		
Apical	Soft	Roaring: $T(14.140) = 2.853$, $p = 0.013$
Middle	Loud	Pulsating: $T(12) = 2.509$, $p = 0.027$
Basal	Loud	Sizzling: $T(11) = 2.279$, $p = 0.044$
		Pulsating: $T(7.633) = 3.601$, $p = 0.008$
HIGH RATE		
Apical	Loud	Hissing: $T(9) = 2.415$, $p = 0.039$
		Pulsating: $T(9) = 2.415$, $p = 0.039$
Middle	Loud	Hissing: $T(4.890) = 3.365$, $p = 0.021$
		Pulsating: $T(4.890) = 3.365$, $p = 0.021$
	Soft	(*Ringing:* $T(11) = -2.589$, $p = 0.025$)
Basal	Loud	Hissing: $T(9) = 4.492$, $p = 0.002$
		Whistling: $T(9) = 2.600$, $p = 0.029$
		Pulsating: $T(9) = 4.492$, $p = 0.002$
	Medium	Pulsating: $T(11) = 2.383$, $p = 0.036$
	Soft	(*Ringing:* $T(9) = -8.435$, $p = 0.000$)

Table 5 | Expected versus actual effectiveness of tinnitus suppression through the CI.

		Research processor		
		Effective	**Not effective**	**Total**
Own speech processor (self-report)	Helpful	5	2	7
	Not helpful	4	2	6
	Total	9	4	13

While this result could be explained by inaccurate reporting by the subjects of actual helpfulness of their CI, it seems less likely that subjects would be oblivious to a significant change to a bothersome percept and more likely that tinnitus suppression achieved using a CI with stimulation parameters ideal for speech understanding may be different from that using a CI optimized for tinnitus suppression. This effect is further clarified in **Figure 6**, which shows this relationship between speech recognition (using their own clinical speech processors) and tinnitus suppression (using research processors) for each subject, with Non-Responders in open diamonds and Responders in filled diamonds. The lack of correlation shown here ($R^2 = 0.02$, $p = 0.68$, Pearson correlation) suggests that optimal stimulation patterns may indeed be distinct for speech understanding and tinnitus suppression needs. Thus, in order to use a CI to manage tinnitus, the clinical speech processor should be programmed not only for speech perception but also by using stimulus parameters optimal for achieving tinnitus suppression in that particular patient.

Furthermore, the two subjects (S4 and S5) who reported that their CI was helpful but did not find relief with our stimuli did find relief from stimulation of the CI, albeit outside the context of our research stimuli. S4 found no relief with any of our 18 stimuli, but reported a "relaxing" and calming effect from the afternoon she got home from our testing until she woke up the next morning. The tinnitus in her implanted ear had disappeared from a "roar into a slight whistle," and the patient felt calm and relaxed with an "unexpected and unusual relief from tinnitus." She had experienced unrelenting tinnitus for 21 years. This was only the third time and by far the longest relief she had ever experienced from her tinnitus; the previous times had lasted only for minutes. This anecdotal report suggests a possible long-term effect of electric stimulation on tinnitus that needs to be explored in the future.

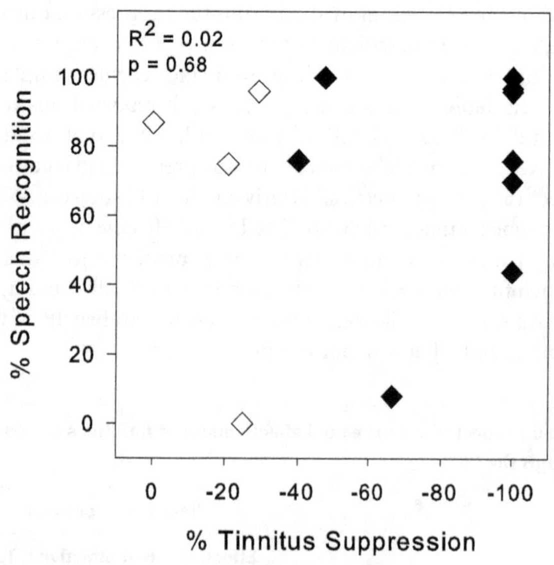

FIGURE 6 | Correlation of speech recognition with tinnitus suppression. The relationship between tinnitus suppression (*x*-axis) and speech recognition scores (*y*-axis) is shown for Responders (filled diamonds) and Non-Responders (open diamonds).

S5 also experienced profound relief of her tinnitus with use of her CI, although her relief is immediate with activation of her implant. With her CIs inactivated, her tinnitus is regularly at a LR 7–8 ("loud but comfortable" to "maximal comfort") loudness. Activation of her CIs (she is a bilateral user) brings her tinnitus down nearly instantaneously to a LR 0, or complete imperceptibility in environments with ambient noise. With CIs activated, her tinnitus does not exceed a LR 2 ("very soft") level even in a sound-attenuating booth; tinnitus suppression via electric cochlear stimulation is clearly effective for this patient. Some subjects may require multiple electrodes to be activated and/or dynamic stimulation to successfully achieve tinnitus suppression, as compared to our single-electrode, fixed stimulation tested here. Of note, 13% (30 of 227) of trials resulting in exacerbation of tinnitus were noted in the conditions tested here. This is consistent with exacerbation of tinnitus associated with CI use that has been noted in a small but notable number of patients (10%) in other studies (Quaranta et al., 2004).

Lastly, we wanted to draw attention to any link between tinnitus and musical hallucinations in acquired deafness, with absence of evidence to suggest epilepsy or psychosis. One individual contacted us with tinnitus, but complaining especially of musical hallucinations. She was not enrolled in the study for unrelated reasons, but upon questioning, two enrolled subjects (one responder and one non-responder) reported musical hallucinations. Reported sounds varied from old Elvis songs to marching band and church bells; interestingly, no individual reported any lyrics or verbal hallucinations. Non-psychotic auditory hallucinations appear to be an underreported phenomenon associated with acquired deafness and especially in the elderly (Griffiths, 2000; Auffarth and Kropp, 2009).

CONCLUSION

Tinnitus suppression is possible via electrical stimulation of the cochlea in a subset of "Responder" subjects. A large variability between subjects, as well as the lack of a "most-effective" stimulus type (with respect to stimuli parameters: rate, place, or level), is indicative of the heterogeneity of the underlying tinnitus pathophysiology and individualized percept. These findings elucidate differences between two populations of individuals with tinnitus, Responders and Non-Responders, who not only respond to their tinnitus differently, but also exhibit different patterns of loudness adaptation to externally presented electric stimuli. These findings support the auditory gain hypothesis of tinnitus and suggest there may be characteristic differences in tinnitus generation between Responder and Non-Responder groups. It should be noted that while this study is to our knowledge the largest of its kind, the study size may nevertheless be relatively small given the grand diversity of tinnitus. Tinnitus suppression appears to be possible, but parameters of effective stimuli for tinnitus suppression may need to be customized for the individual.

ACKNOWLEDGMENTS

The authors would like to thank Essie Fine, Vanessa Rothholtz, and Hamid Djalilian for subject recruitment and data collection in two of the 13 subjects tested. The authors also thank Kelly M. Reavis and Hsin-I Yang for their insightful input and support during data analysis and production of the manuscript. They also are gratefully indebted to all the subjects who participated in this study for their patience, involvement, and time. This work was supported in part by grants from the American Tinnitus Association, National Institutes of Health (P30-DC008369 and T32-DC010775) and Medical Scientist Training Program (T32-GM0862), as well as a fellowship from the Achievement Rewards for College Scientists Foundation.

REFERENCES

American Tinnitus Association. (2011). *Support for Our Vets: One of Our Top Priorities*. Portland: American Tinnitus Association. Available online: http://www.ata.org/action-alliance/support-for-veterans [Accessed 3 January 2011].

Amoodi, H. A., Mick, P. T., Shipp, D. B., Friesen, L. M., Nedzelski, J. M., Chen, J. M., and Lin, V. Y. (2012). Results with cochlear implantation in adults with speech recognition scores exceeding current criteria. *Otol. Neurotol.* 33, 6–12.

Arndt, S., Aschendorff, A., Laszig, R., Beck, R., Schild, C., Kroeger, S., Ihorst, G., and Wesarg, T. (2011). Comparison of pseudobinaural hearing to real binaural hearing rehabilitation after cochlear implantation in patients with unilateral deafness and tinnitus. *Otol. Neurotol.* 32, 39–47.

Auffarth, I. S., and Kropp, S. (2009). Musical hallucination in a patient after cochlear implantation. *J. Neuropsychiatry Clin. Neurosci.* 21, 230–231.

Axelsson, A., and Ringdahl, A. (1989). Tinnitus—a study of its prevalence and characteristics. *Br. J. Audiol.* 23, 53–62.

Baguley, D. M., and Atlas, M. D. (2007). Cochlear implants and tinnitus. *Prog. Brain Res.* 166, 347–355.

Balkany, T., Hodges, A., Menapace, C., Hazard, L., Driscoll, C., Gantz, B., Kelsall, D., Luxford, W., Mcmenomy, S., Neely, J. G., Peters, B., Pillsbury, H., Roberson, J., Schramm, D., Telian, S., Waltzman, S., Westerberg, B., and Payne, S. (2007). Nucleus Freedom North American clinical trial. *Otolaryngol. Head Neck Surg.* 136, 757–762.

Bovo, R., Ciorba, A., and Martini, A. (2010). Tinnitus and cochlear implants. *Auris Nasus Larynx* 38, 14–20.

Coles, R. R. A., Smith, P., and Davis, A. C. (1988). "The relationship between noise-induced hearing loss and tinnitus and its management," in *5th International Congress on Noise as a Public Health Problem*, eds B. Berglund, J. Karlsson, and T. Lindvall, (Stockholm: Swedish Council for Building Research).

Dauman, R., Tyler, R., and Aran, J. (1993). Intracochlear electrical tinnitus reduction. *Acta Otolaryngol.* 113, 291–295.

Eggermont, J. J., and Roberts, L. E. (2004). The neuroscience of tinnitus. *Trends Neurosci.* 27, 676–682.

Friesen, L. M., Shannon, R. V., Baskent, D., and Wang, X. (2001). Speech recognition in noise as a function of the number of spectral channels: comparison of acoustic hearing and cochlear implants. *J. Acoust. Soc. Am.* 110, 1150–1163.

Goodey, R. (2007). Tinnitus treatment: state of the art. *Prog. Brain Res.* 166, 237–246.

Griffiths, T. (2000). Musical hallucinosis in acquired deafness. Phenomenology and brain substrate. *Brain* 123 (Pt 10), 2065–2076.

Hazell, J., McKinney, C., and Aleksy, W. (1995). Mechanisms of tinnitus in profound deafness. *Ann. Otol. Rhinol. Laryngol. Suppl.* 166, 418–420.

House, J., and Brackmann, D. (1981). Tinnitus: surgical treatment. *Ciba Found. Symp.* 85, 204–216.

Ito, J., and Sakakihara, J. (1994). Tinnitus suppression by electrical stimulation of the cochlear wall and by cochlear implantation. *Laryngoscope* 104, 752–754.

Kaltenbach, J. A. (2011). Tinnitus: models and mechanisms. *Hear. Res.* 276, 52–60.

Miyamoto, R., Wynne, M., McKnight, C., and Bichey, B. (1997). Electrical suppression of tinnitus via cochlear implants. *Int. Tinnitus J.* 3, 35–38.

Moore, B. C. (2004). *An Introduction to the Psychology of Hearing*. London: Elsevier, Ltd.

Moore, B. C., Huss, M., Vickers, D. A., Glasberg, B. R., and Alcantara, J. I. (2000). A test for the diagnosis of dead regions in the cochlea. *Br. J. Audiol.* 34, 205–224.

Muhlnickel, W., Elbert, T., Taub, E., and Flor, H. (1998). Reorganization of auditory cortex in tinnitus. *Proc. Natl. Acad. Sci. U.S.A.* 95, 10340–10343.

Nilsson, M., Soli, S. D., and Sullivan, J. A. (1994). Development of the hearing in noise test for the measurement of speech reception thresholds in quiet and in noise. *J. Acoust. Soc. Am.* 95, 1085–1099.

Nondahl, D., Cruickshanks, K., Wiley, T., Klein, R., Klein, B., and Tweed, T. (2002). Prevalence and 5-year incidence of tinnitus among older adults: the epidemiology of hearing loss study. *J. Am. Acad. Audiol.* 13, 323–331.

Norena, A. J. (2011). An integrative model of tinnitus based on a central gain controlling neural sensitivity. *Neurosci. Biobehav. Rev.* 35, 1089–1109.

Pan, T., Tyler, R., Ji, H., Coelho, C., Gehringer, A., and Gogel, S. (2009). Changes in the tinnitus handicap questionnaire after cochlear implantation. *Am. J. Audiol.* 18, 144–151.

Quaranta, N., Wagstaff, S., and Baguley, D. (2004). Tinnitus and cochlear implantation. *Int. J. Audiol.* 43, 245–251.

Roberts, L. E., Eggermont, J. J., Caspary, D. M., Shore, S. E., Melcher, J. R., and Kaltenbach, J. A. (2010). Ringing ears: the neuroscience of tinnitus. *J. Neurosci.* 30, 14972–14979.

Rubinstein, J., Wilson, B., Finley, C., and Abbas, P. (1999). Pseudospontaneous activity: stochastic independence of auditory nerve fibers with electrical stimulation. *Hear. Res.* 127, 108–118.

Rubinstein, J. T., Tyler, R. S., Johnson, A., and Brown, C. J. (2003). Electrical suppression of tinnitus with high-rate pulse trains. *Otol. Neurotol.* 24, 478–485.

Ruckenstein, M. J., Hedgepeth, C., Rafter, K. O., Montes, M. L., and Bigelow, D. C. (2001). Tinnitus suppression in patients with cochlear implants. *Otol. Neurotol.* 22, 200–204.

Salvi, R. J., Wang, J., and Ding, D. (2000). Auditory plasticity and hyperactivity following cochlear damage. *Hear. Res.* 147, 261–274.

Shulman, A., Goldstein, B., and Strashun, A. M. (2009). Final common pathway for tinnitus: theoretical and clinical implications of neuroanatomical substrates. *Int. Tinnitus J.* 15, 5–50.

Souliere, C. J., Kileny, P., Zwolan, T., and Kemink, J. (1992). Tinnitus suppression following cochlear implantation. *A multifactorial investigation. Arch. Otolaryngol. Head Neck Surg.* 118, 1291–1297.

Surr, R. K., Montgomery, A. A., and Mueller, H. G. (1985). Effect of amplification on tinnitus among new hearing aid users. *Ear Hear.* 6, 71–75.

Tang, Q., Liu, S., and Zeng, F. (2006). Loudness adaptation in acoustic and electric hearing. *J. Assoc. Res. Otolaryngol.* 7, 59–70.

Tyler, R., and Kelsay, D. (1990). Advantages and disadvantages reported by some of the better cochlear-implant patients. *Am. J. Otol.* 11, 282–289.

Tyler, R. S. (ed). (2000). *Tinnitus Handbook*. Clifton Park: Delmar, Cengage Learning.

UK Cochlear Implant Study Group. (2004). Criteria of candidacy for unilateral cochlear implantation in postlingually deafened adults I: theory and measures of effectiveness. *Ear Hear.* 25, 310–335.

van de Heyning, P., Vermeire, K., Diebl, M., Nopp, P., Anderson, I., and de Ridder, D. (2008). Incapacitating unilateral tinnitus in single-sided deafness treated by cochlear implantation. *Ann. Otol. Rhinol. Laryngol.* 117, 645–652.

Vernon, J. A. (2000). Masking of tinnitus through a cochlear implant. *J. Am. Acad. Audiol.* 11, 293–294.

Vernon, J. A., and Meikle, M. (2000). "Tinnitus Masking," in *Tinnitus Handbook*, ed R. Tyler (Clifton Park: Delmar, Cengage Learning), 464.

Wilson, B. S., Finley, C. C., Lawson, D. T., Wolford, R. D., Eddington, D. K., and Rabinowitz, W. M. (1991). Better speech recognition with cochlear implants. *Nature* 352, 236–238.

Zeng, F. G. (2004). Trends in cochlear implants. *Trends Amplif.* 8, 1–34.

Zeng, F. G., Rebscher, S., Harrison, W. V., Sun, X., and Feng, H. (2008). Cochlear implants: system design, integration and evaluation.

IEEE Rev. Biomed. Eng. 1, 115–142.

Zeng, F. G., and Shannon, R. V. (1994). Loudness-coding mechanisms inferred from electric stimulation of the human auditory system. *Science* 264, 564–566.

Zeng, F. G., Tang, Q., Dimitrijevic, A., Starr, A., Larky, J., and Blevins, N. H. (2011). Tinnitus suppression by low-rate electric stimulation and its electrophysiological mechanisms. *Hear. Res.* 277, 61–66.

11

Gap prepulse inhibition and auditory brainstem-evoked potentials as objective measures for tinnitus in guinea pigs

Susanne Dehmel[1], Daniel Eisinger[1] and Susan E. Shore[1,2]*

[1] Department of Otolaryngology, Kresge Hearing Research Institute, University of Michigan, Ann Arbor, MI, USA
[2] Department of Molecular and Integrative Physiology, University of Michigan, Ann Arbor, MI, USA

***Correspondence:**
Susan E. Shore, Department of Otolaryngology, Kresge Hearing Research Institute, University of Michigan, Ann Arbor, Rm 5434 MSI, MI 48109-5616, USA.
e-mail: sushore@umich.edu

Tinnitus or ringing of the ears is a subjective phantom sensation necessitating behavioral models that objectively demonstrate the existence and quality of the tinnitus sensation. The gap detection test uses the acoustic startle response elicited by loud noise pulses and its gating or suppression by preceding sub-startling prepulses. Gaps in noise bands serve as prepulses, assuming that ongoing tinnitus masks the gap and results in impaired gap detection. This test has shown its reliability in rats, mice, and gerbils. No data exists for the guinea pig so far, although gap detection is similar across mammals and the acoustic startle response is a well-established tool in guinea pig studies of psychiatric disorders and in pharmacological studies. Here we investigated the startle behavior and prepulse inhibition (PPI) of the guinea pig and showed that guinea pigs have a reliable startle response that can be suppressed by 15 ms gaps embedded in narrow noise bands preceding the startle noise pulse. After recovery of auditory brainstem response (ABR) thresholds from a unilateral noise over-exposure centered at 7 kHz, guinea pigs showed diminished gap-induced reduction of the startle response in frequency bands between 8 and 18 kHz. This suggests the development of tinnitus in frequency regions that showed a temporary threshold shift (TTS) after noise over-exposure. Changes in discharge rate and synchrony, two neuronal correlates of tinnitus, should be reflected in altered ABR waveforms, which would be useful to objectively detect tinnitus and its localization to auditory brainstem structures. Therefore, we analyzed latencies and amplitudes of the first five ABR waves at suprathreshold sound intensities and correlated ABR abnormalities with the results of the behavioral tinnitus testing. Early ABR wave amplitudes up to N3 were increased for animals with tinnitus possibly stemming from hyperactivity and hypersynchrony underlying the tinnitus percept. Animals that did not develop tinnitus after noise exposure showed the opposite effect, a decrease in wave amplitudes for the later waves P4–P5. Changes in latencies were only observed in tinnitus animals, which showed increased latencies. Thus, tinnitus-induced changes in the discharge activity of the auditory nerve and central auditory nuclei are represented in the ABR.

Keywords: prepulse inhibition, gap detection, noise exposure, behavioral model of tinnitus, auditory brainstem responses

INTRODUCTION

Until recently, there were no reliable behavioral models to determine whether or not animals *perceive* the phantom sound known as tinnitus. Recently a test was developed by Turner et al. (Turner et al., 2006) based on the modification of the acoustic startle.

The mammalian acoustic startle response, which is elicited by sudden, loud sound, is characterized by muscle contractions of the face, neck, limb, and back resulting in a crouching posture. The primary startle reflex-eliciting circuit consists of the dorsal and ventral cochlear nucleus (DCN and VCN), cochlear root neurons, and the lateral superior olive, which deliver startle stimulus information to the caudal pontine reticular nucleus that mediates the startle via its projections to relevant muscles (Koch, 1999). The force produced during the startle can be enhanced or suppressed in the course of fear-potentiation via projections from structures such as auditory cortex, thalamus, amygdala, and hippocampus (Koch, 1999; Swerdlow et al., 2001; Li et al., 2009). Preceding the startle stimulus 30–500 ms with a non-startle-eliciting sensory input diminishes the startle amplitude. This "prepulse inhibition" (PPI) of the startle is mediated by a gating pathway comprised of the cochlear nucleus, inferior colliculus (IC), superior colliculus, and pedunculopontine tegmental nucleus, which project to the caudal pontine reticular nucleus.

The tinnitus test developed by Turner et al. (Turner et al., 2006) uses a gap embedded in different narrow gap-carrier bands as a

Abbreviations: ABR, auditory brainstem response; BBN, broad-band noise; DCN, dorsal cochlear nucleus; IC, inferior colliculus; LL, lateral lemniscus; MNTB, medial nucleus of the trapezoid body; PPI, prepulse inhibition; SOC, superior olivary complex; TTS, temporary threshold shift; VCN, ventral cochlear nucleus.

prestimulus (gap-PPI) that reduces the startle amplitude. Animals perceiving tinnitus in a specific frequency band are predicted to have diminished detection of gaps embedded in gap-carrier bands similar to the tinnitus frequency. The ongoing tinnitus thus, masks the gap. This reduces the gating efficiency of the gap, producing a larger startle. This test thus not only detects tinnitus but also reveals its frequency content.

As the test relies on a pre-attentive modification of reflex behavior and the PPI doesn't require learning (Swerdlow et al., 2000; Fendt et al., 2001; Li et al., 2009), it takes less time and effort compared to tests requiring training (Jastreboff et al., 1988; Bauer and Brozoski, 2001; Heffner and Harrington, 2002; Ruttiger et al., 2003; Lobarinas et al., 2004), enabling simultaneous testing of many animals over long time periods. Gap-PPI is not influenced by threshold shifts limited to one ear (Bauer and Brozoski, 2001; Turner et al., 2006), which is important in studies using noise over-exposure to induce tinnitus.

To date, gap-PPI has been reliably used to demonstrate noise- and salicylate-induced tinnitus in rats, mice, and gerbils and has been validated with other conditioning techniques (Bauer and Brozoski, 2001; Turner et al., 2006, 2012; Yang et al., 2007; Turner and Parrish, 2008; Longenecker and Galazyuk, 2011; Nowotny et al., 2011). Here, we apply this test to guinea pigs, which have become a model species for auditory neuroscience because of easier accessibility of their cochleas and auditory brainstems for manipulations and recordings compared to rats and mice. We describe the basic features of the guinea pigs' startle and gating and show that noise exposure results in gap-PPI deficits comparable to that shown in rats.

While ABR's have been used to measure hearing threshold and can detect hearing loss, recent studies show that thresholds can recover after noise exposure even in the face of defective auditory nerve synapses and decreased ABR wave I amplitudes (Kujawa and Liberman, 2009; Lin et al., 2011), which can be one factor in the development of tinnitus. Therefore, changes in the ABRs can be used as an objective measure of tinnitus in addition to the gap detection testing. Furthermore, ABRs could reveal areas of the auditory brainstem that are involved in the tinnitus pathology.

The ABRs recorded here were comprised of five positive and four negative peaks (**Figure 1**) as described previously for guinea pigs and cats (Wada and Starr, 1983a; Simha et al., 1988; Melcher et al., 1996a; Hsu et al., 2008; Gourevitch et al., 2009). In the ongoing discussion about the generators of certain components of the ABR, there is a general consensus that the first wave or P1–N1 is generated by the VIIIth nerve (Wada and Starr, 1983a; Simha et al., 1988; Melcher and Kiang, 1996; Melcher et al., 1996a,b). There is evidence that P2 is generated by the anteroventral and posteroventral cochlear nucleus (Buchwald and Huang, 1975; Simha et al., 1988; Melcher and Kiang, 1996; Melcher et al., 1996a,b). Contribution of the trapezoid body is seen starting with the N2 wave (Wada and Starr, 1983a,b,c; Simha et al., 1988). Wave P3 as well as N3 is attributed to superior olivary complex (SOC) and medial nucleus of the trapezoid body (MNTB) (Achor and Starr, 1980; Gardi and Bledsoe, 1981; Simha et al., 1988; Melcher and Kiang, 1996; Melcher et al., 1996a,b). P4 and N4 have been

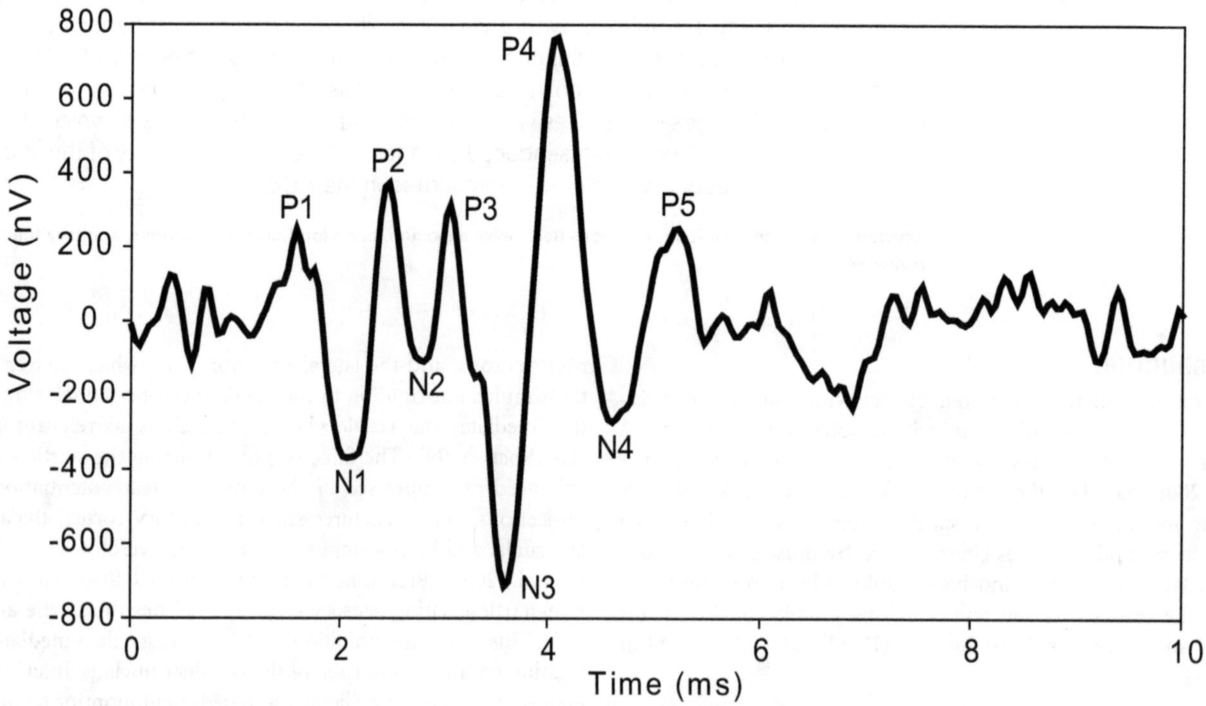

FIGURE 1 | ABR waveform morphology. Typical waveform (12 kHz, 80 dB SPL) illustrating the peaks (P) and troughs (N) of the ABR waves measured in guinea pig.

found to represent SOC and the lateral lemniscus (LL) or the trapezoid body (Buchwald and Huang, 1975; Wada and Starr, 1983b; Simha et al., 1988; Popelar et al., 2008). There is also a general consensus that P5 is generated by the IC and/or the LL (Melcher and Kiang, 1996; Melcher et al., 1996a,b; Popelar et al., 2008).

We recorded ABRs to tonal stimulation (4, 6, 7, 8, 9, 12, 16 kHz) in 10 dB steps up to 90 dB SPL. Latencies as well as interpeak latencies and amplitudes of all five positive and negative waves were measured after recovery from TTS. These parameters were compared between normal, non-exposed animals, and noise exposed animals that had or had not developed tinnitus and this comparison was done for stimulus frequency regions inside and outside the tinnitus frequency region based on the results of the behavioral gap detection testing.

Part of the behavioral test results were used as confirmation of tinnitus occurence in a different study (Dehmel et al., 2012).

METHODS

ANIMALS

Male pigmented guinea pigs from Cady Ridge Farms (270–380 g at study onset; Chelmsford, MA, USA) were used in this study. All procedures were performed in accordance with the National Institutes of Health (NIH) *Guidelines for the Use and Care of Laboratory Animals* (NIH publication no. 80-23) and guidelines provided by the University Committee on Use and Care of Animals of the University of Michigan. The number of animals used differed for the different parts of the presented results, they are indicated in each figure legend and are as follows: 13 animals were used to characterize the TTS following the noise exposure, eight animals were used to characterize the dependence of the startle on the startle pulse level, 14 animals were used to characterize the gap- and noise pulse-PPI, of those seven were noise-exposed and four were sham-exposed and continued gap- and noise pulse-PPI testing after the exposures.

BEHAVIORAL TESTING

A Kinder Behavioral Testing System (Poway, CA, USA) with testing cage and platform enclosed in a 40 × 30 × 35 cm testing chamber with speakers contained in the ceiling was used. The walls were lined with blue-pads to reduce reverberations ensuring that the 15 ms gap was "clean" as judged from an oscillogram. Two testing chambers were placed in a single walled sound booth. The signal spectra outside the gap-carrier/noise pulse bands were between 19 dB SPL and 24 dB SPL for the different frequency bands of the gap-carrier/noise pulse (4–6 kHz: 19 dB SPL, 8–10 kHz, and 12–14 kHz: 23 dB SPL, 16–18 kHz: 24 dB SPL). Gap-carrier/noise pulse bands and startle pulse calibrations were performed using a microphone (B&K ¼ inch 4136 and spectrum analyzer SR760, Stanford research systems) and guinea pig cloth model inside the testing cage with closed chamber and booth.

For the gap-PPI a 15 ms gap (excluding 5 ms offset/onset ramps) was embedded in four different 2 kHz gap-carrier bands (4–6 kHz, 8–10 kHz, 12–14 kHz, 16–18 kHz) and a broad-band noise (BBN) with two levels (60 and 70 dB SPL). The gap-carriers were played before the startle pulse for a variable time starting between 3.1 and 8.1 s to prevent anticipation of the startle pulse (**Figure 2B**). The prepulse in the noise pulse-PPI consisted of a 15 ms pulse (excluding 5 ms rise-fall time) of the same frequency bands as the gap-carrier (**Figure 2A**). The startle pulse (115 dB SPL, BBN, 20 ms) followed the gap onset or noise pulse by 100 ms. The maximum startle response in a time window 250 ms after the startle pulse was recorded.

One block of the test session began with a recording trial with no sound to record the animals' background movement (**Figure 2C**). This was followed by two presentations of the startle pulse alone. At the outset this habituated the startle response to a more stable startle level (Swerdlow et al., 2000). This was followed by alternating trials of each gap-carrier band with gap (in the gap-PPI test) or noise pulse (in the noise pulse-PPI test) preceding the startle pulse and trials with the startle pulse only. For the gap-PPI the trials with 60 and 70 dB SPL background alternated as well as the sequence of gap preceding the startle pulse ("with gap" condition) or no gap preceding the startle pulse ("without gap" condition). Inter-stimulus trial time (without gap-carrier presentation in the gap-PPI session) was pseudorandomly varied (from 0 to 5 s) to prevent startle anticipation and interval-based habituation (**Figures 2A,B**). Together with the variable time length of the gap-carrier this resulted in a separation of the startle pulses between 3.1 and 13.1 s (**Figures 2A,B**). This block of trials containing all stimulus conditions (level and frequency of gap-carrier/noise pulse, trial with or without gap/noise pulse) was repeated 10 times. The sound booth and the testing chamber doors were opened for a short break between the gap-PPI and noise pulse-PPI session. Both sessions lasted about 35 min each.

The gap-PPI and noise pulse-PPI testing was performed throughout the study on two days each week (Monday and Thursday, unless otherwise noted; **Figure 2C**). ABRs and noise exposures were performed on the following day (Tuesdays or Fridays). Baseline gap-PPI and noise pulse-PPI testing were performed for 2–3 weeks before the noise exposure. After the first noise exposure, testing continued for another two weeks until the animals received a second noise or sham exposure ($n = 9$ animals; all of the control animals); two other animals received only one noise exposure (both no-tinnitus animals). After the last noise exposure the gap-PPI and noise pulse-PPI testing continued for 2–3 weeks. Behavioral data after the noise exposure was used only for days after the animals ABR had recovered.

NOISE EXPOSURE

The noise exposure was performed under anesthesia (first dose: 14 mg/kg body weight Xylazine and 110 mg/kg Ketamine; additional dose 2–3 h later, when responses to toe pinch occured: 4 mg/kg Xylazine and 13 mg/kg Ketamine). Body temperature was kept constant with a temperature controlled heating pad. The left ear was exposed for 2 h and the right ear was plugged with pieces of soft, moldable silicon ear plugs. A Beyer DT 48 speaker was enclosed in a custom-made housing that attached to a 3 cm silicon tube that ended in a cone-shaped plastic tip inserted about 2 mm tightly into the ear canal. Pilot experiments showed no influence of the noise on the unexposed ear. The noise was generated with digital signal processing hardware (TDT, Alachua, FL, USA) and Matlab and its spectrum is shown in **Figure 2B**. The noise was calibrated by inserting the plastic tip into a tube attached to a B&K ¼

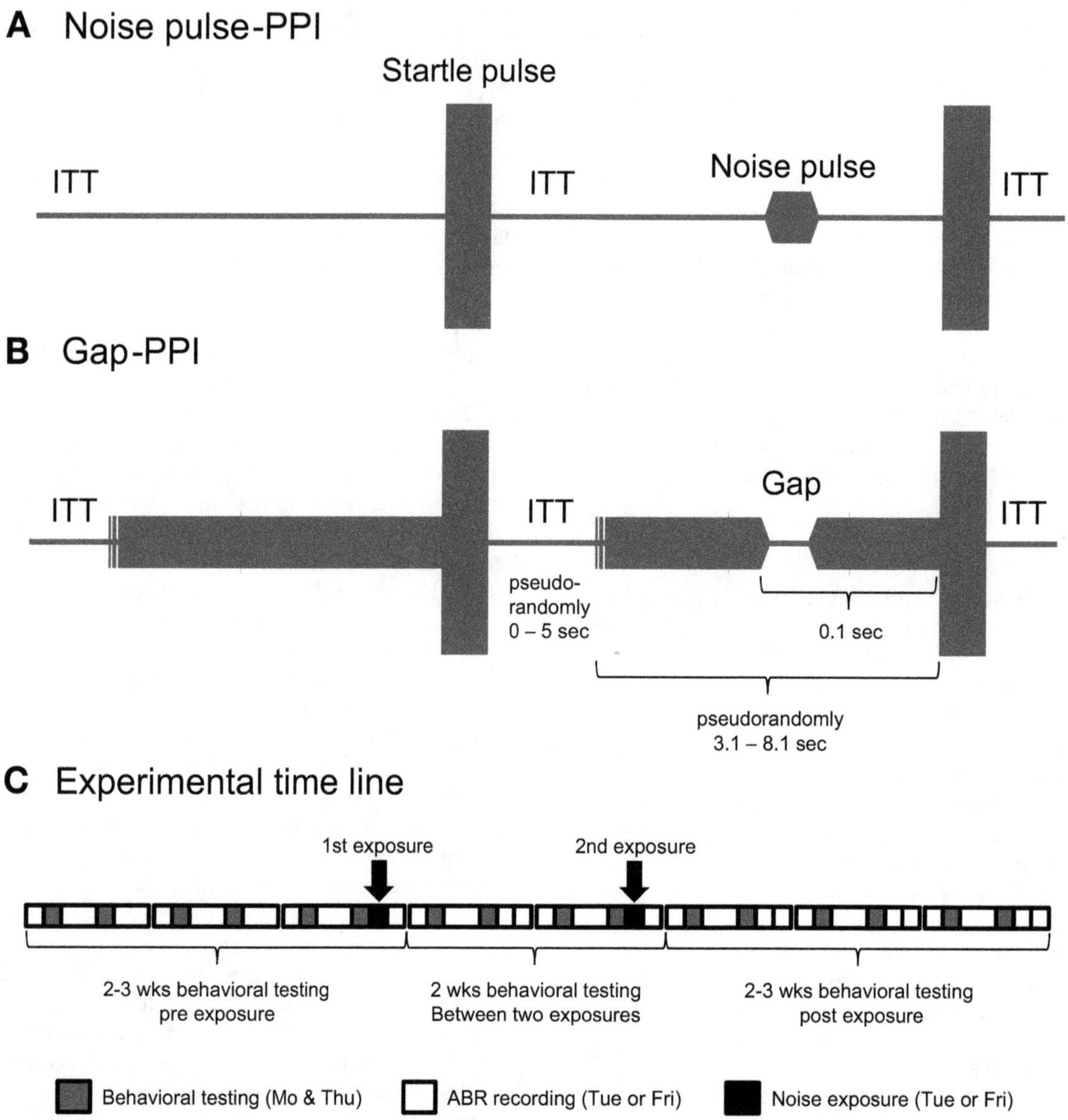

FIGURE 2 | Stimulus structure for the noise pulse-PPI test (A) and Gap-PPI test (B) showing a trial without the prepulse followed by a trial with the prepulse. Note that the timeline is not entirely drawn to scale, because of the comparably long inter-trial interval time (ITT), which was pseudo-randomly varied between 0 and 5 s and the long pseudo-randomly varied time of 3.1–8.1 s between the start of a trial and the presentation of the startle pulse. The experimental timeline is shown in **(C)**. Behavioral testing was done throughout the experiment, including 2–3 weeks before the first, and 2–3 weeks after the last exposure. Note that two of the 11 animals tested received only one noise exposure. The exposures and ABRs were done either on Tuesdays or Fridays for a certain animal; in the example shown in the **(C)** they were done on Fridays.

inch microphone (4136) and spectrum analyzer (SR760 Stanford research systems).

ABR RECORDINGS

Prior to ABR measurements the animals received an injection of antibacterial solution (enrofloxacin, 10 mg/kg body weight, Baytril, Bayer, KS, USA), after the ABR they received an injection of 10 ml saline and antibacterial eardrops (ofloxacin, 0.3%, Floxin Otic, Daiichi Sankyo Inc., Edison, NJ, USA).

ABR recordings were performed using BioSigRP software and RX5/RA4LI hardware (TDT, Alachua, FL, USA). The speaker (Beyer DT 48) calibration and acoustic stimulation were performed with SigGenRP software and RX8/PA5 hardware (TDT, Alachua, FL, USA). The speaker was coupled to the animals' ear canal as described above for the noise. ABRs were recorded immediately before and immediately after the noise exposure. ABRs were performed weekly on days following the behavioral testing after the exposure (Tuesdays, Fridays) under anesthesia (5 or 10 mg/kg body weight Xylazine) (AnaSed Injection, Akorn Inc., Decatur, IL, USA) and 20 or 40 mg/kg body weight Ketamine (Hospira Inc., Lake Forest, IL, USA). Body temperature was kept constant with a temperature controlled heating pad. Sanded 0.6 × 25 mm injection needles placed subdermally at vertex and on each masseter were used for recording, grounding, and reference. ABRs were recorded for 10 ms tone pips (2 ms ramp, 11 stimuli/s) starting with a level of 90 dB SPL, and decremented in 10 dB steps. Each level was repeated 250 times and the lower levels near threshold were re-run to record a second set of 250 presentations. ABR waveforms were visually inspected across levels; threshold was the lowest level of sound that resulted in one or more of the ABR waves being distinguishable by eye from the background noise. The second set of repetitions for the low levels was checked for waveform consistency.

DATA ANALYSIS

Data analysis and plotting were performed with Sigma Plot (Version 11, Systat Software Inc., Chicago, IL, USA) and SPSS (Version 17, SPSS Inc., Chicago, IL, USA). Two-Way repeated measure ANOVAs were performed on the averaged absolute startle data within each gap-carrier band for either the gap-PPI or noise pulse-PPI. Repeated within subject factors were trial type (with or without prepulse) and sound level (60 or 70 dB, **Figure 6**), an additional between subject factor was the animal group (control or exposure group, **Figure 7**; control or "tinnitus" or "no-tinnitus" group, **Figure 9**). *Post-hoc* all pairwise multiple comparisons were done using Holm–Sidak ($p = 0.05$).

ABR's were analyzed without any knowledge of group of animal. All ABR's were analyzed at 4, 6, 7, 8, 9, 12, and 16 kHz and from 90 to 50 dB SPL in decrements of 10 dB. Latency (time in ms at which the positive peak occurred after the stimulus onset) and interpeak latency (time between positive peaks) of each consecutive peak were measured (**Figure 1**). Increased interpeak latencies indicate further shifting of the peak in addition to the shift of P1.

Two types of linear mixed model statistics were used to reveal significant differences in ABR amplitudes and latencies. First, four linear mixed models with wave (P1, N1, etc.), group (control, tinnitus, no-tinnitus) and interaction as fixed effects and a pairwise comparison of groups for each wave were used to investigate significant differences between groups. This was done separately for amplitudes and latencies for ABR frequencies within the tinnitus frequency region (according to the behavioral test) and outside the tinnitus frequency region (results of those tests noted with < and > symbols). Second, linear mixed models with group, dB level, and interaction as fixed effects and pairwise comparison at each dB level revealed significant differences between the groups for single dB levels. This was done separately for each wave amplitude peak (P1, N1, etc.) and wave latency (PL P1, IPL 2–1, etc.) for frequencies with tinnitus and frequencies without tinnitus (results noted with * and ‡ symbols above and below the respective dB levels). Differences were significant at the 0.05 level, adjustment for multiple comparisons with Bonferroni.

RESULTS

TEMPORARY THRESHOLD SHIFT FOLLOWING UNILATERAL NARROW BAND NOISE EXPOSURE

Since noise over-exposure is the most common cause of tinnitus among patients with known tinnitus origin (Davis and Rafaie, 2000; Eggermont, 2005) noise exposure was used to induce tinnitus in guinea pigs. In order to distinguish its effects on auditory thresholds from those on the measured tinnitus, unilateral noise exposure conditions were chosen (1/4 octave noise band centered at 7 kHz; **Figure 3B**) that resulted in a TTS in the exposed ear (**Figure 3A**). A center frequency of 7 kHz was chosen because it is within the central region of the guinea pig audiogram (Heffner et al., 1971; Prosen et al., 1978; Gourevitch et al., 2009), allowing the development of tinnitus within the hearing range of the guinea pig above and below the center of the noise band. The immediate mean threshold shift in the left/exposed ears during the first hour after the exposure was 50 dB centered at 8 kHz

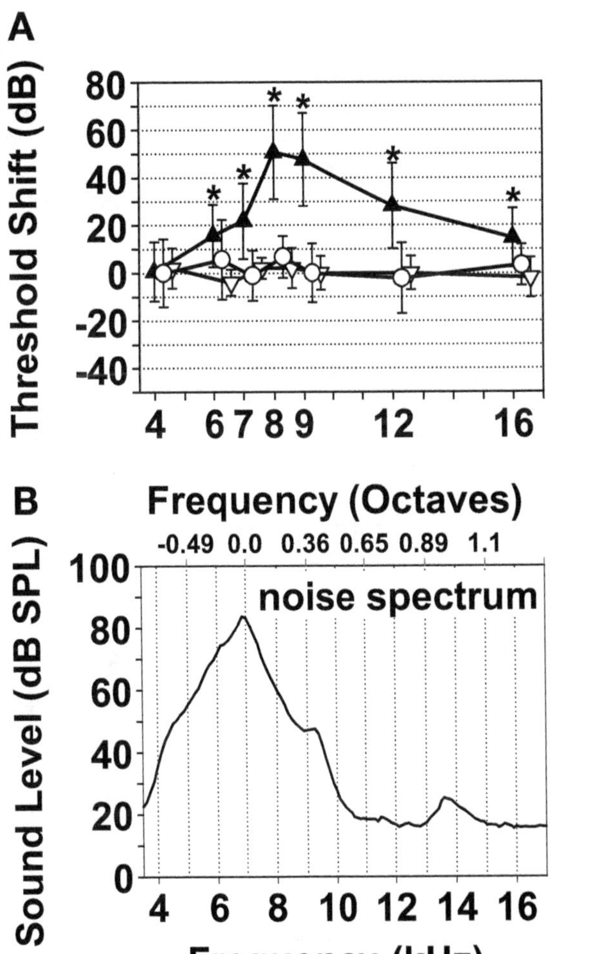

FIGURE 3 | Characterization of the narrow band noise over-exposure protocol leading to TTS. (A) ABR threshold shift pre-exposure vs. immediately after the noise overexposure (black triangles) and one and two weeks after the exposure (white triangles and dots). The mean and standard deviation of the 1st and/or 2nd noise exposures (17 ABRs) of 13 animals are shown for the immediate (1 h) threshold shift (black triangles), one week (three animals/fiveABRs; white triangles) and 11–14 days after the noise exposure (seven animals/nine ABRs; white dots). *Marks significance in one-sample *t*-test against a mean threshold shift equaling 0 performed for each test frequency: $p <= 0.001$. **(B)** Noise Spectrum centered at 7 kHz, bandwidth 6.4–7.6 kHz (1.21 kHz, 1/4 octave band), RMS 97 dB SPL.

(black triangles, **Figure 3A**, $p <= 0.001$). One and two weeks after the exposure, the ABR thresholds of the exposed ears had recovered to their pre-exposure values (white triangles and dots, **Figure 3A**, $p = 0.05$).

THE ACOUSTIC STARTLE RESPONSE IN THE GUINEA PIG

Influence of the startle pulse level

The strength of the startle response was assessed for different startle pulse levels embedded in background noise (**Figure 4**). In this example, pulses embedded in the 12–14 kHz/70 dB SPL background elicited startle responses that increased in amplitude for sound levels above 80 dB SPL. No obvious (across the group of animals tested) and consistent (over the two test days for each animal) saturation of the startle response was observed up to the highest level of 115 dB SPL tested. The average 0.32 N for the startle at a level of 115 dB (**Figure 4**) was clearly not the maximal startle response of guinea pigs, which was dependent on the stimulus parameters (e.g., mean of 0.41 N with the startle pulse embedded in BBN 70 dB SPL; see **Figure 6A**). Therefore, 115 dB SPL was the chosen level for the subsequent gap-PPI and noise pulse-PPI tests to ensure a reliable startle response without presenting unnecessarily loud startle pulses above the saturation point.

Reliability of the startle response

A sufficiently large startle response is a prerequisite for observing its reduction by gaps or noise pulses. However, the startle response amplitude is affected by startle pulse level, stimulus repetition rate, and test session duration. The startle amplitude as well as the general background movement (without sound presentation) over the time course of a test session is shown in **Figure 5**. The decrement in startle response amplitudes over time, commonly described as short-term habituation (black and white circles, **Figure 5**) occurred in conjunction with decrements in the background movement of the animal such as walking, scratching, etc., over time (white triangles, **Figure 5**). The habituation affects the startle responses with and without the preceding gap in a similar way, because the habituation is a characteristic of the startle response itself, not of the circuitry mediating the sensorimotor gating i.e., reduction of the startle response by the gap. Thus, both graphs shifted to lower startle amplitudes in parallel over the time course of the session. Although the normalized startle response was variable, it did not show a clear pattern over time, especially when comparing the responses in the four different gap-carrier bands (gray graphs in the four panels of **Figure 5**; a Two-Way repeated measures ANOVA on ranks of the normalized startle, with the gap-carrier bands and trial number as repeated within subjects factors, revealed a significant effect of the gap-carrier bands but not of the trial number and no significant interaction between bands and trial number, $p = 0.05$). Moreover, the startle responses were clearly larger than the background movements (white triangles, **Figure 5**). These data demonstrate that it is possible to reliably measure the startle behavior of the guinea pig.

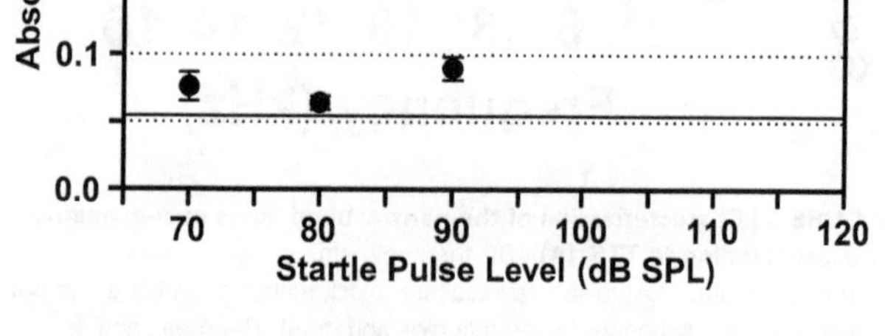

FIGURE 4 | Acoustic startle response amplitude varies with the startle stimulus level and does not saturate up to 115 dB SPL. The startle amplitudes are plotted in response to different intensity pulses embedded in a background noise band of 12–14 kHz/70 dB SPL. Mean ± SEM for eight animals are shown, including two test days per animal. The horizontal line marks the Mean + SEM of the animal's background movement (without sound presentation).

Gap- and noise pulse-salience are indicated by reduced startle responses

A preceding gap reduced the startle response (white circles, **Figure 5**) even in the first trial of a session compared to the "without gap" condition (black filled circles, **Figure 5**). This reduction reflects the ability of the animal to detect the gap, which serves as a prepulse that reduces the startle response without the requirement of learning (Fendt et al., 2001; Li et al., 2009). **Figure 5** also shows that the normalized startle did not increase over the time of the session, suggesting that the length of the gap was sufficiently above detection threshold not to be influenced by attention (Gewirtz and Davis, 1995).

The baseline gap-PPI for gaps in noise and noise pulse-PPI for noise pulses in quiet before noise exposure are shown in **Figure 6**. The results of the noise pulse-PPI test are used to indicate the salience of the same noise band used as a gap-carrier. Thus, a good performance on the noise pulse-PPI task indicates a solid salience of the noise band also used as gap-carrier. This helps to distinguish threshold changes from changes that affect gap detection. The normalized startle (startle "with gap"/"without gap", right Y axis, **Figure 6A**) was smaller for the 70 dB SPL background noise bands (lower panels in **Figure 6A**) compared to the 60 dB SPL noise bands (upper panels in **Figure 6A**), presumably because of the greater gap salience in a louder carrier background i.e., producing a larger reduction of the startle by the gap. The normalized startle decreased as the frequency band of the gap-carrier increased and was smallest for the BBN carrier (0.81 for the 4–6 kHz and 0.49 for the BBN carrier). The reduction of the startle by the gap was significant for both levels and all gap-carrier bands ($p < 0.05$). The size of the absolute startle without the gap (black dots, left Y axis **Figure 6**) decreased from the 60 dB SPL background carrier to the 70 dB SPL background carrier, indicating a greater masking effect of a louder background on the startle pulse. Therefore, when the two levels of the gap-carrier were compared, for the 70 dB SPL level a smaller absolute

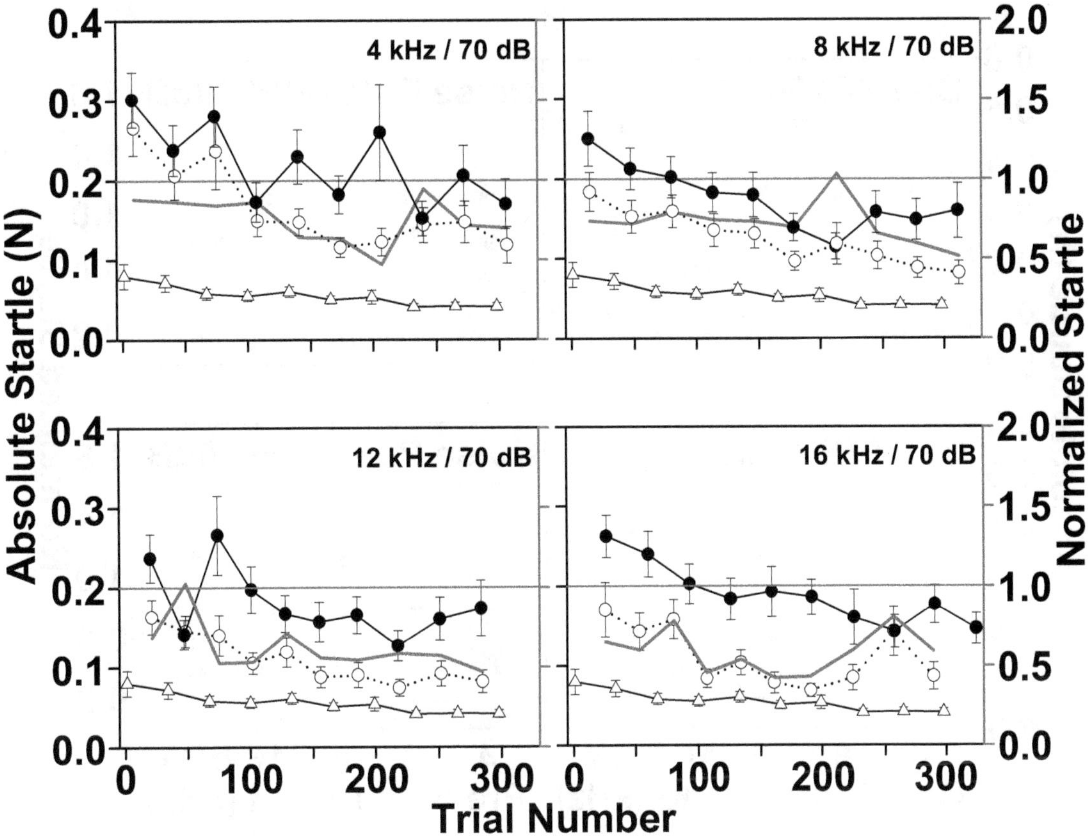

FIGURE 5 | Short-term habituation of the startle responses and decrement of the background movement during a during a gap-PPI test session. Each stimulus condition was repeated 10 times. The mean ± SEM of the responses from 14 animals is shown over four test days (two consecutive weeks, Monday, and Thursday) for different background bands (4–6 kHz, 8–10 kHz, 12–14 kHz, 16–18 kHz, all at 70 dB SPL). Black filled circle graphs designate the absolute responses to a startle pulse without preceding gap; white circle graphs are the responses when the startle pulse follows a 15 ms gap, white triangle graphs indicate the background movement of the animal in intermingled trials without sound presentation (left Y axis). The gray line graphs plot the normalized startle response (startle "with gap"/startle "without gap"; right Y axis with gray labels) derived from the mean startle responses of all days of all animals.

startle was accompanied by a greater reduction of the startle due to the gap. Also in the noise pulse-PPI paradigm the reduction of the startle due to the noise pulse was larger for the 70 dB SPL compared to the 60 dB SPL noise pulse (normalized startle response, bars in upper panel vs. lower panel of **Figure 6B**). The normalized startle response varied for the 70 dB SPL noise pulse between 0.53 for the 4–6 kHz noise pulse and 0.37 for the BBN pulse. These baseline data show that the guinea pigs' ability to detect gaps and noise pulses can be reliably measured by the PPI tests. The 70 dB SPL gap-carrier and noise pulse conditions resulted in larger reductions of the startle response, and thus, are better suited to observe an increase in the normalized startle i.e., decreasing gap or noise pulse detection. We, therefore, concentrated on the gap-PPI and noise pulse-PPI in the 70 dB SPL condition after the noise exposure.

DECREASED GAP DETECTION AFTER NOISE EXPOSURE AS AN INDICATOR OF TINNITUS

After establishing a baseline for the gap- and noise pulse-PPI, seven animals were over-exposed with noise and four animals served as controls, receiving a sham exposure. One to two weeks after noise exposure, after the ABR thresholds had recovered (**Figure 3**), the normalized startles of the noise exposed animals were increased for the gap in the 8–10 kHz gap-carrier band (white bars, **Figure 7A**), the difference between the startle in the "with gap" and "without the gap" condition was not significant. This indicates decreased gap detection for the noise exposed group compared to the control group. In contrast to the gap-PPI, the noise pulse-PPI (**Figure 7B**) showed a significant difference between the "with pulse" and "without pulse" condition indicating a significant detection of the pulses for all frequency bands. Therefore, the decreased gap detection in the 8–10 kHz band after noise exposure was not a result of decreased salience of the gap-carrier. The diminished gap detection after noise exposure in the 8–10 kHz gap-carrier band is hypothesized to be a reflection of tinnitus that develops in the noise exposed animals and is pronounced in this frequency band as it "masks the gap".

Not all patients with abnormal audiograms or noise exposures develop tinnitus (Lockwood et al., 2002; Kaltenbach et al., 2005). Therefore, an analysis based on groups of animals that develop

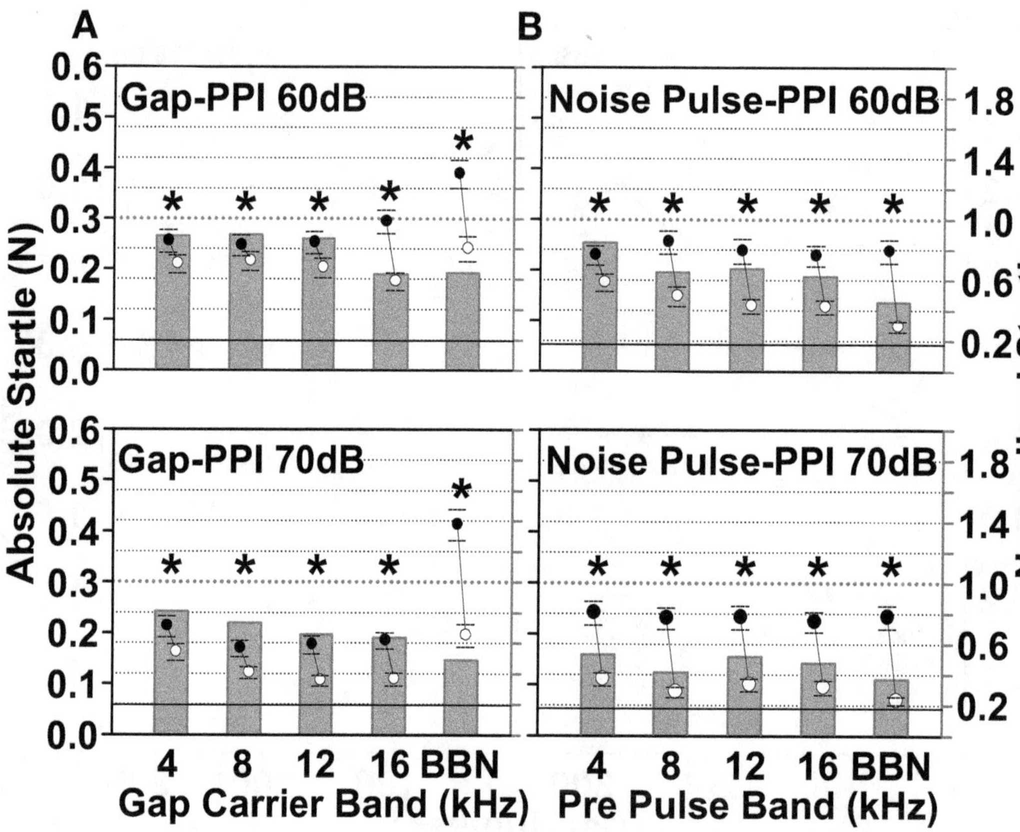

FIGURE 6 | Guinea pigs show significant detection of gaps in background noise and noise pulses of 60 and 70 dB SPL. Baseline gap-PPI **(A)** and noise pulse-PPI **(B)** are shown before noise exposure for five different noise bands of the gap-carrier and noise pulse: 4–6 kHz, 8–10 kHz, 12–14 kHz, 16–18 kHz, and BBN. Top panels show the PPI of a 15 ms gap embedded in a 60 dB SPL gap-carrier and of a 15 ms pre pulse of 60 dB SPL, lower panels show the respective data for 70 dB SPL gap-carrier and noise pulse. The data is from 14 animals, during the three or four test-days per animal directly before the noise exposure (two days per week, Monday and Thursday), for 10 repetitions per stimulus condition. Normalized startle (bars, right Y-axis) was calculated by dividing all trials of all animals with gap **(A)** or noise pulse **(B)** by all trials without gap or noise pulse. The absolute startle response is shown as mean ±95% confidence interval of all trials without and of all trials with the gap or noise pulse (black and white dots and lines, left Y-axis). Gray dotted line at 1 is the startle without the gap or noise pulse preceding (normalized startle, right Y axis). The black line designates the mean +95% confidence interval of responses due to random background movements (recorded without sound presentation). The * marks significance in Two-Way repeated measures ANOVA ($p < 0.05$).

tinnitus vs. those that do not is ideal. The distribution of gap-PPI data for the different gap-carrier bands is shown for individual animals in **Figure 8**. In agreement with the significant increase in the normalized startle across the group of noise exposed animals (**Figure 7**), the distribution of normalized startles for the 8–10 kHz carrier was shifted toward higher values compared to the control animals (black line distribution curve, top panel vs. bottom panel of 8–10 kHz in **Figure 8**). The distribution of the data of single animals for the 8–10 kHz gap-carrier (colors of stacked histogram, top row panels in **Figure 8**) divides the noise exposed group into two subgroups, which mark the extremes of the distribution: animals whose data points are above the mean of the control group ("tinnitus" group, pale, striped bars), and a second group of animals, whose data points are at or below the mean of the control group ("no-tinnitus" group: dark bars). The tinnitus animals were also characterized by increased normalized startle responses compared to their pre-exposure responses. Although there was only a significant difference for the noise exposed vs. the control group as a whole for the 8–10 kHz gap-carrier (**Figure 7**), the "tinnitus" group animals tend to have higher normalized startle values also for the 12–14 kHz, 16–18 kHz gap-carrier bands (pale bars shifted to the right compared to dark bars, top row panels **Figure 8**).

The absolute startles of the gap-PPI and noise pulse-PPI task, together with the resulting normalized startles are shown for the "tinnitus" and "no-tinnitus" groups of animals (classified with **Figure 8**) in comparison to the control group in **Figure 9**. There was no significant difference between the "with gap" and "without gap" condition in the 8–10, 12–14, and 16–18 kHz bands in the tinnitus group (**Figure 9A**), indicating deteriorated gap detection in those bands, whereas the control groups' data showed significant differences in all bands. The difference between the "with prepulse" and "without prepulse" condition (**Figure 9B**) was significant for all three groups of animals in all frequency bands. This

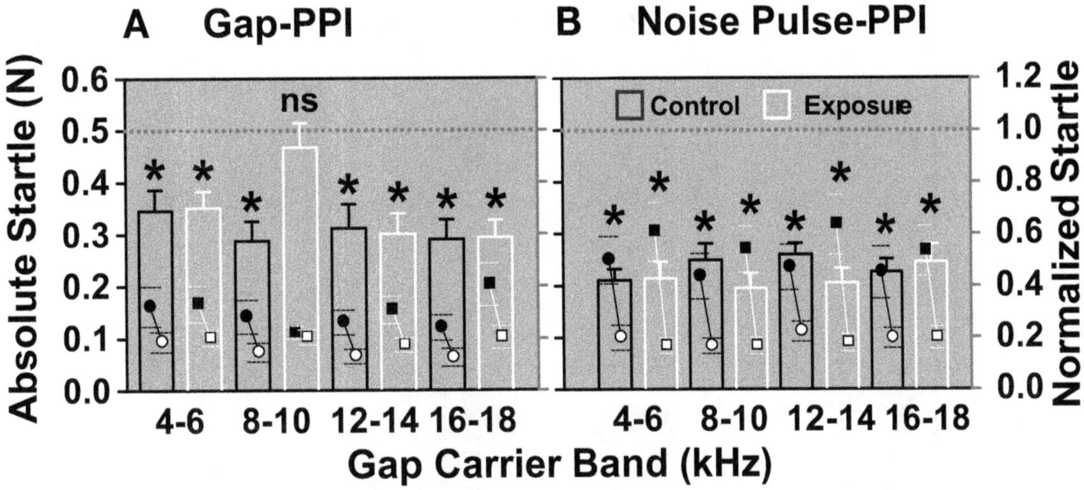

FIGURE 7 | After noise exposure animals cannot detect a gap in the 8–10 kHz band anymore (A), while their noise pulse-PPI (B) is still significant (detectible) in all bands. The normalized startle response (mean + SEM) of exposed animals (white bars; $N = 7$) is shown in comparison with control sham exposed animals (black bars; $N = 4$) for the four different gap-carrier/noise pulse bands. Normalized startle responses were derived from the mean of all trials of one animal for one day with the gap normalized to the mean of all trials of one animal of one day without the gap. *Indicates significance in Two-Way repeated measures ANOVA ($p < 0.05$).

indicates tinnitus residing in the 8–18 kHz bands, which diminishes the gap detection in those bands. Even though the absolute startle "without gap" was decreased for the 8–10 kHz and the 12–14 kHz band in the "tinnitus" group compared to the control group it was still larger than the startle "with gap" in the control group i.e., giving room for further reduction of the startle due to the gap. That means that the failure to decrease the startle by the gap was not caused by a floor effect, further supporting tinnitus as underlying cause for the increased normalized startle.

MODIFICATIONS OF ABR WAVES ACCOMPANYING TINNITUS MANIFESTATION

Amplitudes of all ABR waves for frequencies with and without tinnitus were larger for tinnitus animals and smaller for the no-tinnitus group compared to the control group. The increase in amplitude across all sound levels of the tinnitus animals compared to the control group was significant for the earlier waves N1, P2, and N3 (con < tinn labels, **Figure 10A**), whereas the amplitude decrease across sound levels of the no-tinnitus group was significant for the later waves P4, N4, and P5 (con > notinn labels, **Figure 10A**, $p < 0.05$, Linear mixed model, pairwise comparison of groups for each wave, details see Methods). Significant increases in the tinnitus groups' wave amplitudes were not confined to the frequency range of the tinnitus, but were observed for frequencies with tinnitus (N1), frequencies without tinnitus (P2), and for both frequency ranges (N3). In case of single levels showing significant differences these were observed at the highest levels tested (* and ‡ labels at 80 and 90 dB, **Figure 10A**, $p < 0.05$, Linear mixed model, pairwise comparison at each level for each IPL, details see Methods). ABR wave latencies tended to be longer in tinnitus animals and shorter in no-tinnitus animals. However, while there were no significant changes for the no-tinnitus group, the latency increase for the tinnitus animals was significant for P1, IPL 2–1, IPL 4–3, and IPL 5–4 (con < tinn labels, **Figure 10B**, $p < 0.05$, Linear mixed model, pairwise comparison of groups for each wave, details see Methods). These significant increases in latency for the tinnitus group were specific for frequencies with tinnitus (IPL 2–1 and IPL 5–4) or affected both frequency ranges (PL P1 and IPL 4–3).

DISCUSSION

PPI OF THE ACOUSTIC STARTLE RESPONSE IN THE GUINEA PIG

In rats, startle reductions of 45–50% occur for 15 and 20 ms gaps in a 75 dB SPL BBN background (Wang et al., 2009b; Swetter et al., 2010). The similarity to the data obtained here (reduction of 51% in a 70 dB SPL BBN) underlines the suitability of the gap-PPI test in the guinea pig.

The startle response did not saturate at higher startle pulse levels as in other species (Pilz and Schnitzler, 1996; Plappert and Pilz, 2002; Gaese et al., 2009; Sun et al., 2009). However, we measured the startle response in the presence of background noise used for the gap- and noise pulse-PPI tests. The background masks the startle pulse and reduces the startle, so larger startles and greater saturation occurs without a background noise. Such a masking effect was also seen in the baseline gap-PPI: increasing the background noise from 60 to 70 dB SPL decreased the absolute startle for trials "without gap."

The average startle for the 115 dB SPL startle pulse was 0.32 N, below the maximal startle but above background movements. This is important to avoid ceiling and floor effects when measuring PPI, i.e., a lower startle is more resistant to a further reduction, whereas a higher startle is relatively more reduced (Swerdlow et al., 2000). Baseline gap-PPI showed no relative floor effect: the absolute startle "without gap" in the 70 dB SPL condition was smaller than that in the 60 dB SPL condition, but its reduction was larger. Therefore, the larger startle response reduction in the

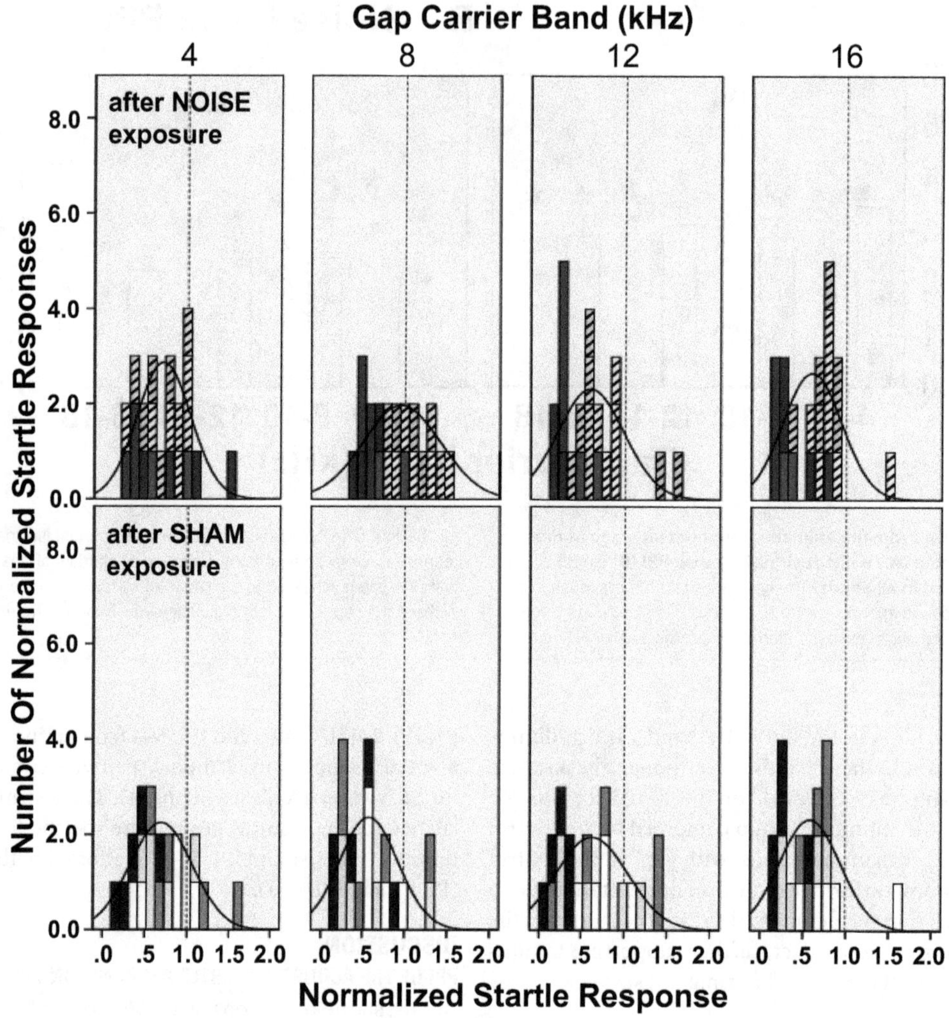

FIGURE 8 | Noise exposure differentially affects gap-PPI in subgroups of noise exposed animals. Normalized startle responses for single days after noise exposure are shown as histograms for the different gap-carrier bands (panel columns), overlaid with the normal distribution curve of the histograms (black graph based on mean and standard deviation). Normalized startle responses were derived from the mean of all trials of one animal for one day with the gap normalized to the mean of all trials of one animal for one day without the gap. Data is included for 2–5 days with recovered ABR thresholds (2, 3, 3, 4, 4, 4 test days in the noise exposed groups and 5 days in the control group). Top row: noise exposed animals ($N = 7$), bottom row: control animals ($N = 4$). The individual animals' data are identified by the color of the stacked histograms. Noise-exposed animals are grouped as "tinnitus" (light, pastel colored striped bars, $N = 4$) or "no tinnitus" (dark colored bars, $N = 3$). "Tinnitus" animals show normalized responses shifted toward higher startle values. The dotted line in each panel marks 1 (100% startle).

70 dB SPL condition can be attributed to greater salience of the gap in a louder carrier.

Short-term habituation of the startle but not of the gap-PPI, as shown previously, suggests that the animals' attention remained constant during the session or that the 15 ms gap length was sufficiently above detection threshold not to be influenced by attention. Decreasing attention results in a reduction of PPI if the prepulses are too close to detection threshold (Wu et al., 1984; Gewirtz and Davis, 1995). Habituation, a proposed correlate of synaptic depression in the caudal pontine reticular nucleus, is specific for the stimulus modality of the prepulse (Simons-Weidenmaier et al., 2006). However, in our dataset the animals' background movement also decreased, suggesting habituation or decreased arousal during the session.

INFLUENCE OF NOISE-INDUCED TEMPORARY THRESHOLD SHIFT ON PPI

After recovery from noise exposure guinea pigs showed significantly diminished gap-PPI but normal noise pulse-PPI in the 8–10 kHz noise band compared to the control group. The absolute startle responses also indicated tinnitus-like behavior in the 12–14 and 16–18 kHz bands in a subgroup of animals. This is interpreted as tinnitus perception in the 8–10/12–14/16–18 kHz frequency bands, which corresponds to the frequency regions that showed TTS immediately after exposure.

Distinguishing tinnitus from other consequences of noise exposure

Gap detection is level-dependent below 20–30 dB SL (Hamann et al., 2004). However, monaural threshold elevation with an

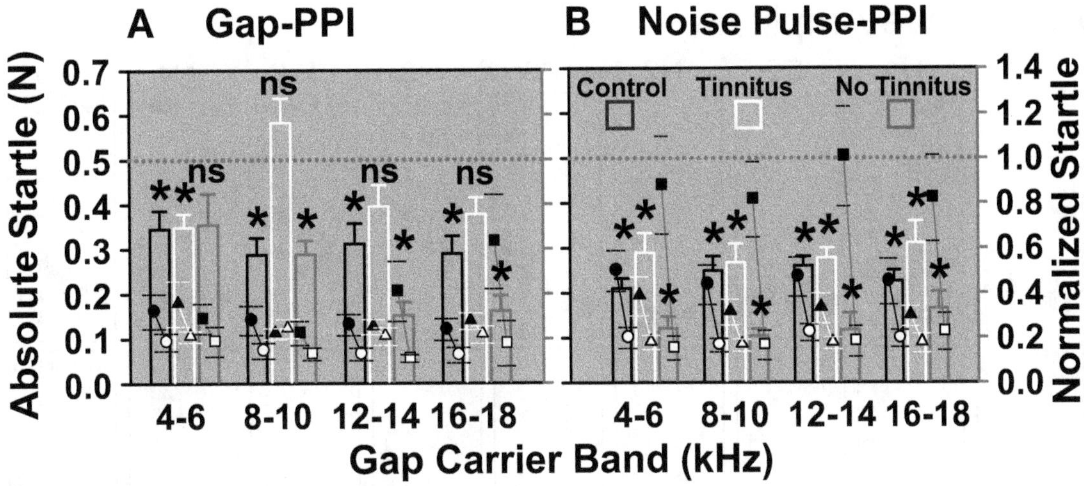

FIGURE 9 | Animals in the tinnitus group show no significant detection of gaps in gap-carrier bands between 8 and 18 kHz. Normalized (bars, right Y axis, mean) and absolute startles (dot plots, left Y axis, mean ±95% confidence interval) are shown for the two noise exposure groups and the control group after the noise/sham exposure. **(A)** Gap-PPI and **(B)** noise pulse-PPI. Black bars and circles: sham exposure control group ($n = 4$), white bars and triangles: "tinnitus" group ($n = 4$), gray bars and squares: "no tinnitus" group ($n = 3$). Black symbols designate the mean of the absolute startles "without gap", white symbols designate the mean of the startles "with gap". Normalized startle responses were derived from the mean of all trials of one animal for one day with the gap normalized to the mean of all trials of one animal of one day without the gap. The *indicates significance in Two-Way repeated measures ANOVA ($p < 0.05$).

earplug does not diminish gap-PPI tested with the present paradigm (Turner et al., 2006). Also, results of the noise pulse-PPI test have been used to argue against hearing loss as a cause for diminished gap-PPI (Yang et al., 2007; Turner and Parrish, 2008). In this and previous studies (Turner et al., 2006; Turner and Parrish, 2008; Wang et al., 2009a) unilateral noise exposures causing TTS were preferred so as to leave one ear undisturbed to accomplish the behavioral task. This will be an important challenge for human studies using the gap-PPI paradigm. Deciding if one ear is undisturbed is difficult based on the knowledge that even with normal thresholds noise exposure can cause deafferentation and loss of hair cells or spiral ganglion cells and other structural and activity changes (Weisz et al., 2006; Zheng et al., 2006, 2007; Bauer et al., 2007; Brozoski et al., 2007; Kujawa and Liberman, 2009; Wang et al., 2009a; Zeng et al., 2009).

Changes in absolute vs. normalized startle—Tinnitus behavior equals increased startle in the "with gap" condition

Changes in PPI after noise exposure reveal changes in both startle behavior, i.e., changes in the pathway mediating the acoustic startle, and in PPI, i.e., the pathway mediating sensorimotor gating (Swerdlow et al., 2000; Yee et al., 2005). Ideally, changes in sensorimotor gating occur because of gap detection deficits due to tinnitus, without concomitant changes in startle behavior. This would be expressed as an increase in the startle "with gap" and no change of the startle "without gap". However, this "ideal case" is unlikely given the unavoidable effects of factors like aging and experience that influence startle behavior and gating (Friedman et al., 2004; Swetter et al., 2010). Changes over time unrelated to noise exposure were taken into account by comparing data for noise-exposed animals with an experience- and age-matched control group and resulted predominantly in a decrease in the startle in trials with and without gaps (not shown). Factors decreasing the startle over time presumably existed also in noise-exposed animals, but here development of tinnitus counteracted the decrease over time and increased the startle in the "with gap" condition only. Factors decreasing the startle over time should also affect noise pulse-PPI. However, the noise pulse-PPI was not diminished after noise exposure, pointing to tinnitus specifically affecting gap-PPI. A comparable absolute startle "without gap" between the control and experimental groups showed that changes in the normalized startle data were not contaminated by "relative floor/ceiling effects" (Swerdlow et al., 2000; Yee et al., 2005), with a higher startle response being more susceptible to a reduction and a smaller startle more susceptible to an enhancement. The difference between groups occurred in the startle response "with gap", which was higher in the "tinnitus" group (**Figure 9A**), consistent with the hypothesis of tinnitus masking the gap.

Tinnitus and hyperacusis

In the present study, hyperacusis would likely result in decreased normalized startle responses for the gap- and noise-pulse PPI test as the gap carrier and noise-pulse are both well above hearing threshold. The startle response without preceding gap or noise-pulse should be increased (Sun et al., 2009). These expectations are met by the no-tinnitus group, which shows decreased normalized startles and increased absolute startles in the gap-PPI and noise pulse-PPI test. Because tinnitus and hyperacusis often co-occur (Anari et al., 1999; Schaaf et al., 2003; Nelson and Chen, 2004; Dauman and Bouscau-Faure, 2005), their effects on normalized startle responses in the gap-PPI test could counteract each other, with tinnitus increasing and hyperacusis decreasing the normalized startle values.

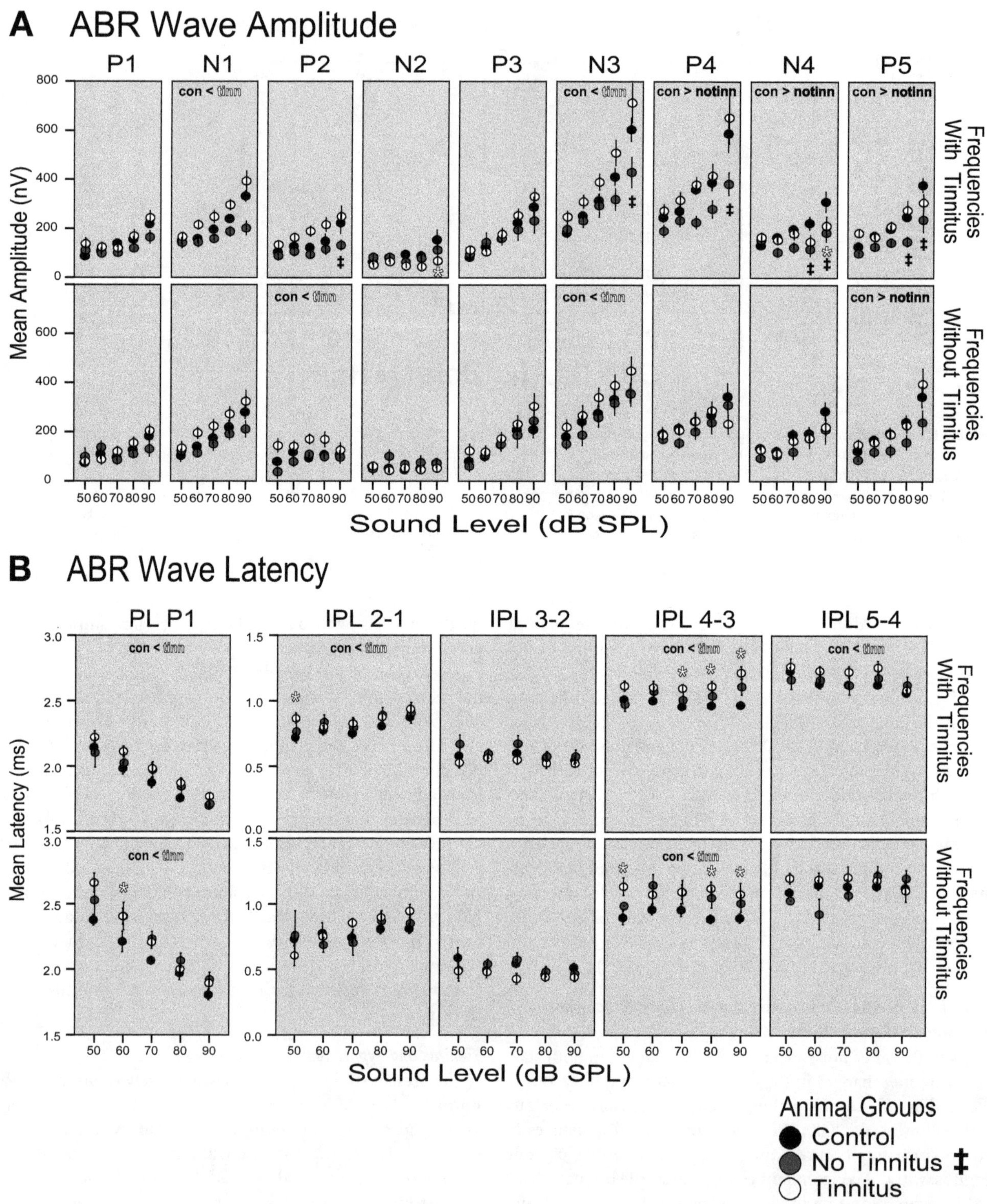

FIGURE 10 | (A) Amplitude and (B) latency of ABRs as functions of sound level. Data was averaged across frequencies "with tinnitus" according to the PPI tests (8, 9, 12, 16 kHz; upper row panels in A and B) and "without tinnitus" (4, 6, 7 kHz; lower row panels). The mean and standard error is shown for the group of control (black dots, $n = 4$ animals), no-tinnitus (gray dots, $n = 3$ animals) and tinnitus animals (white dots, $n = 4$ animals). Significant differences between groups for an ABR parameter are indicated with < or > in the respective panel ($p < 0.05$, linear mixed model statistics with pairwise comparisons of groups across dB level) and significant differences for single levels are indicated with * (tinnitus vs. control group) and with ‡ (no-tinnitus vs. control; $p < 0.05$, linear mixed model statistics with pairwise comparisons at each level). For details see Methods. P1, P2, P3, P4, P5: positive wave peaks, N1, N2, N3, N4: negative wave troughs, PL: peak latency, IPL: interpeak latency, measured between the positive wave peaks.

The site of tinnitus manifestation

Because of the gap-PPI specificity (pulse-PPI is not influenced, **Figures 7, 9**) tinnitus presumably occurs in neuronal groups that are part of the gap-encoding circuitry. The auditory input pathways of the gating circuits mediating the PPI reside in the auditory brainstem and midbrain (Koch, 1999; Li et al., 2009) and neuronal correlates of gap-detection in the IC match behavioral performance (Walton et al., 1997). Still top-down modulation from cortical inputs to the brainstem/midbrain could influence PPI by changed attention to the prepulses (Li et al., 2009; Du et al., 2011) and deficits in gap-PPI have been observed after cortex inactivation (Ison et al., 1991).

Noise-exposure also changes activity levels in structures outside the auditory system. Activity changes in structures as amygdala, hypothalamus, locus coeruleus, and others, have been implicated in tinnitus development (Wallhausser-Franke et al., 2003; Zhang et al., 2003; Mahlke and Wallhausser-Franke, 2004; Wang et al., 2009a; Rauschecker et al., 2010). These structures also play a role in the modulation of the acoustic startle and of the PPI (Koch, 1999; Li et al., 2009). Descending modulation of the gating circuit modifying the effectiveness of a prestimulus for PPI would change the normalized startle. However, changes in the gating circuit would presumably not be specific for the frequency or type of the auditory prepulse. In our data-set gap-PPI changed only for specific gap-carrier bands (8–10 kHz, 12–14 kHz, and 16–18 kHz) but not for the 4–6 kHz gap-carriers. In addition, the pulse-PPI task did not show changes. This argues against changes in descending modulation of the gating circuit underlying the observed tinnitus like behavior supporting the concept that gap encoding of auditory neurons in the primary gating pathway is disturbed due to tinnitus.

CHANGES OF ABRs WITH TINNITUS DEVELOPMENT

The amplitude of the tinnitus groups' ABRs were increased for the earlier waves up to N3, although this was only significant for waves N1, P2, and N3 and not specific for the tinnitus frequency range. The increase in amplitude fits the assumption that tinnitus is caused by hyperactivity and hyper-synchrony in the auditory brainstem and midbrain, i.e., in the auditory nerve (N1), anteroventral and posteroventral cochlear nucleus (P2), and SOC and/or MNTB [N3; (Buchwald and Huang, 1975; Achor and Starr, 1980; Gardi and Bledsoe, 1981; Wada and Starr, 1983a; Simha et al., 1988; Melcher and Kiang, 1996; Melcher et al., 1996a,b)].

This contradicts studies showing reduced wave I and III amplitudes in patients with tinnitus (Lemaire and Beutter, 1995; Schaette and Kempter, 2009; Schaette and McAlpine, 2011), however, corroborates another study showing enlarged wave III amplitudes in tinnitus patients (Attias et al., 1996). Otherwise enlarged waves were only found in middle latency responses, not in the early ABR waves (Gerken et al., 2001; Singh et al., 2011). Hyperactivity in animals with tinnitus in single unit recordings has only been shown in the DCN (Brozoski et al., 2002; Kaltenbach et al., 2004; Dehmel et al., 2012). Hyperactivity after noise exposure has been shown in the VCN (Bledsoe et al., 2009; Vogler et al., 2011). However, hyperactivity after noise exposure in the auditory nerve, VCN, posteroventral cochlear nucleus, and their projection targets in the TB and SOC as suggested by our ABR data would need to be corroborated by unit recordings in animals with tinnitus.

The no-tinnitus animals showed a tendency for a reduction of wave amplitudes, which was significant for waves presumably generated by the SOC, TB, and LL [P4, N4; (Buchwald and Huang, 1975; Wada and Starr, 1983b; Simha et al., 1988; Popelar et al., 2008)] and by the IC and/or LL [P5; (Melcher and Kiang, 1996; Melcher et al., 1996a,b; Popelar et al., 2008)].

The effects seen in the early waves are not detectable in later waves starting with P4. This might result from plastic changes of e.g., synapse efficiency, excitatory-inhibitory balance that counteract the modified input from the lower brainstem.

The discrepancy between the ABR results of our study and the studies with tinnitus patients (Lemaire and Beutter, 1995; Schaette and Kempter, 2009; Schaette and McAlpine, 2011) might result from the longer times between the noise exposure and development of tinnitus in case of the human studies and/or the more diverse or unclear causes of tinnitus in patients compared to the controlled conditions in animal experiments.

There are no other animal ABR studies comparing noise-exposed animals with and without the development of tinnitus, however, in the studies investigating the effect of noise exposure a higher percentage of animals not developing tinnitus might have resulted in decreased wave I amplitudes, as in our no-tinnitus group (Kujawa and Liberman, 2009; Lin et al., 2011). In addition the difference between our study and the studies of Liberman et al. might be caused by the different noise exposure regimes (awake, binaural exposure in Libermans' studies vs. anesthetized, monaural in our model).

An effect on the latency of the ABR waveforms was only observed in the tinnitus group which showed a significant prolongation of the P1 latency and all interpeak latencies except IPL 3–2 for the tinnitus frequency range. These data replicate the prolonged latencies found in tinnitus patients (Lemaire and Beutter, 1995; Rosenhall and Axelsson, 1995; Gerken et al., 2001; Kehrle et al., 2008) and are assumed to indicate the effect of the noise exposure on the auditory nerve and additional conductivity and processing problems along the auditory pathway, which as shown here, lead to tinnitus.

Changes in amplitudes and latencies of the different ABR waves and thus in the gross activity of the respective structures would also change their function as part of the primary startle reflex-eliciting circuit (VCN and lateral superior olive) and of the gating pathway (cochlear nucleus and IC).

ACKNOWLEDGMENTS

This work was supported by the Tinnitus Research Initiative, NIH R01DC004825, and P01 DC00078. We are grateful to Chris Ellinger and Dwayne Vailliencort for the excellent technical assistance with the setup and Beth Hand and Gary Dootz, for expert data collection and analysis. We thank Ben Yates for excellent graphic and editorial assistance and Jeremy Turner for valuable discussions and comments on the manuscript.

REFERENCES

Achor, L. J., and Starr, A. (1980). Auditory brain stem responses in the cat. II. Effects of lesions. *Electroencephalogr. Clin. Neurophysiol.* 48, 174–190.

Anari, M., Axelsson, A., Eliasson, A., and Magnusson, L. (1999). Hypersensitivity to sound. *Scand. Audiol.* 28, 219–230.

Attias, J., Pratt, H., Reshef, I., Bresloff, I., Horowitz, G., Polyakov, A., and Shemesh, Z. (1996). Detailed analysis of auditory brainstem responses in patients with noise-induced tinnitus. *Audiology* 35, 259–270.

Bauer, C. A., and Brozoski, T. J. (2001). Assessing tinnitus and prospective tinnitus therapeutics using a psychophysical animal model. *J. Assoc. Res. Otolaryngol.* 2, 54–64.

Bauer, C. A., Brozoski, T. J., and Myers, K. (2007). Primary afferent dendrite degeneration as a cause of tinnitus. *J. Neurosci. Res.* 85, 1489–1498.

Bledsoe, S. C. Jr., Koehler, S., Tucci, D. L., Zhou, J., Le Prell, C., and Shore, S. E. (2009). Ventral cochlear nucleus responses to contralateral sound are mediated by commissural and olivocochlear pathways. *J. Neurophysiol.* 102, 886–900.

Brozoski, T. J., Bauer, C. A., and Caspary, D. M. (2002). Elevated fusiform cell activity in the dorsal cochlear nucleus of chinchillas with psychophysical evidence of tinnitus. *J. Neurosci.* 22, 2383–2390.

Brozoski, T. J., Ciobanu, L., and Bauer, C. A. (2007). Central neural activity in rats with tinnitus evaluated with manganese-enhanced magnetic resonance imaging (MEMRI). *Hear. Res.* 228, 168–179.

Buchwald, J. S., and Huang, C. (1975). Far-field acoustic response: origins in the cat. *Science* 189, 382–384.

Dauman, R., and Bouscau-Faure, F. (2005). Assessment and amelioration of hyperacusis in tinnitus patients. *Acta Otolaryngol.* 125, 503–509.

Davis, A., and Rafaie, E. A. (2000). "Epidemiology of tinnitus," in *Tinnitus Handbook,* ed R. S. Tyler (San Diego, CA: Singular Publishing Group),1–24.

Dehmel, S., Pradhan, S., Koehler, S., Bledsoe, S., and Shore, S. (2012). Noise over-exposure alters long-term somatosensory-auditory processing in the dorsal cochlear nucleus – possible basis for tinnitus-related hyperactivity? *J. Neurosci.* 32, 1660–1671.

Du, Y., Wu, X., and Li, L. (2011). Differentially organized top-down modulation of prepulse inhibition of startle. *J. Neurosci.* 31, 13644–13653.

Eggermont, J. J. (2005). Tinnitus: neurobiological substrates. *Drug Discov. Today* 10, 1283–1290.

Fendt, M., Li, L., and Yeomans, J. S. (2001). Brain stem circuits mediating prepulse inhibition of the startle reflex. *Psychopharmacology (Berl.)* 156, 216–224.

Friedman, J. T., Peiffer, A. M., Clark, M. G., Benasich, A. A., and Fitch, R. H. (2004). Age and experience-related improvements in gap detection in the rat. *Brain Res. Dev. Brain Res.* 152, 83–91.

Gaese, B. H., Nowotny, M., and Pilz, P. K. (2009). Acoustic startle and prepulse inhibition in the Mongolian gerbil. *Physiol. Behav.* 98, 460–466.

Gardi, J. N., and Bledsoe, S. C. Jr. (1981). The use of kainic acid for studying the origins of scalp-recorded auditory brainstem responses in the guinea pig. *Neurosci. Lett.* 26, 143–149.

Gerken, G. M., Hesse, P. S., and Wiorkowski, J. J. (2001). Auditory evoked responses in control subjects and in patients with problem-tinnitus. *Hear. Res.* 157, 52–64.

Gewirtz, J. C., and Davis, M. (1995). Habituation of prepulse inhibition of the startle reflex using an auditory prepulse close to background noise. *Behav. Neurosci.* 109, 388–395.

Gourevitch, B., Doisy, T., Avillac, M., and Edeline, J. M. (2009). Follow-up of latency and threshold shifts of auditory brainstem responses after single and interrupted acoustic trauma in guinea pig. *Brain Res.* 1304, 66–79.

Hamann, I., Gleich, O., Klump, G. M., Kittel, M. C., and Strutz, J. (2004). Age-dependent changes of gap detection in the Mongolian gerbil (*Meriones unguiculatus*). *J. Assoc. Res. Otolaryngol.* 5, 49–57.

Heffner, H. E., and Harrington, I. A. (2002). Tinnitus in hamsters following exposure to intense sound. *Hear. Res.* 170, 83–95.

Heffner, R., Heffner, H., and Masterton, B. (1971). Behavioral measurements of absolute and frequency-difference thresholds in guinea pig. *J. Acoust. Soc. Am.* 49, 1888–1895.

Hsu, W. C., Wang, J. D., Lue, J. H., Day, A. S., and Young, Y. H. (2008). Physiological and morphological assessment of the saccule in Guinea pigs after noise exposure. *Arch. Otolaryngol. Head Neck Surg.* 134, 1099–1106.

Ison, J. R., O'Connor, K., Bowen, G. P., and Bocirnea, A. (1991). Temporal resolution of gaps in noise by the rat is lost with functional decortication. *Behav. Neurosci.* 105, 33–40.

Jastreboff, P. J., Brennan, J. F., Coleman, J. K., and Sasaki, C. T. (1988). Phantom auditory sensation in rats: an animal model for tinnitus. *Behav. Neurosci.* 102, 811–822.

Kaltenbach, J. A., Zacharek, M. A., Zhang, J., and Frederick, S. (2004). Activity in the dorsal cochlear nucleus of hamsters previously tested for tinnitus following intense tone exposure. *Neurosci. Lett.* 355, 121–125.

Kaltenbach, J. A., Zhang, J., and Finlayson, P. (2005). Tinnitus as a plastic phenomenon and its possible neural underpinnings in the dorsal cochlear nucleus. *Hear. Res.* 206, 200–226.

Kehrle, H. M., Granjeiro, R. C., Sampaio, A. L., Bezerra, R., Almeida, V. F., and Oliveira, C. A. (2008). Comparison of auditory brainstem response results in normal-hearing patients with and without tinnitus. *Arch. Otolaryngol. Head Neck Surg.* 134, 647–651.

Koch, M. (1999). The neurobiology of startle. *Prog. Neurobiol.* 59, 107–128.

Kujawa, S. G., and Liberman, M. C. (2009). Adding insult to injury: cochlear nerve degeneration after "temporary" noise-induced hearing loss. *J. Neurosci.* 29, 14077–14085.

Lemaire, M. C., and Beutter, P. (1995). Brainstem auditory evoked responses in patients with tinnitus. *Audiology* 34, 287–300.

Li, L., Du, Y., Li, N., Wu, X., and Wu, Y. (2009). Top-down modulation of prepulse inhibition of the startle reflex in humans and rats. *Neurosci. Biobehav. Rev.* 33, 1157–1167.

Lin, H. W., Furman, A. C., Kujawa, S. G., and Liberman, M. C. (2011). Primary neural degeneration in the Guinea pig cochlea after reversible noise-induced threshold shift. *J. Assoc. Res. Otolaryngol.* 12, 605–616.

Lobarinas, E., Sun, W., Cushing, R., and Salvi, R. (2004). A novel behavioral paradigm for assessing tinnitus using schedule-induced polydipsia avoidance conditioning (SIP-AC). *Hear. Res.* 190, 109–114.

Lockwood, A. H., Salvi, R. J., and Burkard, R. F. (2002). Tinnitus. *N. Engl. J. Med.* 347, 904–910.

Longenecker, R. J., and Galazyuk, A. V. (2011). Development of tinnitus in CBA/CaJ mice following sound exposure. *J. Assoc. Res. Otolaryngol.* 12, 647–658.

Mahlke, C., and Wallhausser-Franke, E. (2004). Evidence for tinnitus-related plasticity in the auditory and limbic system, demonstrated by arg3.1 and c-fos immunocytochemistry. *Hear. Res.* 195, 17–34.

Melcher, J. R., Guinan, J. J. Jr., Knudson, I. M., and Kiang, N. Y. (1996a). Generators of the brainstem auditory evoked potential in cat. II. Correlating lesion sites with waveform changes. *Hear. Res.* 93, 28–51.

Melcher, J. R., Knudson, I. M., Fullerton, B. C., Guinan, J. J. Jr., Norris, B. E., and Kiang, N. Y. (1996b). Generators of the brainstem auditory evoked potential in cat. I. An experimental approach to their identification. *Hear. Res.* 93, 1–27.

Melcher, J. R., and Kiang, N. Y. (1996). Generators of the brainstem auditory evoked potential in cat. III: Identified cell populations. *Hear. Res.* 93, 52–71.

Nelson, J. J., and Chen, K. (2004). The relationship of tinnitus, hyperacusis, and hearing loss. *Ear Nose Throat J.* 83, 472–476.

Nowotny, M., Remus, M., Kossl, M., and Gaese, B. H. (2011). Characterization of the perceived sound of trauma-induced tinnitus in gerbils. *J. Acoust. Soc. Am.* 130, 2827–2834.

Pilz, P. K., and Schnitzler, H. U. (1996). Habituation and sensitization of the acoustic startle response in rats: amplitude, threshold, and latency measures. *Neurobiol. Learn. Mem.* 66, 67–79.

Plappert, C. F., and Pilz, P. K. (2002). Difference in anxiety and sensitization of the acoustic startle response between the two inbred mouse strains BALB/cAN and DBA/2N. *Genes Brain Behav.* 1, 178–186.

Popelar, J., Grecova, J., Rybalko, N., and Syka, J. (2008). Comparison of noise-induced changes of auditory brainstem and middle latency response amplitudes in rats. *Hear. Res.* 245, 82–91.

Prosen, C. A., Petersen, M. R., Moody, D. B., and Stebbins, W. C. (1978). Auditory thresholds and kanamycin-induced hearing loss in the guinea pig assessed by a positive reinforcement procedure. *J. Acoust. Soc. Am.* 63, 559–566.

Rauschecker, J. P., Leaver, A. M., and Muhlau, M. (2010). Tuning out the noise: limbic-auditory interactions in tinnitus. *Neuron* 66, 819–826.

Rosenhall, U., and Axelsson, A. (1995). Auditory brainstem response latencies in patients with tinnitus. *Scand. Audiol.* 24, 97–100.

Ruttiger, L., Ciuffani, J., Zenner, H. P., and Knipper, M. (2003). A behavioral paradigm to judge acute sodium salicylate-induced sound experience in rats: a new approach for an animal model on tinnitus. *Hear. Res.* 180, 39–50.

Schaaf, H., Klofat, B., and Hesse, G. (2003). Hyperacusis, phonophobia, and recruitment. Abnormal deviations of hearing associated with hypersensitivity to sound. *HNO* 51, 1005–1011.

Schaette, R., and Kempter, R. (2009). Predicting tinnitus pitch from patients' audiograms with a computational model for the development of neuronal hyperactivity. *J. Neurophysiol.* 101, 3042–3052.

Schaette, R., and McAlpine, D. (2011). Tinnitus with a normal audiogram: physiological evidence for hidden hearing loss and computational model. *J. Neurosci.* 31, 13452–13457.

Simha, N., Paquereau, J., Cazals, Y., and Aran, J. M. (1988). Effects of electrolytic lesions of the superior olivary complex and trapezoid body on brainstem auditory-evoked potentials in the guinea pig. I. Vertex-tragus recordings. *Audiology* 27, 279–290.

Simons-Weidenmaier, N. S., Weber, M., Plappert, C. F., Pilz, P. K., and Schmid, S. (2006). Synaptic depression and short-term habituation are located in the sensory part of the mammalian startle pathway. *BMC Neurosci.* 7, 38.

Singh, S., Munjal, S. K., and Panda, N. K. (2011). Comparison of auditory electrophysiological responses in normal-hearing patients with and without tinnitus. *J. Laryngol. Otol.* 125, 668–672.

Sun, W., Lu, J., Stolzberg, D., Gray, L., Deng, A., Lobarinas, E., and Salvi, R. J. (2009). Salicylate increases the gain of the central auditory system. *Neuroscience* 159, 325–334.

Swerdlow, N. R., Braff, D. L., and Geyer, M. A. (2000). Animal models of deficient sensorimotor gating: what we know, what we think we know, and what we hope to know soon. *Behav. Pharmacol.* 11, 185–204.

Swerdlow, N. R., Geyer, M. A., and Braff, D. L. (2001). Neural circuit regulation of prepulse inhibition of startle in the rat: current knowledge and future challenges. *Psychopharmacology (Berl.)* 156, 194–215.

Swetter, B. J., Fitch, R. H., and Markus, E. J. (2010). Age-related decline in auditory plasticity: experience dependent changes in gap detection as measured by prepulse inhibition in young and aged rats. *Behav. Neurosci.* 124, 370–380.

Turner, J., Larsen, D., Hughes, L., Moechars, D., and Shore, S. (2012). Time course of tinnitus development following noise exposure in mice. *J. Neurosci. Res.* 90, 1480–1488.

Turner, J. G., Brozoski, T. J., Bauer, C. A., Parrish, J. L., Myers, K., Hughes, L. F., and Caspary, D. M. (2006). Gap detection deficits in rats with tinnitus: a potential novel screening tool. *Behav. Neurosci.* 120, 188–195.

Turner, J. G., and Parrish, J. (2008). Gap detection methods for assessing salicylate-induced tinnitus and hyperacusis in rats. *Am. J. Audiol.* 17, S185–S192.

Vogler, D. P., Robertson, D., and Mulders, W. H. (2011). Hyperactivity in the ventral cochlear nucleus after cochlear trauma. *J. Neurosci.* 31, 6639–6645.

Wada, S. I., and Starr, A. (1983a). Generation of auditory brain stem responses (ABRs). I. Effects of injection of a local anesthetic (procaine HCI) into the trapezoid body of guinea pigs and cat. *Electroencephalogr. Clin. Neurophysiol.* 56, 326–339.

Wada, S. I., and Starr, A. (1983b). Generation of auditory brain stem responses (ABRs). II. Effects of surgical section of the trapezoid body on the ABR in guinea pigs and cat. *Electroencephalogr. Clin. Neurophysiol.* 56, 340–351.

Wada, S. I., and Starr, A. (1983c). Generation of auditory brain stem responses (ABRs). III. Effects of lesions of the superior olive, lateral lemniscus and inferior colliculus on the ABR in guinea pig. *Electroencephalogr. Clin. Neurophysiol.* 56, 352–366.

Wallhausser-Franke, E., Mahlke, C., Oliva, R., Braun, S., Wenz, G., and Langner, G. (2003). Expression of c-fos in auditory and non-auditory brain regions of the gerbil after manipulations that induce tinnitus. *Exp. Brain Res.* 153, 649–654.

Walton, J. P., Frisina, R. D., Ison, J. R., O'Neill, W. E. (1997). Neural correlates of behavioral gap detection in the inferior colliculus of the young CBA mouse. *J. Comp. Physiol. A* 181, 161–176.

Wang, H., Brozoski, T. J., Turner, J. G., Ling, L., Parrish, J. L., Hughes, L. F., and Caspary, D. M. (2009a). Plasticity at glycinergic synapses in dorsal cochlear nucleus of rats with behavioral evidence of tinnitus. *Neuroscience* 164, 747–759.

Wang, H., Turner, J. G., Ling, L., Parrish, J. L., Hughes, L. F., and Caspary, D. M. (2009b). Age-related changes in glycine receptor subunit composition and binding in dorsal cochlear nucleus. *Neuroscience* 160, 227–239.

Weisz, N., Hartmann, T., Dohrmann, K., Schlee, W., and Norena, A. (2006). High-frequency tinnitus without hearing loss does not mean absence of deafferentation. *Hear. Res.* 222, 108–114.

Wu, M. F., Krueger, J., Ison, J. R., and Gerrard, R. L. (1984). Startle reflex inhibition in the rat: its persistence after extended repetition of the inhibitory stimulus. *J. Exp. Psychol. Anim. Behav. Process.* 10, 221–228.

Yang, G., Lobarinas, E., Zhang, L., Turner, J., Stolzberg, D., Salvi, R., and Sun, W. (2007). Salicylate induced tinnitus: behavioral measures and neural activity in auditory cortex of awake rats. *Hear. Res.* 226, 244–253.

Yee, B. K., Chang, T., Pietropaolo, S., and Feldon, J. (2005). The expression of prepulse inhibition of the acoustic startle reflex as a function of three pulse stimulus intensities, three prepulse stimulus intensities, and three levels of startle responsiveness in C57BL6/J mice. *Behav. Brain Res.* 163, 265–276.

Zeng, C., Nannapaneni, N., Zhou, J., Hughes, L. F., and Shore, S. (2009). Cochlear damage changes the distribution of vesicular glutamate transporters associated with auditory and nonauditory inputs to the cochlear nucleus. *J. Neurosci.* 29, 4210–4217.

Zhang, J. S., Kaltenbach, J. A., Wang, J., and Kim, S. A. (2003). Fos-like immunoreactivity in auditory and nonauditory brain structures of hamsters previously exposed to intense sound. *Exp. Brain Res.* 153, 655–660.

Zheng, Y., Baek, J. H., Smith, P. F., and Darlington, C. L. (2007). Cannabinoid receptor down-regulation in the ventral cochlear nucleus in a salicylate model of tinnitus. *Hear. Res.* 228, 105–111.

Zheng, Y., Seung Lee, H., Smith, P. F., and Darlington, C. L. (2006). Neuronal nitric oxide synthase expression in the cochlear nucleus in a salicylate model of tinnitus. *Brain Res.* 1123, 201–206.

12

Tinnitus does not require macroscopic tonotopic map reorganization

Dave R. M. Langers[1,2]*, Emile de Kleine[1,2] and Pim van Dijk[1,2]

[1] Department of Otorhinolaryngology/Head and Neck Surgery, University Medical Center Groningen, University of Groningen, Groningen, Netherlands

[2] Graduate School of Medical Sciences (Research School of Behavioural and Cognitive Neurosciences), University of Groningen, Groningen, Netherlands

***Correspondence:**
Dave R. M. Langers, Department of Otorhinolaryngology/Head and Neck Surgery, University Medical Center Groningen, University of Groningen, P.O. Box 30.001, 9700 RB Groningen, Netherlands.
e-mail: d.r.m.langers@umcg.nl

The pathophysiology underlying tinnitus, a hearing disorder characterized by the chronic perception of phantom sound, has been related to aberrant plastic reorganization of the central auditory system. More specifically, tinnitus is thought to involve changes in the tonotopic representation of sound. In the present study we used high-resolution functional magnetic resonance imaging to determine tonotopic maps in the auditory cortex of 20 patients with tinnitus but otherwise near-normal hearing, and compared these to equivalent outcomes from 20 healthy controls with matched hearing thresholds. Using a dedicated experimental paradigm and data-driven analysis techniques, multiple tonotopic gradients could be robustly distinguished in both hemispheres, arranged in a pattern consistent with previous findings. Yet, maps were not found to significantly differ between the two groups in any way. In particular, we found no evidence for an overrepresentation of high sound frequencies, matching the tinnitus pitch. A significant difference in evoked response magnitude was found near the low-frequency tonotopic endpoint on the lateral extreme of left Heschl's gyrus. Our results suggest that macroscopic tonotopic reorganization in the auditory cortex is not required for the emergence of tinnitus, and is not typical for tinnitus that accompanies normal hearing to mild hearing loss.

Keywords: functional magnetic resonance imaging, auditory cortex, humans, tinnitus, tonotopy

INTRODUCTION

Subjective tinnitus is a prevalent and presently incurable hearing disorder that is characterized by the perception of sound in the absence of an identifiable sound source. Many people have experienced ephemeral episodes of tinnitus at some point in their life without permanent consequences. However, persisting tinnitus may have a debilitating effect on an individual's state and functioning, leading many chronic tinnitus patients to seek medical attention.

In spite of a growingly useful body of behavioral and neurophysiological research in humans and animals, the pathophysiological mechanism that causes tinnitus still remains to be elucidated (Baguley, 2002; Eggermont, 2007a; Møller, 2007a; Rauschecker et al., 2010; Roberts et al., 2010; Kaltenbach, 2011). An important clue lies in the observation that the perceived tinnitus pitch often coincides with frequency regions in which hearing thresholds are found to be elevated. It is still debated whether tinnitus is most closely associated with the frequency range that covers the hearing loss (Noreña et al., 2002; Roberts et al., 2008) or with the edge-frequency where the audiogram is steepest (König et al., 2006; Moore and Vinay, 2010), but in either case the existence of the association suggests some causal relationship.

Tinnitus is not generated in the ear itself. Presumably, hearing loss results in the sensory deprivation of neural assemblies that are tuned to the affected frequencies, providing an incentive for plasticity to occur. In an effort to upregulate their reduced activity back to normal levels, neurons may change the strength of existing connections or develop new connections. If, through homeostatic plasticity (Burrone and Murthy, 2003), all excitatory synapses are strengthened or all inhibitory synapses are weakened in unison, then neurons may become more susceptible to be activated in response to low incoming levels of spontaneous activity already (Schaette and Kempter, 2006; Noreña, 2011). Alternatively, if inputs from unaffected frequencies are strengthened (or newly grown) and inputs from frequencies with hearing loss are suppressed (or pruned altogether), then a large body of neurons may end up responding to the same limited amount of sensory input, thus enhancing neural synchronicity across the population (Eggermont, 2007b). In the healthy auditory system, spontaneous activity is ubiquitously present, but it tends to be relatively weak and incoherent. Elevated levels of neural activity and synchronicity normally only occur in the presence of a driving stimulus, i.e., a sound source. Therefore, if the spontaneous activity or synchronicity is elevated as a result of functional changes that are induced by hearing loss, this can be perceived as the presence of a phantom sound percept in the absence of a true sound source (Dominguez et al., 2006; Chrostowski et al., 2011).

Research in animals as well as humans supports the theory that tinnitus is a side effect of plastic reorganization in the central auditory system. Some studies suggest that homeostatic mechanisms play a dominant role. In rats that developed behavioral signs of high-frequency tinnitus after exposure to loud noise, down-regulation of inhibitory synapses was observed in neurons that were tuned to high frequencies (Yang et al., 2011). In humans with tinnitus, auditory brainstem responses that originated from the periphery were found to be reduced, but those from more central levels had recovered to normal levels, suggesting an increase in neural gain (Schaette and McAlpine, 2011). At the same time, abnormalities in the tonotopic organization of the auditory cortex have been observed that are consistent with an enlarged representation of sensory input from edge-frequency regions. In various animal studies, neurons that were expected to be tuned to sound frequencies coinciding with the tinnitus pitch on the basis of their location in the tonotopic representation were found to display shifts in characteristic frequency (Rajan and Irvine, 1998; Noreña et al., 2003; Stolzberg et al., 2011). Signs of tinnitus disappeared when the representation was restored, suggesting that the map reorganization is responsible for the tinnitus (Engineer et al., 2011). In humans, magnetoencephalography was used to show deviant spatial source localization of frequency-dependent responses in tinnitus patients as compared to controls (Mühlnickel et al., 1998; Wienbruch et al., 2006). Finally, a number of therapeutical strategies that specifically aim to reestablish the tonotopic representation have been reported to be successful in suppressing tinnitus in humans (Herraiz et al., 2007; Pineda et al., 2008), providing indirect evidence for the importance of tonotopic reorganizations in tinnitus.

Unfortunately, the tonotopic organization in humans is still poorly understood even for normal-hearing subjects. Many studies have consistently shown that low sound frequencies are represented in the distal end of Heschl's gyrus, anterolateral to the high frequencies, which are represented in the proximal root of Heschl's gyrus (Romani et al., 1982; Lauter et al., 1985; Pantev et al., 1989; Wessinger et al., 1997). However, this ignores the existence of multiple functional fields in auditory cortex, many of which may display distinct tonotopic maps. In the last decade, research has started to differentiate between multiple abutting representations in much more detail. Initial results were groundbreaking but appeared somewhat contradictory (Formisano et al., 2003; Talavage et al., 2004). In the last couple of years, however, various studies were published that were in excellent agreement (Woods et al., 2009; Humphries et al., 2010; Da Costa et al., 2011; Langers and van Dijk, 2011; Striem-Amit et al., 2011). Encouraged by these developments, the present study was set up to map the tonotopic representation in tinnitus patients in similar detail. Because we were interested in effects related to tinnitus specifically, we extended our own recent findings to include patients with tinnitus but otherwise normal hearing.

MATERIALS AND METHODS

SUBJECTS

Twenty healthy controls and 20 chronic subjective tinnitus patients participated in this functional magnetic resonance imaging (fMRI) study on the basis of written informed consent, in approved accordance with the requirements of the medical ethical committee at the University Medical Center Groningen in the Netherlands. Subjects were recruited from the hospital's tinnitus outpatient clinic (for the patient group) as well as from advertisements in various media (for the control and patient groups). They reported no history of neurological or psychiatric disorders. The patients were not undergoing tinnitus treatment at the time of the study. **Table 1** summarizes the subjects' gender, handedness, and age.

Except for the presence of tinnitus in the patient group, all subjects were selected to have normal or near-normal hearing up to 8 kHz. Thresholds were determined in a frequency range of 0.25–16 kHz by means of pure-tone audiometry. Furthermore, subjects performed the adaptive categorical loudness scaling (ACALOS) procedure (Brand and Hohmann, 2002). These tests were carried out for the left and right ears separately, but because no notable differences were found results were averaged over both ears.

To characterize the participants' self-reported complaints, all subjects filled out the 14-item hyperacusis questionnaire, relating to the attentional, social, and emotional aspects of auditory hypersensitivity (Khalfa et al., 2002). In addition, all subjects completed the 27-item short symptom checklist that screens for psychiatric symptoms in patients with somatic complaints, and that contains subscales for symptoms of depression, dysthymia, vegetativeness, agoraphobia, sociophobia, and mistrust (Hardt and Gerbershagen, 2001). The tinnitus patients also filled out questionnaires related to their tinnitus, including the Tinnitus Handicap Inventory (THI) that measures tinnitus severity in daily life (Newman et al., 1996), the Tinnitus Reaction Questionnaire (TRQ) that assesses the psychological distress associated with tinnitus (Wilson et al., 1991), and the Tinnitus Coping Style Questionnaire (TCSQ) that quantifies effective as well as maladaptive coping strategies (Budd and Pugh, 1996). All questionnaires were translated into Dutch, and outcome measures were linearly rescaled to obtain a uniform range from 0 to 100.

Tinnitus patients were furthermore asked where they perceived their tinnitus (lateralized toward the left or right ear, or centrally), and whether it was steady or pulsatile. Finally, all patients performed a modified tinnitus spectrum test (Noreña et al., 2002; Roberts et al., 2008). First, some example sounds were played and they were asked which type of sound resembled their tinnitus best: a tonal sound (pure tone), or a ringing or hissing sound (filtered noise with 0.04 or 0.15 octave bandwidths, respectively). Next, the chosen sound was repeatedly played at several center frequencies, and subjects were asked to indicate the subjective "likeness" of the presented sound compared to their tinnitus using a visual analog scale.

IMAGING PARADIGM

During the imaging session, subjects were placed supinely in the bore of a 3.0-T MR system (Philips Intera, Best, the Netherlands), which was equipped with an 8-channel phased-array (SENSE) transmit/receive head coil. The functional imaging session included three 8-min runs, each consisting of a dynamic series of 40 identical high-resolution T_2*-sensitive gradient-echo echo-planar imaging (EPI) volume acquisitions (TR 12.0 s; TA 2.0 s; TE 22 ms; FA 90°; matrix 128 × 128 × 40; resolution 1.5 mm × 1.5 mm × 1.5 mm; interleaved slice order, no slice gap). A sparse, clustered-volume sequence was employed to avoid interference from acoustic scanner noise (Edmister et al., 1999; Hall et al., 1999). The acquisition volume was positioned in an oblique axial orientation, tilted forward parallel to the Sylvian fissure, and approximately centered on the superior temporal sulci. Additional preparation scans were used to achieve stable image contrast and to trigger the start of stimulus delivery, but these were not included

Table 1 | Comparison of subject characteristics between the two subject groups.

Group	Healthy controls ($N = 20$)	Tinnitus patients ($N = 20$)	p
Demographics			
Gender	16 female, 4 male	12 female, 8 male	°
Handedness	17 right, 3 left	19 right, 1 left	°
Age (years)	33 ± 13 (21–60)	46 ± 11 (26–60)	**
Audiometry			
Average threshold (dB HL)	5 ± 5 (−1 to 18)	8 ± 5 (0–23)	°
Loudness range (dB)	98 ± 8 (84–113)	84 ± 14 (56–105)	***
Self-reported symptoms			
Hyperacusis (%)	25 ± 14 (8–51)	59 ± 16 (29–82)	***
Depression (%)	8 ± 9 (0–31)	27 ± 27 (0–100)	**
Dysthymia (%)	18 ± 14 (0–44)	38 ± 24 (0–75)	**
Vegetativeness (%)	9 ± 12 (0–38)	18 ± 16 (0–54)	°
Agoraphobia (%)	5 ± 8 (0–30)	11 ± 14 (0–55)	°
Social phobia (%)	20 ± 16 (0–56)	25 ± 23 (0–69)	°
Mistrust (%)	13 ± 12 (0–44)	18 ± 19 (0–63)	°
Tinnitus effects			
Tinnitus handicap (%)	–	43 ± 22 (6–88)	–
Tinnitus reaction (%)	–	38 ± 21 (0–88)	–
Effective coping (%)	–	52 ± 14 (17–68)	–
Maladaptive coping (%)	–	29 ± 15 (3–60)	–
Tinnitus percept†			
Lateralization	–	8 central, 4 right, 2 left	–
Dynamics	–	16 steady, 3 pulsatile	–
Bandwidth	–	10 tone, 7 hiss, 2 ring	–
Frequency	–	16 high, 2 other, 1 low	–

*For an explanation of the various items, see Section "Subjects" of the Section "Materials and Methods." Numbers indicate mean ± standard deviation (range). For ease of interpretation, all questionnaire scales were expressed to range from 0 to 100 (%). The significance of group differences was based on Fisher's exact test (for gender and handedness) or Student's t-test (for all other comparisons), and classified as: ***$p < 0.001$; **$p < 0.01$; *$p < 0.05$; °$p \geq 0.05$.*

† Numbers do not add up to equal the group size because for some patients not all tinnitus characteristics were obtained.

into the analysis. The scanner coolant pump and fan were turned off during imaging to diminish ambient noise levels.

To control their attentional state, subjects performed an engaging visual/emotional task that comprised 40 trials of 12-s duration per run (Langers and van Dijk, 2011). During the first 5 s of each trial, a fixation cross was presented on a screen. During the next 5 s, a picture was shown that was randomly selected out of 300 images from the International Affective Picture System (Lang et al., 2008). Subjects were instructed to empathize with the depicted scene, and decide whether the picture's affective valence was positive, negative, or neutral. During the final 2 s, coinciding with the EPI acquisitions, subjects could respond by pressing any of three touch buttons on a handheld device. Before the scanning session, the task was clearly explained and demonstrated, and subjects were given the opportunity to practice.

To exclude that the tinnitus percept might have been masked by ambient noise during the scanning session, all patients were asked to rate their tinnitus at various moments before, between, and after the imaging runs on a scale from 0 to 10, where 0 signified that the tinnitus was absent and 10 signified that the tinnitus was maximal. Responses varied but never equaled 0 (the lowest rating encountered was 2) and also never systematically decreased during the session (contrariwise, according to some subjects it systematically increased due to accruing fatigue and stress).

SOUND STIMULI

During the functional runs, sound was presented by means of MR-compatible electrodynamic headphones (MR Confon GmbH, Magdeburg, Germany; Baumgart et al., 1998) that were connected to a standard PC with soundcard. Underneath the headset, subjects wore foam ear plugs to further dampen the acoustic noise produced by the scanner. Subjects were informed beforehand that the presented sound stimuli were irrelevant for the purpose of the visual/emotional task. During the first 10 s of each trial, while the MR-scanner was inactive, a sequence of 50 identical 100-ms tone stimuli was presented at a rate of 5 Hz. The fundamental frequency f_0 of the tones remained the same within a trial, and equaled $f_0 = 0.25$, 0.50, 1.00, 2.00, 4.00, or 8.00 kHz. On top of a constant fundamental, each tone stimulus contained a first overtone that quickly decayed with an e-folding time $\tau = 25$ ms. A windowing function $A(t)$ was used to impose 5-ms linear rise and fall times. The corresponding waveform $w(t)$ is given by the equation $w(t) = A(t)\cdot[\sin(2\pi\cdot f_0\cdot t) + {}^1/_2\cdot e^{-t/\tau}\cdot\sin(2\pi\cdot 2f_0\cdot t)]$. An additional silent waveform $[w(t) = 0]$ was included in the set of stimuli.

All waveforms were digitized and saved as 16-bit 44.1-kHz data files, scaled at two levels that differed by a factor 10 in amplitude. As a result, the louder set of stimuli was precisely 20 dB louder than the softer set of stimuli. The stimuli were played at the same level for all subjects; the corresponding audible intensities were calibrated in a separate session, by determining audiometric thresholds to the presented tone stimuli inside the scanner environment, and comparing those to the corresponding standard audiometric thresholds. For example: if the loud 2-kHz stimulus needed to be attenuated by 40 dB to reach the threshold for that stimulus as determined inside the scanner, and if the standard audiometric threshold at 2 kHz was 5 dB HL, then the loud 2-kHz stimulus was inferred to have been presented at 45 dB HL, and the corresponding soft stimulus at 25 dB HL.

The stimulus frequencies and intensity levels were randomly varied across trials, in an order that differed across runs and subjects, and that was unrelated to the affective valence of the task-related pictures.

DATA ANALYSIS

During data processing, we used Matlab (The MathWorks Inc., Natick, MA, USA), supplemented with processing routines from the SPM8b software package (Wellcome Department of Imaging Neuroscience, http://www.fil.ion.ucl.ac.uk/spm/).

Contrast differences between odd and even slices due to the interleaved slice order were eliminated by interpolating between pairs of adjacent slices, shifting the imaging grid over half the slice thickness. Next, the functional imaging volumes were corrected for motion effects using 3-D rigid body transformations. The anatomical images were coregistered to the functional volumes, and all images were normalized into Montreal Neurological Institute (MNI) stereotaxic space. Images were moderately smoothed using an isotropic 5-mm full-width at half-maximum Gaussian kernel, and resampled to a 2-mm isotropic resolution. A logarithmic transformation was carried out in order to naturally express all derived voxel signal measures in units of percentage signal change relative to the mean. (Given the small relative magnitude of the hemodynamic signal, a truncated Taylor series expansion of the transformed signal $\hat{s}(t) = 100{\cdot}\ln(s(t))$ gives rise to $\Delta\hat{s}(t) = 100{\cdot}\Delta s(t)/S$, indicating that the absolute signal change in $\Delta\hat{s}(t)$ equals the relative signal change in $\Delta s(t)$ expressed as a percentage of its mean S.)

Mass-univariate general linear regression models (GLMs) were constructed and assessed for each subject, including: (i) two regressors modeling the reported affective valences (positive or negative, relative to neutral); (ii) twelve regressors modeling the sound stimulus conditions (6 frequencies $\times$ 2 intensity levels, relative to silence); (iii) translation and rotation parameters in the x-, y- and z-direction, modeling residual motion effects; and (iv) a third-degree polynomial for each run, modeling baseline and drift effects. The estimated sound-evoked response amplitudes were entered into a group-level mixed effects analysis. On a voxel-by-voxel basis, the significance of the response to sound was assessed by means of an omnibus F-test, including the coefficients of all 12 sound-related regressors equally. A region of interest (ROI) was defined comprising the supra-threshold voxels. The 7517 voxels (i.e., 60 cm^3) that remained formed two coherent clusters of approximately equal size, located bilaterally in the superior temporal lobes that contain auditory cortex (see Results). For every subject and for all six stimulus frequencies, the activation levels of these voxels in response to stimuli of a uniform intensity level of 40 dB HL were estimated by linearly interpolating the sound-evoked activity between the two intensities that were presented. The resulting activation levels were collected in an aggregate 300680 $\times$ 6 matrix **B** (40 subjects $\times$ 7517 voxels, 6 frequencies).

From this aggregate activation matrix, two principal components were extracted. Thus, $\mathbf{B} = \mathbf{x}_1 \otimes \mathbf{f}_1 + \mathbf{x}_2 \otimes \mathbf{f}_2 + \epsilon$, where $\mathbf{x}_1$ and $\mathbf{x}_2$ are 300680-element vectors containing spatial response maps (masked by the ROI and aggregated across subjects), $\mathbf{f}_1$ and $\mathbf{f}_2$ are 6-element vectors containing the corresponding frequency response profiles, and ϵ is a matrix containing the residuals that were minimized in least-squares sense. Because the magnitude of the outer products in the decomposition are well-defined, but the magnitudes of the maps or profiles individually are not, the frequency response profiles $\mathbf{f}_1$ and $\mathbf{f}_2$ were constrained to unit root-mean-square amplitude. As a result, the spatial response maps $\mathbf{x}_1$ and $\mathbf{x}_2$ are expressed in common fMRI units of percentage signal change. The aggregate spatial response maps $\mathbf{x}_1$ and $\mathbf{x}_2$ were partitioned into 40 maps corresponding with individual subjects. From these, average maps were computed for each of the two subject groups.

For the purpose of bootstrap permutation testing, all 40 subjects were repeatedly subdivided into two random subgroups of 20 subjects each, and analyzed. On the basis of 1000 such repetitions, null-distributions were derived that were used to estimate the statistical significance of any differences between the groups of healthy controls and tinnitus patients.

RESULTS

SUBJECTS

Figure 1A displays the subjects' hearing thresholds as a function of frequency. Except above 8 kHz, where some hearing loss occurred, average thresholds were normal. Subject groups were well matched with regard to hearing loss. At all frequencies except 4 kHz, the thresholds did not significantly differ; only at 4 kHz, the patients' thresholds were worse by 7 dB on average (nominal $p = 0.003$). **Table 1** includes the mean thresholds across all frequencies at which stimuli were presented in this study, i.e., the octave frequencies from 0.25 to 8.00 kHz. These did not differ significantly between groups. It also lists the dynamic intensity range that corresponded with a loudness ranging from the minimum to the maximum score according to the ACALOS test (i.e., 0–50, corresponding with labels "inaudible" to "too loud"). The intensity range was significantly reduced in tinnitus patients, indicating a diminished tolerance for loud sounds. This finding was confirmed by the hyperacusis questionnaire, which also revealed

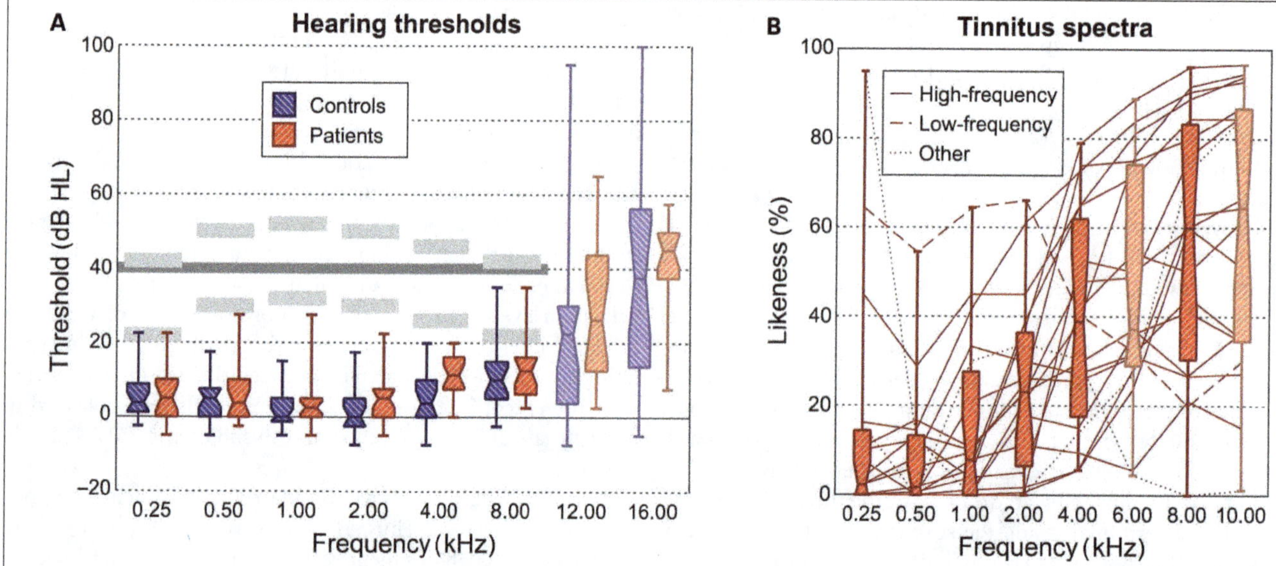

FIGURE 1 | (A) Hearing thresholds were measured at frequencies from 0.25 to 16.00 kHz. Results were averaged over both ears, and shown by means of boxplots (showing inter-quartile ranges). Stimuli were presented at all octave frequencies from 0.25 to 8.00 kHz at two different intensity levels that differed by 20 dB. The light gray bars indicate the approximate presentation levels. In the analysis, the sound-evoked activation levels were interpolated to a uniform intensity level of 40 dB HL, indicated by the dark gray line. **(B)** Patients performed a tinnitus spectrum test in which they indicated the subjective "likeness" to their tinnitus percept of a range of sound stimuli with varying center frequencies. The majority of subjects showed high-frequency tinnitus (solid; likeness increasing with frequency); one subject showed a low-frequency tinnitus (dashed; likeness decreasing with frequency); two subjects showed a spectrum that could not be classified as high- or low-frequency (dotted; with a peak or a dip at intermediate frequencies).

a significantly reduced self-reported tolerance to sound. According to the symptom checklist, patients showed significantly more depressive and dysthymic signs. With respect to the other subscales, the patients also scored worse, but differences remained insignificant. With regard to the specifically tinnitus-related questionnaires, patients showed a wide range of self-reported levels of tinnitus complaints, varying from very mild to very severe. The tinnitus severity according to the THI, the tinnitus-related distress according to the TRQ, and the maladaptive coping level according to the TCSQ were all strongly correlated (pairwise $R > 0.85$). The effective coping level according to the TCSQ did not correlate appreciably with any of these three measures (pairwise $|R| < 0.05$). Finally, **Table 1** tabulates the occurrence of various tinnitus characteristics. Overall, the tinnitus percept was most prevalently perceived centrally in the head, steady over time, and with a high-frequency tone-like character. **Figure 1B** displays the obtained tinnitus spectra, which on average showed a monotonous increase as a function of frequency.

SOUND-EVOKED ACTIVATION

The sound-evoked activation according to a family-wise error (FWE) corrected group-level omnibus F-test is shown in **Figure 2. Figure 2A** shows all significant voxels, assessed across all 40 subjects as a group. A minimum cluster size of 100 voxels was imposed in order to exclude small sub-cortical activation foci. The resulting two extensive activation clusters in the bilateral auditory cortices were used as a ROI. In the lower bar plot, the mean activation levels in this ROI for each of the six frequencies and each of the two subject groups are plotted. Results were linearly interpolated between the two employed stimulus intensities to estimate the activation levels that would be obtained at uniform stimulus intensity levels of 40 dB HL across all frequencies. For instance, the 2-kHz stimuli were presented at approximately 30 and 50 dB HL (see **Figure 1A**), and the two corresponding activations were therefore averaged; at 4 kHz, however, the presented stimulus intensities were approximately 26 and 46 dB HL, and therefore the corresponding activations were weighted at 0.3:0.7. The resulting profiles showed the largest activation levels below 1 kHz, and a gradual decline in activation toward the highest frequency of 8 kHz. No systematic differences between controls and patients were apparent.

Figure 2B shows all locally significant differences in activation between the 20 healthy controls on the one hand and the 20 tinnitus patients on the other hand. Results were thresholded at a confidence level of $p < 0.05$ (FWE-corrected) and a minimum cluster size of 20 voxels. One cluster reached significance, located in the most lateral aspect of the Heschl's gyrus in the left hemisphere, peaking at coordinates $(x, y, z) = (-62, 0, 0)$. The average response profile of these voxels, shown in the bar plot, showed relatively weak activation in the controls and relatively strong activation in the patients. This qualitative difference was found at all frequencies, but it was quantitatively most prominent for the low frequencies.

In **Figure 3A**, the mean activation levels (expressed as a percentage signal change, interpolated to 40 dB HL) across all six stimulus frequencies are mapped for the two subject groups separately. Obviously, in both groups the overall activation tended to decline as the stimulus frequency increased. Additionally, a gradual transition in the activation pattern was visible. At the lowest frequencies, fMRI activation tended to peak in a region centered

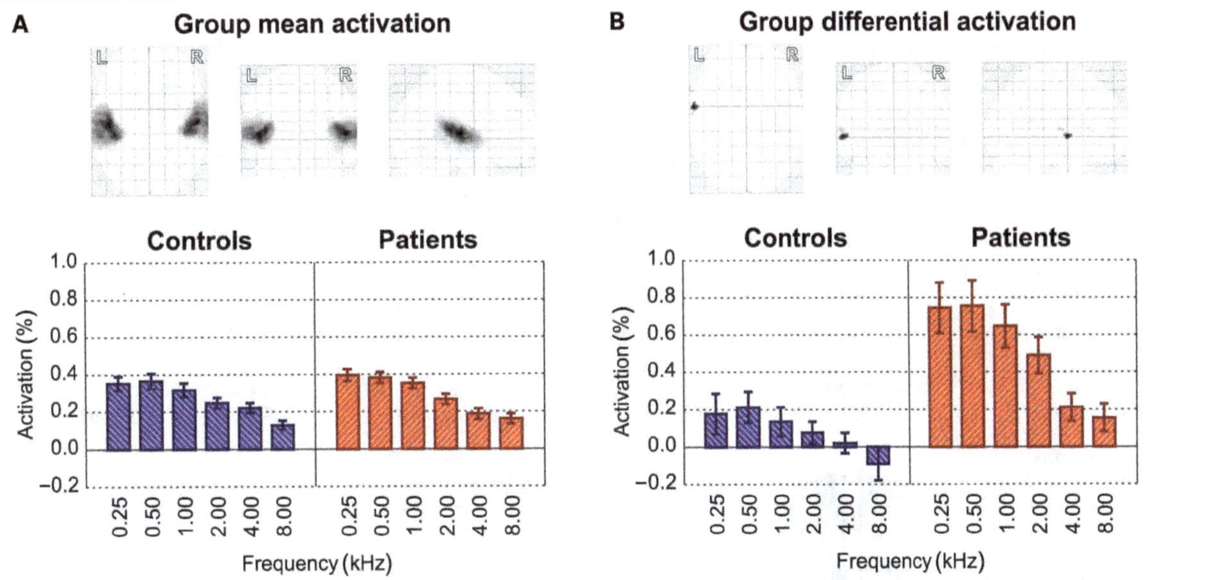

FIGURE 2 | (A) Overall activation to all sound stimuli in the controls and patients combined (thresholded at $p < 0.05$, FWE-corrected, and minimum cluster size of 100 voxels) occurred in the bilateral auditory cortices. Below the glass brain display, the bar plot shows the activation to various frequencies (interpolated to 40 dB HL) for both subject groups separately. Error bars indicate standard errors of the mean across subjects. **(B)** Testing for any differences between groups in the frequency-dependent sound-evoked activation profile (thresholded at $p < 0.05$, FWE-corrected, and minimum cluster size of 20 voxels) revealed one cluster in left lateral Heschl's gyrus. The bar plot shows the mean response levels for this subset of voxels.

on lateral Heschl's gyrus. At the highest frequencies, the activation cluster appeared to have broken up into two clusters, one on the rostral bank of medial Heschl's gyrus, bordering the central sulcus, and one on its caudal bank, bordering the planum temporale. For intermediate frequencies, intermediate patterns were observed. These trends occurred similarly in both hemispheres and in both subject groups.

In order to summarize these activation maps more concisely, principal component analysis was employed. **Figure 3B** shows the first (left) and second (right) principal component's spatial response maps $\mathbf{x}_{1,2}$ (averaged across the controls or patients separately), together with their corresponding frequency response profiles $\mathbf{f}_{1,2}$ (which apply to both groups equally). Unsurprisingly, for the first principal component, the spatial map well summarized the typical activation pattern that was already observed in **Figure 3A**, and the shape of the frequency profile well resembled the ROI average in **Figure 2A**. More interestingly, the second principal component summarized how voxels primarily deviated from that typical behavior. The frequency profile showed a monotonous and gradual increase from negative values (at low frequencies) to positive values (at high frequencies). In the spatial map, positive coefficients were encountered bilaterally on the rostral and caudal banks of medial Heschl's gyrus, and negative values were found on its lateral crest. In combination, this means that the medial endpoints shown in blue tended to respond more strongly to high-frequency stimuli and less strongly to low-frequency stimuli, as compared to the average behavior of all voxels. Contrariwise, in the lateral endpoint shown in red, responses were stronger in response to low-frequency stimuli and weaker in response to high-frequency stimuli. This reflects two tonotopic representations on the rostral and caudal banks of Heschl's gyrus. Comparing the second component's spatial maps, these representations existed in a highly similar form for both subject groups.

PLACE-FREQUENCY MAPS

Because the frequency profile for an individual voxel, as estimated by a combination of the profiles shown in **Figure 3B**, depends on the relative contribution of the first and the second principal component in that voxel (contained in $\mathbf{x}_1$ and $\mathbf{x}_2$, respectively), the ratio x_2/x_1 was calculated for each voxel. **Figure 3C** illustrates the shape of various mixtures of frequency profiles that may be obtained for a number of different ratios. The profile shifts from low to high frequencies as the ratio increases from negative to positive values. Therefore, the ratio x_2/x_1 may serve to quantify a voxel's frequency tuning, where low/negative values indicate low-frequency tuning and high/positive values indicate high-frequency tuning.

Figure 3D displays the resulting ratio map. Qualitatively, the obtained pattern was very similar to that of the second component alone, but results were more pronounced toward the edges of the cluster, where responses were weakest. Moreover, a secondary low-frequency endpoint was more clearly found to exist in lateral planum temporale, posterior to the other low-frequency endpoint in lateral Heschl's gyrus. Again, both groups showed highly similar results overall. Perhaps the most striking difference was observed in the left lateral Heschl's gyrus, where the healthy controls showed highly pronounced low-frequency responses (dark red) whereas the tinnitus patients showed only moderately pronounced low-frequency responses (orange red). This is related to the fact that in this vicinity the first component's spatial map was weaker in the controls than in the patients (see **Figure 3B**; further corroborated

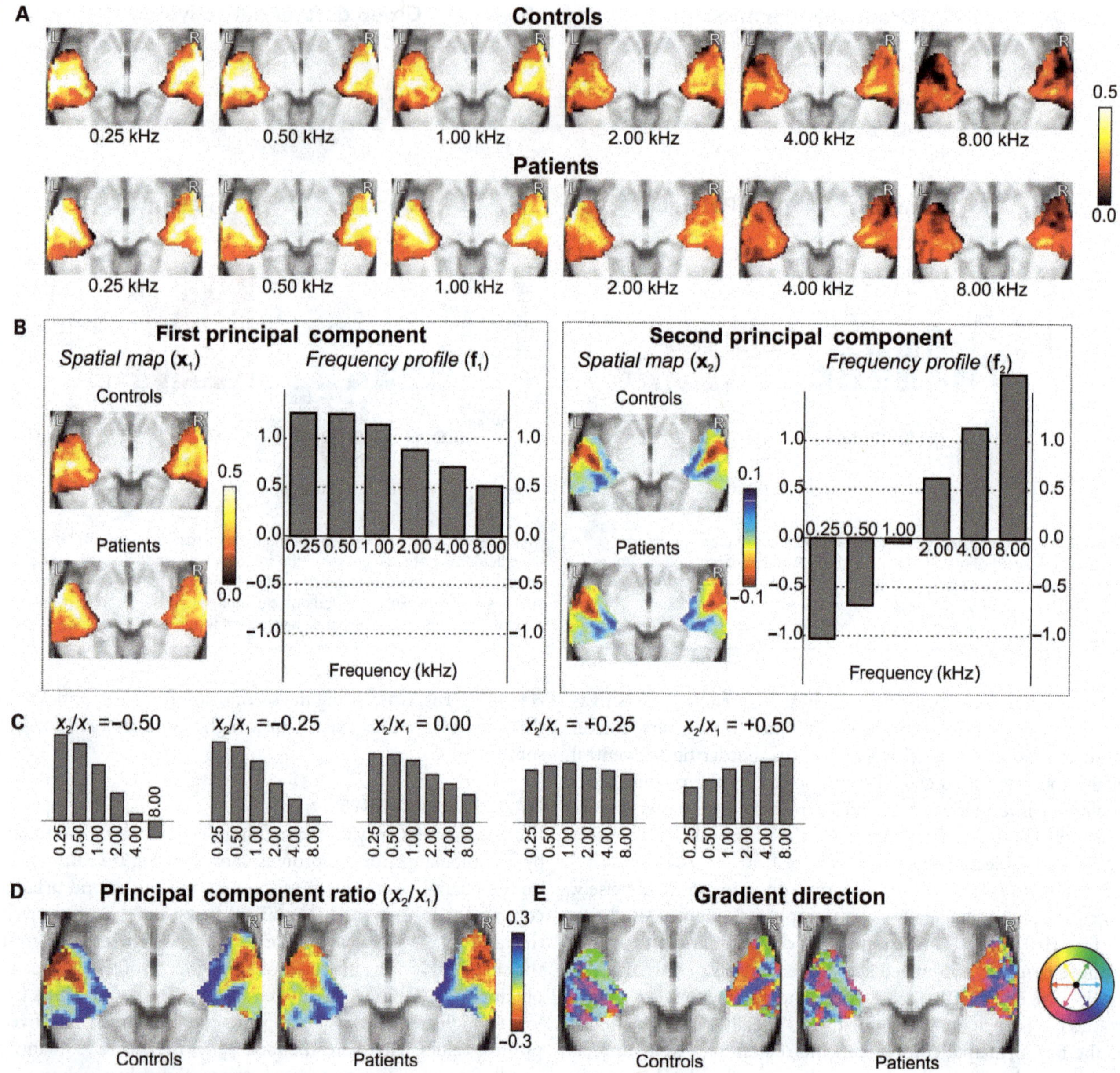

FIGURE 3 | (A) Mean intensity projections of the activation to all sound stimuli (interpolated to 40 dB HL) in the controls and patients separately. **(B)** A principal component decomposition of the frequency-dependent response profiles across all voxels and all subjects resulted in a first component that summarized the general activation levels, and a second component that reflected the frequency-selectivity that differed between voxels. **(C)** For various mixtures of the first and second principal components' frequency response profiles, one may obtain response behaviors that range from low- to high-frequency tuning as the ratio of the coefficients x_2/x_1 increases from negative to positive values. **(D)** Spatial maps of the ratio x_2/x_1 reveal the tonotopic organization of the auditory cortices. **(E)** By color-coding the gradient direction of the maps in **(D)**, multiple parallel strips of cortex are distinguishable.

by **Figure 2B**), whereas the second component's spatial map still showed similar magnitudes.

Finally, the direction of the gradient in the transverse maps of **Figure 3D** is color-coded in **Figure 3E**. In both hemispheres, a series of "strips" of auditory cortex could be distinguished, tentatively corresponding with distinct functional fields in auditory cortex. Fields were aligned more or less parallel to the axis of Heschl's gyrus. On the rostral bank of Heschl's gyrus, the low-to-high tonotopic gradient was homogeneously oriented in an anteromedial direction. Toward the caudal bank of Heschl's gyrus, it showed a sharp transition to another homogeneous region where the gradient was oriented in the posterior direction. Further caudally, on the planum temporale, another gradient reversal was visible, followed possibly by yet another reversal near the temporoparietal junction. Again, comparable results were obtained for both groups.

In an effort to elucidate potential differences regarding the tonotopic organization in the two groups, we plotted the strength of the first component (x_1) versus that of the second component (x_2) in **Figure 4A**. Each voxel contributes one data point. Results are shown separately for the mean maps derived from the controls (left) and patients (right). In **Figure 4B** these data were transformed into a representation where the ratio x_2/x_1, reflecting frequency tuning, was plotted on the horizontal axis, and the value x_1, reflecting the overall activation level, was plotted on the vertical axis. This once more shows that the strongest responses (i.e., high x_1) occurred for voxels that were tuned to the lower frequencies (i.e., negative x_2/x_1). Some differences were visible in the shape of the data cloud of both groups, but the overall distributions were rather similar. To statistically quantify and assess the differences between both groups, we compared these outcomes in various ways. First, in **Figure 4C**, the value x_1 (top) and the ratio x_2/x_1 (bottom) are plotted for one group versus the other. In other words, the response level and frequency tuning, respectively, of a particular voxel in one group is compared to that of the same voxel (i.e., at the same location in stereotaxic space) in the other group. The resulting scatter plots can both be seen to cluster along the diagonal. Any difference in excitability or any shift in frequency tuning would have been visible as a systematic deviation of the data cloud from the diagonal, but apart from stochastic variations hardly any such deviations were observed. Second, in **Figure 4D** we compared the marginal distributions of the scatter plots in **Figure 4B** by plotting the histograms of the value x_1 (top) and the ratio x_2/x_1 (bottom). These plots also include the median and the surrounding 95% confidence intervals for these histograms, obtained by repeatedly sampling 20 random subjects (dashed lines). The overall shape of the distributions differed little, and did not significantly differ from that obtained from any random group. Third, in **Figure 4E**, we plotted the cumulative density function (cdf) of the value x_1 (top) and the ratio x_2/x_1 (bottom) for one group versus the other, as is commonly done in the Kolmogorov–Smirnov test for statistical equality of distributions. If the groups show identical distributions, the result is a straight line along the diagonal. Again, the bootstrapped median and 95% confidence interval are shown by dashed lines. The obtained curves did not significantly deviate from the diagonal anywhere.

In **Figure 5A**, the second principal component's spatial map ($\mathbf{x}_2$) is shown for each subject individually. (For individual subjects we avoided the ratio x_2/x_1 because it resulted in ill-defined values for a large abundance of weakly activated voxels due to "division by zero" divergences when $x_1 \approx 0.0$.) Per group, subjects were sorted in order of decreasing Pearson correlation (R) with the average map over all 40 subjects. In both groups, some subjects were highly representative of the mean ($R > 0.5$), whereas some others were not at all ($R \approx 0.0$). Still, the median correlations ($R = 0.44$ for controls; $R = 0.43$ for patients) were substantial and did not appreciably differ between groups.

Because it is hard to oversee differences between subjects in these map representations, we reduced the dimensional complexity of the data by projecting them onto a two-dimensional "feature space" that was obtained by means of principal component analysis, thus ensuring that a maximal amount of variance was retained (a procedure conceptually analogous to multidimensional scaling). In **Figure 5B**, the loadings of the individual subjects are plotted. The axes are labeled with images that show several mixtures of features that are represented in the various directions. The upward vertical axis, which explains the largest amount of signal power in the maps, well depicts the typical tonotopic layout that was already observed in **Figure 3B** (the downward vertical axis depicts negative loadings, where high- and low-frequency endpoints are therefore reversed). The rightward horizontal axis shows an overall representation of high frequencies (cyan colors) and the leftward horizontal axis shows an overall representation of low frequencies (yellow colors). The further from the origin, the more pronounced these features were represented in individuals. Subjects were typically located in the segments between the 11 o'clock and 2 o'clock positions, and therefore mostly showed a rather similar tonotopic map, with a slight over- or underrepresentation of higher or lower frequencies. The centroids of the two groups were located close to each other, especially when compared with the spread across individuals, indicating that the groups did not significantly differ with respect to these features. Although it is questionable whether these data can be formally assumed to be normally distributed, an F-test indeed confirmed that the groups did not differ significantly ($p = 0.90$).

Finally, to exclude that the obtained outcomes regarding tonotopic maps were dominated by the (stronger) low-frequency responses to such a degree that differences in the (weaker) high-frequency responses were rendered undetectable, we repeated the principal component decomposition and all subsequently described statistical analyses on the basis of only the half of the response data that concerned the 2-, 4-, and 8-kHz stimuli. Again, none of the tests resulted in significant (or nearly significant) outcomes, similarly indicating that the mean tonotopic maps were highly comparable in both groups.

DISCUSSION

In this study, we determined tonotopic representations in the bilateral human auditory cortices. The current stimulus and acquisition paradigm was identical to that in a previous publication (Langers and van Dijk, 2011). There, we reported in more detail on the current control group only, and demonstrated that the employed experimental setup may be used to robustly extract tonotopic maps. For the purpose of the present paper, the subject group was extended to include tinnitus patients that were matched with respect to hearing loss. Our goal was to test the hypothesis that tinnitus results from an abnormal tonotopic organization of the auditory cortex. We did not find supporting evidence for any such reorganization.

TONOTOPIC MAPPING

In spite of the fact that we well reproduced our previous findings in the control group, the analyses that we currently performed differed from our earlier report in two respects that are worth noting.

Firstly, instead of detailing the activation in response to the louder and softer set of sound stimuli separately, we interpolated our data to uniform intensity levels of 40 dB HL. The reason for this was that, unlike in our previous report, we currently did not mean to study the spread of activation that increasingly occurs at higher intensity levels. Because sound-evoked activation

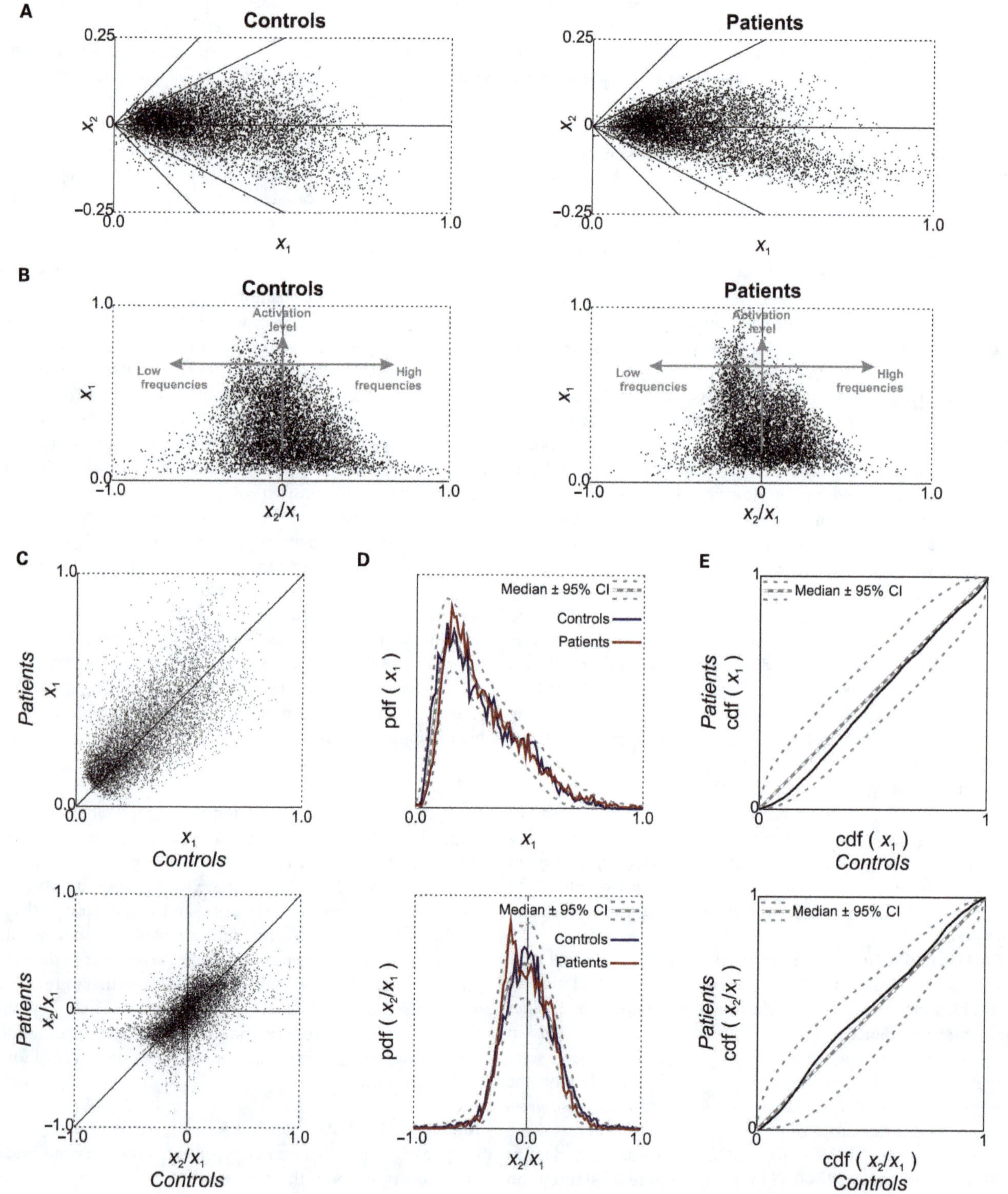

FIGURE 4 | (A) The coefficients in the first and second components' spatial response maps (see **Figure 3B**) were plotted against each other. Each data point corresponds with one voxel. The diagonal lines show where the ratio x_2/x_1 remains constant. **(B)** Transforming the representation in **(A)**, the ratio of the first and second components' coefficients was plotted against the coefficient of the first component. The vertical coordinate of a voxel's data point reflects its sound-evoked activation level, and the horizontal coordinate reflects its frequency tuning. **(C)** A plot of the sound-evoked activation level (top) and frequency tuning (bottom), as quantified by the value x_1 and ratio x_2/x_1, respectively, comparing healthy controls and tinnitus patients. **(D)** The probability density function (pdf) of the value x_1 (top) and ratio x_2/x_1 (bottom) is plotted in the form of a histogram. Dashed lines indicate the median and 95% confidence intervals as obtained from a bootstrap procedure. **(E)** The corresponding cumulative density function (cdf) in both groups are plotted against each other. Again, dashed lines indicate the bootstrap median and 95% confidence intervals.

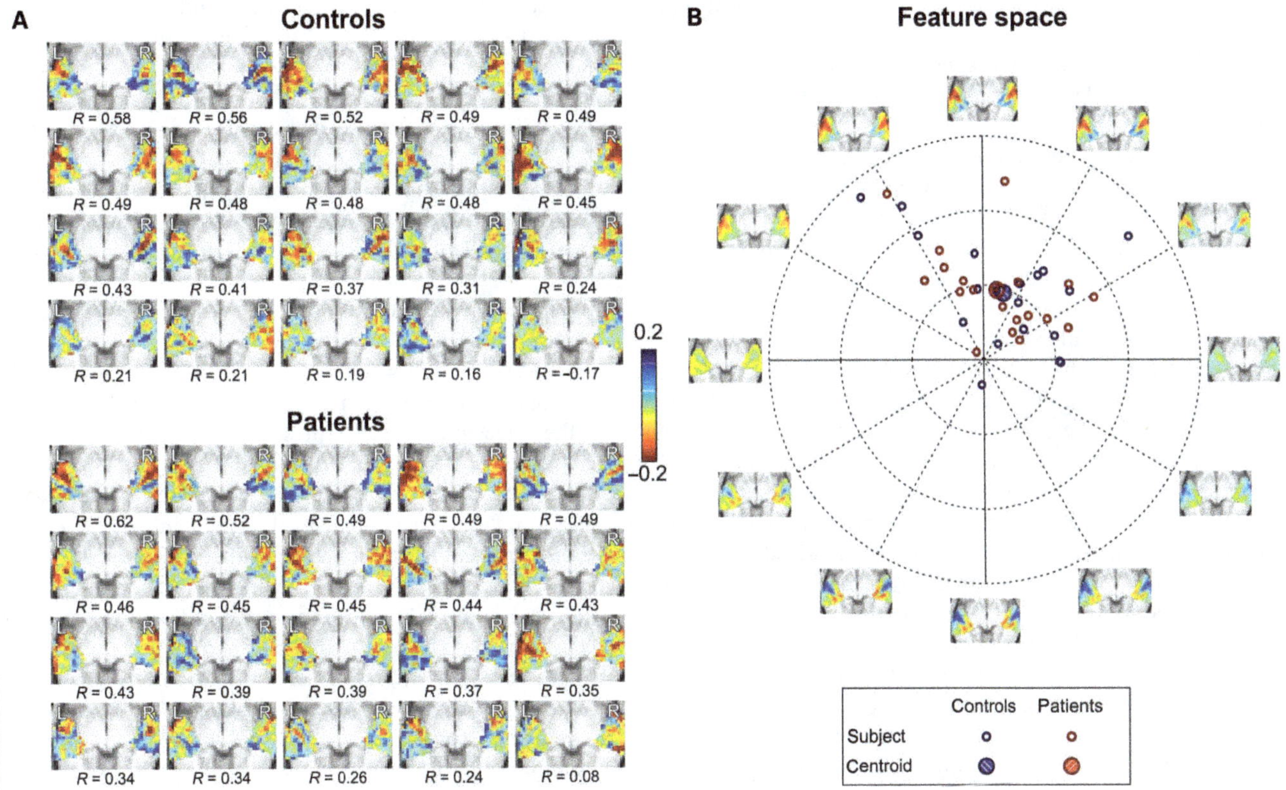

FIGURE 5 | (A) Individual spatial response maps of the second principal component $\mathbf{x}_2$ for all subjects in the two groups, arranged in order of decreasing similarity with the mean map of all subjects (as quantified by Pearson correlations *R*). **(B)** The detailed but complex representations in **(A)** were projected onto a two-dimensional feature space that still captured a maximal amount of variance by means of principal component analysis. Each subject is represented by a colored symbol at coordinates that reflect the loading on the two features. The axes are labeled with images that display the spatial response maps corresponding with the dimensions of the feature space, as are various mixtures along diagonals in between. The further from the origin, the more pronounced a feature is represented in a subject.

in primary auditory cortex as measured by fMRI increases more or less linearly with the stimulus intensity level in normal hearing subjects (Hall et al., 2001; Brechmann et al., 2002; Langers et al., 2007), the employed interpolation enabled us to largely account for differences in the presentation level across stimulus frequencies. We still observed a decline of the overall activation level as a function of frequency. This may partly be attributed to the small amount of hearing loss at the highest presentation frequencies.

Secondly, instead of simply averaging the response data across subjects for the purpose of principal component decomposition, we concatenated all data to obtain a single data matrix (**B**). The resulting data reduction method has been analogously incorporated in independent component analyses (Svensén et al., 2002). In contrast to our previous report, the present approach does not assume spatial response characteristics (including tonotopic representations) to be identical across subjects or groups. Instead, for each principal component, individual spatial response maps were obtained that were still identically interpretable across subjects due to the fact that they shared the same frequency response profile. This allowed us to statistically test for differences between the two subject groups in a data-driven but unbiased manner.

GROUP DIFFERENCES

Using a conventional linear regression model, we found significantly stronger activation in the patients than in the controls in the vicinity of the low-frequency endpoint of the tonotopic map in left lateral Heschl's gyrus (see **Figure 2B**). Note that the low-frequency preference of this cortical region does not agree with the typical high-pitched tinnitus percept. However, the lateral extreme of Heschl's gyrus has also been proposed to subserve pitch processing in humans (Patterson et al., 2002; Penagos et al., 2004; Puschmann et al., 2010). Although high and low pitches may be processed in different ways (Oxenham et al., 2004) and the precise role of this area remains obscure (Hall and Plack, 2009; Barker et al., 2011), this interpretation suggests that the abnormal activity in tinnitus patients may be related to pitch extraction. Ongoing anomalous activity in such a center can easily be conceived to induce the percept of a continuous tone-like sound. The observed activity can be argued to result from tinnitus, since the ongoing presence of a tone-like phantom percept that is generated lower in the auditory pathway may well induce abnormal activity in an area that is dedicated to the assessment of pitch. Alternatively, this hyperactivity may be construed to underlie the cause of tinnitus itself. In either case, one expects elevated activity during silence in the presence of tinnitus, which would diminish rather than enlarge the contrast with the activation that occurs during the perception of true sound. Yet, at the same time, an intrinsically hyperexcitable pitch processing center may respond excessively to true sound as well. The latter effect would be consistent with our findings.

Interestingly, due to the superficial location of this area in the brain, it forms an accessible target for non-invasive therapeutic interventions. Our finding may therefore help explain the reported success of some recently developed transcranial magnetic stimulation (TMS) therapies that target left auditory cortex (Burger et al., 2011; Chung et al., 2012).

Hyperexcitability might also clarify why tinnitus is commonly accompanied by hyperacusis (Baguley, 2003; Møller, 2007b). Our patient group showed evidence for hyperacusis, both objectively in the form of a reduced dynamic range of audible but tolerable sound intensities, and subjectively on the basis of self-reported complaints in a hyperacusis questionnaire. It has been forwarded that hyperacusis forms a confound in fMRI and abnormal activity levels that are ascribed to tinnitus might actually be due to hyperacusis, particularly for the subcortical auditory nuclei (Gu et al., 2010). In the present study, we found only limited elevations in cortical sound-evoked response levels, since activation was not significantly different between groups in most of the auditory cortex. This suggests that hyperacusis did not play a dominant role, possibly as a result of the low sound presentation levels that were employed. However, this equality can also be argued to result from two opposing effects that happen to cancel each other: an increase in activation related to hyperacusis (due to hyperexcitability), and a concomitant decrease in activation due to tinnitus itself (for instance due to elevated levels of activity during baseline already). Because we are unable to disentangle these two subtle effects, their possible extent and magnitude presently remains speculative.

Apart from the aforementioned significant focal difference, we found remarkably few discrepancies between the control subjects and the tinnitus patients. In particular, the tonotopic maps that were extracted from both groups looked highly similar at first glance. Various detailed comparisons across voxels (**Figure 4**) and across subjects (**Figure 5**) subsequently indeed confirmed that any differences that did occur between the two groups could be completely ascribed to chance. We therefore found no evidence for macroscopic tonotopic reorganization in tinnitus patients. In particular, we found no signs of a systematic overrepresentation of the moderate to high sound frequencies that corresponded with the tinnitus pitch itself or its spectral edge. Nevertheless, a number of practical limitations should be kept in mind.

LIMITATIONS

A first important limitation is that the fact that our data did not result in the rejection of the null-hypothesis should not be interpreted as proof that the null-hypothesis is true. If tonotopic reorganization takes place in a subtle form (for instance if it induces only a weak shift in the measurable best frequencies, or if it is confined to a small subregion of auditory cortex only), then the statistical power of our study may have been inadequate and our methodology insufficiently sensitive to detect it. However, the cortical tonotopic reorganizations that have been observed in animal studies are far from subtle, as response characteristics have been found to show changes that are immediately obvious and that extend over multiple octaves in the tonotopic map (Stolzberg et al., 2011; Yang et al., 2011). Although it is difficult to formulate and test a precise alternative hypothesis that would correspond with these animal data, the comparison in **Figure 3D** does not indicate any such large-scale reorganizations.

Moreover, our analyses were able to detect differences between the tonotopic organizations in individuals, as becomes clear from **Figure 5**. We do not attribute this variability to inaccuracies in the measurement method alone (i.e., "noise"). Within subjects, the detected tonotopic representations were still organized into large-scale patterns that exceeded the inherent resolution of the data. Therefore, we believe that the observed inter-subject variations reflect actual differences in the individual cortical organization. Then our inability to distinguish between healthy controls and tinnitus patients on the basis of their tonotopic organization is not a limitation of our paradigm, but an inherent characteristic of these populations instead. Although perhaps differences between the means of the two groups might have turned out significant if substantially larger numbers of subjects had been considered, these would then still have been clinically insignificant: the macroscopic tonotopic organization cannot serve as a practical criterion to objectify tinnitus in individuals.

A second limitation is related to the nature of the measurements that we performed. Functional MRI relies on hemodynamic changes in the volume and oxygenation of the brain's local blood supply that occur as a result of variations in the tissue's metabolic demand. These variations have been shown to be related to neuronal firing as well as synaptic events like the release and reuptake of excitatory and inhibitory neurotransmitters (Logothetis et al., 2001; Logothetis, 2008). However, importantly, fMRI has a limited temporal and spatial resolution. Functional MRI may be completely insensitive to the synchronicity of neuronal discharges, and the measured signal at best forms a correlate of the integrated activity over a large collection of neurons. If tonotopic reorganization is expressed only as a change in synchronicity or as a change in the fine-grained distribution of neural activity across microscopic cortical columns, for instance, then this will have remained undetected in this study. Other techniques (like electro- and magnetoencephalography, or electrophysiological recordings) may prove sensitive to some of these changes (Mühlnickel et al., 1998; Wienbruch et al., 2006), but these have so far been less successful in mapping the detailed cortical tonotopy in humans either because of their limited ability to distinguish activity from numerous sites simultaneously or because of their invasive nature.

A third limitation of this study may be related to the subject group. We deliberately included tinnitus patients with normal hearing thresholds over most of the range of audible frequencies in order to be able to attribute any detectable deviations specifically to the presence of tinnitus but not hearing loss. Although near-normal hearing is not entirely uncommon, tinnitus patients typically show substantially elevated thresholds at moderate frequencies already. Even in tinnitus patients with allegedly normal hearing thresholds, high-frequency hearing loss may occur that has been missed due to the fact that standard audiometry often does not extend beyond 8 kHz. Of particular importance in the comparison with previous results from animal studies, tinnitus in animals is often induced by acoustic trauma and can be accompanied by hearing loss in excess of 40 dB (Noreña et al., 2003; Yang et al., 2011). In contrast, for sufficiently small damage to the peripheral hearing organ, the balance between excitation and inhibition was shown not to change, suggesting that tonotopic maps are not required to shift under such circumstances (Rajan, 2001). Therefore, this study may inadvertently have considered a special subgroup in which tonotopic reorganization plays no role (Barnea et al., 1990), whereas this mechanism may still remain important in the patient population as a whole. Or, perhaps tonotopic reorganizations in these patients occurred only in areas tuned to frequencies beyond 8 kHz, where some hearing loss was observed, but which exceeded the highest presentation frequency in this study.

Still, except for a relative lack of hearing loss, this subpopulation of patients is surprisingly typical. This may be argued for our subjects in particular based on the data in **Table 1**, but it has been independently pointed out for a much larger subject group previously (Sanchez et al., 2005). On average, tinnitus patients with normal hearing thresholds are younger (likely causing better thresholds) and less burdened (likely as a result of better thresholds) than the tinnitus population as a whole, but the perceived acoustic attributes of their tinnitus percept are remarkably similar. This raises the possibility that perhaps these patients have a type of hearing loss that conventional tone-audiometry is insensitive to. For instance, substantial loss of neurons in the cochlear nerve (especially neurons with high thresholds and low spontaneous activity) and even loss of inner hair cells may remain unnoticed if, in contrast to dead regions, such losses occur sparsely spread across a range of audible frequencies. Alternatively, the plastic changes may have been induced by temporary hearing loss that later recovered without reverting the tonotopic map back to normal. In conclusion, even though peripheral damage was not proven in our subject group, except at extreme frequencies, it is still conceivable that similar mechanisms may have occurred at the central level, resulting in tinnitus (Weisz et al., 2006; Kujawa and Liberman, 2009; Schaette and McAlpine, 2011).

IMPLICATIONS FOR PATHOPHYSIOLOGICAL MODELS

We conclude by comparing our findings with models that attribute tinnitus to cortical plasticity, either homeostatic plasticity through upregulation of central gain or tonotopic plasticity through shifts in characteristic frequency. **Figure 6A** shows a highly simplified diagram of how sound information is normally transmitted from the periphery to the auditory cortex along numerous frequency channels in parallel. Of course, in reality complex signal transformations take place in several intermediate processing stages that comprise cross-channel integration of afferent as well as efferent information, and we do not mean to claim that these cannot play a role in tinnitus, but for the sake of clarity these intricacies will be presently overlooked.

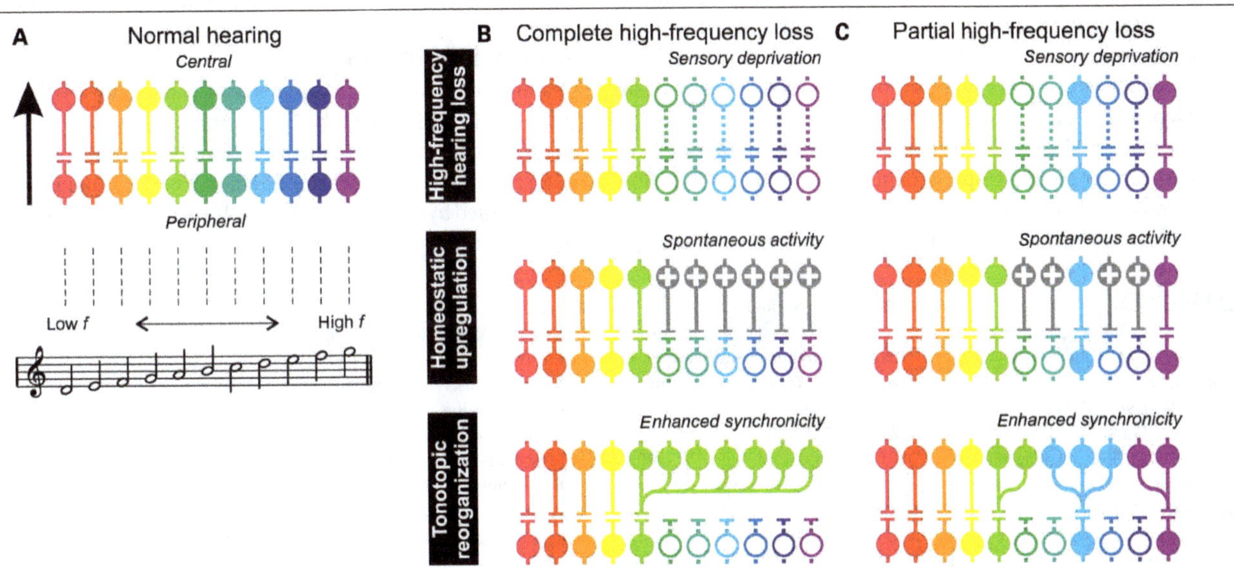

FIGURE 6 | (A) A simplified diagram showing transmission of acoustic information from the peripheral to the central auditory system across multiple parallel channels. The colors represent frequency tuning. **(B)** After complete high-frequency hearing loss (top panel), sensory deprivation leads to permanently reduced activity in the affected channels (symbolized by dotted lines and open circles). Following homeostatic upregulation (middle panel), neurons with increased gain (indicated with plusses) respond even to low levels of spontaneous activity. Alternatively, following tonotopic reorganization (bottom panel), large numbers of neurons receive input from the edge-frequency region. **(C)** In the present study, high-frequency hearing thresholds were largely normal, suggesting that sufficient hair cells and neurons in the affected frequency regions remained intact. Homeostatic upregulation or tonotopic reorganization would then be limited to the interspersed deprived neurons only, but would still lead to elevated activity or enhanced synchronicity, respectively, resulting in the presence of a tinnitus percept.

The top panel in **Figure 6B** illustrates what may happen after complete loss of hearing at high frequencies. Various channels are deprived from sensory input and their activity will permanently drop (indicated by the dotted lines and open circles). This provides a strong incentive for plasticity to occur, as depicted in the lower panels. Homeostatic upregulation may reinstate a normal rate of activity by increasing the gain in the affected channels. The model predicts that this induces elevated levels of spontaneous activity, which would be perceived as a high-pitched tinnitus. Alternatively, tonotopic reorganization may entice the high-frequency channels to start responding to input from the nearest frequency regions that still retain normal input, i.e., from the edge-frequency region. Thus, high-frequency regions in the central auditory system become massively tuned to a limited amount of sensory input that originates from a small tonotopic region in the periphery. This induces enhanced synchronicity across the high-frequency region, which could be similarly perceived as a high-pitched tinnitus. The fact that we found normal tonotopic representations in tinnitus patients would at first sight contradict the model that involves tonotopic reorganization.

However, our patients showed normal thresholds in much of the high-frequency range, suggesting that sensory deprivation may have been partial, and some fraction of neurons with intact input may have survived throughout the tonotopic axis. These may suffice in order to detect the presence of sound (explaining the normal thresholds), but there would still be loss of input such that plastic reorganization can occur (explaining the tinnitus). This situation is schematically depicted in **Figure 6C**. The model involving homeostatic upregulation would predict that elevated levels of spontaneous activity still occur for the deprived subpopulation of neurons, similarly leading to tinnitus as in the condition with complete loss. The model involving tonotopic reorganization might now predict negligible shifts in characteristic frequency, because neurons can still obtain input from intact nearby channels. Depending on the scale at which losses are clustered this might lead to a slightly coarser, more granular representation, but the macroscopic tonotopic organization would survive. Still, large numbers of neurons would be excited by a small number of inputs, thus increasing neural synchronicity, again leading to tinnitus. Following this argument, even though we exclude that large-scale macroscopic tonotopic reorganization is required for tinnitus to arise, our results can still be brought into agreement with a model based on tonotopic reorganization. However, it should be realized then that abnormalities can be limited to microscopic dimensions, and the resulting enhanced synchronicity is a more direct correlate of tinnitus than the reorganization itself.

Finally, we note that our data also showed little evidence for homeostatic changes in central gain. As far as elevated levels of excitability were observed, they occurred in low-frequency regions in the left hemisphere. This is hard to reconcile with the prediction that neural gain would be upregulated in the high-frequency regions where the tinnitus pitch was found. In contrast, in high frequency regions, no significant elevations in activity were found. However, for this model as well, our findings might be explained to some degree if the elevation in spontaneous activity would happen to equal the elevation in evoked activity. Because fMRI is sensitive only to the contrast between these conditions, such an overall effect might remain unobservable.

CONCLUSION

In conclusion, our findings strongly suggest that macroscopic tonotopic reorganization is not required for tinnitus to arise, at least in patients with normal hearing or mild hearing loss only. Although this observation can be reconciled with prevailing models regarding the pathophysiology of tinnitus in the central auditory system, it sheds a new and subtle light on how these mechanisms may naturally take shape. We plan to extend this study to subjects with hearing loss, both with and without tinnitus, in an effort to further unravel tinnitus pathophysiology in humans.

ACKNOWLEDGMENTS

The author Dave R. M. Langers was funded by VENI research grant 016.096.011 from the Netherlands organization for scientific research (NWO) and the Netherlands organization for health research and development (ZonMw). Further financial support was provided by the Heinsius Houbolt Foundation. We thank Eline Deenen for the audiometric evaluation of all subjects.

REFERENCES

Baguley, D. M. (2002). Mechanisms of tinnitus. *Br. Med. Bull.* 63, 195–212.

Baguley, D. M. (2003). Hyperacusis. *J. R. Soc. Med.* 96, 582–585.

Barker, D., Plack, C. J., and Hall, D. A. (2011). Reexamining the evidence for a pitch-sensitive region: a human fMRI study using iterated ripple noise. *Cereb. Cortex.* doi: 10.1093/cercor/bhr065 [Epub ahead of print].

Barnea, G., Attias, J., Gold, S., and Shahar, A. (1990). Tinnitus with normal hearing sensitivity: extended high-frequency audiometry and auditory-nerve brain-stem-evoked responses. *Audiology* 29, 36–45.

Baumgart, F., Kaulisch, T., Tempelmann, C., Gaschler-Markefski, B., Tegeler, C., Schindler, F., Stiller, D., and Scheich, H. (1998). Electrodynamic headphones and woofers for application in magnetic resonance imaging scanners. *Med. Phys.* 25, 2068–2070.

Brand, T., and Hohmann, V. (2002). An adaptive procedure for categorical loudness scaling. *J. Acoust. Soc. Am.* 112, 1597–1604.

Brechmann, A., Baumgart, F., and Scheich, H. (2002). Sound-level-dependent representation of frequency modulations in human auditory cortex: a low-noise fMRI study. *J. Neurophysiol.* 87, 423–433.

Budd, R. J., and Pugh, R. (1996). Tinnitus coping style and its relationship to tinnitus severity and emotional distress. *J. Psychosom. Res.* 41, 327–335.

Burger, J., Frank, E., Kreuzer, P., Kleinjung, T., Vielsmeier, V., Landgrebe, M., Hajak, G., and Langguth, B. (2011). Transcranial magnetic stimulation for the treatment of tinnitus: 4-year follow-up in treatment responders – a retrospective analysis. *Brain Stimul.* 4, 222–227.

Burrone, J., and Murthy, V. N. (2003). Synaptic gain control and homeostasis. *Curr. Opin. Neurobiol.* 13, 560–567.

Chrostowski, M., Yang, L., Wilson, H. R., Bruce, I. C., and Becker, S. (2011). Can homeostatic plasticity in deafferented primary auditory cortex lead to travelling waves of excitation? *J. Comput. Neurosci.* 30, 279–299.

Chung, H.-K., Tsai, C.-H., Lin, Y.-C., Chen, J.-M., Tsou, Y.-A., Wang, C.-Y., Lin, C.-D., Jeng, F.-C., Chung, J.-G., and Tsai, M.-H. (2012). Effectiveness of theta-burst repetitive transcranial magnetic stimulation for treating chronic tinnitus. *Audiol. Neurootol.* 17, 112–120.

Da Costa, S., van der Zwaag, W., Marques, J. P., Frackowiak, R. S. J., Clarke, S., and Saenz, M. (2011). Human primary auditory cortex follows the shape of Heschl's gyrus. *J. Neurosci.* 31, 14067–14075.

Dominguez, M., Becker, S., Bruce, I., and Read, H. (2006). A spiking neuron model of cortical correlates of sensorineural hearing loss: spontaneous firing, synchrony, and tinnitus. *Neural Comput.* 18, 2942–2958.

Edmister, W. B., Talavage, T. M., Ledden, P. J., and Weisskoff, R. M. (1999).

Improved auditory cortex imaging using clustered volume acquisitions. *Hum. Brain Mapp.* 7, 89–97.

Eggermont, J. J. (2007a). Pathophysiology of tinnitus. *Prog. Brain Res.* 166, 19–35.

Eggermont, J. J. (2007b). Correlated neural activity as the driving force for functional changes in auditory cortex. *Hear. Res.* 229, 69–80.

Engineer, N. D., Riley, J. R., Seale, J. D., Vrana, W. A., Shetake, J. A., Sudanagunta, S. P., Borland, M. S., and Kilgard, M. P. (2011). Reversing pathological neural activity using targeted plasticity. *Nature* 470, 101–104.

Formisano, E., Kim, D. S., Di Salle, F., van de Moortele, P. F., Ugurbil, K., and Goebel, R. (2003). Mirror-symmetric tonotopic maps in human primary auditory cortex. *Neuron* 40, 859–869.

Gu, J. W., Halpin, C. F., Nam, E.-C., Levine, R. A., and Melcher, J. R. (2010). Tinnitus, diminished sound-level tolerance, and elevated auditory activity in humans with clinically normal hearing sensitivity. *J. Neurophysiol.* 104, 3361–3370.

Hall, D. A., Haggard, M. P., Akeroyd, M. A., Palmer, A. R., Summerfield, A. Q., Elliott, M. R., Gurney, E. M., and Bowtell, R. W. (1999). "Sparse" temporal sampling in auditory fMRI. *Hum. Brain Mapp.* 7, 213–223.

Hall, D. A., Haggard, M. P., Summerfield, A. Q., Akeroyd, M. A., Palmer, A. R., and Bowtell, R. W. (2001). Functional magnetic resonance imaging measurements of sound-level encoding in the absence of background scanner noise. *J. Acoust. Soc. Am.* 109, 1559–1570.

Hall, D. A., and Plack, C. J. (2009). Pitch processing sites in the human auditory brain. *Cereb. Cortex* 19, 576–585.

Hardt, J., and Gerbershagen, H. U. (2001). Cross-validation of the SCL-27: a short psychometric screening instrument for chronic pain patients. *Eur. J. Pain* 5, 187–197.

Herraiz, C., Diges, I., and Cobo, P. (2007). Auditory discrimination therapy (ADT) for tinnitus management. *Prog. Brain Res.* 166, 467–471.

Humphries, C., Liebenthal, E., and Binder, J. R. (2010). Tonotopic organization of human auditory cortex. *Neuroimage* 50, 1202–1211.

Kaltenbach, J. A. (2011). Tinnitus: models and mechanisms. *Hear. Res.* 276, 52–60.

Khalfa, S., Dubal, S., Veuillet, E., Perez-Diaz, F., Jouvent, R., and Collet, L. (2002). Psychometric normalization of a hyperacusis questionnaire. *ORL J. Otorhinolaryngol. Relat. Spec.* 64, 436–442.

König, O., Schaette, R., Kempter, R., and Gross, M. (2006). Course of hearing loss and occurrence of tinnitus. *Hear. Res.* 221, 59–64.

Kujawa, S. G., and Liberman, M. C. (2009). Adding insult to injury: cochlear nerve degeneration after "temporary" noise-induced hearing loss. *J. Neurosci.* 29, 14077–14085.

Lang, P. J., Bradley, M. M., and Cuthbert, B. N. (2008). *International Affective Picture System (IAPS): Affective Ratings of Pictures and Instruction Manual. Technical Report A-8.* Gainesville, FL: University of Florida.

Langers, D. R. M., and van Dijk, P. (2011). Mapping the tonotopic organization in human auditory cortex with minimally salient acoustic stimulation. *Cereb. Cortex.* doi: 10.1093/cercor/bhr282 [Epub ahead of print].

Langers, D. R. M., van Dijk, P., Schoenmaker, E. S., and Backes, W. H. (2007). fMRI activation in relation to sound intensity and loudness. *Neuroimage* 35, 709–718.

Lauter, J. L., Herscovitch, P., Formby, C., and Raichle, M. E. (1985). Tonotopic organization in human auditory cortex revealed by positron emission tomography. *Hear. Res.* 20, 199–205.

Logothetis, N. K. (2008). What we can do and what we cannot do with fMRI. *Nature* 453, 869–878.

Logothetis, N. K., Pauls, J., Augath, M., Trinath, T., and Oeltermann, A. (2001). Neurophysiological investigation of the basis of the fMRI signal. *Nature* 412, 150–157.

Møller, A. R. (2007a). The role of neural plasticity in tinnitus. *Prog. Brain Res.* 166, 37–45.

Møller, A. R. (2007b). Tinnitus: presence and future. *Prog. Brain Res.* 166, 3–16.

Moore, B. C. J., and Vinay, S. N. (2010). The relationship between tinnitus pitch and the edge frequency of the audiogram in individuals with hearing impairment and tonal tinnitus. *Hear. Res.* 261, 51–56.

Mühlnickel, W., Elbert, T., Taub, E., and Flor, H. (1998). Reorganization of auditory cortex in tinnitus. *Proc. Natl. Acad. Sci. U.S.A.* 95, 10340–10343.

Newman, C. W., Jacobson, G. P., and Spitzer, J. B. (1996). Development of the Tinnitus Handicap Inventory. *Arch. Otolaryngol. Head Neck Surg.* 122, 143–148.

Noreña, A., Micheyl, C., Chéry-Croze, S., and Collet, L. (2002). Psychoacoustic characterization of the tinnitus spectrum: implications for the underlying mechanisms of tinnitus. *Audiol. Neurootol.* 7, 358–369.

Noreña, A. J. (2011). An integrative model of tinnitus based on a central gain controlling neural sensitivity. *Neurosci. Biobehav. Rev.* 35, 1089–1109.

Noreña, A. J., Tomita, M., and Eggermont, J. J. (2003). Neural changes in cat auditory cortex after a transient pure-tone trauma. *J. Neurophysiol.* 90, 2387–2401.

Oxenham, A. J., Bernstein, J. G. W., and Penagos, H. (2004). Correct tonotopic representation is necessary for complex pitch perception. *Proc. Natl. Acad. Sci. U.S.A.* 101, 1421–1425.

Pantev, C., Hoke, M., Lütkenhöner, B., and Lehnertz, K. (1989). Tonotopic organization of the auditory cortex: pitch versus frequency representation. *Science* 246, 486–488.

Patterson, R. D., Uppenkamp, S., Johnsrude, I. S., and Griffiths, T. D. (2002). The processing of temporal pitch and melody information in auditory cortex. *Neuron* 36, 767–776.

Penagos, H., Melcher, J. R., and Oxenham, A. J. (2004). A neural representation of pitch salience in nonprimary human auditory cortex revealed with functional magnetic resonance imaging. *J. Neurosci.* 24, 6810–6815.

Pineda, J. A., Moore, F. R., and Viirre, E. (2008). Tinnitus treatment with customized sounds. *Int. Tinnitus J.* 14, 17–25.

Puschmann, S., Uppenkamp, S., Kollmeier, B., and Thiel, C. M. (2010). Dichotic pitch activates pitch processing centre in Heschl's gyrus. *Neuroimage* 49, 1641–1649.

Rajan, R. (2001). Plasticity of excitation and inhibition in the receptive field of primary auditory cortical neurons after limited receptor organ damage. *Cereb. Cortex* 11, 171–182.

Rajan, R., and Irvine, D. R. (1998). Neuronal responses across cortical field A1 in plasticity induced by peripheral auditory organ damage. *Audiol. Neurootol.* 3, 123–144.

Rauschecker, J. P., Leaver, A. M., and Mühlau, M. (2010). Tuning out the noise: limbic-auditory interactions in tinnitus. *Neuron* 66, 819–826.

Roberts, L. E., Eggermont, J. J., Caspary, D. M., Shore, S. E., Melcher, J. R., and Kaltenbach, J. A. (2010). Ringing ears: the neuroscience of tinnitus. *J. Neurosci.* 30, 14972–14979.

Roberts, L. E., Moffat, G., Baumann, M., Ward, L. M., and Bosnyak, D. J. (2008). Residual inhibition functions overlap tinnitus spectra and the region of auditory threshold shift. *J. Assoc. Res. Otolaryngol.* 9, 417–435.

Romani, G. L., Williamson, S. J., and Kaufman, L. (1982). Tonotopic organization of the human auditory cortex. *Science* 216, 1339–1340.

Sanchez, T. G., de Medeiros, I. R. T., Levy, C. P. D., da Rosa Oiticica Ramalho, J., and Bento, R. F. (2005). Tinnitus in normally hearing patients: clinical aspects and repercussions. *Braz. J. Otorhinolaryngol.* 71, 427–431.

Schaette, R., and Kempter, R. (2006). Development of tinnitus-related neuronal hyperactivity through homeostatic plasticity after hearing loss: a computational model. *Eur. J. Neurosci.* 23, 3124–3138.

Schaette, R., and McAlpine, D. (2011). Tinnitus with a normal audiogram: physiological evidence for hidden hearing loss and computational model. *J. Neurosci.* 31, 13452–13457.

Stolzberg, D., Chen, G.-D., Allman, B. L., and Salvi, R. J. (2011). Salicylate-induced peripheral auditory changes and tonotopic reorganization of auditory cortex. *Neuroscience* 180, 157–164.

Striem-Amit, E., Hertz, U., and Amedi, A. (2011). Extensive cochleotopic mapping of human auditory cortical fields obtained with phase-encoding fMRI. *PLoS ONE* 6, e17832. doi: 10.1371/journal.pone.0017832

Svensén, M., Kruggel, F., and Benali, H. (2002). ICA of fMRI group study data. *Neuroimage* 16, 551–563.

Talavage, T. M., Sereno, M. I., Melcher, J. R., Ledden, P. J., Rosen, B. R., and Dale, A. M. (2004). Tonotopic organization in human auditory cortex revealed by progressions of frequency sensitivity. *J. Neurophysiol.* 91, 1282–1296.

Weisz, N., Hartmann, T., Dohrmann, K., Schlee, W., and Norena, A. (2006). High-frequency tinnitus without hearing loss does not mean absence of deafferentation. *Hear. Res.* 222, 108–114.

Wessinger, C. M., Buonocore, M. H., Kussmaul, C. L., and Mangun, G. R. (1997). Tonotopy in human auditory cortex examined with functional magnetic resonance imaging. *Hum. Brain Mapp.* 5, 18–25.

Wienbruch, C., Paul, I., Weisz, N., Elbert, T., and Roberts, L. E. (2006). Frequency organization of the 40-Hz auditory steady-state response in normal hearing and in tinnitus. *Neuroimage* 33, 180–194.

Wilson, P. H., Henry, J., Bowen, M., and Haralambous, G. (1991). Tinnitus Reaction Questionnaire: psychometric properties of a measure of distress associated with tinnitus. *J. Speech Hear. Res.* 34, 197–201.

Woods, D. L., Stecker, G. C., Rinne, T., Herron, T. J., Cate, A. D., Yund, E. W., Liao, I., and Kang, X. (2009). Functional maps of human auditory cortex: effects of acoustic features and attention. *PLoS ONE* 4, e5183. doi: 10.1371/journal.pone.0005183

Yang, S., Weiner, B. D., Zhang, L. S., Cho, S.-J., and Bao, S. (2011). Homeostatic plasticity drives tinnitus perception in an animal model. *Proc. Natl. Acad. Sci. U.S.A.* 108, 14974–14979.

13

Neural plasticity expressed in central auditory structures with and without tinnitus

Larry E. Roberts*, Daniel J. Bosnyak and David C. Thompson

Department of Psychology, Neuroscience, and Behaviour, McMaster University, Hamilton, ON, Canada

Correspondence:
Larry E. Roberts, Department of Psychology, Neuroscience, and Behaviour, McMaster University, 1280 Main Street West, Hamilton, ON L8S 4K1, Canada.
e-mail: roberts@mcmaster.ca

Sensory training therapies for tinnitus are based on the assumption that, notwithstanding neural changes related to tinnitus, auditory training can alter the response properties of neurons in auditory pathways. To assess this assumption, we investigated whether brain changes induced by sensory training in tinnitus sufferers and measured by electroencephalography (EEG) are similar to those induced in age and hearing loss matched individuals without tinnitus trained on the same auditory task. Auditory training was given using a 5 kHz 40-Hz amplitude-modulated (AM) sound that was in the tinnitus frequency region of the tinnitus subjects and enabled extraction of the 40-Hz auditory steady-state response (ASSR) and P2 transient response known to localize to primary and non-primary auditory cortex, respectively. P2 amplitude increased over training sessions equally in participants with tinnitus and in control subjects, suggesting normal remodeling of non-primary auditory regions in tinnitus. However, training-induced changes in the ASSR differed between the tinnitus and control groups. In controls the phase delay between the 40-Hz response and stimulus waveforms reduced by about 10° over training, in agreement with previous results obtained in young normal hearing individuals. However, ASSR phase did not change significantly with training in the tinnitus group, although some participants showed phase shifts resembling controls. On the other hand, ASSR amplitude increased with training in the tinnitus group, whereas in controls this response (which is difficult to remodel in young normal hearing subjects) did not change with training. These results suggest that neural changes related to tinnitus altered how neural plasticity was expressed in the region of primary but not non-primary auditory cortex. Auditory training did not reduce tinnitus loudness although a small effect on the tinnitus spectrum was detected.

Keywords: tinnitus, neural plasticity, auditory system, sensory training, EEG

INTRODUCTION

Tinnitus is a phantom sound (ringing of the ears) that affects quality of life for millions around the world and is a major challenge for health systems because effective medical treatments are lacking. Most cases are associated with hearing impairment detected by the audiogram (Henry and Meikle, 2000) or more sensitive measures (Weisz et al., 2006; Kujawa and Liberman, 2009; Schaette and McAlpine, 2011). One of the neural changes consequent on hearing loss is tonotopic map reorganization in which neurons in the hearing loss region of primary auditory cortex (A1) begin to express the tuning preferences of their unaffected neighbors, thereby augmenting the representation of neighboring frequencies in the cortical place map (Rajan and Irvine, 1998; Noreña et al., 2003). Map reorganization, which has been documented in human tinnitus sufferers with hearing loss (Wienbruch et al., 2006), suggests that pre-existing inputs on lateral connections to neurons in the hearing loss region now have a stronger influence on these neurons than do surviving inputs from thalamocortical pathways (Eggermont and Roberts, 2004). Other hearing loss-induced changes include shifts in the balance of excitation and inhibition in auditory cortical networks (Scholl and Wehr, 2008), increased spontaneous activity of neurons in central auditory structures (Noreña and Eggermont, 2003; Kaltenbach et al., 2004), increased burst firing in some of these structures (Finlayson and Kaltenbach, 2009), and increased synchronous activity among cortical neurons affected by hearing loss (Seki and Eggermont, 2003). Although the contribution of these changes to tinnitus percepts is not fully understood, enhanced neural synchrony is a likely proximal neural correlate because it is largely confined to the hearing loss frequencies (Noreña and Eggermont, 2003) where in human subjects tinnitus percepts also localize (Noreña et al., 2002; Roberts et al., 2008).

Forms of neural plasticity are believed to contribute to these neural changes following hearing impairment. Cochlear damage in an animal model of hearing loss is followed within two weeks by an upregulation of somatosensory inputs to auditory neurons in the dorsal cochlear nucleus (DCN), one of the early processing stages in subcortical auditory pathways (Zeng et al., 2009). This change is believed to reflect compensatory homeostatic plasticity that acts to preserve the global firing rates of deafferented auditory neurons within a prescribed dynamic range (Turrigiano and Nelson, 2004; Pozo and Goda, 2010). Homeostatic plasticity may explain why wave I of the auditory brain stem response (ABR) is reduced in tinnitus sufferers with normal audiograms, implying diminished auditory nerve activity consequent undetected cochlear damage, but wave V is not reduced (Schaette and McAlpine, 2011) suggesting compensatory changes in intervening central auditory structures. At the cortical level an undesirable consequence of compensatory change may be an increase in the spontaneous and driven activity of auditory neurons setting the stage for the development of tinnitus and hyperacusis which is reported by many tinnitus sufferers (Noreña, 2011). Increased neural synchrony is a further neural correlate of tinnitus that may result from neuroplastic mechanisms (Seki and Eggermont, 2003; Weisz et al., 2007). Following hearing loss and diminished feedforward inhibition, cortical neurons are likely to discharge in phase-locked patterns mediated by their lateral connections. Subsequently such activity may be forged into stable and larger functional assemblies by spike-timing dependent plasticity in the hearing loss region (cf. Yao and Dan, 2001), giving rise to persistent tinnitus sounds. These examples represent possible maladaptive consequences of neural plasticity operating in auditory regions affected by hearing loss. However, it has been proposed that therapeutic sensory training regimens may prevent or reverse maladaptive remodeling after hearing loss. In support of this hypothesis, prolonged exposure to low-level, complex high frequency sounds covering the region of threshold (TH) shift prevents cortical map reorganization in cats subjected to noise trauma (Noreña and Eggermont, 2005) and has been reported to rescale loudness growth in human hyperacusis patients (Noreña and Chery-Croze, 2007). Improvements in peripheral hearing consequent on therapeutic sound appear to contribute to map preservation after noise trauma (Noreña and Eggermont, 2005), but rescaling of loudness growth in hyperacusis patients appears to depend on central adaptive mechanisms (Formby et al., 2003). Effects of therapeutic sound have been more variable applied to tinnitus percepts. Distress behavior associated with tinnitus is typically reduced following sensory training therapies, but effects on psychoacoustic measurements of tinnitus are inconsistent and have not been strongly realized (see Roberts and Bosnyak, 2010a; Hoare et al., 2011 for reviews).

Sensory training therapies are based on the assumption that the response properties of auditory neurons can be manipulated by neuroplastic mechanisms in the tinnitus brain, as is the case in normal hearing individuals. However, it is also possible that neural changes underlying tinnitus (for example, spontaneous or synchronous activity propagated by intact centrifugal pathways) may impede cortical remodeling in tinnitus sufferers. To address this question, we investigated whether brain changes induced by sensory training in individuals with tinnitus and measured by the electroencephalogram (EEG) are similar to those induced in age and hearing level matched individuals without tinnitus trained on the same auditory task. Training was given for a sound that was amplitude-modulated (AM) at 40 Hz, which enabled extraction from the EEG of (1) the 40 Hz auditory steady-state response (ASSR) generated by cortical sources in posterior-medial Heschl's gyrus (A1; Brugge et al., 2009), and (2) the P2 transient response, which is believed to arise from distributed sources centered in non-primary (A2) auditory cortex (Picton et al., 1999). We thus gained a picture of changes occurring in both cortical regions from the same data-set (Bosnyak et al., 2004; Gander et al., 2010b). In previous research ASSR phase (the time delay between zero-crossings in the stimulus and response waveforms) and P2 amplitude have been found to be highly plastic revealing, respectively, changes in temporal population activity in A1 (Bosnyak et al., 2004; Gander et al., 2010b) and expansion of auditory representations in the region A2 (Tremblay et al., 2001; Reinke et al., 2003; Bosnyak et al., 2004; Sheehan et al., 2005; Ross and Tremblay, 2009; Gander et al., 2010b). In the current study auditory training was given for a sound in the tinnitus frequency region, to ensure that tinnitus networks were engaged in tinnitus subjects and to assess whether such training modified the tinnitus percept itself. Our goal was to determine whether tinnitus-related neural activity would affect the expression of plasticity in individuals with tinnitus compared to controls, and if neural plasticity was demonstrated in the tinnitus group, whether the tinnitus percept would be modulated.

Participants with chronic tinnitus ($n = 11$) and age and hearing-level matched controls ($n = 11$) participated in seven sessions of auditory training each separated by 1–3 days. Audiometric THs were measured for all participants in an initial session one week before auditory training commenced. Measurements of tinnitus spectra and loudness by the Tinnitus Tester method of Roberts et al. (2008) and tinnitus distress by the Tinnitus Handicap Questionnaire (THQ; Kuk et al., 1990) were taken in this session and repeated in a follow-up session one week after auditory training had ended. The stimulus for auditory training was a 5 kHz pure tone of 976 ms duration AM with a 40.96 Hz sinusoid (called 40 Hz herein, 100% modulation depth). This carrier frequency was chosen because it is typically judged by tinnitus subjects to be in the tinnitus spectrum (Roberts et al., 2008; see **Figure 2B**). Sound level was matched by all participants to a 2 kHz 40-Hz AM reference tone presented at 65 dB SPL used in prior research (Gander et al., 2010b), so that findings could be contrasted across studies with perceived loudness controlled. The training procedure was identical to that of Gander et al. (2010b) except for the change in carrier frequency. During training (see **Figure 1A**) auditory stimuli were separated by an intertrial interval (ITI) of approximately 1900 ms during which behavioral responses were recorded. Approximately 2/3 of the stimuli contained a single 40-Hz AM pulse of variably increased amplitude (bracketing the TH of detection) that occurred randomly at times commencing 415 ms after stimulus onset (target). On active blocks participants pressed one of two mouse buttons after each trial indicating whether a target had or had not occurred (feedback for correctness was given). On passive blocks subjects ceased behavioral responding and ignored the auditory cues. Active and passive blocks alternated in sessions 1, 4, and 7 of auditory training during which the EEG was recorded. The remaining sessions were identical except that EEG was not recorded and all blocks were now active blocks. In all sessions, participants in the tinnitus group indicated using a slider their tinnitus "awareness" and "loudness" on a Borg CR100 scale (Borg and Borg, 2001) immediately before, at the midpoint, and the end of training (**Figure 1B**). ASSR amplitude and phase were extracted from the unmodeled data recorded by 128 EEG sensors using the method shown in **Figure 1C** (for further details see the Materials and Methods

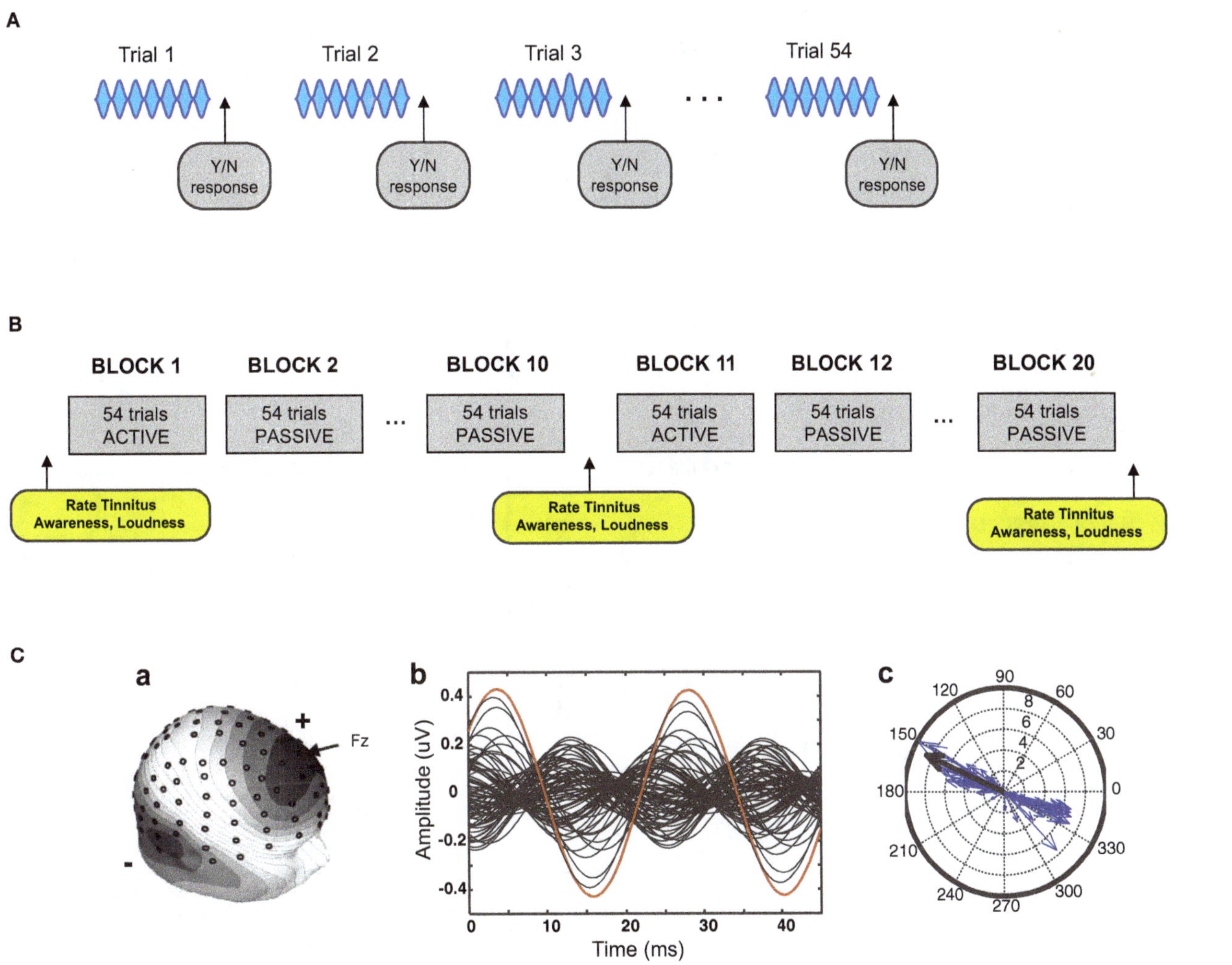

FIGURE 1 | Experimental design. (A) Stimulus procedure. The stimulus was a 5 kHz 40-Hz AM pure tone of 976 ms duration. Approximately 2/3 of the stimuli contained a single 40 Hz AM pulse of variable increased amplitude (target) that occurred randomly in an interval commencing 415 ms after sound onset. Participants pressed one of two mouse buttons after each trial to indicate whether a target had or had not occurred. Four trials are depicted here in simplified form (each trial contained 40 AM pulses), with a target illustrated on the third trial. **(B)** Training procedure. Sessions consisted of 20 blocks of trials each block containing 54 trials. Tinnitus awareness and loudness were probed within sessions as shown. On days on which the EEG was recorded (sessions 1, 4, and 7) blocks alternated between active and passive conditions. On the remaining days (sessions 2, 3, 5, and 6) all blocks were active blocks. **(C)** Analysis of EEG from a representative participant. The left panel shows the digitized location of the 128 electrodes and the voltage map of the ASSR. In the middle panel the 128-channel data were collapsed to two modulation cycles of the ASSR. A compass plot of the 40-Hz component of the FFT of the two-cycle waveform is shown in the right panel. The length of each vector gives ASSR amplitude at one electrode and the angle gives ASSR phase. Vectors determined by an algorithm to contribute 50% of the 40-Hz total power with the smallest angle were used to compute ASSR phase (see Materials and Methods). The single red trace in the middle panel, corresponding to the single black arrow in the right panel, is electrode Fz.

section). P2 and other transient responses were extracted by low pass filtering of the continuous EEG file and recorded at their amplitude maxima. In previous research we found that results obtained with these methods based on the unmodeled data concurred closely with results obtained when the cortical sources of ASSR and P2 responses were modeled in source space (Gander et al., 2010a,b).

RESULTS

Table 1 reports the mean age and age range of the tinnitus and control groups, their sound THs at 2 and 5 kHz determined by clinical audiometry, and the sound level of the training stimulus delivered to each group. No significant group differences were found on any of these measures (all p's > 0.37). Both groups experienced low to moderate hearing loss between 3 and 6 kHz and deeper losses above this range (see **Figure 2A**), but no group differences were found at any frequency (main effect of frequency and group by frequency interaction F's < 1). On average participants reported chronic tinnitus 11.7 years duration. All were bilateral cases with the majority reporting a narrow band "tonal" tinnitus and the remainder a tinnitus of greater bandwidth ("ringing" or "hissing") when comparing their tinnitus to

Table 1 | Group information.

	Tinnitus Group	Control Group
CHARACTERISTICS OF PARTICIPANTS		
Number (male)	11 (7)	11 (6)
Age in Years Mean (SE)	48.6 (4.75)	53.9 (5.86)
Age Range in Years	22–68	22–76
AUDIOMETRIC DATA AND SOUND LEVELS		
Mean (SE) threshold @ 2 kHz Left Ear (dB HL)	10.0 (4.54)	15.9 (4.54)
Mean (SE) threshold @ 2 kHz Right Ear (dB HL)	9.6 (2.77)	7.7 (2.77)
Mean (SE) threshold @ 5 kHz Left Ear (dB HL)	29.4 (7.65)	28.4 (7.65)
Mean (SE) threshold @ 5 kHz Right Ear (dB HL)	27.3 (5.68)	23.0 (5.68)
Mean (SE) Training stimulus loudness (dB SPL)[a]	60.0 (2.05)	58.5 (2.01)
TINNITUS CHARACTERISTICS		
Mean (SE) duration in years	11.7 (3.03)	
Mean (SE) loudness rating Borg CR100 Scale[b]	57.1 (6.21)	
Mean (SE) loudness match (1 kHz tone, dB SPL)[b]	53.9 (6.32)	
Tinnitus Bandwidth (number of participants)[b]		
Tonal	6	
Ringing	2	
Hissing	3	
Tinnitus Ear		
Bilateral	11	
Left	0	
Right	0	

[a]*Participants matched the 5 kHz 40-Hz AM training stimulus to the loudness of a 2 kHz 40-Hz AM 65 dB SPL sound used in earlier research with young normal hearing subjects Gander et al. (2010b).*

[b]*Before auditory training.*

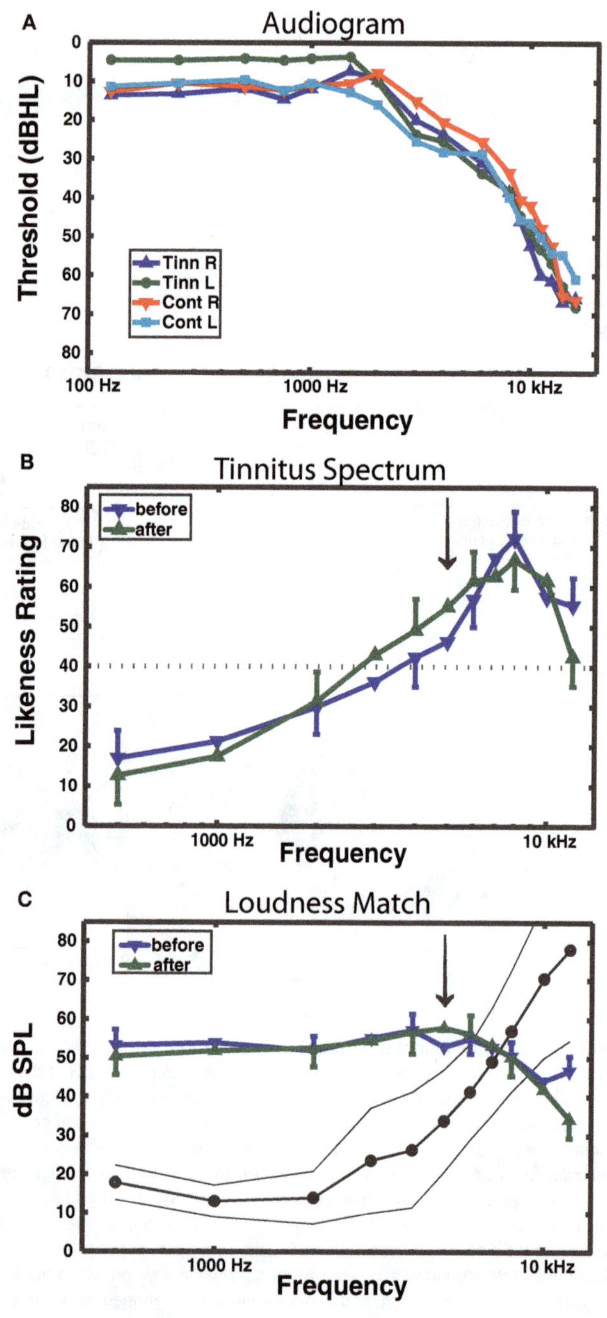

FIGURE 2 | Audiometric and psychoacoustic measures. (A) Audiogram for each group, right and left ears shown separately. For clarity, error bars are omitted (group main effect $F < 1$). **(B)** Tinnitus spectrum (likeness ratings) before and after training in the tinnitus group, from the Tinnitus Tester software (Roberts et al., 2008). A likeness rating of 40 (broken line) corresponds to sounds beginning to resemble the individual's tinnitus (the lower boundary of the tinnitus spectrum; Roberts et al. (2008). The arrow denotes the 5 kHz training frequency. **(C)** Loudness matches from the Tinnitus Tester, before and after training. The line connected by dots denotes the group averaged audiogram converted from dB HL to dB SPL (thin lines denote between-subject 95% confidence limits). The difference between the audiogram and the loudness matches gives an approximate estimate of the loudness of the tinnitus in dB SL (Roberts et al., 2008). Error bars shown in panels **(B)** and **(C)** are the mean within-subject standard error (1 SE).

sound files delivered by the Tinnitus Tester (Roberts et al., 2008). At the outset of training participants rated their tinnitus loudness at 57.1 (SE = 6.21) on the Borg CR100 scale of the Tinnitus Tester, which is near the midpoint between of "Loud" and "Very Loud" on this scale. The mean tinnitus spectrum and loudness matches of the participants measured by the Tinnitus Tester are reported in **Figures 2B** and **2C**, respectively. The training frequency of 5 kHz was 1.5 octaves above the audiometric edge of 2 kHz and in the range of the tinnitus frequency spectrum for this group.

BEHAVIORAL PERFORMANCE

Psychophysical functions determined for sessions 1, 4, and 7 from the collapsed data of the tinnitus and control groups are presented for each group in **Figure 3A**. Performance improved rapidly from the first to the fourth session, with smaller improvements occurring in the later sessions. THs determined from psychophysical functions calculated for each participant and session confirmed this trend (**Figure 3B**) giving a main effect of

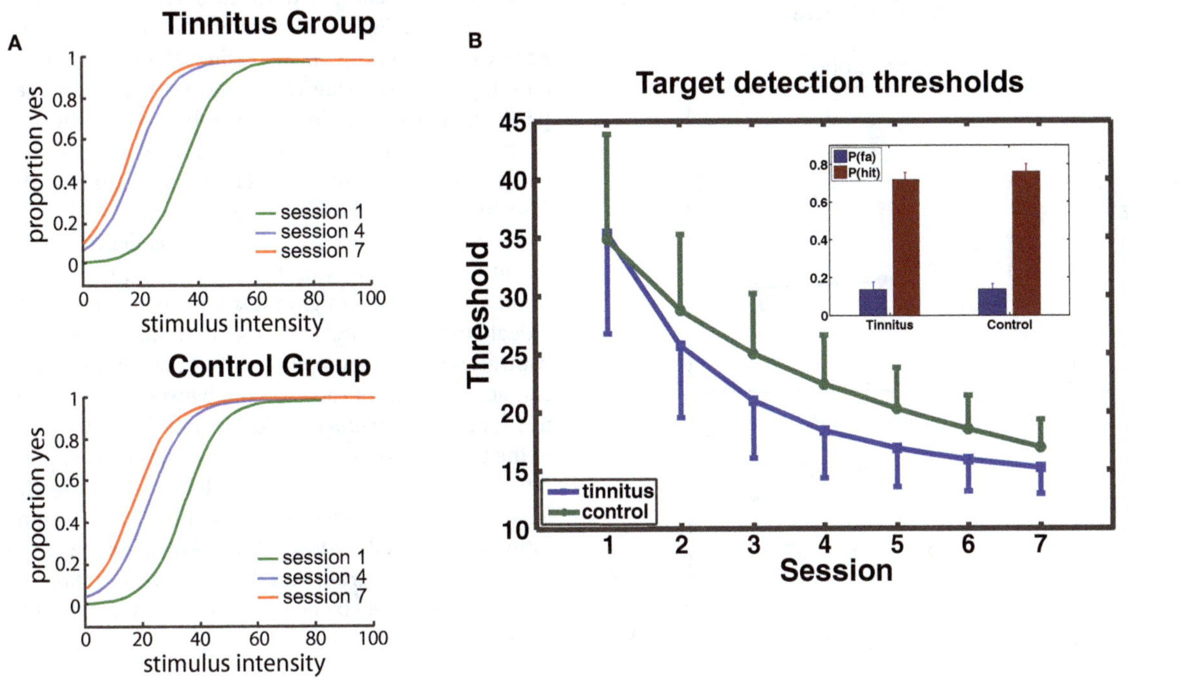

FIGURE 3 | Behavioral performance. (A) Group averaged psychophysical functions are shown for sessions 1, 4, and 7, separately for each group. **(B)** Changes in target detection THs over sessions for each group. The model used for curve fitting of each participant's data applied a negative exponential (direction determined by the data; see Materials and Methods). Error bars give the mean within-subject standard error (1 SE). The inset shows the mean hit and false alarm rates for each group.

sessions [$F_{(6, 114)} = 11.7, p = 0.00$] while factors involving group were not significant (p's > 0.68). P(Hit) exceeded P(FA) for every participant [$F_{(1, 20)} = 289, p < 0.0001$] with no group difference on either measure (see inset, **Figure 3B**).

ASSR PHASE

ASSR phase for all participants on the first passive block fell within an arc of 123° centered at 161.9° with respect to the zero-crossing in the stimulus waveform. Individual differences in ASSR phase were reliable giving a test–re-test correlation between passive blocks on days 1 and 7 of $r = 0.91$ in the tinnitus group and $r = 0.83$ in controls ($r = 0.86$ overall, $p < 0.01$). Mean phase in the tinnitus group on the first passive block (168.6°, SD = 34.2) did not differ significantly from that of controls (155.2°, SD = 19.3).

Changes in ASSR phase across sessions are depicted separately for the tinnitus and control groups in **Figure 4A**. Following Gander et al. (2010b) phase was normalized within each group by dividing the data of each subject by their respective group mean for the passive blocks of day 1, giving a common reference point (1.0) from which to evaluate effects of training and active/passive blocks. In the control group ASSR phase decreased progressively over training sessions [$F_{(2, 20)} = 6.54, p = 0.006$], in agreement with results obtained previously for young normal hearing subjects trained by Gander et al. (2010b) with a 2 kHz 40-Hz AM sound. The phase change in the control group (reflecting a shortened time delay between zero-crossings in the stimulus and response waveforms) was more pronounced on active blocks, but neither the main effect of block ($p = 0.35$) nor its interaction with sessions ($p = 0.60$) reached significance. The phase shift averaged −10.1° on active blocks, which is similar to mean shifts of −14.7° and −12.9° on these blocks observed in Groups E and C, respectively, of Experiment 2 by Gander et al. (2010b). On the other hand, neither the main effect of sessions [$F_{(2, 20)} = 1.63, p = 0.22$] or blocks [$F_{(1, 10)} = 1.31, p = 0.28$] nor their interaction [$F_{(2, 20)} = 0.79, p = 0.46$] were significant in the tinnitus group. When the tinnitus and control groups were entered into the same analysis a main effect of sessions was found [$F_{(2, 40)} = 5.08, p = 0.011$], but the interaction of group with sessions did not reach significance ($p = 0.20$). However, the phase shift seen in tinnitus participants on active blocks (mean difference day 7 – day 1 = −2.1°) was significantly smaller when contrasted to that of the three above mentioned non-tinnitus groups (mean shifts of −10.1, −14.7, and −12.9°, respectively, $t_{(38)} = 2.43, p = 0.019$). These results suggest that the presence of tinnitus may have interfered with normal remodeling of ASSR phase by the training procedure.

Two further analyses were undertaken to assess performance in the tinnitus group. In the first analysis, the before/after change in ASSR phase (day 7 – day 1) was determined for each tinnitus and control subject on active blocks and are rank ordered by magnitude in **Figure 4B**. Several tinnitus subjects expressed phase shifts overlapping with those of control subjects; however, phase shifts in the control group were less variable and for each

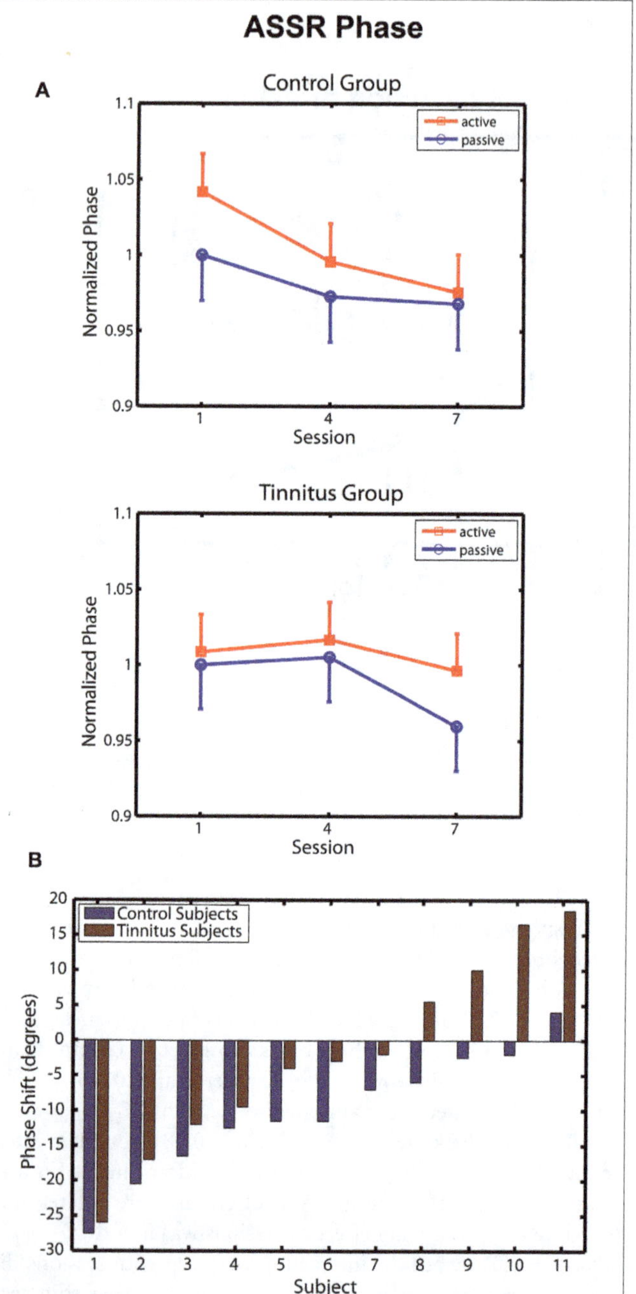

FIGURE 4 | ASSR phase. (A) Change in ASSR phase over training sessions in the Control (top panel) and Tinnitus (bottom panel) groups. Phase is normalized in each group to their baseline on passive blocks of the first session. Negative shifts denote advances of the 40-Hz response waveform toward the zero-crossing of the 40-Hz stimulus waveform. Bars are 1 within-subject standard error. **(B)** Changes in phase (session 7 – Session 1, active blocks) are shown for each participant in the active and control groups. Phase changes are shown in degrees. Subjects within each group are ordered by the magnitude of the phase shift.

pairwise comparison were in the direction of a phase decrease for controls relative to individuals with tinnitus. Overall ASSR phase decreased in 91% (10/11) of the control subjects of this study and in 90% (18/20) of normal hearing subjects reported by Gander et al. (2010b), compared to 63% (7/11) of tinnitus subjects reported here. **Figure 4B** further shows that the group difference was affected by an increasing delay between the response and stimulus waveforms (phase increases) that were seen in some participants with tinnitus. It may be noteworthy that the peak of the tinnitus spectrum in these participants (mean = 8.0 kHz) tended to be closer to the 5 kHz training stimulus than was the case for subjects showing phase decreases (mean = 8.71 kHz; $r = -0.59$, $p < 0.06$). Except for this tendency, no correlate was found (hearing THs, stimulus levels, other tinnitus attribute, or brain response) that might explain the performance of these individual tinnitus subjects. In a second analysis, we attempted to contrast within-session phase shifts between the first two and last two active blocks of each session, between our tinnitus and control groups. On average phase decreased −7.50° within sessions in the control group compared to a phase increase of 2.65° in tinnitus subjects, but this difference did not reach significance ($p = 0.34$). Thus, within the limits of this analysis (signal-to-noise ratio is greatly reduced in sub-block analyses) it did not appear that the tinnitus group displayed phase decreases within sessions that were reset by neural activity related to tinnitus between sessions.

ASSR AMPLITUDE

ASSR amplitude measured as total field power (128 electrodes) varied widely across subjects from 467 μV^2 to 22,132 μV^2, averaging 1871 μV^2 (SD = 1074) in the tinnitus group and 4192 μV^2 (SD = 6081) in controls on the passive blocks of the first session. Although mean field power was thus 2.2 times larger in the control group than in the tinnitus group on passive blocks, this difference did not reach significance [$t(20) = 1.25$, $p = 0.22$]. However, individual differences in ASSR amplitude were highly reliable giving test–re-test correlations between sessions 1 and 7 of $r = 0.99$ and 1.0 in the tinnitus and control groups, respectively, in agreement with unpublished observations by Gander et al. (2010b). These differences likely reflect individual variation in the anatomy of Heschl's gyrus, the orientation of ASSR generators in this region, and the summed neural activity of ASSR sources across reversing tonotopic maps sharing a low frequency border situated laterally in A1 (Kaas and Hackett, 2000; Formisano et al., 2003).

Changes in ASSR amplitude across sessions are depicted separately for the tinnitus and control groups in **Figure 5A**. Following Gander et al. (2010b) ASSR amplitude was normalized by dividing the data of each subject by their respective group mean for the passive blocks of day 1. In agreement with previous findings (Gander et al., 2010b) ASSR amplitude was larger on active blocks where subjects performed the task than on passive blocks where they did not, in the control group [$F_{(1, 10)} = 4.85$, $p = 0.05$] as well as in the tinnitus condition [$F_{(1, 10)} = 5.09$, $p = 0.03$]. In controls no further effects were found, which is consistent with Gander et al. (2010b) where ASSR amplitude did not increase over four sessions of training with EEG measurement although an increase was detected in a concluding tenth session where EEG was again measured. The picture in the tinnitus group was different. Here ASSR amplitude increased over sessions, first on

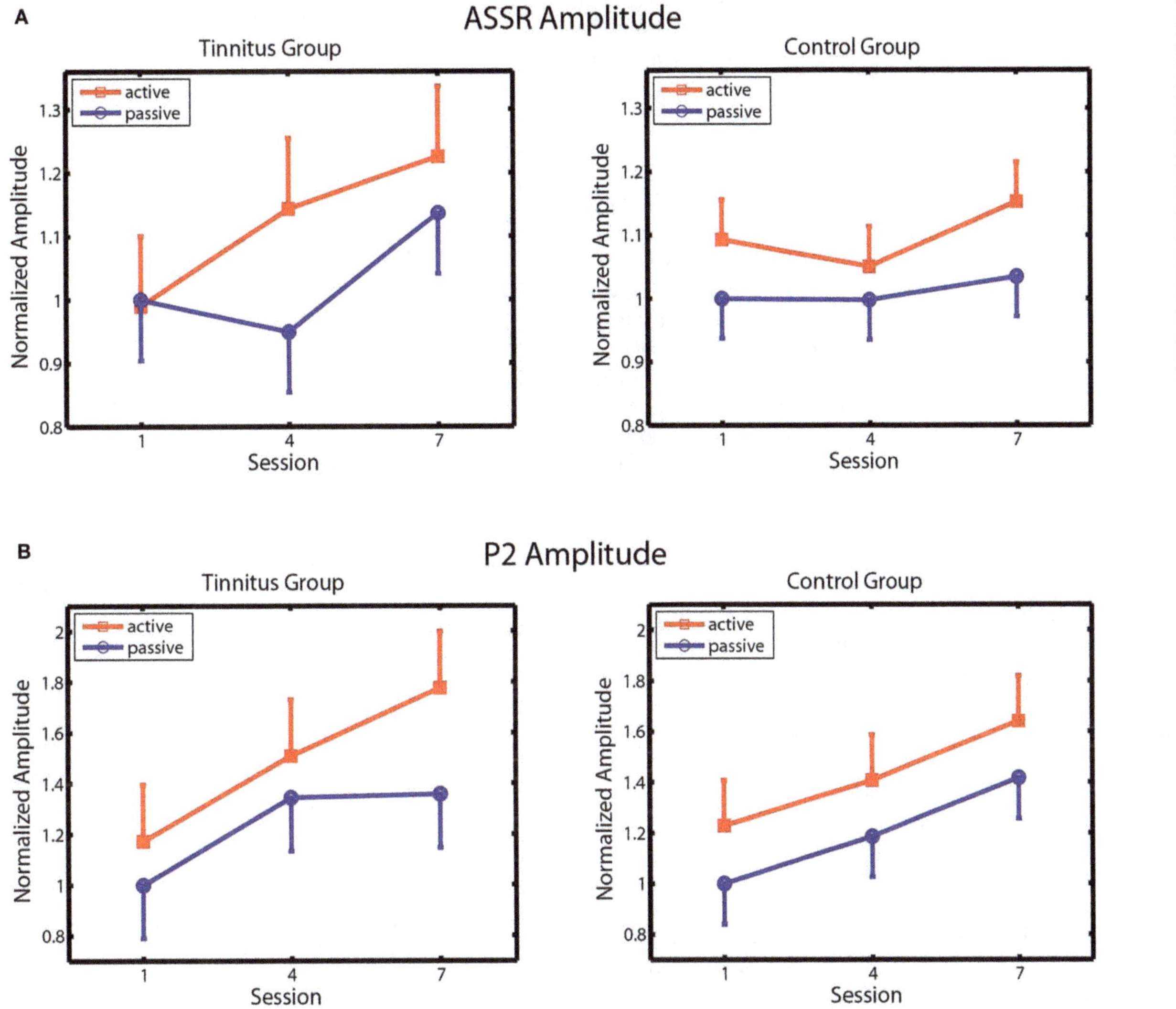

FIGURE 5 | ASSR amplitude and P2 amplitude. (A) Changes in ASSR amplitude over training in the Tinnitus (left panel) and Control (right panel) groups, on active and passive blocks. **(B)** Changes in P2 amplitude are similarly depicted. Response amplitude is normalized within each group to amplitude on passive blocks of the first session. Bars denote 1 within-subject standard error.

active and then on active and passive blocks, giving an interaction of sessions with block [$F_{(2, 20)} = 4.68$, $p = 0.022$] as well as the main effect of block mentioned above. *Post-hoc* contrasts found that ASSR amplitude was larger on the active and passive blocks of session 3 compared to the corresponding blocks of session 1, and on the active blocks of session 2 compared to the active and passive blocks of session 1 (all p's < 0.006, LSD tests). When the tinnitus and control groups were entered in the same analysis a main effect of block was found [$F_{(1, 20)} = 10.84$, $p = 0.003$] as well as a three-way interaction of session, block, and group [$F_{(2, 40)} = 4.56$, $p = 0.016$] which reflected the growth of ASSR amplitude preferentially on active trials in the tinnitus group. Thus, ASSR amplitude was larger on active than passive blocks in both groups but increased over seven sessions of auditory training only in the tinnitus condition.

P2 AMPLITUDE

P2 amplitude ranged from $-1.87\,\mu V$ to 2.57 across all participants, averaging $0.48\,\mu V$ (SD $= 0.89$) in the tinnitus group and $0.57\,\mu V$ (SD $= 1.17$) in controls (group difference not significant). Individual differences were reliable across active blocks on days 1 and 7 within the control group ($r = 0.84$, $p < 0.05$) but less so in the tinnitus group ($r = 0.31$, not significant) although the preceding N1 response was reliable in both groups ($r = 0.65$ and 0.70 in controls and tinnitus, respectively, both r's $p < 0.05$).

Changes in P2 amplitude across sessions are depicted separately for the tinnitus and control groups in **Figure 5B**. Again, amplitude was normalized by dividing the data of each subject by their respective group mean for the passive blocks of Day 1. P2 amplitude increased progressively over training sessions in both groups on active and passive blocks, with larger P2 amplitude seen on active trials in each group. Main effects of session were found in both the control [$F_{(2, 20)} = 7.61$, $p = 0.003$] and tinnitus [$F_{(2, 20)} = 7.67$, $p = 0.003$] groups, confirming a training effect on P2 amplitude. The main effect of block was also significant in the control group [$F_{(2, 20)} = 5.35$, $p = 0.04$] and nearly so in the tinnitus group [$F_{(1, 20)} = 3.23$, $p = 0.10$]. Analysis of the combined groups revealed a main effect of sessions [$F_{(2, 40)} = 14.8$, $p = 0.00001$] and of block [$F_{(1, 20)} = 7.80$, $p = 0.011$] and no other effects. Thus, P2 amplitude remodeled normally in tinnitus subjects, equaling the performance of their age and hearing matched controls. The changes observed in these groups are comparable to those reported in studies by Gander et al. (2010b) and others (Tremblay et al., 2001; Reinke et al., 2003; Bosnyak et al., 2004; Sheehan et al., 2005; Alain et al., 2007; Ross and Tremblay, 2009) showing increased P2 amplitude after auditory training in normal hearing individuals. No main effects or interactions involving group, sessions, or block were found for P2 latency, which averaged 203.9 ms overall (SD = 15.2 ms) on active blocks of the first session.

OTHER TRANSIENT RESPONSES

The transient responses P1 (mean latency 47.4 ms), N1 (mean latency 109.8 ms), N2 (mean latency 326.0 ms), and the auditory sustained response (SR) (350–900 ms) were also analyzed for each subject and group. No effects involving sessions, block or group were found on the latency of P1, N1, and P2 transient responses. Neither did the amplitude of P1, N1, and N2 responses or the SR change significantly over sessions in either group. On the other hand, P1 amplitude and N2 amplitude were significantly larger on active compared to passive blocks in both groups, as was the SR in the tinnitus group; main effects of block were found for each response when the groups were combined ($p < 0.004$, 0.008, and 0.001, respectively, for P1, N2, the SR). N1 amplitude was also larger on active than passive blocks, but only in the control group (block by group interaction $p = 0.041$). When passive blocks alone were considered where participants performed no task, N1 tended to be larger in tinnitus subjects ($-3.02\,\mu V$) than in controls ($-2.26\,\mu V$; $p = 0.077$, LSD test).

EFFECTS OF TRAINING ON TINNITUS

Four measurements of tinnitus were taken from tinnitus participants in the present study, namely; (i) ratings of tinnitus awareness and loudness recorded three times within each training session; (ii) psychoacoustic measurements of tinnitus loudness (by sound level matching) and the tinnitus spectrum taken by the Tinnitus Tester of Roberts et al. (2008) before and after training; (iii) ratings of tinnitus loudness on a Borg CR100 scale by the Tinnitus Tester; and (iv) measurement of the participant's reaction to tinnitus by the THQ before and after training.

The first of these measures is reported in **Figure 6**. Tinnitus awareness (panel A) diminished across the three measurements taken within each session (main effect of measurement [$F_{(2, 20)} = 5.45$, $p < 0.037$]. The interaction of measurement with sessions was also significant [$F_{(12, 120)} = 4.28$, $p < 0.00001$], reflecting the larger within-session change seen on the first day of training.

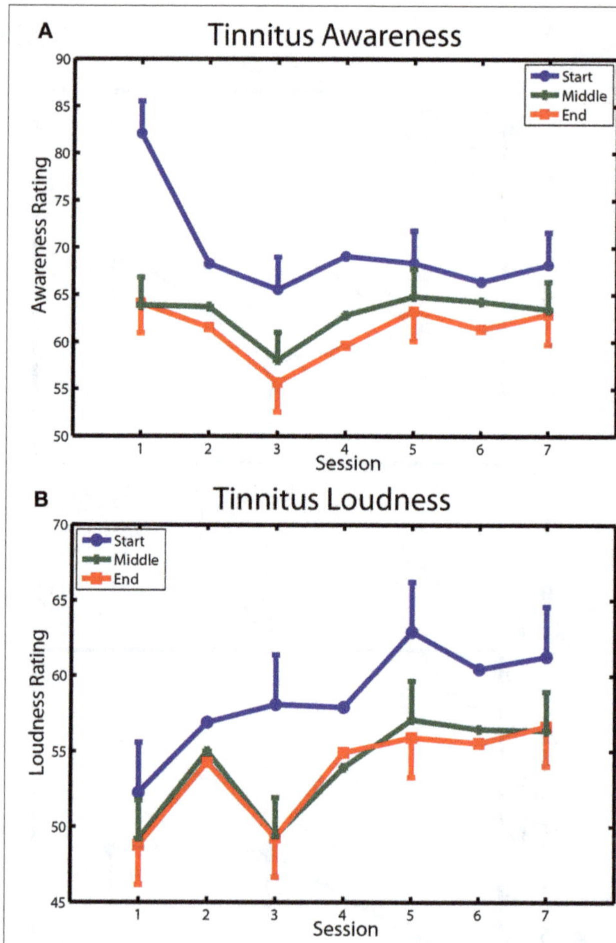

FIGURE 6 | Changes in tinnitus awareness and loudness over training. **(A)** Ratings of tinnitus awareness are shown for each within-session measurement over the seven sessions of training. **(B)** Ratings of tinnitus loudness are similarly depicted. Bars denote 1 within-subject standard error.

Tinnitus awareness averaged over measurements of the last session was 64.8 (SD = 19.4), which was above the midpoint between "Aware" and "Very Aware" on the rating scale used for these measurements. Tinnitus loudness (bottom panel) decreased non-significantly within sessions ($p = 0.17$) but over days showed an upward trend that approached significance (main effect of sessions $p = 0.09$). The overall mean loudness rating of 58.1 (SD = 20.4) on the last day of training corresponded to a rating between "Loud" and "Very Loud" on the Borg CR 100 scale used for these ratings.

Figure 2B shows the tinnitus spectrum (likeness ratings) and **Figure 2C** tinnitus loudness matches taken before and after training by the Tinnitus Tester. For the likeness ratings a significant a main effect was found for frequency [$F_{(10, 100)} = 14.7, p = 0.000$] confirming earlier results that sound frequencies in the region of hearing loss are typically judged to resemble tinnitus percepts (Noreña et al., 2002; Roberts et al., 2008; Sereda et al., 2011; Zhou et al., 2011). The main effect of before/after was not significant, but the interaction of frequency with before/after came close [$F_{(10, 100)} = 1.77$, $p = 0.074$] and was significant when the frequencies of 5 kHz (the training frequency) and 8 kHz were used for the analysis [$F_{(1, 10)} = 10.7$, $p = 0.008$]. The same analyses applied to the loudness matches revealed no significant effects. Thus, while auditory training had no effect on loudness matches, the tinnitus spectrum was affected, with 5 kHz rated more highly and 8 kHz less highly as a component of tinnitus after training than before training. **Figure 2C** also includes the mean audiogram of the tinnitus participants converted from dB HL to dB SPL. Tinnitus loudness matches referenced to the audiogram before training (which gives an approximation of initial tinnitus loudness in dB SL) revealed a significant effect of frequency [$F_{(10, 100)} = 21.3$, $p = 0.000$], confirming previous reports (Henry and Meikle, 2000; Roberts et al., 2008) that tinnitus loudness matches are greater when the sound frequencies used for matching are below rather than in the spectrum of the tinnitus (in the present data, 40.8 dB SL at 1 kHz compared to 3.9 dB SL at 7 kHz).

The effect of auditory training on the THQ, and on loudness ratings on the Borg CR100 scale included in the Tinnitus Tester, are summarized in **Table 2**, where measurements taken before and after auditory training are contrasted. For completeness, this table also reports before/after loudness matches to the 1 kHz sound taken from the Tinnitus Tester (in dB SPL, these data from **Figure 2C**) and ratings of tinnitus loudness and awareness taken within sessions 1 and 7 of auditory training (these data from **Figures 6B** and **6A**, respectively). Correlations between the first (Before) and second (After) measurements for each variable are reported in the last column of **Table 2** and give a conservative estimate of test–re-test reliability for each measure, keeping in mind that effects of auditory training (if present) could attenuate them. The correlations ranged from 0.49 to 0.98 and in most instances were statistically significant indicating the presence of reliable individual variability. Nonetheless only Factor 2 of the THQ showed a significant change, in this case indicating that difficulties of hearing in noise were reported to be slightly worse after auditory training than before. Other measures (total score on the THQ, Factors 1 and 3 of the THQ, the tinnitus rating and loudness match from the Tinnitus Tester, and tinnitus awareness assessed by the Borg CR100 scale within sessions) were in the direction of a beneficial effect of auditory training on tinnitus, but none of these differences reached significance.

CORRELATIONS AMONG EEG RESPONSES AND THEIR RELATION TO HEARING FUNCTION AND TINNITUS

Two between-subject correlational analyses were conducted. The first analysis examined relationships among training-induced changes in ASSR amplitude, ASSR phase, and P2 amplitude, and the relationship of these changes to the effects of active and passive blocks on the responses. When the tinnitus and control groups were combined, changes in ASSR amplitude produced by training and by active versus passive blocks were correlated with baseline ASSR amplitude on the passive blocks ($r = 0.65$ and 0.79, respectively, $p < 0.05$), reflecting larger contributions to these effects by participants with larger ASSR baseline amplitudes. This pattern was evident within each group separately. In the tinnitus group changes in P2 amplitude with training correlated with changes in ASSR amplitude ($r = 0.781$, $p < 0.05$), but changes in P2 amplitude with training did not correlate with ASSR amplitude changes in the control group or with any other brain measure in either group.

The second analysis examined the relationship of changes in EEG responses to (1) the loudness of the training stimuli and to hearing THs at 5 kHz in the tinnitus and control groups separately and in the combined sample, and (2) to the tinnitus measures of **Table 2** in the tinnitus group. **Table 1** shows that the tinnitus and control groups were well matched for hearing THs at 2 kHz and 5 kHz and for stimulus level (no group differences were found on these measures). ASSR amplitude, ASSR phase, and P2 amplitude measured during the passive baseline did not correlate with sound THs at 2 kHz or 5 kHz or with stimulus level, nor did changes in these brain responses over training correlate significantly with sound THs or stimulus level within each group separately or in the combined sample. Sound THs at 2 kHz and 5 kHz increased with age ($r = 0.83$ and 0.92, respectively, both $p < 0.05$), but age did not correlate with effects of training or of active/passive blocks on any brain response and did not differ significantly between the tinnitus and control groups (see **Table 1**). Correlations between changes in ASSR amplitude, ASSR phase, and P2 amplitude over training and changes in the tinnitus measurements of **Table 2** were not significant.

Table 2 | Tinnitus Handicap Questionnaire and Tinnitus Loudness.

	Before	After	Difference	Correlation
THQ SCORES				
THQ Total score	48.9 (6.66)	46.4 (7.48)	−2.4 (3.12)	0.90*
Factor 1 (Physical, emotional, social consequences of tinnitus)	51.1 (7.63)	46.1 (8.84)	−4.9 (4.26)	0.89*
Factor 2 (Tinnitus effects on hearing abilities)	40.8 (8.71)	45.8 (8.52)	5.1 (2.06)**	0.98*
Factor 3 (Patient's views on tinnitus)	56.8 (5.00)	48.7 (4.38)	−8.1 (4.57)	0.59†
TINNITUS LOUDNESS AND AWARENESS				
Loudness rating from Tinnitus Tester (Borg CR100 scale)	57.1 (6.21)	52.6 (7.13)	−4.6 (3.09)	0.91*
Loudness match to 1 kHz sound from Tinnitus Tester (dB SPL)	53.9 (6.32)	51.8 (4.51)	−2.1 (3.46)	0.85*
Loudness rating Session 1 and Session 7 (Borg CR100 scale)	50.1 (6.10)	58.1 (6.28)	8.0 (4.36)	0.75*
Awareness rating Session 1 and Session 7 (Borg CR100 scale)	70.0 (5.18)	64.9 (5.86)	−5.2 (5.60)	0.49

*$p < 0.01$; **$p < 0.05$; †$p < 0.10$.

DISCUSSION

Sensory training therapies for tinnitus are based on the assumption that, notwithstanding neural changes related to tinnitus, auditory training can alter the response properties of neurons in auditory pathways, as has been demonstrated in normal hearing individuals (Gander et al., 2010b). To address this question, we investigated whether brain changes induced by sensory training in tinnitus sufferers and measured by EEG are similar to those induced in age and hearing level matched individuals without tinnitus trained on the same auditory task. Auditory training was given using a sound that was in the tinnitus frequency region of the tinnitus subjects. We found that P2 amplitude increased with training equally in participants with tinnitus and in control subjects, suggesting normal remodeling non-primary (A2) auditory regions in tinnitus. However, training-induced changes in the 40 Hz ASSR, which localizes to sources in posterior-medial Heschl's gyrus (A1), differed between the tinnitus and control groups. Training-induced changes ASSR phase which reflect changes in temporal population activity expressed in A1 were normal in control participants; the time delay between the response and stimulus waveforms decreased by about $-10°$ in this group. However, ASSR phase did not change significantly with training in the tinnitus group. On the other hand, ASSR amplitude increased with training in the tinnitus group, whereas in controls no changes were seen in this response attribute over training. Effects of auditory training on tinnitus loudness were not significant, although an effect on the tinnitus spectrum was detected.

These results suggest that neural changes related to tinnitus altered how neural plasticity was expressed in A1 but not A2 auditory cortex. We discuss auditory plasticity in normal hearing individuals and then consider how the presence of tinnitus may have affected the expression of neural plasticity in auditory pathways. In a concluding section limitations on our findings are discussed.

AUDITORY REMODELING IN NORMAL HEARING

The first reported study of auditory training using the 40 Hz ASSR (Bosnyak et al., 2004) required that normal hearing subjects discriminate between a standard stimulus consisting of a 40 Hz AM 2 kHz carrier frequency and comparison stimuli using carriers that were either 200 Hz higher or lower than the standard. The phase delay between the ASSR response and stimulus waveforms shortened in a brief interval (150–400 ms) following stimulus onset over 15 sessions of training, and was greater for the trained standard stimulus (2 kHz) than for untrained comparison stimuli. However, no change was detected in ASSR amplitude even though behavioral performance improved over the lengthy training experience. Because competitive interactions among the different carrier frequencies during frequency discrimination may have prevented expansion of the tonotopic representation for the standard sound (Kilgard et al., 2001), the stimulus procedure of the current study was designed to deliver extensive experience of only a single carrier frequency over training, and to deliver target events randomly in the second half of the stimulus so that sustained attention was required. Using this procedure Gander et al. (2010b) found that the magnitude of the phase change increased over ten sessions of training, expressed throughout the duration of the training stimulus, and correlated with behavioral performance over the training sessions. Effects on ASSR amplitude were, however, more variable. An increase in this response was not observed until the tenth session of training, and the change in ASSR amplitude over sessions did not correlate with behavioral performance while the phase shift did. No increase in ASSR amplitude was seen in a control group that received two sessions of training separated by six weeks, although the ASSR phase shift occurred in this group dissociating the two measures in agreement with previous findings.

A further difference between ASSR phase and ASSR amplitude in the research of Gander et al. (2010a,b) concerned the effects of task attention (active and passive sound exposure) on the two response attributes. ASSR amplitude was larger on active blocks than on passive blocks in the Gander et al. (2010b) studies, as was true in the tinnitus and control groups of the present study. Parallel research disambiguating the effects of auditory attention from button pressing and correctness feedback on active blocks showed that attention to the trained sounds was the source of the ASSR amplitude increase (Gander et al., 2010a). However, attention was found to have no effect on ASSR phase in these studies. Gander et al. (2010b, Experiment 1) also found that changes in phase with auditory training appeared in equal magnitude in a group that performed the task for two sessions under conditions of attention as in a group that heard the same 40-Hz AM sounds presented passively while they watched a silent video with no knowledge of the auditory task. Thus, while attention increases ASSR amplitude (Ross et al., 2004; Gander et al., 2010a), it has no effect on ASSR phase and does not appear to be required for changes in this response attribute with auditory experience.

In order to explain these findings, Gander et al. (2010b) suggested that the ASSR phase shift may reflect stimulus-driven changes in temporal activity that occur in subcortical auditory structures during auditory experience and are inherited by the cortical sources of the ASSR in A1 with little involvement of attention. The temporal response properties of subcortical auditory neurons are known to be modified by experience with complex speech and musical sounds (Song et al., 2008; Tzounopoulos and Kraus, 2009) indicating that neural plasticity is expressed in these structures. In subsequent research with the same stimulus procedure, Baynton (2010, unpublished results) obtained phase shifts that were as evident in children aged 5–8 years as in older age cohorts aged 18–25 years, consistent with an early form of stimulus-driven plasticity operating in auditory pathways. ASSR amplitude did not increase with training in any age group in this study, but this variable increased during auditory attention (active compared to passive blocks) in cohorts aged 13–15 years and older although not at younger ages. It has been suggested (Gander et al., 2010b) that increases in ASSR amplitude on active blocks may reflect activation of the basal forebrain cholinergic system that performs some of the functions of attention (Sarter et al., 2005) by distributing acetylcholine to the neocortical mantle thus making cortical neurons more sensitive to their afferent inputs (Metherate and Ashe, 1993). Animal data indicate that this system does not mature until puberty (Kiss and Patel, 1992), which aligns with Baynton's results where modulation of ASSR amplitude by active and passive blocks did not reach significance until age 13–15 years.

AUDITORY REMODELING IN TINNITUS

To allow comparison with earlier results obtained from normal hearing subjects trained with a 2 kHz 40-Hz AM sound, the current study used the training method of Gander et al. (2010b) substituting a 5 kHz 40-Hz AM sound which was in the tinnitus frequency region of the tinnitus subjects. Individuals with tinnitus and control subjects of comparable age and TH hearing function were studied. The results from the control group with regard to ASSR phase and amplitude were in agreement with earlier findings (Gander et al., 2010b) and are consistent with the interpretation suggested for those findings. However, the results from participants with tinnitus were different, and invite interpretation from current knowledge regarding neural changes associated with hearing loss and tinnitus.

One interpretation of impaired phase plasticity in the tinnitus group is that remodeling of phase occurred normally within sessions, but that persisting neural changes associated with tinnitus (these not present in controls) reset the phase changes between sessions in the tinnitus group. However, within the limits of our data, analyses of within-session phase shifts in the tinnitus and control groups did not support this interpretation. Alternatively, neural population activity associated with tinnitus may have interfered with the processing that occurs in A1 or in subcortical structures projecting to this region, in the tinnitus group. This possibility received limited but provocative support from the observation that phase shifts opposite to the normal phase change occurred in participants whose dominant tinnitus frequency was comparatively closer to the trained 5 kHz sound ($r = -0.59$, $p < 0.06$). This relationship could reflect an interaction between tinnitus-related synchronous neural activity occurring in the dominant tinnitus frequency region (Weisz et al., 2007) and synchronous neural activity driven by the 5 kHz 40-Hz AM training stimulus. A third possibility is that because ASSR amplitude increased over training in the tinnitus subjects suggesting an increased cortical representation in A1 for the trained sound, it may be considered that this effect obstructed changes in ASSR phase in this group. The relationship of changes in ASSR amplitude to changes in ASSR phase between tinnitus subjects was in the direction of such an effect ($r = -0.328$) but did not reach significance. It is of interest that ASSR amplitude increased significantly with training in the tinnitus group, but not in the control group of this study. Enhanced remodeling of ASSR amplitude could be consequent on inhibitory deficits that occur in central auditory structures with hearing loss (Scholl and Wehr, 2008) and tinnitus (Wang et al., 2009), which could permit additional neurons to be recruited into a representation for the trained sound. If this hypothesis is provisionally accepted, it implies that similar inhibitory changes were absent in controls who did not have tinnitus although they had a similar level of hearing loss. The absence of tinnitus in controls could signal comparatively better preserved inner hair cell function in these individuals despite outer hair cell damage contributing to their TH shifts (Kujawa and Liberman, 2009).

In contrast to group differences in remodeling of ASSR phase and amplitude, which reflect group differences in neural processing expressed in the region of A1, P2 amplitude (reflecting neural activity in non-primary regions) increased normally over training in both groups. The amplitude of the preceding N1 response did not change with training, indicating an effect specific to the P2 component of the N1/P2 waveform in agreement with earlier findings (e.g., Bosnyak et al., 2004; Ross and Tremblay, 2009). P2 amplitude was also larger on active compared to passive blocks pointing to its modulation by attention, but this effect did not interact with groups or with the effect of training on P2. The effect of attentional performance on P2 amplitude seen here agrees with observations by Gander et al. (2010b), although modulation of P2 amplitude by attention on other types of task is not always seen (cf. Hillyard et al., 1973; Carpenter et al., 2002) possibly relating to procedural variables and their effect on the preceding polarity-opposite N1. In contrast, enhancement of P2 amplitude by auditory training is a robust finding reported by many studies cited above. Changes in P2 amplitude induced by training in the control group of the present study and in earlier research by Gander et al. (2010b) were uncorrelated between-subjects with changes in ASSR amplitude, suggesting that these two responses reflect independent events occurring in auditory pathways. In contrast, in the tinnitus group of the present experiment these effects were correlated between-subjects ($r = 0.78$, $p < 0.05$). These findings suggest that neural activity in A1 (reflected by increased ASSR amplitude in the tinnitus group) may modulate P2 cortical sources in A2, but P2 sources can change independently of events occurring in the auditory core region via parallel thalamocortical projections or top-down pathways.

EFFECTS OF AUDITORY REMODELING ON TINNITUS

The stimulus procedure of this study was adopted from previous research so that we could compare neural plasticity in individuals with tinnitus and their aged-matched controls with results obtained from normal hearing subjects trained with the same method. There were, however, reasons to suggest that training with sounds in the tinnitus frequency region might also alter tinnitus. In earlier research (Roberts and Bosnyak, 2010a) we found that ASSR amplitude evoked by a 5 kHz 40-Hz AM sound in the tinnitus frequency region was reduced in individuals with tinnitus compared to hearing level matched controls, while masking in this region (which yielded residual inhibition) restored ASSR amplitude to control levels suggesting modified neural activity in or projecting to A1. Because ASSR amplitude increased during residual inhibition, we were interested to learn whether auditory training with a 5 kHz 40-Hz AM sound could increase ASSR amplitude in our tinnitus subjects, and if so, diminish their tinnitus percept in the 5 kHz region. For this reason we conducted a thorough assessment of tinnitus before, during, and after training. Consistent with results reported by Roberts and Bosnyak (2010b), non-normalized ASSR amplitude evoked by the 5 kHz 40-Hz AM sound tended to be lower in the tinnitus group compared to controls under passive conditions. However, even though training increased ASSR amplitude in the tinnitus group, the tinnitus percept (likeness rating) did not decrease at 5 kHz but showed an increase relative to 8 kHz instead (**Figure 2B**). On-line ratings of tinnitus loudness also tended to increase over sessions (**Figure 6B**). However, changes in ASSR amplitude with training did not correlate between-subjects with changes in either of these attributes of tinnitus. Alternatively, changes in the tinnitus spectrum after auditory training could reflect greater familiarity with the dimension of pitch after training. Noreña et al. (2002) observed changes in the shape of the spectrum in a single participant who was trained to discriminate among frequencies around four standard stimuli between 3279 and 6500 Hz. After training the contribution of frequencies above 8 kHz to the tinnitus percept was significantly reduced. Whether this effect reflected a reduction in cortical representation for the untrained sounds or greater familiarity with the trained stimuli could not be decided.

Sound therapies are based on the premise that neural plasticity can be harnessed to ameliorate phantom sound. Our results suggest that the presence of tinnitus may itself affect how neural activity is modified by auditory training in the tinnitus frequency region. Although we did not observe meaningful improvements in tinnitus, it remains possible that sounds with wider bandwidth trained for longer periods could be beneficial. In support of this possibility, treatment studies using the Neuromonics procedure (Davis et al., 2008), which delivers complex low-level sounds covering the tinnitus frequency (hearing loss) region, have reported reductions in tinnitus as well as improved minimum masking and loudness tolerance levels for a subset of tinnitus patients. Long-term exposure to low-level background sound also rescales loudness growth functions in normal hearing individuals (Formby et al., 2003) and, when engineered to cover the hearing loss region, improves loudness tolerance in hyperacusis patients (Noreña and Chery-Croze, 2007). These findings for tinnitus and hyperacusis are congruent with animal research showing that passive exposure to band-pass filtered low-level sound for weeks or longer suppresses neural activity and cortical representations in the exposure frequency band (Pienkowski and Eggermont, 2010).

LIMITATIONS AND QUESTIONS FOR FURTHER STUDY

Several limitations of the present results for understanding auditory plasticity in normal hearing and in tinnitus remodeling should be noted. One limitation that is the mechanism (or mechanisms) underlying the ASSR phase shift in normal hearing and in tinnitus are not presently known. In a further analysis of results from normal hearing participants, Gander et al. (2010b, Experiment 1) applied inverse modeling to the data of each subject in order to evaluate effects of attention and training on ASSR phase and amplitude in each hemisphere separately. ASSR amplitude was larger in the right than the left hemisphere in agreement with earlier reports (Ross, 2008), and increased with attention in both hemispheres but more so in the right hemisphere. In contrast, ASSR phase changed in unison in both hemispheres and did not differ between the hemispheres. ASSR phase was not affected by attention, but shifted toward the stimulus waveform with training while ASSR amplitude remained unchanged, underscoring the independence of the response attributes. These findings suggest that interhemispheric interactions between amplitude and phase are not likely to have contributed to changes in the responses with attention or auditory experience, although such analyses have yet to be carried out on the present data.

Changes in ASSR phase and amplitude within trials are also relevant to understanding experience-induced effects. ASSR phase is a circular variable, but the nature of the phase changes (whether large or small delays or advances) can be disambiguated by referencing the ASSR response in the time domain to the onset of sound. Within trial analyses by Gander et al. (2010b) showed that during the 976 ms of sound stimulation the ASSR waveform shifted gradually away from the time of stimulus onset toward the zero-crossing in the stimulus waveform, stabilizing with respect to the zero-crossing after about 300 ms in broad agreement with fine grained analyses reported by Ross et al. (2002). Auditory training added a further shift toward the zero-crossing as the response waveform moved closer to the stimulus waveform over sessions. The training effect on ASSR phase (a latency increase with respect to sound onset) was fully expressed over the initial 488 ms of the stimulus which was free of target events and persisted without diminution until stimulus offset. The latter result suggests that changes in ASSR phase resulting from auditory experience were not affected by resets of the ASSR that can be evoked when salient stimuli (for example, an unexpected change in carrier frequency or a noise burst) are delivered during auditory tasks (Rohrbaugh et al., 1990a; Ross et al., 2005; Bosnyak et al., 2007). We have not observed reset responses to target stimuli in our studies, likely because the target stimuli were close to the TH of detection and did not alter the AM rhythm or its carrier frequency. It should be noted that reset responses shift the ASSR waveform back toward stimulus onset (a latency decrease; Ross et al., 2005) which is opposite the phase change observed during auditory training. Reset responses are also larger when behavioral responding is required (Rohrbaugh et al., 1989), vanish as the TH of detection is approached (Ross, 2008), and have been associated with behavioral orienting or similar change detection processes (Rohrbaugh et al., 1990b; Ross et al., 2005). These findings suggest that experience-induced phase shifts and reset responses may reflect different underlying mechanisms. However, Rohrbaugh et al. (1990b) found that reset responses showed adaptation when measured in a second session. If the processes that underlie development of the ASSR after reset are the same as those responsible for its development with sound onset (Ross et al., 2005), reset responses and phase shifts with auditory training could reflect one and the same mechanism. Additional experiments will be required to uncover the mechanisms responsible for changes in ASSR phase induced by auditory experience and to explore the neural basis of such effects.

A further gap in our knowledge concerns the role of attention in modulating auditory plasticity in humans. Because our procedures involved active performance, we have for convenience described them as training procedures. However, it has shown that passive exposure to the 40-Hz AM training sound without task knowledge is by itself sufficient to change ASSR phase (Gander et al., 2010b, Experiment 1). Remodeling by passive exposure has also been reported for P2 amplitude by Sheehan et al. (2005), Ross and Tremblay (2009), and Gander et al. (2010b), while Tremblay et al. (2010) observed differential effects of attended performance on P2 amplitude recorded over the vertex compared to temporal-parietal regions. In our studies ASSR phase changes over sessions have tended to be greater on active blocks than on passive blocks, although interactions with block have not reached significance (Gander et al., 2010b). When collapsed over experiments (Bosnyak et al., 2004; Gander et al., 2010a,b, and the present findings) our results suggest that a stimulus exposure totaling 40 min (however, distributed in time) may be sufficient to yield a phase shift of up to 18° (depending on carrier frequency) in individuals without tinnitus, that persists up to six weeks without intervening experience. This raises the possibility that procedures more efficient than the current ones (which descended from animal studies of auditory neural plasticity) could be devised to investigate effects of attention, mechanisms of ASSR phase shifts, and how experience-induced changes in ASSR phase are modified by neural changes related to tinnitus.

Looking ahead, the present findings offer only a first glimpse into how neural changes in tinnitus alter the expression of neural plasticity in auditory pathways. It is well established that tinnitus spectra (Noreña et al., 2002; Roberts et al., 2008) and residual inhibition functions (Roberts et al., 2008) overlap the region of auditory TH shift. These results have been interpreted to suggest that what neurons in the tinnitus frequency region do generates tinnitus, and stopping what they do suppresses it (Roberts et al., 2010). This line of reasoning suggests that shifts in ASSR phase may remodel normally in individuals with tinnitus, if training is given for sounds below the tinnitus frequency region. Were this result to be obtained, additional evidence of an interaction of auditory training with frequency-specific activity in tinnitus expressed in A1 would be revealed. It is also of interest to determine how ASSR amplitude evoked by probes presented to the tinnitus frequency region is affected by training below the tinnitus spectrum, and how tinnitus percepts are modulated by such training. Training with multiple frequencies outside of the tinnitus frequency region has been reported to reverse tonotopic map distortion and reduce behavioral evidence of tinnitus in rats subjected to noise trauma (Engineer et al., 2011). Similarly, passive exposure to background sound sparing the tinnitus frequency region has been reported to reduce tinnitus in humans (Okamoto et al., 2010; Teismann et al., 2011), putatively by distributing lateral inhibition to the tinnitus generating neurons. However, as noted above, passive exposure to background sound covering the tinnitus frequency/hearing loss region for weeks to months has been also reported to reduce tinnitus in humans (Davis et al., 2008) and to rescale loudness growth in individuals experiencing hyperacusis (Noreña and Chery-Croze, 2007).

MATERIALS AND METHODS

PARTICIPANTS

Subjects with tinnitus ($n = 12$) were recruited by advertisements in the local newspaper, from the university ENT clinic, and our laboratory archive. Control participants ($n = 12$) were recruited from family and friends of the tinnitus subjects or from the local community. Controls reported no history of tinnitus or ear diseases. No subjects were receiving medication at the time of the study. Informed consent was obtained by procedures consistent with the Declaration of Helsinki and approved by the Research Ethics Board of McMaster University. One control participant withdrew after two sessions of auditory training owing to the occurrence of an unrelated medical illness. One tinnitus participant withdrew after the first auditory training session expressing concern that training might worsen his tinnitus. The remaining 22 participants completed training without incident. Participants were reimbursed for their parking fees and received an honorarium of $160 for completing the study.

DESIGN AND PROCEDURE

Intake session

Participants in the tinnitus group completed a structured interview which collected detailed information on the nature and personal history of their tinnitus. The THQ was administered to assess with a standardized procedure the impact of tinnitus on quality of life (Kuk et al., 1990). Audiological measurements included an otoscopic examination, compliance testing, and measurement of THs to the limit of hearing using a GSI 61 audiometer with Telephonics 296D200 (0.125–8.0 kHz) and Sennheiser HDA 200 (8.0–16 kHz) headphones (pulsed-tone method). Psychoacoustic properties of tinnitus were assessed by self-directed, computer-based tools (Roberts et al., 2008) that reported the ear of the tinnitus, its bandwidth (tonal, ringing, or hissing), loudness match for 11 sounds between 0.5 and 12.0 kHz, tinnitus frequency spectrum (likeness rating) over this same range, and a brief test for residual inhibition. Control participants completed the same intake procedure given to tinnitus subjects except for the omission of items pertaining to tinnitus.

Follow-up session

Tinnitus subjects returned one week after their last auditory training session for follow-up tinnitus measurements. The procedure was identical to their intake session except the intake questionnaire and audiological tests (audiogram, compliance) were omitted. Five tinnitus subjects did not complete the THQ in the follow-up session (the other measurements were completed) but provided their scores by mail afterwards.

AUDITORY STIMULUS

The stimulus for auditory training was a 5 kHz pure tone AM with a 40.96 Hz sinusoid (called 40 Hz above, 100% modulation depth following the modulation wave). Stimulus duration was 976.56 ms, allowing 40 AM pulses per stimulus (each stimulus constituting a "trial"). To determine sound level, each subject matched the loudness of the 5 kHz training stimulus to that of a 2 kHz 40-Hz AM reference tone presented at 65 dB SPL. The reference tone was identical to the training stimulus used in earlier research on normal hearing subjects (Gander et al., 2010b) permitting comparison of results across studies with sound level controlled. Matching also controlled for the possibility of abnormal loudness growth (recruitment) above 2 kHz where for some subjects in the tinnitus and control groups a degree of TH shift was present (**Table 1** and **Figure 2A**). Stimuli were generated by a digital signal processor (Tucker–Davis RP2.1) and presented binaurally via ear inserts (Etymotic Research ER-2).

TRAINING PROCEDURE

During auditory training participants sat in a chair placed 1.4 m in front of a computer monitor in a sound attenuated (ambient noise level 16 dBA SPL), electrically shielded booth. Auditory stimuli were presented successively separated by an ITI in which behavioral responses were recorded (**Figure 1A**). Approximately 2/3 of the stimuli (determined randomly) contained a single amplitude-enhanced 40-Hz pulse occurring randomly at 415 ms, 610 ms, or 805 ms after stimulus onset (target). On active blocks (**Figure 1B**) the word "Listen" appeared in a text box on the computer screen, instructing the participant to listen for a target event. At stimulus offset the word "Listen" on the computer screen was replaced by text asking "Did you hear a target?" Instructions beneath this text instructed the participant to press a right mouse button if a target had occurred ("yes") and a left mouse button if one had not ("no"). If the response was correct (hit or correct rejection), the text box turned green for 400 ms (feedback cue); if the response was incorrect (miss or false alarm) the text box turned red for 400 ms. A variable ITI between 1400 and 1600 ms commenced with each behavioral response, giving an average ITI (including the feedback cue) of about 1900 ms depending on behavioral response latency. The computer screen remained blank after the feedback cue and changed to read "Listen" when the next trial commenced.

EEG was recorded on the first, fourth, and seventh session of auditory training, always on the same week day and time of day for each subject. In each of these sessions participants received 20 blocks of trials, each block about 2.5 min long and containing 54 stimuli (see **Figure 1B**). On alternate blocks participants performed the training task described above (active blocks) or were instructed by text on the computer screen ("Stop responding and ignore stimulus") to cease attending and wait until the next training block (passive blocks). Each session began with an active block. Sessions without EEG contained the same total number of trials as sessions with EEG except that all blocks were now active blocks.

Target events varied in the magnitude of their amplitude increase bracketing the TH of detection, so that a psychophysical function could be determined. Immediately prior to the first training session, a staircase procedure consisting of 80 successively presented stimuli (commencing with a 200% amplitude enhancement known to be detectable by inexperienced subjects) was used to measure the target detection TH for each participant. This TH was used to generate an individual stimulus set (TH, TH ±5%, TH ±10%, and TH + 20%) suitable for learning. During training an adaptive procedure was followed in which if two targets were detected more than 95% of the time, TH was reduced by 5% and the remaining targets adjusted accordingly. On the last day of training the target values bracketing the detection TH measured at their amplitude peak averaged 1.57, 1.90, 2.25, 2.58, 2.90, and 3.51 dB above the prevailing steady-state signal. The first two of these targets were below TH and usually not detectable.

In the tinnitus group, the participant's awareness of tinnitus and its perceived loudness were probed immediately before, at the midpoint, and immediately after each training session (see **Figure 1B**). For each measurement, two questions appeared successively on the computer screen, each positioned above a horizontally oriented slider. The first question asked "How aware are you of your tinnitus at this moment?", and the second "How loud is your tinnitus at this moment?" Using a Powermate Controller (Griffin Technologies), subjects moved the slider to give their rating on a Borg CR100 scale with values ranging from 0 to 100 (Borg and Borg, 2001). On this scale a rating of 5 corresponded to "Almost Unaware" or "Extremely Soft," 30 to "Moderately Unaware" or "Moderate" loudness, 50 to "Aware" or "Loud," 70 to Very Aware" or "Very Loud," and 95 to "Extremely Aware" or "Extremely Loud." Subjects practiced moving the slider without any reference to tinnitus before the training session commenced.

ELECTROPHYSIOLOGICAL RECORDING

The EEG was sampled at 2048 Hz (DC to 417 Hz) using a 128-channel Biosemi ActiveTwo amplifier (Cortech Solutions, Wilmington, NC). The electrode array was digitized for each participant (Polhemus Fastrak) prior to recording. EEG data were stored as continuous data files referenced to the vertex electrode.

SIGNAL PROCESSING OF EEG DATA

Eye blink artifacts were removed from the raw continuous data files by the spatial filtering option of BESA (version 5.1.8, MEGIS Software GmbH, Gräfelfing, Germany). EEG responses (128 channels) were then epoched including 200 ms pre- and post-stimulus baselines.

Transient responses

EEG responses for ~75% of trials (rejecting trials with surviving artifacts >150 μV) were used for analysis of transient responses. The data were averaged and interpolated to the 81-channel "reference free" average reference montage of BESA using each participant's digitized electrode array. Subsequent filtering (0.2–20 Hz, zero phase) extracted P1, N1, P2, and N2 transient responses and the auditory SR. Responses were measured at electrode Fz where they reached their amplitude maxima. Peak amplitude and the corresponding latency were recorded for the latency windows 30–85 ms (P1), 85–140 ms (N1), 140–230 ms (P2), and 250–350 ms (N2).

40-Hz steady-state response

EEG responses for ~90% of trials (rejecting trials with amplitude changes >100 μV) were averaged for analysis of the ASSR, and filtered 40–42 Hz (zero phase) after conversion to average reference. The scalp topography of the ASSR and a digitized 128 electrode array are shown in **Figure 1C** (left panel) for a representative participant. The 128-channel data for each participant for the interval 244–952 ms were collapsed into a two-pulse wide waveform (**Figure 1C**, middle panel) and ASSR amplitude and phase determined at 40 Hz for each electrode by FFT (**Figure 1C**, right panel). Collapsing enhanced the signal-to-noise ratio and was adopted here and in previous research because changes in ASSR changes attributable to training or attention were found to be expressed throughout the stimulus interval (Gander et al., 2010b). ASSR amplitude was calculated as the total field power at 40 Hz summed over 128 electrodes. For calculation of ASSR phase a search algorithm, moving in steps of 0.5°, found the minimum angle width, encompassing electrodes on both sides of the dipolar field pattern, comprising 50% of the total 40 Hz power across the array. The value (in degrees) in the middle of that width was taken as the phase of the ASSR (**Figure 1C**). In infrequent cases where the absolute phase change between conditions was greater than π, phase was unwrapped by adding or subtracting 2π to minimize the phase difference. Phase determined by this method was very close to lines determined by spatial principal component analysis but was not influenced by noisy electrodes and spurious data that do not represent the ASSR. These methods of analysis had the advantage of using all of the unmodeled data available from each participant. In previous research we found that results obtained with these methods concurred with those obtained when ASSR amplitude and phase were analyzed at electrode Fz where the ASSR typically reaches its amplitude maximum (Gander et al., 2010a,b). The results also concurred with those obtained by inverse modeling of the ASSR field patterns (Gander et al., 2010a,b).

Because P2 amplitude was negative for some subjects reflecting their preceding polarity-opposite N1 response, P2 data were linear transformed by adding 1.9 to each data point prior to normalization, to remove negative values and prevent division by zero (after Gander et al., 2010a).

STATISTICAL EVALUATION

Repeated measures ANOVAS were performed using the General Linear Model of Statistica (version 6.0). Repeated measures having more than two levels were Greenhouse–Geisser corrected. Unless stated otherwise, significance level was set at $\alpha = 0.05$ (two-tailed). Least significant difference (LSD) tests were used to describe significant main effects and interactions.

Behavioral data

Behavioral performance was evaluated for each participant by calculating the mean probability of a hit [*P*(Hit), a target reported when one was present] collapsed over target amplitudes and sessions, and the mean probability of a false alarm [*P*(FA), a target reported when target amplitude was zero] collapsed over sessions. The difference between these probabilities was used to assess group performance. A psychophysical function was also constructed for each participant and session by plotting *P*(Hit) as a function of target amplitude and fitting a logistic [$f_{(x)} = 0.5/\{1 + \exp[-\text{slope} \times (\text{amp increase} - \text{threshold})]\} + 0.5$] using a maximum likelihood method with the *Palamedes* psychophysics toolbox for Matlab (Prins and Kingdom, 2009). Changes in TH (the amplitude increase corresponding to 75% correct) over sessions were assessed for the tinnitus and control groups separately. These changes were modeled for each participant assuming that the slopes followed an exponential decay but allowing bidirectional changes such that the results were driven by the data (Prins and Kingdom, 2009).

It should be noted that the TH for target detection determined prior to training by the staircase procedure that was administered to each participant gave values (mean TH = 68% for tinnitus, 74% for controls, difference not significant) that were high compared to earlier experiments where young normal hearing subjects were trained with a 2 kHz 40-Hz AM sound (mean TH = 31%, Gander et al., 2010b). The reason for this difference may relate to the carrier frequency used in the present study and the presence of some degree of hearing loss at 5 kHz in tinnitus and control participants (**Table 1**). However, in the first training session most (but not all) of the targets calculated from each participant's TH quickly became detectable, giving THs determined from individual psychophysical functions (TH = 35.1% on day 1 of **Figure 3B**) that were closer to previous results for normal hearing subjects. Changes in THs over sessions gave a coherent picture of discrimination performance during training, but changes in slope did not, because for many subjects slopes were uncommonly steep in the initial training sessions. Therefore, we relied on TH changes to depict changes in performance over sessions (**Figure 3B**). It was also possible to construct a psychophysical function from the collapsed data of each group on sessions (**Figure 3A**).

EEG data

Because individual differences in ASSR amplitude are large, likely reflecting stable anatomical differences among subjects in the orientation and strength of ASSR generators and their summation across tonotopic maps in Heschl's gyrus, ASSR amplitude for each subject was normalized by dividing each participant's data by the mean of the passive block of their respective group on day 1 (after Gander et al., 2010b). This step referenced the effects of training and task to a common passive baseline within each group. For purposes of comparison ASSR phase and P2 amplitude were normalized by the same method, although these measures are typically less variable between-subjects than ASSR amplitude.

ACKNOWLEDGMENTS

Support from a grant by the Tinnitus Research Initiative is gratefully acknowledged. Additional funding was provided by the Natural Sciences and Engineering Research Council of Canada. We thank Victoria Mosher for assistance and our participants for undertaking the study.

REFERENCES

Alain, C., Snyder, J. S., He, Y., and Reinke, K. S. (2007). Changes in auditory cortex parallel rapid perceptual learning. *Cereb. Cortex* 17, 1074–1084.

Borg, G., and Borg, E. (2001). A new generation of scaling methods: level anchored ratio scaling. *Psychologica* 28, 15–45.

Baynton, S. (2010). *The Development of Neural Plasticity in the Human Auditory System*. Unpublished MSc thesis (preview available at www.hnplab.mcmaster.ca).

Bosnyak, D. J., Eaton, R. A., and Roberts, L. E. (2004). Distributed auditory cortical representations are modified when non-musicians are trained at pitch discrimination with 40 Hz amplitude modulated tones. *Cereb. Cortex* 14, 1088–1099.

Bosnyak, D. J., Stevens, S., Gander, P. E., and Roberts, L. E. (2007). "Phase dynamics in the 40hz auditory steady state response," in *New Frontiers in Biomagnetism*, eds D. Cheyne, B. Ross, G. Stroink, and H. Weinberg, International Congress Series (Amsterdam: Elsevier), 29–32.

Brugge, J. F., Nourski, K. V., Oya, H., Reale, R. A., Kawasaki, H., Steinschneider, M., and Howard, M. A. (2009). Coding of repetitive transients by auditory cortex on heschl's gyrus. *J. Neurophysiol.* 102, 2358–2374.

Carpenter, M., Cranford, J. L., Hymal, M. R., DeChicchis, A. R., and Holbert, D. (2002). Electrophysiologic signs of attention versus distraction in a binaural listening task. *J. Clin. Neurophysiol.* 19, 55–60.

Davis, P. B., Wilde, R. A., Steed, L. G., and Hanley, P. J. (2008). Treatment of tinnitus with a customized acoustic neural stimulus: a controlled clinical study. *Ear Nose Throat J.* 87, 330–339.

Eggermont, J. J., and Roberts, L. E. (2004). The neuroscience of tinnitus. *Trends Neurosci.* 27, 676–682.

Engineer, N. D., Riley, J. R., Seale, J. D., Vrana, W. A., Shetake, J. A., Sudanagunta, S. P., Borland, M. S., and Kilgard, M. P. (2011). Reversing pathological neural activity using targeted plasticity. *Nature* 470, 101–104.

Finlayson, P. G., and Kaltenbach, J. A. (2009). Alterations in the spontaneous discharge patterns of single units in the dorsal cochlear nucleus following intense sound exposure. *Hear. Res.* 256, 104–117.

Formby, C., Sherlock, L. P., and Gold, S. L. (2003). Adaptive plasticity of loudness induced by chronic attenuation and enhancement of the acoustic background. *J. Acoust. Soc. Am.* 114, 55–58.

Formisano, E., Kim, D. S., Di Salle, F., van de Moortele, P. F., Ugurbil, K., and Goebel, R. (2003). Mirror-symmetric tonotopic maps in human primary auditory cortex. *Neuron* 40, 859–869.

Gander, P. E., Bosnyak, D. J., and Roberts, L. E. (2010a). Evidence for modality-specific but not frequency-specific modulation of human primary auditory cortex by attention. *Hear. Res.* 268, 213–226.

Gander, P. E., Bosnyak, D. J., and Roberts, L. E. (2010b). Acoustic experience but not attention modifies neural population phase expressed in human primary auditory cortex. *Hear. Res.* 269, 81–94.

Hillyard, S. A., Hink, R. F., Schwent, V. L., and Picton, T. W. (1973). Electrical signs of selective attention in the human brain. *Science* 182, 177–180.

Henry, J. A., and Meikle, M. B. (2000). Psychoacoustic measures of tinnitus. *J. Am. Acad. Audiol.* 11, 138–155.

Hoare, D. J., Kowalkowski, V. L., Kang, S., and Hall, D. A. (2011). Systematic review and meta-analyses of randomized controlled trials examining tinnitus management. *Laryngoscope* 121, 1555–1564.

Kaltenbach, J. A., Zacharek, M. A., Zhang, J., and Frederick, S. (2004). Activity in the dorsal cochlear nucleus of hamsters previously tested for tinnitus following intense tone exposure. *Neurosci. Lett.* 355, 121–125.

Kilgard, M. P., Pandya, P. K., Vazquez, J., Gehi, A., Schreiner, C. E., and Merzenich, M. M. (2001). Sensory input directs spatial and temporal plasticity in primary auditory cortex. *J. Neurophysiol.* 86, 326–338.

Kaas, J. H., and Hackett, T. A. (2000). Subdivisions of auditory cortex and processing streams in primates. *Proc. Natl. Acad. Sci. U.S.A.* 97, 11793–11799.

Kiss, J., and Patel, A. J. (1992). Development of the cholinergic fibres innervating the cerebral cortex of the rat. *Int. J. Dev. Neurosci* 10, 153–170.

Kujawa, S. G., and Liberman, M. C. (2009). Adding insult to injury: cochlear nerve degeneration after "temporary" noise-induced hearing loss. *J. Neurosci.* 29, 14077–14085.

Kuk, F. K., Tyler, R. S., Russell, D., and Jordan, H. (1990). The psychometric properties of a tinnitus handicap questionnaire. *Ear Hear.* 11, 434–445.

Metherate, R., and Ashe, J. H. (1993). Nucleus basalis stimulation facilitates thalamocortical synaptic transmission in the rat auditory cortex. *Synapse* 14, 132–143.

Noreña, A. J. (2011). An integrative model of tinnitus based on a central gain controlling neural sensitivity. *Neurosci. Biobehav. Rev.* 35, 1089–1090.

Noreña., A. J., and Chery-Croze, S. (2007). Enriched acoustic environment rescales auditory sensitivity. *Neuroreport* 18, 1251–1255.

Noreña, A. J., and Eggermont, J. J. (2003). Changes in spontaneous neural activity immediately after an acoustic trauma: implications for neural correlates of tinnitus. *Hear. Res.* 183, 137–153.

Noreña, A., and Eggermont, J. J. (2005). Enriched acoustic environment after noise trauma reduces hearing loss and prevents cortical map reorganization. *J. Neurosci.* 25, 699–705.

Noreña, A., Micheyl, C., Chéry-Croze, S., and Collet, L. (2002). Psychoacoustic characterization of the tinnitus spectrum: implications for the underlying mechanisms of tinnitus. *Audiol. Neurootol.* 7, 358–369.

Noreña, A. J., Tomita, M., and Eggermont, J. J. (2003). Neural changes in cat auditory cortex after a transient pure-tone trauma. *J. Neurophysiol.* 90, 2387–2401.

Okamoto, H., Stracke, H., Stoll, W., and Pantev, C. (2010). Listening to tailor-made notched music reduces tinnitus loudness and tinnitus-related auditory cortex activity. *Proc. Natl. Acad. Sci. U.S.A.* 107, 1207–1210.

Picton, T. W., Alain, C., Woods, D. L., John, M. S., Scherg, M., Valdes-Sosa, P., Bosch-Bayard, J., and Trujillo, N. J. (1999). Intracerebral sources of human auditory-evoked potentials. *Audiol. Neurootol.* 4, 64–79.

Pienkowski, M., and Eggermont, J. J. (2010). Passive exposure of adult cats to moderate-level tone pip ensembles differentially decreases AI and AII responsiveness in the exposure frequency range. *Hear. Res.* 268, 151–162.

Pozo, K., and Goda, Y. (2010). Unraveling mechanisms of homeostatic synaptic plasticity. *Neuron* 66, 337–351.

Prins, N., and Kingdom, F. A. A. (2009). Palamedes: matlab routines for analyzing psychophysical data. Available online at http://www.palamedestoolbox.org

Rajan, R., and Irvine, D. R. F. (1998). Neuronal responses across cortical field A1 in plasticity induced by peripheral auditory organ damage. *Audiol. Neurootol.* 3, 123–144.

Reinke, K. S., He, Y., Wang, C., and Alain, C. (2003). Perceptual learning modulates sensory evoked response during vowel segregation. *Cogn. Brain Res.* 17, 781–791.

Roberts, L. E., and Bosnyak, D. J. (2010a). "Auditory training in tinnitus," in *The Textbook of Tinnitus*, eds A. Møller, T. Kleinjung, B. Langguth, and D. de Ridder (New York, NY: Springer), 563–574.

Roberts, L. E., and Bosnyak, D. J. (2010b). Evidence for depression of auditory cortical synapses in tinnitus and its reversal in residual inhibition. *Soc. Neurosci.* 170.22.

Roberts, L. E., Eggermont, J. J., Caspary, D. C., Shore, S. E., Melcher, J. R., and Kaltenbach, J. A. (2010). Ringing ears: the neuroscience of tinnitus. *J. Neurosci.* 30, 14980–14986.

Roberts, L. E., Moffat, G., Baumann, M., Ward, L. M., and Bosnyak, D. J. (2008). Residual inhibition functions overlap tinnitus spectra and the region of auditory threshold shift. *J. Assoc. Res. Otolaryngol.* 9, 417–435.

Rohrbaugh, J. W., Varner, J. L., Paige, S. R., Eckardt, M. J., and Ellingson, R. J. (1989). Event-related perturbations in an electrophysiological measure of auditory function: a measure of sensitivity during orienting? *Biol. Psychol.* 29, 247–271.

Rohrbaugh, J. W., Varner, J. L., Paige, S. R., Eckardt, M. J., and Ellingson, R. J. (1990a). Auditory and visual event-related perturbations in the 40 Hz auditory steady-state response. *Electroencephaloqr. Clin. Neurophysiol.* 76, 148–164.

Rohrbaugh, J. W., Varner, J. L., Paige, S. R., Eckardt, M. J., and Ellingson, R. J. (1990b). Event-related perturbations in an electrophysiological measure of auditory sensitivity: effects of probability, intensity and repeated sessions. *Int. J. Psychophysiol.* 10, 17–32.

Ross, B. (2008). A novel type of auditory responses: temporal dynamics of 40-Hz steady-state responses induced by changes in sound localization. *J. Neurophysiol.* 100, 1265–1277.

Ross, B., Herdman, A. T., and Pantev, C. (2005). Stimulus induced desynchronization of human auditory 40-Hz steady-state responses. *J. Neurophysiol.* 94, 4082–4093.

Ross, B., Picton, T. W., Herdman, A. T., and Pantev, C. (2004). The effect of attention on the auditory steady-state response. *Neurol. Clin. Neurophysiol.* 22. November 30.

Ross, B., Picton, T. W., and Pantev, C. (2002). Temporal integration in the human auditory cortex as represented by the development of the steady-state magnetic field. *Hear. Res.* 165, 68–84.

Ross, B., and Tremblay, K. (2009). Stimulus experience modifies auditory neuromagnetic responses in young and older listeners. *Hear. Res.* 248, 48–59.

Sarter, M., Hasselmo, M. E., Bruno, J. P., and Givens, B. (2005). Unraveling the attentional functions of cortical cholinergic inputs: interactions between signal-driven and cognitive modulation of signal detection. *Brain Res. Rev.* 48, 98–111.

Schaette, R., and McAlpine, D. (2011). Tinnitus with a normal audiogram: physiological evidence for hidden hearing loss and computational model. *J. Neurosci.* 31, 13452–13457.

Scholl, B., and Wehr, M. (2008). Disruption of balanced cortical excitation and inhibition by acoustic trauma. *J. Neurophysiol.* 100, 646–656.

Seki, S., and Eggermont, J. J. (2003). Changes in spontaneous firing rate and neural synchrony in cat primary auditory cortex after localized tone-induced hearing loss. *Hear. Res.* 180, 28–38.

Sereda, M., Hall, D. A., Bosnyak, D. J., Edmondson-Jones, M., Roberts, L. E., Adjamian, P., and Palmer, A. R. (2011). Re-examining the relationship between audiometric profile and tinnitus pitch. *Int. J. Audiol.* 50, 303–312.

Sheehan, K. A., McArthur, G. M., and Bishop, D. V. (2005). Is discrimination training necessary to cause changes in the P2 auditory event-related brain potential to speech sounds? *Cogn. Brain Res.* 25, 547–553.

Song, J. H., Skoe, E., Wong, P. C. M., and Kraus, N. (2008). Plasticity in the adult human auditory brainstem following short-term linguistic learning. *J. Cogn. Neurosci.* 20, 1892–1902.

Teismann, H., Okamoto, H., and Pantev, C. (2011). Short and intense tailor-made notched music training against tinnitus: the tinnitus frequency matters. *PLoS ONE* 6:e24685. doi: 10.1371/journal.pone.0024685

Tremblay, K., Kraus, N., McGee, T., Ponton, C., and Otis, B. (2001). Central auditory plasticity: changes in the N1-P2 complex after speech-sound training. *Ear Hear.* 22, 79–90.

Tremblay, K. L., Inoue, K., McClannahan, K., and Ross, B. (2010). Repeated stimulus exposure alters the way sound is encoded in the human brain. *PLoS ONE* 5:e10283. doi: 10.1371/journal.pone.0010283

Turrigiano, G. G., and Nelson, S. B. (2004). Homeostatic plasticity in the developing nervous system. *Nat. Rev. Neurosci.* 5, 97–107.

Tzounopoulos, T., and Kraus, N. (2009). Learning to encode timing: mechanisms of plasticity in the auditory brainstem. *Neuron* 62, 463–469.

Wang, H. N., Brozoski, T. J., Turner, J. G., Ling, L. L., Parrish, J. L., Hughes, L. F., and Caspary, D. M. (2009). Plasticity at glycinergic synapses in the dorsal cochlear nucleus of rats with behavioral evidence of tinnitus. *Neuroscience* 164, 747–759.

Weisz, N., Hartmann, T., Dohrmann, K., Schlee, W., and Noreña, A. (2006). High-frequency tinnitus without hearing loss does not mean absence of deafferentation. *Hear. Res.* 222, 108–114.

Weisz, N., Müller, S., Schlee, W., Dohrmann, K., Hartmann, T., and Elbert, T. (2007). The neural code of auditory phantom perception. *J. Neurosci.* 26, 1479–1484.

Wienbruch, C., Paul, I., Weisz, N., Elbert, T., and Roberts, L. E. (2006). Frequency organization of the 40-Hz auditory steady-state response in normal hearing and in tinnitus. *Neuroimage* 33, 180–194.

Yao, H., and Dan, Y. (2001). Stimulus timing-dependent plasticity in cortical processing of orientation. *Neuron* 32, 315–323.

Zeng, C., Nannapaneni, N., Zhou, J., Hughes, L. F., and Shore, S. (2009). Cochlear damage changes the distribution of vesicular glutamate transporters associated with auditory and nonauditory inputs to the cochlear nucleus. *J. Neurosci.* 29, 4210–4217.

Zhou, X., Henin, S., Long, G. R., and Parra, L. C. (2011). Impaired cochlear function correlates with the presence of tinnitus and its estimated spectral profile. *Hear. Res.* 277, 107–116.

14

Predictors for rTMS response in chronic tinnitus

Astrid Lehner[1]*, Martin Schecklmann[1], Michael Landgrebe[1], Peter M. Kreuzer[1], Timm B. Poeppl[1], Elmar Frank[1], Veronika Vielsmeier[2], Tobias Kleinjung[2,3], Rainer Rupprecht[1] and Berthold Langguth[1]

[1] Department of Psychiatry and Psychotherapy, University of Regensburg, Regensburg, Germany
[2] Department of Otorhinolaryngology, University of Regensburg, Regensburg, Germany
[3] Department of Otorhinolaryngology, University of Zuerich, Zuerich, Switzerland

Correspondence:
Astrid Lehner, Department of Psychiatry and Psychotherapy, University of Regensburg, Universitaetsstraße 84, 93053 Regensburg, Germany.
e-mail: astrid.lehner@medbo.de

Background: Repetitive transcranial magnetic stimulation (rTMS) has been studied as a treatment option for chronic tinnitus for almost 10 years now. Although most of these studies have demonstrated beneficial effects, treatment results show high interindividual variability and yet, little is known about predictors for treatment response. **Methods:** Data from 538 patients with chronic tinnitus were analyzed. Patients received either low-frequency rTMS over the left temporal cortex ($n = 345$, 1 Hz, 110% motor threshold, 2000 stimuli/day) or combined temporal and frontal stimulation ($n = 193$, 110% motor threshold, 2000 stimuli at 20 Hz over left dorsolateral prefrontal cortex plus 2000 stimuli at 1 Hz over temporal cortex). Numerous demographic, clinical, and audiological variables as well as different tinnitus characteristics were analyzed as potential predictors for treatment outcome, which was defined as change in the tinnitus questionnaire (TQ) score. **Results:** Both stimulation protocols resulted in a significant decrease of TQ scores. Effect sizes were small, however. In the group receiving combined treatment, patients with comorbid temporomandibular complaints benefited more from rTMS than patients without those complaints. In addition, patients with higher TQ scores at baseline had more pronounced TQ reductions than patients with low TQ baseline scores. Also, patients who had already improved from screening to baseline benefited less than patients without initial improvement. **Conclusions:** The results from this large sample demonstrate that rTMS shows only small but clinically significant effects in the treatment of chronic tinnitus. There are no good demographic or clinical predictors for treatment outcome.

Keywords: rTMS, transcranial magnetic stimulation, chronic tinnitus, neuromodulation

INTRODUCTION

Subjective tinnitus is defined as a perception of sound that is not linked to an internal or external sound source. It is considered a common symptom affecting about 10–15% of adults (Hoffman and Reed, 2004) some of which are considerably impaired in their everyday lives. Chronic tinnitus is often accompanied by hearing loss, comorbid depression, sleeping problems, anxiety, and psychological stress (Halford and Anderson, 1991; Langguth, 2011). Tinnitus sufferers are considered a heterogeneous group of patients which might be divisible into several subgroups with different underlying pathophysiologies and thus benefiting from different treatment options (Landgrebe et al., 2010). Various criteria for subtyping have been proposed based both on clinical experience (Levine et al., 2008; Lindblad et al., 2011) and on empirical data (Tyler et al., 2008; Vielsmeier et al., 2011). However, it still remains a major challenge to identify useful criteria for identifying clinically relevant subtypes.

Studies using positron emission tomography (PET) and functional magnetic resonance imaging (fMRI) indicate altered neuronal activity in the central auditory system in patients with chronic tinnitus (for a review see Lanting et al., 2009). These alterations supposedly result from reorganization processes in the central nervous system that occurs as a consequence of abnormal auditory input (Eggermont, 2005). Furthermore, altered activity has also been found in non-auditory areas such as the frontal cortex or the amygdalohippocampal area (for a review see Adjamian et al., 2009). As repetitive transcranial magnetic stimulation (rTMS) is able to modify cortical excitability, it has been introduced as a new treatment option for chronic tinnitus. rTMS is a non-invasive technique applying magnetic fields for the purpose of modulating neural activity. These magnetic fields are produced by a pulsed electrical current flowing through a coil which is placed on the scalp. The magnetic fields pass through the skull and induce an electrical current in the underlying cortical neurons. If applied repetitively, long lasting changes in the excitability of directly stimulated cortical neurons as well as in functionally connected areas can be obtained. It depends on stimulation parameters if those changes act in an inhibitory or excitatory way (Ridding and Rothwell, 2007). Studies on the motor cortex revealed that low-frequency rTMS ($\leq$1 Hz) inhibits neural activity whereas high-frequency rTMS ($\geq$5 Hz) increases cortical excitability (Fitzgerald et al., 2006). As rTMS turned out to be effective in other hyperexcitability disorders like auditory hallucinations (Hoffman and Cavus, 2002), several studies investigated the effectiveness of low-frequency rTMS over auditory cortical areas in patients with chronic tinnitus (Kleinjung et al., 2005;

Plewnia et al., 2007b; Smith et al., 2007; Khedr et al., 2008). Recently, the frontal cortex was examined as an additional target area as well (Kleinjung et al., 2008; Kreuzer et al., 2011). While the majority of those studies reported beneficial effects of rTMS on tinnitus severity, treatment outcomes varied highly across patients (Langguth et al., 2008a; Frank et al., 2010; Plewnia, 2011). It would, therefore, be of high clinical relevance to find out, which patient characteristics are predictive for treatment outcome as it would then be possible to offer rTMS more systematically to those patients who will most likely show positive response. Moreover, the mechanisms by which rTMS exerts beneficial effects on tinnitus are still incompletely understood (Langguth et al., 2008a; Mennemeier et al., 2011). More detailed knowledge about clinical and demographic characteristics of treatment responders may also shed light on the neurobiological mechanisms of rTMS in the treatment of tinnitus.

Some previous studies which examined the effect of rTMS on chronic tinnitus already reported an influence of clinical characteristics on treatment outcome. Tinnitus duration was found to have an effect on treatment response in studies using single sessions (De Ridder et al., 2005; Plewnia et al., 2007a) and repeated sessions of rTMS (Kleinjung et al., 2007; Khedr et al., 2008, 2010) showing that patients with shorter tinnitus duration improve more than patients with longer tinnitus duration. Some studies also indicate that patients with normal hearing develop better treatment response than patients with hearing loss (Fregni et al., 2006; Kleinjung et al., 2007) and that patients with left or bilateral tinnitus benefit more from left-sided rTMS than patients with right-sided tinnitus (Frank et al., 2010). Still, these results are debatable as there are just as many studies suggesting that tinnitus duration (Folmer et al., 2006; Rossi et al., 2007; Burger et al., 2011) or tinnitus laterality (Kleinjung et al., 2007; Rossi et al., 2007; Khedr et al., 2008) do not have any influence on treatment outcome, or that rTMS contralateral to the tinnitus side is most efficient (Khedr et al., 2010). In addition to these diverging results, most of the mentioned studies investigated only small samples and examined only the influence of demographical data, tinnitus side, and tinnitus duration on treatment outcome. Although there are studies which have taken additional characteristics into account (Kleinjung et al., 2007; Frank et al., 2010; Burger et al., 2011), there are many variables left which have not been considered yet. The aim of the current study is, therefore, to identify predictors for treatment outcome, including a larger amount of clinical and demographic variables as potential predictors. In order to identify the possible existence of different predictors for treatment with temporal and for combined frontal plus temporal rTMS, both treatment protocols were examined separately. The analysis has been conducted on pooled data stored in the database of the tinnitus research initiative (TRI) (Landgrebe et al., 2010), providing large sample sizes and thus allowing generalization of results.

MATERIALS AND METHODS

SUBJECTS

Taken as a whole, data from 538 patients with chronic tinnitus were analyzed. 345 (248 men, 97 women; mean age 50.14 ± 13.10 years) patients were treated with left temporal rTMS. The remaining 193 patients (135 men and 58 women, mean age 51.12 ± 11.91 years) received a combined frontal and temporal treatment. rTMS was either done in the course of different clinical trials (Kleinjung et al., 2005, 2008, 2009b, 2011; Langguth et al., 2006b, 2008b) or as compassionate use treatment between 2003 and January 2011. As the studies of Kleinjung et al. (2009b, 2011) revealed no enhancing effect of Levodopa or Bupropion on rTMS outcome, data of those studies were included in the current analysis. All participants were treated at the Tinnitus Center at the University of Regensburg, Germany and gave written informed consent after comprehensive explanation of the procedures. Patient data was kept confidential throughout all analyses, which have been approved by the local ethics committee. Patients with a history of epilepsy, cardiac pacemakers or other contraindications to TMS were excluded from treatment.

CLINICAL ASSESSMENT AND OUTCOME MEASUREMENT

Demographical and clinical characteristics were assessed by using the Tinnitus Sample Case History Questionnaire (Langguth et al., 2007a). Characteristics of both patient groups are given in **Table 1**. As not every variable was available for every patient, the table provides sample sizes for each variable separately. For calculation of the hearing level [dB HL], all thresholds measured in pure-tone audiogram from 125 Hz to 8 kHz and from both sides were averaged. If hearing was too bad to assess a threshold, the value was set to 110 dB. Tinnitus pitch was defined as the geometric mean of the lower and upper bound frequency [Hz] measured during the audiological examination.

Assessment of treatment effects was performed using standardized procedures as established in the TRI database (Landgrebe et al., 2010). This follows the consensus for patient assessment and outcome measurement approved by tinnitus experts from many countries during an international tinnitus conference in 2006 (Langguth et al., 2007a).

REPETITIVE TRANSCRANIAL MAGNETIC STIMULATION

Patients were treated with rTMS on 10 consecutive working days, receiving one of two possible treatment protocols. Either low-frequency rTMS was applied over the left temporal cortex (1 Hz, 2000 stimuli/day) or a combined stimulation over the left temporal (1 Hz, 2000 stimuli/day) and left dorsolateral prefrontal cortex (20 Hz, 40 trains with 50 stimuli and an intertrain interval of 25 s) was performed. As both protocols differ substantially with respect to stimulation sites and number of stimuli, data from the 1 Hz and 20 + 1 Hz treatment were analyzed separately. For both protocols, stimulation intensity was set at 110% of the individual resting motor threshold but never higher than 60% of maximal stimulator output. Motor threshold was defined as the minimal intensity sufficient to produce motor-evoked potentials of at least 50 μV in the left thenar muscle in five out of 10 trials. Localization of the stimulated areas was either done with a neuronavigational system or by using a standard procedure based on the 10–20 system (Langguth et al., 2006b). As there is no evidence for neuronavigation being superior to the 10–20 system (Langguth et al., 2010), data were pooled without taking the localization method into account. For all patients, a Medtronic system with a figure-of-eight coil (90 mm outer diameter; Alpine

Table 1 | Demographical data and clinical characteristics for both treatment groups.

	n	**Temporal rTMS**	*n*	**Frontal + Temporal rTMS**
Gender	345	M (72%) F (28%)	193	M (70%) F (30%)
Age (years)	345	50.14 ± 13.10	193	51.12 ± 11.91
Handedness	334	Right (86%) Left (6%) Both Sides (8%)	186	Right (79%) Left (9%) Both Sides (12%)
Hearingthreshold (dB)	224	20.19 ± 12.68	157	21.26 ± 13.98
Hearing loss (left/right)	205	0–20 dB (21%/23%) 21–60 dB (62%/56%) >60 dB (17%/21%)	146/148	0–20 dB (23%/24%) 21–60 dB (57%/52%) >60 dB (20%/24%)
BDI	221	9.88 ± 7.98	181	13.67 ± 8.65
Motor threshold	345	43.14 ± 8.50	192	42.52 ± 8.11
TQ baseline	345	38.49 ± 17.60	193	45.25 ± 17.84
TQ difference (baseline – screening)	285	−1.99 ± 9.48	166	−1.43 ± 9.58
Tinnitus laterality	335	Right (14%) Left (18%) Both ears worse left (16%) Both ears worse right (16%) Both ears equally (29%) Inside the head (7%)	188	Right (11%) Left (15%) Both ears worse left (21%) Both ears worse right (18%) Both ears equally (24%) Inside the head (11%)
Tinnitus duration (years)	328	7.75 ± 7.43	181	7.62 ± 8.73
Tinnitus pitch	104	6780.62 ± 3662.23	97	6712.60 ± 3484.62
Tinnitus pitch (patient rating)	205	Very high frequency (22%) High frequency (60%) Medium frequency (16%) Low frequency (2%)	176	Very high frequency (29%) High frequency (57%) Medium frequency (13%) Low frequency (1%)
Tinnitus quality	202	Tone (67%) Noise (8%) Crickets (19%) Other (6%)	173	Tone (57%) Noise (14%) Crickets (19%) Other (10%)
Event-related to tinnitus onset	206	Loud blast of sound (4%) Whiplash (0%) Change in hearing (14%) Stress (19%) Head trauma (0%) Others (37%) More than one event (26%)	163	Loud blast of sound (5%) Whiplash (2%) Change in hearing (6%) Stress (22%) Head trauma (1%) Others (33%) More than one event (31%)
Pulsating tinnitus	181	No (84%) Yes with heart beat (10%) Yes, different from heart beat (6%)	166	No (79%) Yes with heart beat (9%) Yes, different from heart beat (12%)
Tinnitus manifestation	235	Intermittent (11%) Constant (89%)	171	Intermittent (9%) Constant (91%)
Varying Tinnitus loudness	189	No (40%) Yes (60%)	167	No (32%) Yes (68%)
Tinnitus reduced by music or sounds	269	No (24%) Yes (65%) I don't know (11%)	170	No (24%) Yes (62%) I don't know (14%)
Loud noise makes tinnitus worse	205	No (24%) Yes (60%) I don't know (16%)	169	No (19%) Yes (59%) I don't know (22%)
Neck movement affects tinnitus	185	No (67%) Yes (33%)	169	No (63%) Yes (37%)
Stress influences tinnitus	187	No (29%) Yes (71%)	162	No (72%) Yes (28%)

(Continued)

Table 1 | (Continued)

	n	Temporal rTMS	n	Frontal + Temporal rTMS
Suffer from headache	188	No (68%) Yes (32%)	168	No (53%) Yes (47%)
Suffer from vertigo	326	No (71%) Yes (29%)	181	No (63%) Yes (37%)
Temporomandibular complaints	287	No (80%) Yes (20%)	171	No (75%) Yes (25%)
Suffer from neck pain	310	No (50%) Yes (50%)	174	No (37%) Yes (63%)

Biomed, Minneapolis, MN, USA) was used with the handle of the coil pointing upwards.

DATA ANALYSIS

Statistical analysis was performed with PASW statistics 18 (SPSS Inc, Chicago, IL). All analyses were conducted separately for the 1 Hz and the 20 + 1 Hz group. The data analysis was based on data of the TRI Database. Data management was conducted according to the Data Handling Plan (TRI-DHP V07, 09.05.2011). Data analysis for the combined frontal and temporal group was conducted according to the Standard Operating Procedure (TRI-SA V01, 09.05.2011) thereby following a study-specific Statistical Analysis Plan (SAP) that was written according to the SAP template (TRI-SAP 005, 26.10.2011). Data from the temporal group were analyzed analogously. All documents are to be found under http://database.tinnitusresearch.org/. Tinnitus severity was assessed at four time points using the German Version of the tinnitus questionnaire (TQ; Goebel and Hiller, 1994): before rTMS treatment ("screening," "baseline"), after the last treatment session ("day 12") and after a follow-up period of three months ("day 90"). Screening data were collected when patients visited the Tinnitus Center for the first time (generally during tinnitus consultation hours), whereas baseline data were collected immediately before treatment started. To test for changes in tinnitus severity from baseline to day 12 as well as from baseline to day 90, paired t-tests were used. Responder rates were calculated with responders defined as patients having improved by five points or more in the TQ score (Kleinjung et al., 2007; Frank et al., 2010). To identify predictors for treatment outcome, all variables listed in **Table 1** were included as potential predictors. Besides demographical data and hearing loss, several tinnitus characteristics and selected somatic disorders like headache or neck pain were analyzed. Differences of TQ scores between baseline and day 12 as well as between baseline and day 90 were used as variables for treatment outcome. As the baseline score was used as subtrahend, negative values describe an improvement in tinnitus severity whereas positive values describe a worsening of tinnitus.

In a first step, correlations between the dependent variables and all predictors were conducted. Dependent on levels of measurement, product-moment correlations, point biserial correlations, or eta were used. ε^2 is a measure of explained variance and thus indicates, how much of the dependent variable's variance can be explained by the independent variable. In a second step, those predictors showing significant correlations with the independent variables were analyzed in a multiple regression analysis. All statistical tests were two-tailed, unadjusted for multiple comparisons and a value of $p < 0.05$ was used to determine statistical significance. In correlation analyses, pair-wise deletion of missing values was applied. In regression analysis, missing values were deleted list-wisely. Data in the text are given as mean ± standard deviation.

RESULTS

rTMS was well tolerated, no serious adverse effects were observed. Paired t-tests revealed a significant change of tinnitus severity at day 12 for both temporal [$T(332) = 6.54$, $p < 0.001$, $d = 0.36$] and combined treatment [$T(180) = 3.61$, $p < 0.001$, $d = 0.27$]. At day 90, tinnitus severity was still significantly decreased in patients receiving combined stimulation [$T(154) = 2.35$, $p = 0.012$, $d = 0.20$] whereas in patients receiving temporal stimulation the effect did not reach significance any more [$T(291) = 1.88$, $p = 0.061$, $d = 0.11$] (see **Figure 1**). Both groups showed similar responder rates which were stable over time: among the patients receiving temporal stimulation, 37% improved by five points or more on the TQ score at day 12 and 36% at day 90. In the group treated with temporal plus frontal stimulation, 38% of patients were classified as responders at day 12 and 38% at day 90.

Only some of the predictors were significantly correlated with treatment outcome and these correlations were, though statistically significant, only weak to moderate ones (see **Table 2**). In both groups, TQ difference from screening to baseline and treatment outcome on both day 12 and day 90 were negatively correlated. This means that those patients in which the TQ score increased from screening to baseline benefited more from treatment with rTMS than patients with improvement from screening to baseline. Furthermore, in both treatment groups, the TQ score on baseline was negatively correlated with treatment outcome on day 12 and day 90. Accordingly, patients with higher TQ scores at baseline had more pronounced TQ reductions after rTMS than patients with low TQ baseline scores. A similar result appeared for the BDI score on baseline: the higher the score on baseline, the more decrease in tinnitus severity was observed. However, this latter result is only true for treatment outcome on day 12 and only in the group receiving temporal stimulation.

In the group receiving combined treatment more investigated variables had a significant effect on treatment outcome. First, tinnitus manifestation (constant vs. intermittent) was correlated with treatment outcome on day 12 with patients with

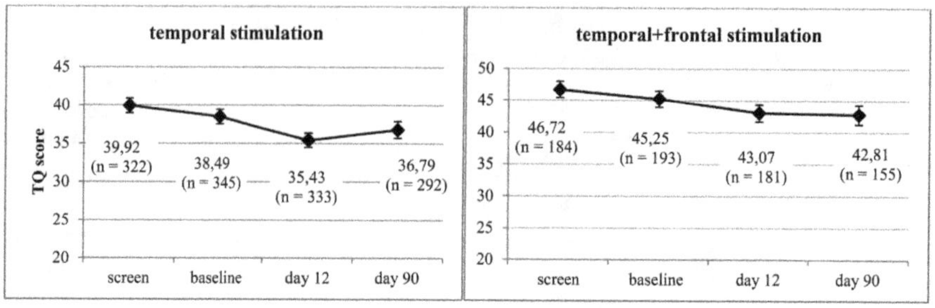

FIGURE 1 | Line chart including mean values and standard errors of TQ scores before ("screen," "baseline") and after ("day 12," "day 90") rTMS treatment for both treatment groups.

Table 2 | Correlations between treatment outcome and predictors for both treatment groups.

	Temporal rTMS		Frontal + Temporal rTMS	
	Treatment outcome day 12	**Treatment outcome day 90**	**Treatment outcome day 12**	**Treatment outcome day 90**
PRODUCT MOMENT CORRELATION *r*				
TQ difference (baseline – screen)	−0.187**	−0.229**	−0.231**	−0.183*
TQ baseline	−0.313**	−0.230**	−0.189*	−0.170*
Age (years)	0.017	−0.037	−0.025	0.001
Motor threshold	0.005	−0.035	0.010	0.014
BDI	−0.240**	−0.127	−0.067	−0.060
Hearing threshold	−0.034	0.007	0.009	0.086
Tinnitus duration (years)	0.043	0.032	−0.113	0.102
Tinnitus pitch	−0.080	−0.146	0.088	−0.013
POINT BISERIAL CORRELATION *r*				
Gender	−0.051	−0.053	−0.131	0.002
Tinnitus manifestation	0.030	0.070	−0.169*	−0.067
Varying tinnitus loudness	−0.059	0.039	0.010	0.010
Neck movement affects tinnitus	0.028	−0.025	0.036	0.036
Stress influences tinnitus	0.064	0.006	0.147	0.025
Suffer from headache	0.032	0.087	0.085	−0.015
Suffer from vertigo	−0.048	−0.067	0.001	0.117
Temporomandibular complaints	−0.042	−0.032	−0.184*	−0.187*
Suffer from neck pain	−0.099	−0.064	−0.045	0.014
ε^2				
Handedness	0.003	0.002	0.004	0.008
Hearing loss (left/right)	0.000/0.005	0.001/0.011	0.006/0.010	0.010/0.006
Tinnitus laterality	0.006	0.017	0.025	0.013
Tinnitus pitch (patient rating)	0.058	0.026	0.020	0.018
Tinnitus quality	0.017	0.025	0.026	0.005
Event-related to tinnitus onset	0.047	0.011	0.049	0.034
Pulsating tinnitus	0.012	0.039	0.010	0.013
Tinnitus reduced by music or sounds	0.015	0.010	0.003	0.023
Loud noise makes tinnitus worse	0.017	0.014	0.007	0.021

*$\alpha < 0.05$.
**$\alpha < 0.001$.

constant tinnitus benefiting more from rTMS than patients with intermittent tinnitus. This effect could not be depicted for data on day 90 though. Finally, a significant influence of comorbid temporomandibular complaints on treatment outcome was found. Patients suffering from temporomandibular complaints experienced more benefit from rTMS than patients without temporomandibular complaints.

As can be seen in **Table 2**, ε^2 was quite low with 5.8% being the highest value. Those 5.8% are explained by "tinnitus pitch." However, the category being responsible for this minimal correlation is "low pitch." Since the sample sizes of the "low pitch" groups are very small (see **Table 1**) the result is assumed to be an idiosyncratic effect of the small samples. The same is true for the variable "event related to onset of tinnitus." All remaining correlations did not reach statistical significance.

Regression analysis was conducted separately for both treatment groups and time points. Only variables significantly correlated with treatment outcome were included in the analyses. Consequently, each analysis contained a different number of independent variables. In all analyses, the TQ difference from screening to baseline proved to be a significant predictor for treatment outcome. For the group receiving temporal stimulation, TQ score at baseline appeared as an additional predictor for treatment outcome on day 90 but did not reach statistical significance in the remaining analyses (see **Table 3**). BDI score on baseline, which was only included in one regression model (temporal stimulation, day 12), was detected as a significant predictor in this model. Furthermore, in the group receiving combined stimulation, temporomandibular complaints predicted treatment outcome on both day 12 and day 90, whereas tinnitus manifestation (intermittent vs. continuous) did not serve as a relevant predictor for treatment outcome any more. The coefficients for determination in the different models range from 0.065 to 0.111.

DISCUSSION

The current results from a large sample indicate that rTMS significantly decreases tinnitus severity in tinnitus patients. Owing to the large sample size, the rather small change in TQ scores (between 4–10%) reaches statistical significance while the effect sizes are only small to moderate. Of course, the question arises if this small decrease in tinnitus severity can be considered not only statistically significant but also clinically relevant. It has to be taken into account that—apart from behavioral therapy (Hesser et al., 2011b)—there are no therapeutic tools for chronic tinnitus available for which the evidence of efficacy has already been clearly provided by metaanalyses. Facing this lack of highly effective therapeutic alternatives, the observed improvement of at least 5 points in the TQ score in 36–38% of all treated patients is a remarkable result, which represents—at least for these responders—a clinically relevant tinnitus reduction. Although the mean TQ score reduction and the effect size of rTMS are small, it brings improvement to patients who would otherwise have no real therapeutic alternatives. The small effect sizes should, therefore, not lead to the conclusion that rTMS is not efficient enough to be examined in future studies. The small effect sizes rather point to the potential of rTMS, but also to the need for future studies to further improve treatment outcome by applying rTMS over new stimulation sites or by changing stimulation frequencies (Kleinjung and Langguth, 2009a).

Regarding the stimulation protocol, both temporal and combined stimulation resulted in a decrease of tinnitus severity on day 12, but significant improvement on day 90 was only observable in the patients receiving combined stimulation. This result is consistent with the finding of Kleinjung et al. (2008) suggesting that combined stimulation has longer lasting effects on chronic tinnitus than temporal stimulation only.

Regarding predictors for treatment outcome, some of the characteristics analyzed were significantly correlated with treatment outcome. These correlations have to be interpreted with caution however, as they are only weak to moderate ones. Two parameters were significantly correlated to treatment outcome in both treatment groups: the change of tinnitus severity from screening to baseline and the tinnitus severity at baseline. Furthermore, in the group receiving combined stimulation, patients with comorbid temporomandibular complaints benefited more from rTMS than patients without temporomandibular complaints. Additionally, depressivity at baseline (assessed by the BDI score) was significantly correlated with treatment outcome on day 12 in patients receiving temporal stimulation. In the group receiving combined stimulation, patients with constant tinnitus showed more improvement on day 12 compared to patients with intermittent tinnitus. However, those latter results were not found for treatment outcome on day 90 indicating that neither depressivity nor tinnitus manifestation exert considerable influence on long-term effects of rTMS. This assumption is supported by regression analysis which reveals that only two of the parameters mentioned remain as significant predictors of treatment outcome: change of tinnitus severity from screening to baseline and suffering from temporomandibular disorder (for patients receiving combined treatment only).

In detail, the changing TQ score from screening to baseline is the strongest predictor for treatment outcome, reaching statistical

Table 3 | Results of multiple regression analyses for both treatment groups: standardized regression coefficients (β).

	Temporal rTMS		Frontal + Temporal rTMS	
	Treatment outcome day 12	**Treatment outcome day 90**	**Treatment outcome day 12**	**Treatment outcome day 90**
Tinnitus manifestation	–	–	−0.141	–
Temporomandibular complaints	–	–	−0.189*	−0.190*
TQ difference (baseline−screen)	−0.169*	−0.176**	−0.244**	−0.215*
TQ baseline	−0.122	−0.159*	−0.078	−0.068
BDI	−0.184*	–	–	–
corr. R^2	0.111	0.067	0.110	0.065

*$\alpha < 0.05$.

**$\alpha < 0.001$.

significance for both treatment groups and both day 12 and day 90. This robust finding is remarkable since the time interval between screening and baseline was not standardized and varied across patients. Patients worsening from screening to baseline benefited more from rTMS than patients who had improved between screening and the beginning of rTMS treatment. A similar relationship has been observed in a recent rTMS study (Kreuzer et al., 2011). Other earlier rTMS studies did not analyze whether changes of tinnitus severity before treatment start has an influence on treatment effects. Several explanations can be provided for this relative robust finding of an influence of the pre-treatment changes on treatment effects. The change between screening and baseline may reflect anticipation effects which are known from waiting list control groups (Hesser et al., 2011a). Thus, the inverse relationship between score changes before treatment and score changes during treatment could be explained by anticipation alone. Those patients, who improved already before treatment because of anticipation show less further improvement during treatment, because they have to catch up the anticipation effect first, whereas those who increase with their score between screening and baseline, have a more pronounced reduction during treatment since they realized, that their worries about the coming rTMS treatment, which might have caused the increase of the scores, were unwarranted.

From a more neurobiological approach the observed effect can be explained by the known dependency of rTMS effects on the history of synaptic activity of the stimulated brain area.

It has been shown that priming of cortical excitability with transcranial direct current stimulation modulates the effects of rTMS both over the motor cortex (Lang et al., 2004; Siebner et al., 2004) and to a lesser extent over the visual cortex (Lang et al., 2007). Based on these findings it has been suggested that effects of rTMS depend critically on the history of neuronal activity. Clinical effects can then be interpreted as normalization of pathologically increased activity (Siebner et al., 2004) providing an explanation why effects from healthy controls cannot be extrapolated on effects on patients with pathologically enhanced activity.

Thus, if we assume that the change in the tinnitus score before begin of TMS is reflected by changes of neuronal excitability in the stimulated area (van der Loo et al., 2009), then the observed inverse relation between changes before and during treatment could be explained as an rTMS induced enhancement of homeostatic mechanisms. Further studies should use neuroimaging methods for assessing neuronal activity at different time points before, during and after rTMS to further identify to which extent changes of neuronal activity before treatment beginning influence treatment effects. Moreover, it is strongly recommended that future clinical trials include multiple baseline assessments to identify the potential influence of pre-treatment dynamics on treatment effects and to rule out individual tinnitus oscillation patterns possibly interfering with treatment effects.

Although tinnitus severity at baseline was no significant predictor in the regression analysis, it correlates significantly with treatment outcome—a result that is consistent with previous studies reporting a negative relation between tinnitus severity at baseline and treatment outcome as well (Frank et al., 2010; Burger et al., 2011). Patients with a higher TQ score on baseline showed stronger reductions in TQ scores than patients who had low scores at the beginning. As Frank et al. (2010) already conjectured, this might be partly due to the fact that treatment outcome was defined as the difference between the TQ score on baseline and day 12/day 90. This approach assumes that a reduction of five points is of comparable clinical relevance no matter if this reduction is from a score of 65 to 60 (7.7% improvement) or from 25 to 20 (20% improvement). This is probably not the case and it remains a matter of debate whether the actual improvement perceived by the patient is better expressed by the percentaged change of TQ scores or by the difference of TQ scores (Zeman et al., 2011). Future studies should try to bring clarity to this issue.

Apart from tinnitus severity itself, only one additional characteristic had an important influence on treatment outcome: the presence or absence of temporomandibular complaints. Patients with temporomandibular complaints benefited significantly more from combined frontal and temporal rTMS than patients without these complaints. It has been suggested that in tinnitus patients with temporomandibular complaints, abnormal somatosensoric input from the trigeminal nerve may be critically involved in the pathophysiology of tinnitus (Levine et al., 2008; Vielsmeier et al., 2011). Moreover in patients with so-called somatic tinnitus treatment interventions aiming at normalizing afferent somatic input have shown benefit (Bezerra Rocha et al., 2008; Biesinger et al., 2008).

In addition to its effect on cortical neurons rTMS always exerts an effect on peripheral nerves and muscles. Peripheral effects of rTMS have been shown to reduce pain perception (Zunhammer et al., 2011) and it has also been suggested that the peripheral effects of rTMS may be involved in tinnitus reduction after single sessions of rTMS (Vanneste et al., 2011). Thus, one could speculate that in patients with comorbid temporomandibular problems tinnitus might be especially sensitive for modulation of sensory input resulting in tinnitus reduction via peripheral effects of rTMS on the temporal muscle.

However, the ability to modulate tinnitus by jaw-, head-, or neckmovements was not related to treatment success, contradicting the explanation that patients who are especially sensitive to somatosensoric input benefit more from rTMS.

Beyond that, it is not directly evident why the effect of temporomandibular complaints is only seen in the group of patients who received combined stimulation whereas those complaints had no effect on treatment outcome in patients treated with temporal stimulation only. It seems somewhat implausible that frontal stimulation is crucial for the improvement in patients with temporomandibular complaints, since it is much more likely to reach the temporal muscle and the trigeminal nerve through temporal stimulation. Theoretically, left frontal rTMS might have had a beneficial effect on temporomandibular complaints, similar like on experimental pain (Fierro et al., 2010; Brighina et al., 2011). Unfortunately, current data contain no information about improvement of temporomandibular complaints after rTMS. It is, therefore, uncertain if improvement of temporomandibular complaints and tinnitus co-occur or if only tinnitus improves while temporomandibular complaints remain unchanged.

Thus, replication of the current exploratory results is needed to rule out the possibility that the effect of temporomandibular complaints on treatment outcome is—though being statistically significant—a random effect only observable in the present sample of patients.

None of the remaining characteristics (see **Table 1**) are suitable predictors for treatment outcome. Consequently, previous results indicating that tinnitus duration (Khedr et al., 2008, 2010; Kleinjung et al., 2007), hearing loss (Fregni et al., 2006; Kleinjung et al., 2007), or tinnitus laterality (Frank et al., 2010) may predict treatment outcome are not supported. The current study used a large sample of patients with chronic tinnitus. It is, therefore, highly improbable that the failure to identify a clear set of reliable predictors is due to insufficient statistical power. Consequently, there are only three possible factors which might have caused these results: the outcome measures, the predictors or the relationship between them. This means that the TQ (and the use of its difference between two time points, respectively) might not be a suitable outcome measure. Perhaps, a rating scale for tinnitus loudness, the tinnitus handicap inventory or any other measure might have given different results. The TQ was used as it is a well-known standard measure for tinnitus severity. Future research should analyze however, if the TQ shows enough sensitivity to change or if another outcome measure should be preferred. Furthermore, although numerous clinical variables were included as predictors for treatment outcome, it is possible that we still missed relevant characteristics. No previous study reported that rTMS might be particularly effective in patients with temporomandibular complaints—maybe just because those complaints were not measured. The same could be the case with other variables we simply did not ask for. This assumption is supported by the finding that the predictors entered into regression analyses explain only between 6.5% and 11.1% of variability in rTMS outcome. Another possibility is that clinical characteristics are less relevant for treatment outcome than neurophysiological or neuroimaging characteristics. Since the neurobiological mechanisms induced by rTMS are known to depend on the neuronal activity of the stimulated brain area, neuroimaging and electrophysiological methods may be better suitable for predicting rTMS effects (Langguth et al., 2006a, 2007b; Plewnia et al., 2007b). In this context it may be of relevance that there is only a relatively weak correlation between clinical characteristics and imaging data (Schecklmann et al., 2011a). Finally, the possibility cannot be ignored that there might be no further associations between predictors and treatment outcome—an interpretation which suggests that in many patients, it might not be rTMS specific effects which are responsible for treatment response but rather unspecific effects caused by regular physician contact and counseling. It should not be neglected, however, that several placebo-controlled studies already controlled for those effects and proved that rTMS is superior to placebo in the treatment of patients with chronic tinnitus (Kleinjung et al., 2005; Plewnia et al., 2007b; Rossi et al., 2007; Marcondes et al., 2010). Another placebo-controlled non-crossover study with an adequate sample size should try to bring further clarity to this issue (Landgrebe et al., 2008).

The most important conclusion that can be drawn from our results is that rTMS shows only small effects in the treatment of chronic tinnitus. These effects are considered clinically significant, however. There are no good demographic or clinical predictors for treatment outcome. The observed inverse relationship between changes before treatment beginning and during treatment argues for the use of multiple baseline assessments in future clinical trials. The finding that patients suffering from temporomandibular complaints benefit more from a treatment with rTMS than patients without temporomandibular complaints suggests that the effects by which rTMS exerts clinical effects may also involve the peripheral nervous system. If the clicking sounds produced during rTMS treatment are additionally taken into account (Schecklmann et al., 2011b), the influence of rTMS on chronic tinnitus might be the sum of central, somatosensoric, and auditory stimulation processes. A closer insight into this interplay may help to refine the treatment of chronic tinnitus with rTMS.

ACKNOWLEDGMENTS

We thank Helene Niebling and Sandra Pfluegl for their technical assistance in administering rTMS and collecting data. Parts of this study were funded by a grant from the Tinnitus Research Initiative (TRI).

REFERENCES

Adjamian, P., Sereda, M., and Hall, D. A. (2009). The mechanisms of tinnitus: perspectives from human functional neuroimaging. *Hear. Res.* 253, 15–31.

Bezerra Rocha, C. A., Sanchez, T. G., and Tesseroli de Siqueira, J. T. (2008). Myofascial trigger point:a possible way of modulating tinnitus. *Audiol. Neurootol.* 13, 153–160.

Biesinger, E., Reisshauer, A., and Mazurek, B. (2008). The role of the cervical spine and the craniomandibular system in the pathogenesis of tinnitus. Somatosensory tinnitus. *HNO* 56, 673–677.

Brighina, F., De Tommaso, M., Giglia, F., Scalia, S., Cosentino, G., Puma, A., Panetta, M., Giglia, G., and Fierro, B. (2011). Modulation of pain perception by transcranial magnetic stimulation of left prefrontal cortex. *J. Headache Pain* 12, 185–191.

Burger, J., Frank, E., Kreuzer, P., Kleinjung, T., Vielsmeier, V., Landgrebe, M., Hajak, G., and Langguth, B. (2011). Transcranial magnetic stimulation for the treatment of tinnitus: 4-year follow-up in treatment responders–a retrospective analysis. *Brain Stimul.* 4, 222–227.

De Ridder, D., Verstraeten, E., Van der Kelen, K., De Mulder, G., Sunaert, S., Verlooy, J., van de Heyning, P., and Moller, A. (2005). Transcranial magnetic stimulation for tinnitus: influence of tinnitus duration on stimulation parameter choice and maximal tinnitus suppression. *Otol. Neurotol.* 26, 616–619.

Eggermont, J. J. (2005). Tinnitus: neurobiological substrates. *Drug Discov. Today* 10, 1283–1290.

Fierro, B., De Tommaso, M., Giglia, F., Giglia, G., Palermo, A., and Brighina, F. (2010). Repetitive transcranial magnetic stimulation (rTMS) of the dorsolateral prefrontal cortex (DLPFC) during capsaicin-induced pain: modulatory effects on motor cortex excitability. *Exp. Brain Res.* 203, 31–38.

Fitzgerald, P. B., Fountain, S., and Daskalakis, Z. J. (2006). A comprehensive review of the effects of rTMS on motor cortical excitability and inhibition. *Clin. Neurophysiol.* 117, 2584–2596.

Folmer, R. L., Carroll, J. R., Rahim, A., Shi, Y., and Hal Martin, W. (2006). Effects of repetitive transcranial magnetic stimulation (rTMS) on chronic tinnitus. *Acta Otolaryngol. Suppl.* (556), 96–101.

Frank, G., Kleinjung, T., Landgrebe, M., Vielsmeier, V., Steffenhagen, C., Burger, J., Frank, E., Vollberg, G., Hajak, G., and Langguth, B. (2010). Left temporal low-frequency rTMS for the treatment of tinnitus: clinical predictors of treatment outcome–a retrospective study. *Eur. J. Neurol.* 17, 951–956.

Fregni, F., Marcondes, R., Boggio, P. S., Marcolin, M. A., Rigonatti, S. P., Sanchez, T. G., Nitsche, M. A., and Pascual-Leone, A. (2006). Transient tinnitus suppression induced by repetitive transcranial magnetic stimulation and transcranial direct current stimulation. *Eur. J. Neurol.* 13, 996–1001.

Goebel, G., and Hiller, W. (1994). The tinnitus questionnaire. A standard instrument for grading the degree of tinnitus. Results of a multicenter study with the tinnitus questionnaire. *HNO* 42, 166–172.

Halford, J. B., and Anderson, S. D. (1991). Anxiety and depression in tinnitus sufferers. *J. Psychosom. Res.* 35, 383–390.

Hesser, H., Weise, C., Rief, W., and Andersson, G. (2011a). The effect of waiting: a meta-analysis of wait-list control groups in trials for tinnitus distress. *J. Psychosom. Res.* 70, 378–384.

Hesser, H., Weise, C., Westin, V. Z., and Andersson, G. (2011b). A systematic review and meta-analysis of randomized controlled trials of cognitive-behavioral therapy for tinnitus distress. *Clin. Psychol. Rev.* 31, 545–553.

Hoffman, H. J., and Reed, G. W. (2004). "Epidemiology of tinnitus," in *Tinnitus: Theory and Management*, ed. J. B. Snow (Lewiston, NY: BC Decker Inc), 16–41.

Hoffman, R. E., and Cavus, I. (2002). Slow transcranial magnetic stimulation, long-term depotentiation, and brain hyperexcitability disorders. *Am. J. Psychiatry* 159, 1093–1102.

Khedr, E. M., Abo-Elfetoh, N., Rothwell, J. C., El-Atar, A., Sayed, E., and Khalifa, H. (2010). Contralateral versus ipsilateral rTMS of temporoparietal cortex for the treatment of chronic unilateral tinnitus: comparative study. *Eur. J. Neurol.* 17, 976–983.

Khedr, E. M., Rothwell, J. C., Ahmed, M. A., and El-Atar, A. (2008). Effect of daily repetitive transcranial magnetic stimulation for treatment of tinnitus: comparison of different stimulus frequencies. *J. Neurol. Neurosurg. Psychiatry* 79, 212–215.

Kleinjung, T., Eichhammer, P., Landgrebe, M., Sand, P., Hajak, G., Steffens, T., Strutz, J., and Langguth, B. (2008). Combined temporal and prefrontal transcranial magnetic stimulation for tinnitus treatment: a pilot study. *Otolaryngol. Head Neck Surg.* 138, 497–501.

Kleinjung, T., Eichhammer, P., Langguth, B., Jacob, P., Marienhagen, J., Hajak, G., Wolf, S. R., and Strutz, J. (2005). Long-term effects of repetitive transcranial magnetic stimulation (rTMS) in patients with chronic tinnitus. *Otolaryngol. Head Neck Surg.* 132, 566–569.

Kleinjung, T., and Langguth, B. (2009a). Strategies for enhancement of transcranial magnetic stimulation effects in tinnitus patients. *Int. Tinnitus J.* 15, 154–160.

Kleinjung, T., Steffens, T., Landgrebe, M., Vielsmeier, V., Frank, E., Burger, J., Strutz, J., Hajak, G., and Langguth, B. (2011). Repetitive transcranial magnetic stimulation for tinnitus treatment: no enhancement by the dopamine and noradrenaline reuptake inhibitor bupropion. *Brain Stimul.* 4, 65–70.

Kleinjung, T., Steffens, T., Landgrebe, M., Vielsmeier, V., Frank, E., Hajak, G., Strutz, J., and Langguth, B. (2009b). Levodopa does not enhance the effect of low-frequency repetitive transcranial magnetic stimulation in tinnitus treatment. *Otolaryngol. Head Neck Surg.* 140, 92–95.

Kleinjung, T., Steffens, T., Sand, P., Murthum, T., Hajak, G., Strutz, J., Langguth, B., and Eichhammer, P. (2007). Which tinnitus patients benefit from transcranial magnetic stimulation? *Otolaryngol. Head Neck Surg.* 137, 589–595.

Kreuzer, P. M., Landgrebe, M., Schecklmann, M., Poeppl, T. B., Vielsmeier, V., Hajak, G., Kleinjung, T., and Langguth, B. (2011). Can temporal repetitive transcranial magnetic stimulation be enhanced by targeting affective components of tinnitus with frontal rTMS? A randomized controlled pilot trial. *Front. Syst. Neurosci.* 5, 88: doi: 10.3389/fnsys.2011.00088

Landgrebe, M., Binder, H., Koller, M., Eberl, Y., Kleinjung, T., Eichhammer, P., Graf, E., Hajak, G., and Langguth, B. (2008). Design of a placebo-controlled, randomized study of the efficacy of repetitive transcranial magnetic stimulation for the treatment of chronic tinnitus. *BMC Psychiatry* 8, 23.

Landgrebe, M., Zeman, F., Koller, M., Eberl, Y., Mohr, M., Reiter, J., Staudinger, S., Hajak, G., and Langguth, B. (2010). The Tinnitus Research Initiative (TRI) database: a new approach for delineation of tinnitus subtypes and generation of predictors for treatment outcome. *BMC Med. Inform. Decis. Mak.* 10, 42.

Lang, N., Siebner, H. R., Chadaide, Z., Boros, K., Nitsche, M. A., Rothwell, J. C., Paulus, W., and Antal, A. (2007). Bidirectional modulation of primary visual cortex excitability: a combined tDCS and rTMS study. *Invest. Ophthalmol. Vis. Sci.* 48, 5782–5787.

Lang, N., Siebner, H. R., Ernst, D., Nitsche, M. A., Paulus, W., Lemon, R. N., and Rothwell, J. C. (2004). Preconditioning with transcranial direct current stimulation sensitizes the motor cortex to rapid-rate transcranial magnetic stimulation and controls the direction of aftereffects. *Biol. Psychiatry* 56, 634–639.

Langguth, B. (2011). A review of tinnitus symptoms beyond 'ringing in the ears': a call to action. *Curr. Med. Res. Opin.* 27, 1635–1643.

Langguth, B., de Ridder, D., Dornhoffer, J. L., Eichhammer, P., Folmer, R. L., Frank, E., Fregni, F., Gerloff, C., Khedr, E., Kleinjung, T., Landgrebe, M., Lee, S., Lefaucheur, J. P., Londero, A., Marcondes, R., Moller, A. R., Pascual-Leone, A., Plewnia, C., Rossi, S., Sanchez, T., Sand, P., Schlee, W., Pysch, D., Steffens, T., van de Heyning, P., and Hajak, G. (2008a). Controversy: does repetitive transcranial magnetic stimulation/ transcranial direct current stimulation show efficacy in treating tinnitus patients? *Brain Stimul.* 1, 192–205.

Langguth, B., Eichhammer, P., Kreutzer, A., Maenner, P., Marienhagen, J., Kleinjung, T., Sand, P., and Hajak, G. (2006a). The impact of auditory cortex activity on characterizing and treating patients with chronic tinnitus–first results from a PET study. *Acta Otolaryngol. Suppl.* (556), 84–88.

Langguth, B., Goodey, R., Azevedo, A., Bjorne, A., Cacace, A., Crocetti, A., Del Bo, L., De Ridder, D., Diges, I., Elbert, T., Flor, H., Herraiz, C., Ganz Sanchez, T., Eichhammer, P., Figueiredo, R., Hajak, G., Kleinjung, T., Landgrebe, M., Londero, A., Lainez, M. J., Mazzoli, M., Meikle, M. B., Melcher, J., Rauschecker, J. P., Sand, P. G., Struve, M., van de Heyning, P., van Dijk, P., and Vergara, R. (2007a). Consensus for tinnitus patient assessment and treatment outcome measurement: Tinnitus Research Initiative meeting, Regensburg, July 2006. *Prog. Brain Res.* 166, 525–536.

Langguth, B., Kleinjung, T., Frank, E., Landgrebe, M., Sand, P., Dvorakova, J., Frick, U., Eichhammer, P., and Hajak, G. (2008b). High-frequency priming stimulation does not enhance the effect of low-frequency rTMS in the treatment of tinnitus. *Exp. Brain Res.* 184, 587–591.

Langguth, B., Kleinjung, T., Landgrebe, M., de Ridder, D., and Hajak, G. (2010). rTMS for the treatment of tinnitus: the role of neuronavigation for coil positioning. *Neurophysiol. Clin.* 40, 45–58.

Langguth, B., Kleinjung, T., Marienhagen, J., Binder, H., Sand, P. G., Hajak, G., and Eichhammer, P. (2007b). Transcranial magnetic stimulation for the treatment of tinnitus: effects on cortical excitability. *BMC Neurosci.* 8, 45.

Langguth, B., Zowe, M., Landgrebe, M., Sand, P., Kleinjung, T., Binder, H., Hajak, G., and Eichhammer, P. (2006b). Transcranial magnetic stimulation for the treatment of tinnitus: a new coil positioning method and first results. *Brain Topogr.* 18, 241–247.

Lanting, C. P., de Kleine, E., and van Dijk, P. (2009). Neural activity underlying tinnitus generation: results from PET and fMRI. *Hear. Res.* 255, 1–13.

Levine, R. A., Nam, E. C., and Melcher, J. (2008). Somatosensory pulsatile tinnitus syndrome: somatic testing identifies a pulsatile tinnitus subtype that implicates the somatosensory system. *Trends Amplif.* 12, 242–253.

Lindblad, A. C., Hagerman, B., and Rosenhall, U. (2011). Noise-induced tinnitus: a comparison between four clinical groups without apparent hearing loss. *Noise Health* 13, 423–431.

Marcondes, R. A., Sanchez, T. G., Kii, M. A., Ono, C. R., Buchpiguel, C. A., Langguth, B., and Marcolin, M. A. (2010). Repetitive transcranial magnetic stimulation improve tinnitus in normal hearing patients: a double-blind controlled, clinical and neuroimaging outcome study. *Eur. J. Neurol.* 17, 38–44.

Mennemeier, M., Chelette, K. C., Allen, S., Bartel, T. B., Triggs, W., Kimbrell, T., Crew, J., Munn, T., Brown, G. J., and Dornhoffer, J. (2011). Variable changes in PET activity before and after rTMS treatment for tinnitus. *Laryngoscope* 121, 815–822.

Plewnia, C. (2011). Brain stimulation: new vistas for the exploration and treatment of tinnitus. *CNS Neurosci. Ther.* 17, 449–461.

Plewnia, C., Reimold, M., Najib, A., Brehm, B., Reischl, G., Plontke, S. K., and Gerloff, C. (2007a). Dose-dependent attenuation of auditory phantom perception (tinnitus) by PET-guided repetitive transcranial magnetic stimulation. *Hum. Brain Mapp.* 28, 238–246.

Plewnia, C., Reimold, M., Najib, A., Reischl, G., Plontke, S. K., and Gerloff, C. (2007b). Moderate therapeutic efficacy of positron emission tomography-navigated repetitive transcranial magnetic stimulation for chronic tinnitus: a randomised, controlled pilot study. *J. Neurol. Neurosurg. Psychiatry* 78, 152–156.

Ridding, M. C., and Rothwell, J. C. (2007). Is there a future for therapeutic use of transcranial magnetic stimulation? *Nat. Rev. Neurosci.* 8, 559–567.

Rossi, S., De Capua, A., Ulivelli, M., Bartalini, S., Falzarano, V., Filippone, G., and Passero, S. (2007). Effects of repetitive transcranial magnetic stimulation on chronic tinnitus: a randomised, crossover, double blind, placebo controlled study. *J. Neurol. Neurosurg. Psychiatry* 78, 857–863.

Schecklmann, M., Landgrebe, M., Poeppl, T. B., Kreuzer, P., Männer, P., Marienhagen, J., Wack, D. S., Kleinjung, T., Hajak, G., and Langguth, B. (2011a). Neural correlates of tinnitus duration and distress: a positron emission tomography study. *Hum. Brain Mapp.* [Epub ahead of print].

Schecklmann, M., Volberg, G., Frank, G., Hadersdorfer, J., Steffens, T., Weisz, N., Landgrebe, M., Hajak G., Greenlee, M., Classen, J., and Langguth, B. (2011b). Paired associative stimulation of the auditory system: a proof-of-principle study. *PLoS One* 6:e27088. doi: 10.1371/journal.pone.0027088

Siebner, H. R., Lang, N., Rizzo, V., Nitsche, M. A., Paulus, W., Lemon, R. N., and Rothwell, J. C. (2004). Preconditioning of low-frequency repetitive transcranial magnetic stimulation with transcranial direct current stimulation: evidence for homeostatic plasticity in the human motor cortex. *J. Neurosci.* 24, 3379–3385.

Smith, J. A., Mennemeier, M., Bartel, T., Chelette, K. C., Kimbrell, T., Triggs, W., and Dornhoffer, J. L. (2007). Repetitive transcranial magnetic stimulation for tinnitus: a pilot study. *Laryngoscope* 117, 529–534.

Tyler, R., Coelho, C., Tao, P., Ji, H., Noble, W., Gehringer, A., and Gogel, S. (2008). Identifying tinnitus subgroups with cluster analysis. *Am. J. Audiol.* 17, S176–S184.

van der Loo, E., Gais, S., Congedo, M., Vanneste, S., Plazier, M., Menovsky, T., Paul Van de Heyning, P., and De Ridder, D. (2009). Tinnitus intensity dependent gamma oscillations of the contralateral auditory cortex. *PLoS One* 4:e7396. doi: 10.1371/journal.pone.0007396

Vanneste, S., Langguth, B., and De Ridder, D. (2011). Do tDCS and TMS influence tinnitus transiently via a direct cortical and indirect somatosensory modulating effect? A combined TMS-tDCS and TENS study. *Brain Stimul.* 4, 242–252.

Vielsmeier, V., Kleinjung, T., Strutz, J., Burgers, R., Kreuzer, P. M., and Langguth, B. (2011). Tinnitus with temporomandibular joint disorders: a specific entity of tinnitus patients? *Otolaryngol. Head Neck Surg.* 145, 748–752.

Zeman, F., Koller, M., Figueiredo, R., Aazevedo, A., Rates, M., Coelho, C., Kleinjung, T., de Ridder, D., Langguth, B., and Landgrebe, M. (2011). Tinnitus handicap inventory for evaluating treatment effects: which changes are clinically relevant? *Otolaryngol. Head Neck Surg.* 145, 282–287.

Zunhammer, M., Busch, V., Griesbach, F., Landgrebe, M., Hajak, G., and Langguth, B. (2011). rTMS over the cerebellum modulates temperature detection and pain thresholds through peripheral mechanisms. *Brain Stimul.* 4, 210–217.e211.

15

Imaging the neural correlates of tinnitus: A comparison between animal models and human studies

Jason W. Middleton [1,2,3]* ***and Thanos Tzounopoulos*** [1,2,3]

[1] *Department of Otolaryngology, University of Pittsburgh, Pittsburgh, PA, USA*
[2] *Department of Neurobiology, University of Pittsburgh, Pittsburgh, PA, USA*
[3] *Center for the Neural Basis of Cognition, University of Pittsburgh, Pittsburgh, PA, USA*

Tinnitus is the perception of a sound, a so-called "phantom sound," in the absence of a physical sound. The phantom perception persists after transection of the auditory nerve, indicating that the site of tinnitus manifestation is in the central nervous system. Imaging studies in tinnitus sufferers have revealed increased neuronal activity—hyperactivity—in subcortical and cortical auditory centers. These studies have demonstrated that non-auditory brain areas, such as the limbic system, are involved in the neural basis of tinnitus, Finally human imaging studies have led to novel hypotheses for the generation of tinnitus, such as the thalamocortical dysrhythmia hypothesis. Imaging in animal models of tinnitus exhibit similarities to results from human studies and have revealed hyperexcitability of auditory brain centers as a neural correlate of tinnitus. We propose that the comparison between animal model and human studies will aid in the design of appropriate experimental paradigms aimed at elucidating the cellular and circuit mechanisms underlying tinnitus.

***Correspondence:**
Jason W. Middleton, Department of Otolaryngology, University of Pittsburgh, Pittsburgh, PA 15213, USA.
e-mail: jmiddlet@pitt.edu

Keywords: tinnitus, imaging, fMRI, PET, flavoproteins autofluorescence, auditory, limbic

INTRODUCTION

Tinnitus sufferers perceive sounds in the absence of any physical auditory stimulus. Tinnitus can be caused by head and neck injuries (Chan and Reade, 1994), chemotherapy (Bokemeyer et al., 1998), ototoxic drugs such as salicylate (Stypulkowski, 1990) but, most frequently, tinnitus is caused by intense sound exposure (Passchier-Vermeer and Passchier, 2000). The various causes of tinnitus generate a diverse range of tinnitus percepts (Eggermont and Roberts, 2004). Some patients with chronic tinnitus are constantly aware of the phantom perception, but cope very effectively with this disturbance. For some patients, however, tinnitus is more than just a minor annoyance—these patients report that tinnitus causes extreme feelings of desperation and in some cases results in suicidal thoughts (Dobie, 2003). Despite the increasing numbers of tinnitus sufferers—due to increasing risks from occupational and recreational sources as well as the increased awareness of the disease—a basic understanding of the neural basis of tinnitus is lacking.

Mechanistically, tinnitus had been considered for many years as a peripheral disorder; a disorder of the external ear. This view has changed as sectioning of the eighth cranial nerve was an ineffective surgical treatment of tinnitus (House and Brackmann, 1981; Barrs and Brackmann, 1984) and collateral sectioning of the auditory nerve with tumor removal surgery even caused tinnitus in some patients (Berliner et al., 1992; Baguley et al., 2006). These results indicate that it is the auditory central nervous system—and not the periphery—that maintains the percept of tinnitus.

Recently developed animal models of noise-induced tinnitus have provided a unique opportunity for determining the neural mechanisms underlying the induction and the expression mechanisms of tinnitus (Eggermont and Roberts, 2004). These studies have uncovered many forms of aberrant plasticity that result in marked changes in the cellular and molecular properties of the auditory system of animals with tinnitus compared to healthy animals. An emerging hypothesis for the cellular mechanisms underlying tinnitus involves reduced activity of the auditory nerve—as a result of the noise-exposure or other injury (Liberman and Kiang, 1978; Mulheran, 1999; Muller et al., 2003)—and subsequent development of hyperactivity of neurons in central auditory brain centers. This hyperactivity is thought to arise from a central down regulation of inhibition to compensate for reduced peripheral afferent drive (Suneja et al., 1998a,b; Wang et al., 2009; Middleton et al., 2011). An alternative hypothesis suggests the up-regulation of excitatory inputs as a contributor to tinnitus-related hyperactivity (Dehmel et al., 2012). Tinnitus-related hyperexcitability has been observed in several auditory centers throughout the ascending auditory pathway. (Jastreboff and Sasaki, 1986; Chen and Jastreboff, 1995; Ochi and Eggermont, 1997; Eggermont and Komiya, 2000; Kaltenbach and Afman, 2000; Kaltenbach et al., 2000; Brozoski et al., 2002; Chang et al., 2002; Norena and Eggermont, 2003). While the establishment of hyperactivity neural activity as a correlate of tinnitus has advanced the understanding of the mechanistic basis for tinnitus, the features of neural activity that specifically underlie the perception of tinnitus remain elusive. One hypothesis proposes that aberrant thalamocortical rhythms—thalamocortical dysrhythmia—emerge as a plastic maladaptation to peripheral injury (Llinas et al., 2005). These rhythms may act to promote coherent high-frequency (gamma) oscillations and thus generate the conscious perception of tinnitus.

Imaging studies in humans have sought to pinpoint the neural correlates of tinnitus, however, they do not allow for the dissection of the cellular mechanisms underlying tinnitus. On the other hand, imaging studies in animal models of tinnitus offer a reduced, better-controlled experimental environment that will facilitate the discovery of the underlying physiological remodeling that leads to tinnitus. Here we will review and compare studies that have employed different imaging modalities to examine the neural correlates of tinnitus in animal models and in humans. We will also discuss how imaging in animal models may help address specific hypotheses about the persistent basis of tinnitus in the central nervous system. Further experimental and conceptual linking between human studies and studies in animal models of tinnitus will facilitate the discovery of the etiology and the cure of tinnitus.

IMAGING TECHNIQUES

Traditional methods of recording electrophysiological brain activity present significant problems that prohibit their usage in human studies. The most important issue being that extracellular electrode recordings require craniotomies, which are untenable for non-critical patients. Imaging techniques offer an alternative means of accessing physiological parameters in a non-invasive manner. Imaging of human patients has gained widespread usage in both clinical and research settings. In particular, positron emission tomography (PET) and functional magnetic resonance imaging (fMRI) are now commonly used to study the physiological basis of tinnitus in human sufferers.

Neural imaging involves monitoring changes in the level of cerebral blood flow or glucose metabolism in areas of the central nervous system. Subjects in PET studies are injected with radioactive tracer isotopes attached to a biologically active compound. These compounds are introduced to the bloodstream and, depending on the biological compound tethered to the isotope, can be used for detecting changes in blood flow, oxygen metabolism or glucose metabolism as a result of brain activity (Fox et al., 1986). fMRI can be used to image the oxygenation state of cerebral blood, and thus provides an indirect measure of neural activity. Hemoglobin in the oxygenated state is more susceptible to the brief magnetic pulses produced by fMRI scanners, thus enabling this technique to specifically measure the contrast of blood oxygenation level dependence (BOLD) (Ogawa et al., 1990). fMRI typically has a finer spatial resolution and faster temporal resolution than PET imaging. However, since the BOLD signal also arises from non-neural sources, baseline neural activity cannot be inferred using fMRI. Instead, relative changes in the BOLD signal must be used as a secondary indicator of changes in neural activity. Both imaging methods described, PET and fMRI, have limitations compared to traditional recording techniques: (1) they indicate blood flow or metabolic state and thus are only indirectly linked to neural activity, (2) their temporal resolution is slower than recording techniques that directly measure neural activity (i.e., electrical recordings, voltage, or calcium-sensitive dyes), and (3) their spatial resolution is limited to the scale of millimeters. This last point is the factor that most limits the usage of these techniques in animal studies of tinnitus. In particular, it becomes difficult to resolve signals from auditory brainstem nuclei in rodent models of tinnitus since their volume is typically smaller than a cubic millimeter.

Other non-invasive recording techniques, such as electroencephalograms (EEGs) and magentoencephalograms (MEGs), provide alternates to PET and fMRI imaging. The electric fields measured by EEGs are the result of extracellular currents that are oriented perpendicular to the cortical surface from synchronously firing neurons (Nunez and Srinivasan, 1981). MEGs likely arise from the synaptic currents that are generated by apical dendrites across synchronously activated neurons (Hillebrand and Barnes, 2002). The skull and scalp attenuate EEGs, but are transparent to magnetic fields, thus MEGs offer better spatial resolution than EEGs. The spatial resolution of MEGs is only limited by the number of neurons that must be synchronously active to generate sufficiently strong signals for detection.

HUMAN IMAGING STUDIES

In this section, we will briefly review several imaging studies that show patterns of activation that are consistent with physiological studies of animal models and some results that point to the involvement of non-auditory brain centers in tinnitus. PET imaging has revealed increased regional cerebral blood flow (rCBF) in the contralateral auditory cortex of patients with tinnitus in one ear (Lockwood et al., 2002). Some patients have the ability to modulate the experience of perceived tinnitus with orofacial manipulations (Lockwood et al., 1998). In the cases where manipulations decreased tinnitus perception, there was a significant reduction of rCBF in the auditory cortex and also in the contralateral hippocampus. This further supports the hypothesis that the basis of tinnitus is centrally located and that internal perceptions can be modulated by the top-down influence of voluntary orofacial movements.

Measuring changes in hemodynamics in tinnitus patients with fMRI has revealed increased activation of inferior colliculus (IC) to sound stimuli compared to control subjects (**Figure 1**) (Melcher et al., 2009). This study is consistent with animal studies showing increased activation of IC in different animal models of tinnitus (Bauer et al., 2008) (see next section). Another fMRI study shows that auditory cortex hyperexcitability correlates with tinnitus while hyperexcitability of subcortical brainstem regions is more directly linked with the occurrence of hyperacusis, or diminished sound level tolerance (Gu et al., 2010).

One recent discovery emerging from human imaging studies is the involvement of the limbic system in tinnitus. Tinnitus-related functional and structural changes are observed in the hippocampus and in the amygdala, (Lockwood et al., 1998; De Ridder et al., 2006; Landgrebe et al., 2009). More recently, strong correlation was shown between structural and functional changes in the auditory system and limbic system in tinnitus patients (Leaver et al., 2011). Specifically, fMRI revealed hyperactivity in the nucleus accumbens (NAc) and primary auditory cortex when tinnitus patients were presented acoustic stimuli matched to their perceived tinnitus frequency (**Figure 2A**). No functional

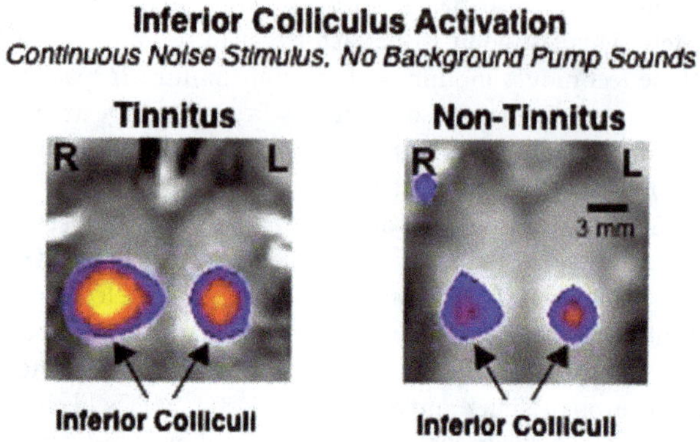

FIGURE 1 | A PET imaging study reveals larger sound-evoked activation of the inferior colliculus in patients with tinnitus (left) compared to control subjects (right). The color scale indicates the significance of the difference of activation between on and off stimulus periods. Figure adapted from Melcher et al. (2009).

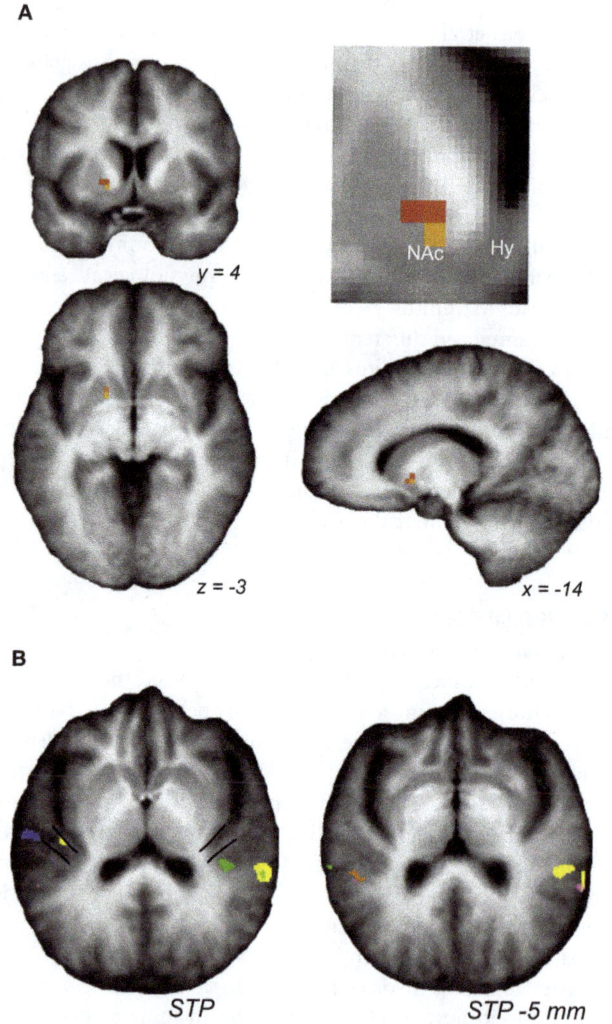

FIGURE 2 | Auditory and limbic brain centers exhibit sound-evoked hyperactivity. Stimuli matched for perceived tinnitus frequency evoked significantly higher activity, as measured by fMRI, in **(A)** the nucleus accumbens (NAc) and **(B)** medial Hershel's gyrus (mHG), the presumed site of primary auditory cortex. Figure adapted from Leaver et al. (2011).

changes were observed in the prefrontal cortex, however, structural changes were uncovered using voxel-based morphometry (VBM) on high resolution structural MRI. The ventromedial prefrontal cortex (vmPFC) of tinnitus patients had increased gray matter and decreased white matter concentrations. The degree of structural changes in vmPFC was significantly correlated with functional changes in NAc and auditory cortex (**Figure 2B**). Because the limbic system is involved in modulating and maintaining emotional state it has previously been hypothesized to play a role in the neural basis of tinnitus (Rauschecker et al., 2010). However, it remains unclear whether the limbic dysfunction is involved in the establishment of tinnitus or whether it is a secondary consequence of the emotional distress tinnitus caused by tinnitus. Furthermore, the recent finding of correlated structural and functional changes in the limbic and auditory systems suggest a widespread alteration in the limbic corticostriatal pathway, which is thought to assess stimulus relevance and filter out undesirable stimuli (Leaver et al., 2011). The compromise of the limbic system may play a role in gating the persistent representation of phantom stimuli in the auditory cortex.

BOLD signals reveal auditory stimulus-induced activity relative to baseline. It is not clear whether the perception of tinnitus is linked to stimulus-induced activity or properties of spontaneous neural activity alone, however, there is evidence that auditory stimulus related changes in the cortical BOLD signal are specifically correlated with the presence of tinnitus (Gu et al., 2010). While the intrinsic, synaptic and circuit mechanisms underlying tinnitus-related hyperactivity or tinnitus-related enhanced evoked activity are not well understood (Tzounopoulos, 2008), it is likely that similar mechanisms may mediate both spontaneous and stimulus-evoked changes.

MEG recordings from tinnitus sufferers have also contributed important insights into the neurobiology of tinnitus. MEG recordings from human sufferers of tinnitus demonstrated a redistribution of the tonotopic axis in A1 in human tinnitus patients (Muhlnickel et al., 1998). MEG signals for the presumed tinnitus frequency occupied more cortical space at the expense of other frequencies. Animal models of noise-induced tinnitus corroborate these findings as they demonstrate tonotopic reorganization (Norena and Eggermont, 2005, 2006). This reorganization can be prevented by enriched acoustic environments (Norena and Eggermont, 2005, 2006) and even reversed by pairing vagus nerve stimulation with pure tone stimulation (Engineer et al., 2011). Despite the evidence that tonotopic reorganization can result from noise-induced tinnitus, human fMRI studies suggest that tonotopic reorganization may not be necessary for the conscious perception of tinnitus (Langers et al., 2012). The interpretation that tinnitus does not require tonotopic reorganization is further supported by the possibility that increased MEG signals may also reflect changes in neural synchrony.

An alternative hypothesis for the neural basis of tinnitus proposes that reduced thalamic input—due to sound-exposure driven deafferentation—leads to thalamocortical dysrhythmia (Llinas et al., 1999). MEG recordings of spontaneous neural activity from tinnitus patient's exhibit pronounced cortical activity peaks in the theta range (4–8 Hz; **Figure 3**). Rhythms in this range were reduced when the patients were presented masking auditory stimuli (Llinas et al., 2005). Tinnitus patients also exhibit MEG activity that has broad-spectrum gamma rhythms with elevated power compared to MEGs from control subjects. Cortical gamma rhythms are hypothesized to bind together activity of neural populations to form the substrate of conscious perception (Fries et al., 2007). A potential causal link between aberrant theta rhythms and aberrant gamma rhythms has been suggested by *in vitro* experiments (Llinas et al., 2005). It was shown that 40 Hz (gamma) stimulation of cortical tissue evokes focal responses while stimulation with 4 Hz (theta) evoked more widespread responses. Furthermore, mixing of theta and gamma-evoked responses promotes the spread of gamma oscillatory activity into neighboring cortical regions. This so-called edge effect provides an attractive mechanistic explanation for the basis of certain forms of tinnitus where patients exhibit abnormally high theta rhythms in MEG signals.

Gamma oscillations have been linked with behaviorally relevant perceptual tasks. In humans and monkeys, the latency of detection of visual stimulus changes is reduced when gamma power in visual cortex is increased (Womelsdorf et al., 2006; Hoogenboom et al., 2010). Correlated activity between different brain regions that is associated with perception can arise through rhythmic gamma activity (Womelsdorf et al., 2007). Thus, noise-induced intracortical gamma-mediated signaling, arising from thalamocortical dysrhythmia, could contribute to the perception of tinnitus.

Tinnitus generation via increases of gamma-band activity at the edge frequency may not be relevant for all forms of tinnitus. The edge effect that we described above may arise from the functional lesion of a very small range of frequencies; such a lesion may lead to increased gamma activity and to subsequent tinnitus perception at the predicted "edge area." However, functional damage of a broader range of cochlear frequencies is expected to lead to a more global cortical reorganization, thus leading to tinnitus that involves perception of broader spectrum of frequencies.

The underlying cellular and molecular causes of aberrant thalamocortical dysrhythmia are unclear, but the relevance of this model is supported by a clinical study showing that a group of patients with therapy-resistant tinnitus exhibited theta frequency bursting of neurons in the medial thalamus (Jeanmonod et al., 1996). This type of bursting pattern is associated with the de-inactivation of low-threshold calcium currents (Llinas and Jahnsen, 1982). Surgical removal of the medial thalamus has suggested a reduced perception of phantom noises associated with tinnitus (Jeanmonod et al., 1996). Despite the appeal of the dysrhythmia hypothesis the mechanism underlying the initiation of pathological bursting in the thalamus remains poorly understood.

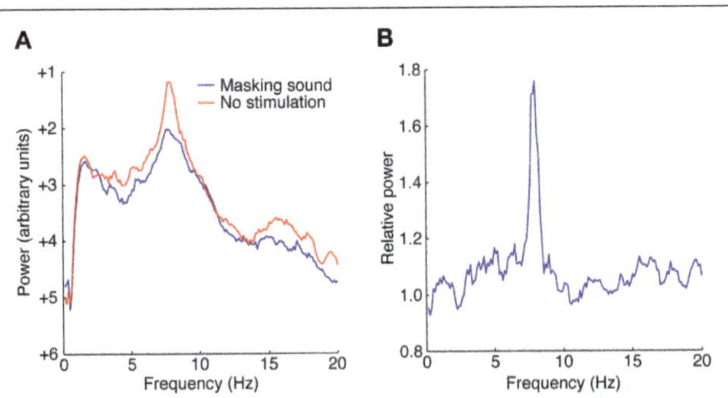

FIGURE 3 | Magnetoencephalograms (MEGs) reveal abnormal rhythmicity in the auditory cortex of tinnitus patients. (A) MEGs of spontaneous neural activity from tinnitus patients show a distinct peak in the theta range (*red*) that is suppressed when a masking sound is presented (*blue*). **(B)** The relative power of these two conditions reveals a strong coherent theta rhythm under spontaneous conditions. Figure adapted from Llinas et al. (2005).

ANIMAL IMAGING STUDIES: FORMING A LINK BETWEEN ANIMAL MODEL PHYSIOLOGY AND HUMAN IMAGING STUDIES

Electrophysiological studies in animal models of tinnitus have contributed significantly to the understanding of the neural basis of tinnitus. These studies have uncovered physiological signatures of tinnitus in different processing centers of the auditory system. In the dorsal cochlear nucleus (DCN) elevated firing rates are observed after exposure to intense sound (Kaltenbach et al., 1998; Brozoski et al., 2002; Chang et al., 2002). In the IC increased firing rates are observed after application of large doses of salicylate (Jastreboff and Sasaki, 1986; Chen and Jastreboff, 1995). Salicylate also results in long lasting increases in firing rates of neurons in cat auditory cortex (Zhang et al., 2011). Noise trauma results in hyperactivity at the auditory cortex (Eggermont and Komiya, 2000; Seki and Eggermont, 2003). The trauma induces increases in both spontaneous firing rates and in peak neuronal cross-correlations (Norena and Eggermont, 2003, 2006). How the neural correlates of tinnitus observed in animal studies relate to the neural correlates of tinnitus revealed by imaging brain activity in human sufferers is not entirely clear. Recent studies that involve imaging techniques applied to animal models of tinnitus have begun to provide these missing connections.

Relatively few animal studies have imaged the neural correlates of tinnitus *in vivo*. One notable study employed the use of micro positron emission tomography (μPET) to image baseline spontaneous activity in rat auditory nuclei (Paul et al., 2009). Rats were injected with a radioactive fluorescent tracer fluorine-18 fluoro-2-deoxyglucose (FDG) and serial reconstructions of relative metabolic activity were made from measurements using a PET scanner. This study showed that metabolic activity signals were higher in IC and auditory cortex, but not significantly increased in the thalamus of rats with salycilate-induced tinnitus. An important aspect of this study is the reproducibility of response magnitudes in successive imaging sessions of control subjects. This allows for the measurement of an absolute baseline signal enabling the assessment of both spontaneous and evoked responses. Altogether, this paper—in agreement with electrophysiological studies—demonstrates that *in vivo* imaging techniques reveal hyperactivity as a neural correlate of tinnitus.

Plastic maladaptive changes in inhibitory neurotransmission in different auditory nuclei are thought to play a role in establishing the neural basis of tinnitus. GABAergic and glycinergic release are altered in auditory brainstem nuclei after cochlear ablation (Suneja et al., 1998b; Wang et al., 2009); GABAergic activity is altered in the IC in a salicylate model of tinnitus (Bauer et al., 2000). Importantly, pharmaceutical treatments that enhance the action of GABAergic systems restore the physiological function of the auditory system in animals with behavioral evidence of tinnitus (Bauer and Brozoski, 2001; Brozoski et al., 2007).

A recent imaging study revealed the role of different excitatory and inhibitory neurotransmitter systems in mediating the observed tinnitus-related hyperactivity. In this study a novel imaging paradigm has been applied; flavoprotein autofluorescence (FA) imaging (Middleton et al., 2011). FA imaging was used to monitor stimulus-evoked activity in DCN brain slices. Flavoproteins are mitochondrial proteins that become oxidized and reduced in the electron transport chain of cellular metabolism (Shibuki et al., 2003; Reinert et al., 2007). In the oxidized state, flavoproteins absorb blue light (~480 nm) and emit green light (~540 nm). Using FA imaging in DCN slices, electrical stimulation of the molecular cell layer of the DCN (**Figure 4A**) reveals that the spread of the FA signal is proximal to the stimulation site in control mice (**Figure 4B1**). Similar stimulation in mice with behavioral evidence of tinnitus revealed FA signals that extend over a much broader region of the DCN (**Figure 4B2**). Analysis of the center (stimulation site) and surround regions of the DCN slice show that the surround/center ratio is significantly larger in the DCN from tinnitus mice (**Figure 4C**). To determine which neurotransmitter system mediates the increased FA signal in tinnitus mice, the impact of a series of neurotransmitter receptor antagonists on FA signals was assessed (**Figures 4D,E**). Application of SR-95531 (GABAergic inhibition antagonist) caused a larger increase in the surround signal of control slices in tinnitus slices (**Figure 4E**). Successive application of blockers of excitation caused similar reductions in the relative FA response in control and tinnitus DCN slices. These results indicate that GABAergic inhibition plays a role in maintaining focal responses in normally functioning DCN. Moreover these results indicate that decreased GABAergic inhibition leads to hyperactive DCN circuits in mice with behavioral evidence of tinnitus. The impairment of GABAergic inhibition provides a mechanism for the neural basis of tinnitus-related hyperexcitability in the DCN in addition to the known role of impaired glycinergic inhibition after cochlear injury (Suneja et al., 1998a,b; Wang et al., 2009), Together, these studies demonstrate the applicability of imaging techniques—that are analogous to human imaging studies—to study the underlying mechanisms of tinnitus neural correlates.

DISCUSSION

The growing prevalence of tinnitus has made it imperative to better understand the mechanistic development of the neurological basis of tinnitus. Animal studies have contributed greatly to this understanding. However, the connection between the underlying physiology in animal models and the functional imaging patterns in human studies remains unclear.

The imaging methods discussed have their own respective advantages and disadvantages. The methods directly related to cellular metabolism, and thus indirectly related to neural activity (PET and fMRI) are somewhat limited in their ability to measure single cell activity and specific microcircuit activation. Metabolic signals may be used to develop models describing the dynamics of neural populations and how they change with tinnitus-related plasticity. However, any such model would be under constrained as there are multiple cell-types contributing to the metabolic signal, and many different combinations of subpopulation activity could lead to the same observable signal.

In order to understand how cellular and circuit based plasticity underlies altered BOLD responses in tinnitus patients one must be able to assess cellular and circuit properties underlying the bold response. A better understanding of the mechanistic link between circuit-based plasticity and the altered BOLD responses in tinnitus patients may be furthered through combined imaging and physiological studies in animal models of tinnitus. One technique that may allow for this powerful combination involves the use c-fos/green fluorescent protein (GFP) constructs to identify subsets of neurons that have been activated by sensory stimulation (Barth et al., 2004). C-fos is an early immediate gene whose expression is dependent on neural activity (Gall et al., 1998). When used in animal models, it is an ideal marker of neural populations that have been recently active in *in vivo* contexts. In a previous immunohistochemical study, levels of c-fos were visualized several hours after animals were exposed to loud narrowband noise or given salycilate injections (Mahlke and Wallhausser-Franke, 2004). In this study, immunoreactive neurons were found in the auditory cortex as well as the amygdala. A previous study showed differences in c-fos activation in the DCN: c-fos expression was increased with noise exposure but not salycilate injections (Wallhausser-Franke et al., 2003). Both of these findings have interesting implications for the different modes of tinnitus induction.

In order to understand the circuit-based mechanisms underlying the BOLD signal or other *in vivo* imaging signals, imaging experiments could be performed on c-fos/EGFP mice that have been given tinnitus-inducing manipulations. These mice could be taken immediately after imaging sessions so that brain slices may be prepared for *in vitro* recording experiments. What this technique will potentially reveal is the identities of the neurons that previously contributed to increased metabolic signals from *in vivo* imaging experiments. These fluorescent neurons may then be targeted for the characterization of changes in intrinsic physiological characteristics allowing for an increased understanding of the cellular and network basis for altered functional imaging signals in sufferers of tinnitus.

One interesting finding from imaging studies in tinnitus sufferers is the involvement of the limbic system in the neural basis of tinnitus (Lockwood et al., 1998; Mahlke and Wallhausser-Franke, 2004; Leaver et al., 2011). These studies revealed hyperactivity in the hippocampus (Lockwood et al., 1998), amygdala

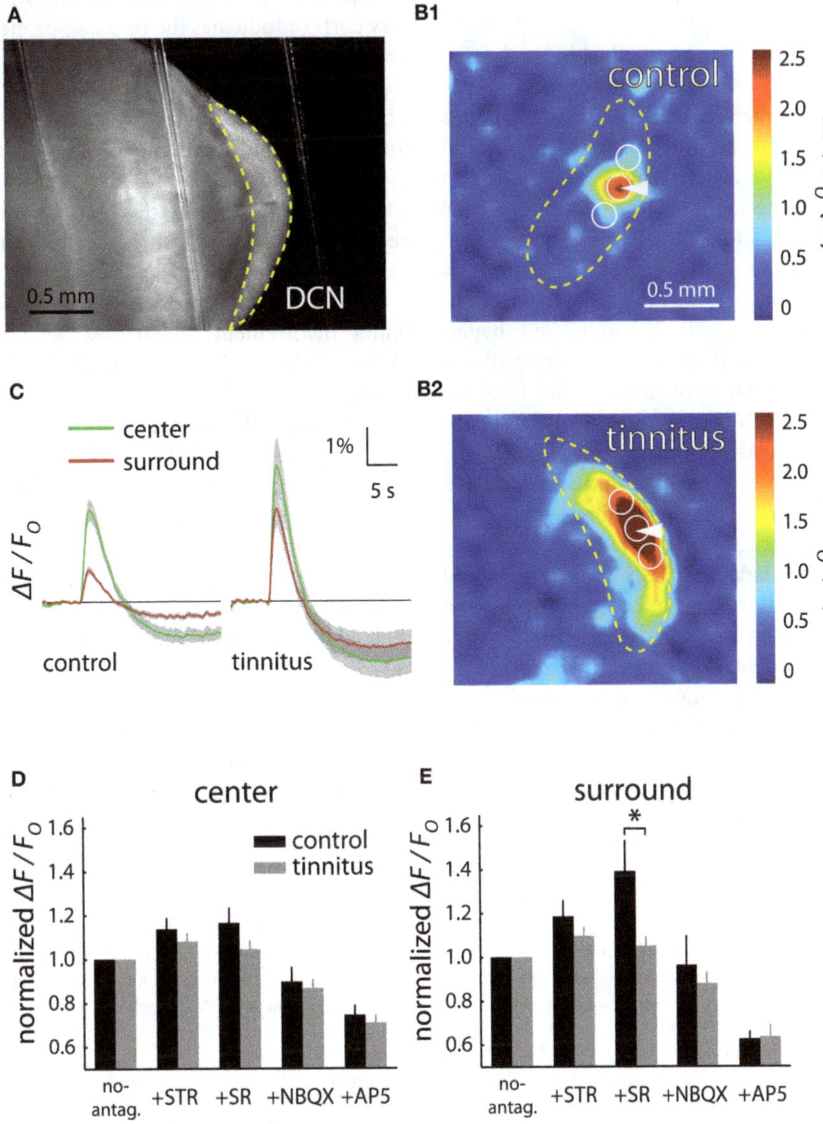

FIGURE 4 | Flavoprotein autofluorescent (FA) imaging reveals GABAergic related hyperactivity in the dorsal cochlear nucleus (DCN) of mice with behavioral evidence of tinnitus. Electrical stimulation of the DCN brain slices **(A)** leads to a spatially concise excitatory response in control animals **(B1)** and a spatially extended response in tinnitus animals **(B2)**. The center region is defined as the area at the stimulation electrode while the surround regions flank the center on either side along the fusiform cell layer. The size of surround responses relative to the stimulation center response is significantly larger in tinnitus brain slices **(C)**. Pharmacological blockade of inhibitory and excitatory neurotransmitters has similar effects on the center signal of control and tinnitus mice **(D)** while the GABAergic antagonist SR causes a larger relative increase in the surround of control brain slices **(E)**. Figure adapted from Middleton et al. (2011).

(Mahlke and Wallhausser-Franke, 2004) and prefrontal cortex (Leaver et al., 2011). These findings point to the need for increased focus on the cellular and circuit properties of neurons in affected limbic areas in animal models of tinnitus. The role of the structural changes in prefrontal cortex and/or other limbic structures could be assessed by stimulating these regions while performing concurrent imaging or electrophysiological recordings of auditory cortical regions in intact animal models of tinnitus.

Human MEG studies support the idea that a low frequency thalamocortical dysrhythmia may form the neurological substrate for long lasting tinnitus in the cortex. This theory hinges on the assumption that thalamic relay neurons are excessively hyperpolarized as a result of partial de-afferentation. Local hyperpolarization disinhibits T-type, burst-promoting calcium channels. The aberrant opening of these channels at the frequency areas where de-afferentation occurs would promote increased cortical gamma band activity in nearby frequency bands: abnormal silence in one area promotes sound generation in a neighboring area (edge effect, Llinas et al., 2005). This is an attractive model for explaining tonal tinnitus. *In vitro* imaging and electrophysiological studies, especially in T-type channel knockout mice will be essential in proving or disproving this hypothesized tinnitus generation mechanism.

While frequency-specific deafferentation at the level of the thalamus would account for burst promoting activation of T-type calcium channels, much evidence from animal studies points to hyperactivity in subthalamic auditory centers (Eggermont and Roberts, 2004). We propose an alternative hypothesis that involves the reciprocally connected excitatory-inhibitory loop between thalamus and the thalamic reticular nucleus (TRN). Sensory nuclei in the thalamus send excitatory collaterals to neurons in TRN, which in turn project inhibitory connections back to the thalamus (Crabtree, 1999). If subthalamic hyperactivity acts to strengthen the feedforward excitatory pathway (MGN → TRN) during early stages of tinnitus, the feedback inhibitory pathway (TRN → MGN) may be upregulated to maintain physiological levels of corticothalamic activity. If subthalamic hyperactivity subsides during later stages of tinnitus, the residual inhibition from TRN may persist thus providing a physiological mechanism for hyperpolarization-activated theta bursting in thalamus. This putative maladaptive TRN inhibition would thus promote thalamocortical dysrhythmia. Longitudinal animal imaging studies are necessary to test this hypothesis to verify whether there are time-dependent changes in hyperexcitability of subthalamic auditory nuclei. Additionally, joint recordings of neurons from MGN and TRN would help support or refute this hypothesis.

Anatomical studies have demonstrated top-down connections from layers 5 and 6 of auditory cortex to the IC, the olivary complex and the cochlear nucleus (Doucet et al., 2003). Activation of top-down pathways in a specific frequency region of auditory cortex modulates the response properties and the number of brainstem neurons preferentially responding to similar frequencies (Yan and Ehret, 2002; Yan et al., 2005; Luo et al., 2008). Therefore, noised-induced modification of top-down modulatory inputs could also play a role in the induction of tinnitus. This hypothesis could be addressed by ablating corticofugal neurons (Bajo et al., 2010) or electrically stimulating them in rodent models of tinnitus while measuring the resulting changes in brainstem neuron receptive field properties.

Another alternative theory, consistent with the discovery of limbic involvement is that NAc activity, which is elevated in tinnitus patients (Leaver et al., 2011), drives the TRN via serotonergic synapses (O'Donnell et al., 1997), and would thus indirectly increase the inhibition to MGN. The resulting increased inhibitory drive that TRN provides to auditory thalamus would provide the necessary hyperpolarization to activate T-type calcium currents and consequently promote aberrant thalamocortical rhythms as described above.

Ultimately, we believe that imaging studies, both in tinnitus sufferers and in animal models of tinnitus, are invaluable for their ability to connect non-invasively measured neural correlates and compare those to similarly measured quantities in animal models. Together with behavioral diagnostic techniques and *in vitro* intrinsic and network characterization of neurons that contributed to increased metabolic activity *in vivo*, imaging studies will increase the understanding of induction and maintenance of tinnitus and aid in the development of therapeutic strategies to improve hearing deficits for human sufferers of tinnitus.

REFERENCES

Baguley, D. M., Phillips, J., Humphriss, R. L., Jones, S., Axon, P. R., and Moffat, D. A. (2006). The prevalence and onset of gaze modulation of tinnitus and increased sensitivity to noise after translabyrinthine vestibular schwannoma excision. *Otol. Neurotol.* 27, 220–224.

Bajo, V. M., Nodal, F. R., Moore, D. R., and King, A. J. (2010). The descending corticocollicular pathway mediates learning-induced auditory plasticity. *Nat. Neurosci.* 13, 253–260.

Barrs, D., and Brackmann, D. (1984). Translabyrinthine nerve section: effect on tinnitus. *J. Laryngol. Otol. Suppl.* 9, 287–293.

Barth, A. L., Gerkin, R. C., and Dean, K. L. (2004). Alteration of neuronal firing properties after *in vivo* experience in a FosGFP transgenic mouse. *J. Neurosci.* 24, 6466–6475.

Bauer, C. A., and Brozoski, T. J. (2001). Assessing tinnitus and prospective tinnitus therapeutics using a psychophysical animal model. *J. Assoc. Res. Otolaryngol.* 2, 54–64.

Bauer, C. A., Brozoski, T. J., Holder, T. M., and Caspary, D. M. (2000). Effects of chronic salicylate on GABAergic activity in rat inferior colliculus. *Hear. Res.* 147, 175–182.

Bauer, C. A., Turner, J. G., Caspary, D. M., Myers, K. S., and Brozoski, T. J. (2008). Tinnitus and inferior colliculus activity in chinchillas related to three distinct patterns of cochlear trauma. *J. Neurosci. Res.* 86, 2564–2578.

Berliner, K. I., Shelton, C., Hitselberger, W. E., and Luxford, W. M. (1992). Acoustic tumors: effect of surgical removal on tinnitus. *Am. J. Otol.* 13, 13–17.

Bokemeyer, C., Berger, C. C., Hartmann, J. T., Kollmannsberger, C., Schmoll, H. J., Kuczyk, M. A., and Kanz, L. (1998). Analysis of risk factors for cisplatin-induced ototoxicity in patients with testicular cancer. *Br. J. Cancer* 77, 1355–1362.

Brozoski, T. J., Bauer, C. A., and Caspary, D. M. (2002). Elevated fusiform cell activity in the dorsal cochlear nucleus of chinchillas with psychophysical evidence of tinnitus. *J. Neurosci.* 22, 2383–2390.

Brozoski, T. J., Spires, T. J., and Bauer, C. A. (2007). Vigabatrin, a GABA transaminase inhibitor, reversibly eliminates tinnitus in an animal model. *J. Assoc. Res. Otolaryngol.* 8, 105–118.

Chan, S. W., and Reade, P. C. (1994). Tinnitus and temporomandibular pain-dysfunction disorder. *Clin. Otolaryngol. Allied Sci.* 19, 370–380.

Chang, H., Chen, K., Kaltenbach, J. A., Zhang, J., and Godfrey, D. A. (2002). Effects of acoustic trauma on dorsal cochlear nucleus neuron activity in slices. *Hear. Res.* 164, 59–68.

Chen, G. D., and Jastreboff, P. J. (1995). Salicylate-induced abnormal activity in the inferior colliculus of rats. *Hear. Res.* 82, 158–178.

Crabtree, J. W. (1999). Intrathalamic sensory connections mediated by the thalamic reticular nucleus. *Cell. Mol. Life Sci.* 56, 683–700.

De Ridder, D., Fransen, H., Francois, O., Sunaert, S., Kovacs, S., and van de Heyning, P. (2006). Amygdalohippocampal involvement in tinnitus and auditory memory. *Acta. Otolaryngol. Suppl.* 566, 50–53.

Dehmel, S., Pradhan, S., Koehler, S., Bledsoe, S., and Shore, S. (2012). Noise overexposure alters long-term somatosensory-auditory processing in the dorsal cochlear nucleus–possible basis for tinnitus-related hyperactivity? *J. Neurosci.* 32, 1660–1671.

Dobie, R. A. (2003). Depression and tinnitus. *Otolaryngol. Clin. North Am.* 36, 383–388.

Doucet, J. R., Molavi, D. L., and Ryugo, D. K. (2003). The source of corticocollicular and corticobulbar projections in area Te1 of the rat. *Exp. Brain Res.* 153, 461–466.

Eggermont, J. J., and Komiya, H. (2000). Moderate noise trauma in juvenile cats results in profound cortical topographic map changes in adulthood. *Hear. Res.* 142, 89–101.

Eggermont, J. J., and Roberts, L. E. (2004). The neuroscience of tinnitus. *Trends Neurosci.* 27, 676–682.

Engineer, N. D., Riley, J. R., Seale, J. D., Vrana, W. A., Shetake, J. A., Sudanagunta, S. P., Borland, M. S., and Kilgard, M. P. (2011). Reversing pathological neural activity using targeted plasticity. *Nature* 470, 101–104.

Fox, P. T., Mintun, M. A., Raichle, M. E., Miezin, F. M., Allman, J. M., and van Essen, D. C. (1986). Mapping human visual cortex with positron emission tomography. *Nature* 323, 806–809.

Fries, P., Nikolic, D., and Singer, W. (2007). The gamma cycle. *Trends Neurosci.* 30, 309–316.

Gall, C. M., Hess, U. S., and Lynch, G. (1998). Mapping brain networks engaged by, and changed by, learning. *Neurobiol. Learn. Mem.* 70, 14–36.

Gu, J. W., Halpin, C. F., Nam, E. C., Levine, R. A., and Melcher, J. R. (2010). Tinnitus, diminished sound-level tolerance, and elevated auditory activity in humans with clinically normal hearing sensitivity. *J. Neurophysiol.* 104, 3361–3370.

Hillebrand, A., and Barnes, G. R. (2002). A quantitative assessment of the sensitivity of whole-head MEG to activity in the adult human cortex. *Neuroimage* 16, 638–650.

Hoogenboom, N., Schoffelen, J. M., Oostenveld, R., and Fries, P. (2010). Visually induced gamma-band activity predicts speed of change detection in humans. *Neuroimage* 51, 1162–1167.

House, J. W., and Brackmann, D. E. (1981). Tinnitus: surgical treatment. *Ciba Found. Symp.* 85, 204–216.

Jastreboff, P. J., and Sasaki, C. T. (1986). Salicylate-induced changes in spontaneous activity of single units in the inferior colliculus of the guinea pig. *J. Acoust. Soc. Am.* 80, 1384–1391.

Jeanmonod, D., Magnin, M., and Morel, A. (1996). Low-threshold calcium spike bursts in the human thalamus. Common physiopathology for sensory, motor and limbic positive symptoms. *Brain* 119(Pt 2), 363–375.

Kaltenbach, J. A., and Afman, C. E. (2000). Hyperactivity in the dorsal cochlear nucleus after intense sound exposure and its resemblance to tone-evoked activity: a physiological model for tinnitus. *Hear. Res.* 140, 165–172.

Kaltenbach, J. A., Godfrey, D. A., Neumann, J. B., McCaslin, D. L., Afman, C. E., and Zhang, J. (1998). Changes in spontaneous neural activity in the dorsal cochlear nucleus following exposure to intense sound: relation to threshold shift. *Hear. Res.* 124, 78–84.

Kaltenbach, J. A., Zhang, J., and Afman, C. E. (2000). Plasticity of spontaneous neural activity in the dorsal cochlear nucleus after intense sound exposure. *Hear. Res.* 147, 282–292.

Landgrebe, M., Langguth, B., Rosengarth, K., Braun, S., Koch, A., Kleinjung, T., May, A., de Ridder, D., and Hajak, G. (2009). Structural brain changes in tinnitus: grey matter decrease in auditory and non-auditory brain areas. *Neuroimage* 46, 213–218.

Langers, D. R., de Kleine, E., and van Dijk, P. (2012). Tinnitus does not require macroscopic tonotopic map reorganization. *Front. Syst. Neurosci.* 6:2. doi: 10.3389/fnsys.2012.00002

Leaver, A. M., Renier, L., Chevillet, M. A., Morgan, S., Kim, H. J., and Rauschecker, J. P. (2011). Dysregulation of limbic and auditory networks in tinnitus. *Neuron* 69, 33–43.

Liberman, M. C., and Kiang, N. Y. (1978). Acoustic trauma in cats. Cochlear pathology and auditory-nerve activity. *Acta. Otolaryngol. Suppl.* 358, 1–63.

Llinas, R., and Jahnsen, H. (1982). Electrophysiology of mammalian thalamic neurones *in vitro*. *Nature* 297, 406–408.

Llinas, R. R., Ribary, U., Jeanmonod, D., Kronberg, E., and Mitra, P. P. (1999). Thalamocortical dysrhythmia: a neurological and neuropsychiatric syndrome characterized by magnetoencephalography. *Proc. Natl. Acad. Sci. U.S.A.* 96, 15222–15227.

Llinas, R., Urbano, F. J., Leznik, E., Ramirez, R. R., and van Marle, H. J. (2005). Rhythmic and dysrhythmic thalamocortical dynamics: GABA systems and the edge effect. *Trends Neurosci.* 28, 325–333.

Lockwood, A. H., Salvi, R. J., and Burkard, R. F. (2002). Tinnitus. *N. Engl. J. Med.* 347, 904–910.

Lockwood, A. H., Salvi, R. J., Coad, M. L., Towsley, M. L., Wack, D. S., and Murphy, B. W. (1998). The functional neuroanatomy of tinnitus: evidence for limbic system links and neural plasticity. *Neurology* 50, 114–120.

Luo, F., Wang, Q., Kashani, A., and Yan, J. (2008). Corticofugal modulation of initial sound processing in the brain. *J. Neurosci.* 28, 11615–11621.

Mahlke, C., and Wallhausser-Franke, E. (2004). Evidence for tinnitus-related plasticity in the auditory and limbic system, demonstrated by arg3.1 and c-fos immunocytochemistry. *Hear. Res.* 195, 17–34.

Melcher, J. R., Levine, R. A., Bergevin, C., and Norris, B. (2009). The auditory midbrain of people with tinnitus: abnormal sound-evoked activity revisited. *Hear. Res.* 257, 63–74.

Middleton, J. W., Kiritani, T., Pedersen, C., Turner, J. G., Shepherd, G. M., and Tzounopoulos, T. (2011). Mice with behavioral evidence of tinnitus exhibit dorsal cochlear nucleus hyperactivity because of decreased GABAergic inhibition. *Proc. Natl. Acad. Sci. U.S.A.* 108, 7601–7606.

Muhlnickel, W., Elbert, T., Taub, E., and Flor, H. (1998). Reorganization of auditory cortex in tinnitus. *Proc. Natl. Acad. Sci. U.S.A.* 95, 10340–10343.

Mulheran, M. (1999). The effects of quinine on cochlear nerve fibre activity in the guinea pig. *Hear. Res.* 134, 145–152.

Muller, M., Klinke, R., Arnold, W., and Oestreicher, E. (2003). Auditory nerve fibre responses to salicylate revisited. *Hear. Res.* 183, 37–43.

Norena, A. J., and Eggermont, J. J. (2003). Changes in spontaneous neural activity immediately after an acoustic trauma: implications for neural correlates of tinnitus. *Hear. Res.* 183, 137–153.

Norena, A. J., and Eggermont, J. J. (2005). Enriched acoustic environment after noise trauma reduces hearing loss and prevents cortical map reorganization. *J. Neurosci.* 25, 699–705.

Norena, A. J., and Eggermont, J. J. (2006). Enriched acoustic environment after noise trauma abolishes neural signs of tinnitus. *Neuroreport* 17, 559–563.

Nunez, P. L., and Srinivasan, R. (1981). *Electric Fields of the Brain: The Neurophysics of EEG*. Oxford: Oxford University Press.

O'Donnell, P., Lavin, A., Enquist, L. W., Grace, A. A., and Card, J. P. (1997). Interconnected parallel circuits between rat nucleus accumbens and thalamus revealed by retrograde transynaptic transport of pseudorabies virus. *J. Neurosci.* 17, 2143–2167.

Ochi, K., and Eggermont, J. J. (1997). Effects of quinine on neural activity in cat primary auditory cortex. *Hear. Res.* 105, 105–118.

Ogawa, S., Lee, T. M., Kay, A. R., and Tank, D. W. (1990). Brain magnetic resonance imaging with contrast dependent on blood oxygenation. *Proc. Natl. Acad. Sci. U.S.A.* 87, 9868–9872.

Passchier-Vermeer, W., and Passchier, W. F. (2000). Noise exposure and public health. *Environ. Health Perspect.* 108, 123–131.

Paul, A. K., Lobarinas, E., Simmons, R., Wack, D., Luisi, J. C., Spernyak, J., Mazurchuk, R., Abdel-Nabi, H., and Salvi, R. (2009). Metabolic imaging of rat brain during pharmacologically-induced tinnitus. *Neuroimage* 44, 312–318.

Rauschecker, J. P., Leaver, A. M., and Muhlau, M. (2010). Tuning out the noise: limbic-auditory interactions in tinnitus. *Neuron* 66, 819–826.

Reinert, K. C., Gao, W., Chen, G., and Ebner, T. J. (2007). Flavoprotein autofluorescence imaging in the cerebellar cortex *in vivo*. *J. Neurosci. Res.* 85, 3221–3232.

Seki, S., and Eggermont, J. J. (2003). Changes in spontaneous firing rate and neural synchrony in cat primary auditory cortex after localized tone-induced hearing loss. *Hear. Res.* 180, 28–38.

Shibuki, K., Hishida, R., Murakami, H., Kudoh, M., Kawaguchi, T., Watanabe, M., Watanabe, S., Kouuchi, T., and Tanaka, R. (2003). Dynamic imaging of somatosensory cortical activity in the rat visualized by flavoprotein autofluorescence. *J. Physiol.* 549, 919–927.

Stypulkowski, P. H. (1990). Mechanisms of salicylate ototoxicity. *Hear. Res.* 46, 113–145.

Suneja, S. K., Benson, C. G., and Potashner, S. J. (1998a). Glycine receptors in adult guinea pig brain stem auditory nuclei: regulation after unilateral cochlear ablation. *Exp. Neurol.* 154, 473–488.

Suneja, S. K., Potashner, S. J., and Benson, C. G. (1998b). Plastic changes in glycine and GABA release and uptake in adult brain stem auditory nuclei after unilateral middle ear ossicle removal and cochlear ablation. *Exp. Neurol.* 151, 273–288.

Tzounopoulos, T. (2008). Mechanisms of synaptic plasticity in the dorsal cochlear nucleus: plasticity-induced changes that could underlie tinnitus. *Am. J. Audiol.* 17, S170–S175.

Wallhausser-Franke, E., Mahlke, C., Oliva, R., Braun, S., Wenz, G., and Langner, G. (2003). Expression of c-fos in auditory and non-auditory brain regions of the gerbil after manipulations that induce tinnitus. *Exp. Brain Res.* 153, 649–654.

Wang, H., Brozoski, T. J., Turner, J. G., Ling, L., Parrish, J. L., Hughes, L. F., and Caspary, D. M. (2009). Plasticity at glycinergic synapses in dorsal cochlear nucleus of rats with behavioral evidence of tinnitus. *Neuroscience* 164, 747–759.

Womelsdorf, T., Fries, P., Mitra, P. P., and Desimone, R. (2006). Gamma-band synchronization in visual cortex predicts speed of change detection. *Nature* 439, 733–736.

Womelsdorf, T., Schoffelen, J. M., Oostenveld, R., Singer, W., Desimone, R., Engel, A. K., and Fries, P. (2007). Modulation of neuronal interactions through neuronal synchronization. *Science* 316, 1609–1612.

Yan, J., and Ehret, G. (2002). Corticofugal modulation of midbrain sound processing in the house mouse. *Eur. J. Neurosci.* 16, 119–128.

Yan, J., Zhang, Y., and Ehret, G. (2005). Corticofugal shaping of frequency tuning curves in the central nucleus of the inferior colliculus of mice. *J. Neurophysiol.* 93, 71–83.

Zhang, X., Yang, P., Cao, Y., Qin, L., and Sato, Y. (2011). Salicylate induced neural changes in the primary auditory cortex of awake cats. *Neuroscience* 172, 232–245.

16

Stress and tinnitus—from bedside to bench and back

Birgit Mazurek[1,2]*, Heidemarie Haupt[1], Heidi Olze[2,3] and Agnieszka J. Szczepek[1,2]*

[1] Molecular Biology Research Laboratory, Department of Otorhinolaryngology, Charité - Universitätsmedizin Berlin, Campus Charité Mitte, Berlin, Germany
[2] Tinnitus Center, Charité - Universitätsmedizin Berlin, Campus Charité Mitte, Berlin, Germany
[3] Department of Otorhinolaryngology, Charité - Universitätsmedizin Berlin, Campus Virchow Klinikum, Berlin, Germany

The aim of this review is to focus the attention of clinicians and basic researchers on the association between psycho-social stress and tinnitus. Although tinnitus is an auditory symptom, its onset and progression often associates with emotional strain. Recent epidemiological studies have provided evidence for a direct relationship between the emotional status of subjects and tinnitus. In addition, studies of function, morphology, and gene and protein expression in the auditory system of animals exposed to stress support the notion that the emotional status can influence the auditory system. The data provided by clinical and basic research with use of animal stress models offers valuable clues for an improvement in diagnosis and more effective treatment of tinnitus.

Keywords: tinnitus, HPA axis, emotional stress, neurotransmitter, corticosteroid, gene expression

***Correspondence:**
Birgit Mazurek, Tinnitus Center, Charité - Universitätsmedizin Berlin, Charitéplatz 1, D-10117 Berlin, Germany.
e-mail: birgit.mazurek@charite.de
Agnieszka J. Szczepek, Molecular Biology Research Laboratory, Charité - Universitätsmedizin Berlin, Charitéplatz 1, D-10117 Berlin, Germany.
e-mail: agnes.szczepek@charite.de

INTRODUCTION

The term "stress" was originally used in physics to define a pressure causing deformation of a physical body. In biology and medicine, the term "stress" is used to describe a reaction of an organism to a stressor. Stressors can be of physical or psychosocial nature (**Figure 1**). Generally speaking, stress is a positive reaction because it increases the chance of survival by initiating adaptation and coping with new situation (Lupien et al., 2009). Changes provoked by stress can be presented as a chain of reactions involving alarm stage, and—if the stressor is not removed—resistance, and exhaustion (Tsigos and Chrousos, 2002). Another, allostatic model of stress-induced reactions is introduced below.

Stress stimulates neuroendocrine axes such as hypothalamus-pituitary-thyroid axis (Mebis and van den Berghe, 2009), hypothalamus-pituitary-gonadal axis (Whirledge and Cidlowski, 2010) and hypothalamus-pituitary-adrenal axis (HPA axis) (Lupien et al., 2007). Further, stress can also activate sympathetic nervous system (Ulrich-Lai and Herman, 2009). Adaptation of neuronal system to stress-induced condition is reflected by *neuronal plasticity*. Neuronal plasticity is not only essential for learning and memory formation but also for the induction of mood illnesses (Berlucchi and Buchtel, 2009; Calabrese et al., 2009). The process of coping with conditions altered by stress is called *allostasis* and means a change from the usual, homeostatic status into a status, in which the organism can adapt to changes (McEwen and Gianaros, 2011). Abuse or chronic deregulation of allostatic processes (such as prolonged or repeated stress) may lead to so-called *allostatic load*, which is a negative physiological and behavioral effect of stress (**Figure 2**) (McEwen and Wingfield, 2003). Allostatic load can affect various tissues and organs and include neuronal atrophy, impaired immunity, atherosclerosis, obesity, bone demineralization and mood disorders (McEwen, 2003).

Tinnitus is a subjective perception of sound without external acoustic signal caused by inappropriate activation of auditory cortex. This activation has been documented in tinnitus patients by using either positron emission tomography (PET) or functional magnetic resonance imagining (fMRI) (Lanting et al., 2009). The results of animal and human studies have helped to determine various possible causes of inappropriate activation of auditory cortex leading to neuronal plasticity. These causes include changes in spontaneous firing rate, increased gamma band reflecting synchronous firing of auditory cortex and tonotopic reorganization (Nava and Roder, 2011).

Tinnitus can be induced by a variety of pathological conditions *via* modification of the middle or inner ear functions (e.g., otosclerosis, chronic otitis media, labirintitis, ototoxicity, noise, genetic defects), or by affecting directly or indirectly neurons in the auditory pathway (e.g., multiple sclerosis, acoustic neuroma/vestibular schwannomas, meningiomas, stroke, hemorrhage, head trauma). Accumulating evidence suggests that changes induced by these diverse conditions may result in similar phenotype, which is inappropriate activation of the auditory cortex.

In this review, we will describe some of HPA axis-mediated effects induced by stress and will discuss their possible influence

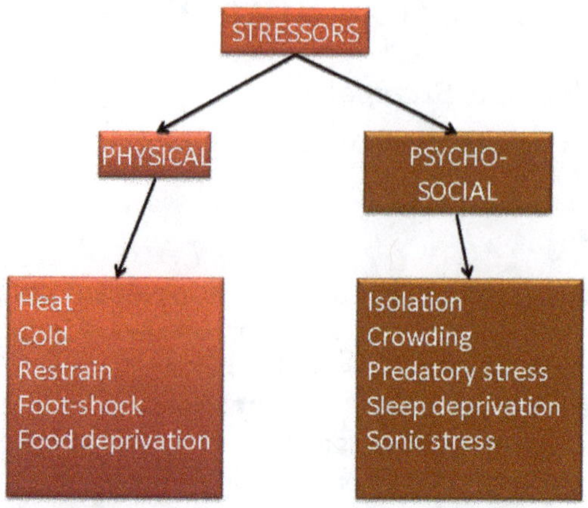

FIGURE 1 | Schematic representation of two main types of stress and different stress models used in basic research.

on the auditory system with special focus on tinnitus. In addition, we will attempt to transfer some of the *in vitro* knowledge into a clinical practice.

STRESS: MECHANISMS (HPA AXIS), MODELS, AND AUDITORY SYSTEM

THE HYPOTHALAMIC-PITUITARY-ADRENAL AXIS (HPAa)

Stress induces secretion of corticotropin-releasing hormone (CRH) from hypothalamus. CRH stimulates in turn the secretion of adrenocorticothropin (ACTH) from pituitary gland. Finally, release of ACTH to blood causes secretion of stress hormones from the adrenal glands (Lupien et al., 2007). Stress hormones comprise glucocorticoids (corticosterone, cortisol) and mineralocorticoids (aldosterone) (de Kloet et al., 2005). Cortisol (corticosterone in rodents)—is released not only upon exposure to stress but also in a circadian rhythm (Weitzman et al., 1971) and regulates in genomic and non-genomic way a variety of processes, from inflammation to behavioral changes (Amsterdam and Sasson, 2002; Amsterdam et al., 2002; Kudielka et al., 2004; de Kloet et al., 2005). Corticosteroids act *via* respective receptors: *mineralocorticoid receptor* (aldosterone receptor, MR) and *glucocorticoid receptor* (GR) and elicit two types of reactions: genomic and non-genomic (**Figure 3**). The genomic reactions occur due to the fact that both GRs and mineralcorticoid receptors are cytoplasmic, ligand-activated transcription factors (Funder, 1997). Binding of steroids to GRs or mineralcorticoid receptors induces translocation of the ligand-receptor complex to the nucleus, where the transcription of selected genes is either induced or suppressed (Datson et al., 2008). The genomic response is relatively slow and on average takes few hours. Non-genomic responses induced by corticosteroids and mineralocorticoids are extremely rapid (seconds to minutes) and are not mediated by a cytoplasmic but by a minor, membrane-bound form of GRs or mineralcorticoid receptors (Groeneweg et al., 2012). Both receptors were shown to be localized to the lipid rafts—more precisely to caveolae on a cell surface. Caveolae are rich in signaling proteins such as G-proteins and kinases, thus, they support formation of various signalosomes. The precise signaling pathways induced by corticosteroids and mineralocorticoids remain to be confirmed but

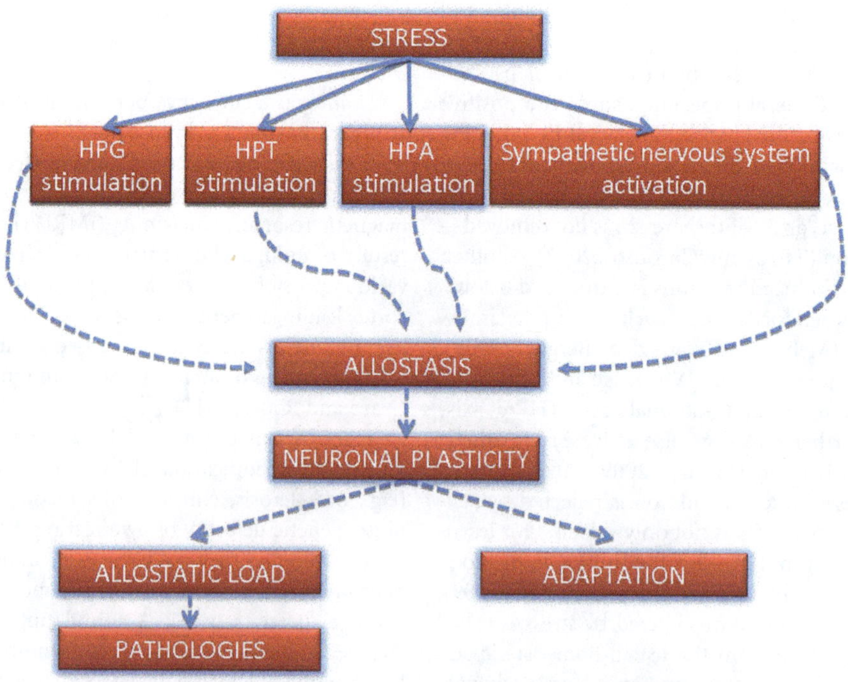

FIGURE 2 | Most representative stress-induced pathways and hypothetical involvement in the induction of allostatic load. HPT, hypothalamus-pituitary-thyroid axis; HPG, hypothalamus-pituitary-gonadal axis; HPA, hypothalamus-pituitary-adrenal axis.

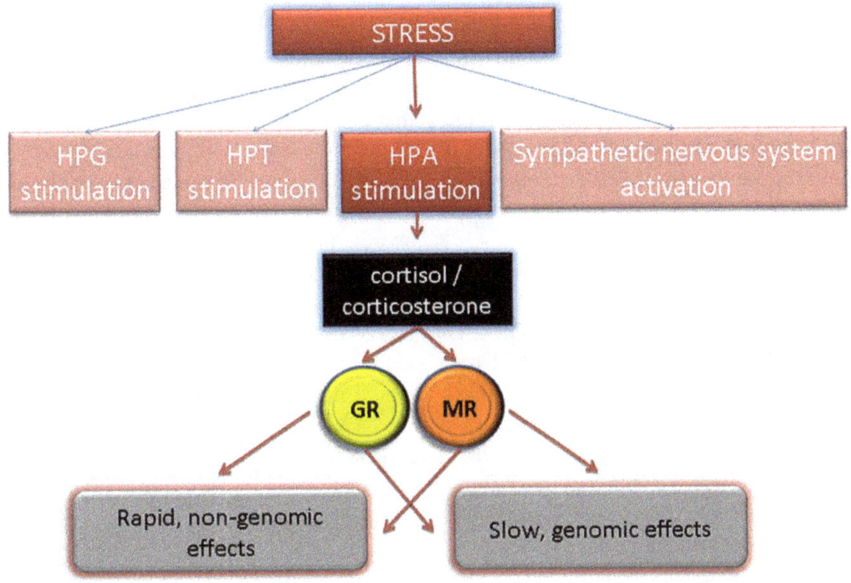

FIGURE 3 | HPA-induced stress hormone release and their signaling via respective receptors induce genomic (slow) and non-genomic (rapid) changes. GR, glucocorticoid receptor; MR, mineralcorticoid receptor.

it is already apparent that the kinase pathways are predominant (Groeneweg et al., 2012).

HYPOTHALAMIC-PITUITARY-ADRENAL AXIS AND AUDITORY SYSTEM

HPA-induced steroids signal trough their respective receptors: glucocorticoid and mineralcorticoid receptors. In contrast to ubiquitously expressed GRs, expression of mineralcorticoid receptors is restricted to selected tissues including brain, eye, intestine, kidney, mammary gland, pancreas, pituitary gland, and the inner ear. In fact, analyses of expressed sequence tag profile in mice demonstrated the highest expression level of mineralcorticoid receptor mRNA in the inner ear, as compared to other tissues (NCBI accession number: Mm.324393). Expression of mineralcorticoid receptors is not incidental—it denotes aldosterone-sensitive tissues, in which mineralcorticoid receptors regulate the ionic and water transports (mainly the epithelial sodium channel, Na^+/K^+ pump, serum, and glucocorticoid-induced kinase or SGK1) resulting in the re-absorption of sodium and an excretion of potassium (Thomas and Harvey, 2011).

Presence and localization of mineralcorticoid and glucocorticoid receptors was studied in the rat cochlea and their expression was positively confirmed (Zuo et al., 1995; Yao and Rarey, 1996). Not surprisingly, mineralcorticoid receptor was found to be predominantly localized in stria vascularis and in the spiral ganglion neurons (Furuta et al., 1994). Hyperactivation of mineralcorticoid receptors in the inner ear could lead to improper potassium-sodium balance in the scala tympani and was, in fact, suspected to play a crucial role in the vertigo and tinnitus/deafness attacks in the Ménière's disease. In a clinical study, where the concentration of aldosterone was measured in plasma of Ménière's patients obtained between the attacks, no abnormal fluctuation was found, suggesting that this hormone does not contribute to the sickness symptomes (Mateijsen et al., 2001). However, the question if aldosterone concentration is being altered *during* active periods of Ménière's disease remains open. On the other hand, Ménière's patients have elevated concentration of cortisol in blood (van Cruijsen et al., 2005), which could contribute to Ménière's symptoms but could also be a secondary marker of stress perceived by the patients.

Recently, local HPA-equivalent signaling system was discovered in the cochlea of mice (Graham et al., 2010; Graham and Vetter, 2011). This local HPA system is independent of the systemic HPA signaling. It consists of locally produced corticotropin-releasing factor (CRF), CRF1-receptor and ACTH. Interestingly, deletion of CRF1-receptor gene resulted in auditory impairment of knock-out animals (Graham and Vetter, 2011). This impairment was accompanied by reduced expression of glutamine synthetase together with abnormal innervation features and was attributed to the developmental role that CRFR1 potentially plays in the inner ear. Future experiments should determine the connection between cochlear and systemic HPA systems.

STRESS AND THE HPA AXIS-INDUCED NEURONAL PLASTICITY

Both acute and chronic stress were demonstrated to influence the *glutamate neurotransmission* and in this way contribute to the *neuronal plasticity* (Krugers et al., 2010; Popoli et al., 2011). Induction of neuronal plasticity was shown to be possible by generation of changes on a pre-synaptic (synthesis, transport, release) and/or post-synaptic level (glutamate recycling, binding, and signaling *via* glutamate receptors).

Glutamate is an abandoned neurotransmitter in CNS and is involved in the process of memory, learning, and also in the auditory processing. Special feature of glutamate circuits is their involvement in the process of plasticity, for the reason that glutamate and glutamate receptors NMDAR (*N*-methyl-D-aspartate receptor) and AMPAR (α-amino-3-hydroxy-5-methyl-4-isoxazolepropionic acid receptor) regulate the strength and function of neuronal synapses. To date, mechanisms determined as responsible for the synaptic plasticity are glutamate receptors (NMDAR)—related long-term potentiation (LTP) and long-term depression (LTD). In addition, changes in AMPAR composition and density on the synapses were shown to be essential for the plasticity process.

Pre-synaptic neuronal plasticity can be mediated by changes in glutamate transport. Predominant type of glutamate transporter present in the organ of Corti (in the supporting cells) is GLAST/EAAT1 (Ruel et al., 2007). Upregulation of GLAST/EAAT1 was demonstrated in astrocytes of animals subjected to chronic physical stress (Madrigal et al., 2003). However, the influence of stress or glucocorticoids on cochlear GLAST/EAAT1 is still unknown.

Post-synaptic neuronal plasticity can be induced by changes in the expression and trafficking of glutamate receptors AMPAR. AMPAR are multimers composed of various subunits, quantity, and ratio of which influences the synaptic strength. The mechanism that mediates HPA-induced changes in AMPA receptors trafficking is attributed to the *genomic* and *non-genomic effects* of glucocorticoids (**Figure 4**). In the prefrontal cortex, stress has been demonstrated to activate in a non-genomic way the glucocorticoid-inducible kinase SGK (Popoli et al., 2011). SGK1 is also expressed in stria vascularis, spiral ligament, spiral limbus, organ of Corti, Reissner's membrane and in the spiral ganglion of rats (Zhong and Liu, 2009) but role of SGK1 in the inner ear has not yet been experimentally addressed. The rapid, non-genomic effects of stress are attributed to the presence of mineralcorticoid receptor (Karst et al., 2005; Groeneweg et al., 2012), which is also expressed in the cochlea (Furuta et al., 1994; Yao and Rarey, 1996).

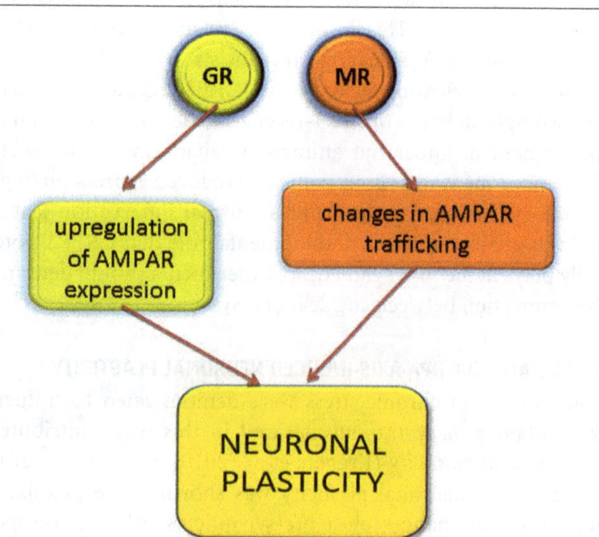

FIGURE 4 | Glucocorticoids induce neuronal plasticity via respective receptors. AMPAR, α-amino-3-hydroxy-5-methyl-4-isoxazolepropionic acid receptor; GR, glucocorticoid receptor; MR, mineralcorticoid receptor.

An example of slow, genomic effects of glucocorticoids is the cortisol/corticosterone-induced increase in transcription and translation of GluA2 AMPA receptor subunit (Krugers et al., 2010). In the auditory system, the expression of GluA2 was demonstrated in the cochlear nucleus and in the medial nucleus of the trapezoid body (Hermida et al., 2010; Wang et al., 2011) but the stress-induced changes in its expression were not yet studied.

Taken together, peripheral and central auditory systems express molecules, which are modulated by stress in the limbic, memory, and learning centers of CNS. This modulation is responsible for neuronal plasticity in above areas. If stress and activated HPA axis could induce plastic changes in the auditory pathway *via* modification of glutamate neurotransmission, remains to be established.

STRESS MODELS

Extended presence of stressor such as inability to escape from a stressing situation (*chronic stress*) or a high impact stressor (*acute stress*) may induce allostatic load reflected by pathological reactions or conditions. However, the outcome of allostatic load not only depends on *duration* and *category* of stress but also on *age*, *gender* and the *genetic makeup* of stressed organism (Joels and Baram, 2009).

To date, research has concentrated mainly on the stress-induced changes in learning, memory, cognition, and on morphological and molecular modifications in the respective brain structures (Lupien et al., 2007; Joels and Baram, 2009). Majority of stress research requiring information regarding histology, molecular or cell biology has been preformed with use of different animal stress models. The goal of animal stress models is to mimic and study stress experienced by people under certain conditions. Therefore, various physical or psycho-social stressors are used (**Figure 1**). To the *physical stress models* belongs between many others the immersion in cold water, restrain, cold-water restrain, electric foot shock, and food deprivation. *Psycho-social stress models* use as stressors neonatal isolation (isolation of off-spring from mother), isolation, crowding (too many animals per cage), predatory (exposure of mice or rats to cat or any substance having its smell), sleep deprivation and sonic stress (harmful or non-harmful to the auditory system) (Quarcoo et al., 2009; Jaggi et al., 2011; Vicario et al., 2012).

Psycho-social stress is quite different in nature than physical stress. In fact, psycho-social stress was shown to induce changes in some areas of brain that were not affected by physical stress (Nakagawa et al., 1981; Iimori et al., 1982). In addition to the type of stress, important is also stress duration. In acute settings, the stressor is used for a short time. In chronic settings, the stressor is applied from 24 h to up to 40 days. Lastly, there are models that mix different types of acute and chronic stress in an unpredictable way (Jaggi et al., 2011).

Taken together, caution needs to be taken when designing, interpreting, and comparing experiments that use various animal stress models.

STRESS MODELS IN AUDITORY RESEARCH

In the auditory research, influence of stress on the auditory processing was often studied using *physical acute* stress. Severe pain (tracheotomy and bladder catheterization performed without general anesthetics) used in guinea pigs as stressors was demonstrated to induce auditory threshold shift, which was later explained by a cochlear hypoxia (Muchnik et al., 1980; Hildesheimer et al., 1985). Sprague-Dawley rats subjected to restraint stress for 10 days, 2 h per day (*physical stressor; chronic stress*) have developed auditory impairment and significant atrophy of inferior colliculus (Dagnino-Subiabre et al., 2005) and of medial geniculate nucleus (Bose et al., 2010). The mechanisms mediating atrophic degeneration in the auditory pathway have not been fully clarified, but it is apparent that degeneration is auditory tissues-specific, since the visual system (e.g., the superior colliculus adjacent to the inferior colliculus) is not affected by stress. From the perspective of allostatic model, one could postulate that *chronic physical stress may induce the allostatic load in auditory pathway*.

Stress (e.g., heat or restraint) was found not only to damage but also to *protect the hearing* (Yoshida et al., 1999; Wang and Liberman, 2002). Physical type of stressor (restraint) in the acute settings (4 h of duration) increased the concentration of corticosterone in blood and as a consequence, protected the animals form the noise-induced trauma. Similar protective effects had the administration of glucocorticoid-based drugs prior to acoustic trauma (reviewed in Meltser and Canlon, 2011). From the perspective of allostatic model, one could hypothesize that the *acute physical stress is unable to induce allostatic load in auditory pathway*. On the contrary, activation of HPA axis resulting in the production of corticosteroids protects the auditory system against the noise trauma. This endogenous corticosteroid protection is comparable to the application of synthetic corticosteroids, used in therapy of acute hearing loss (Meltser and Canlon, 2011).

Under special circumstances, the administration of corticosteroids can also have adverse effects on the auditory system. Prenatal, long-term administration of glucocorticoids, increased the susceptibility of the of the Sprague-Dawley offspring rats to noise trauma (Canlon et al., 2003). However, these findings could not be reproduced by other group in Wistar rats, possibly reflecting inter-strain genetic differences in stress and corticosteroid susceptibility (Hougaard et al., 2007).

In addition to physical stress, psycho-social stress model was also used in the auditory research. Wistar rats subjected to 24 h of stress (non-harmful sonic stress: sound pressure level 61–65 dB, sound frequency 300 Hz, 1 s sound in intervals of 15 s) have developed temporary but significant reduction of the ABR thresholds in all frequencies tested and of the DPOAE thresholds in low frequencies, consistent with auditory hypersensitivity (Mazurek et al., 2010). This implies that *chronic, psycho-social stress may influence the function of auditory pathway*. Long-term consequences of such influence remain to be determined.

STRESS AND TINNITUS

There is a bulk of evidence supporting the view that *tinnitus induces stress* in patients. However, little is known about the other side of this interaction—that is about *stress inducing tinnitus*. It has been a frequent observation made by otologists and audiologists that many tinnitus patients complain of psycho-social distress *prior to* or during the onset and progression of tinnitus. One of the earliest published observations connecting the onset of tinnitus with psycho-social distress was made by John Harrison Curtis, the surgeon of the Royal Dispensary for Diseases of the Ear in London (the first hospital in England offering specialized care for ear diseases, est. 1817). Dr. Curtis has noticed that in two of five cases, affected patients attributed the beginning of tinnitus to a psycho-social strain caused by death in immediate family (Curtis, 1841).

Hundred and seventy years later, two large-scale studies provided epidemiological information about the association of psycho-social stress with tinnitus (Baigi et al., 2011; Hasson et al., 2011). The first study demonstrated that the probability of developing tinnitus is approximately the same for highly stressed persons as it is for persons exposed to occupational noise (Baigi et al., 2011). Importantly, the authors also have noticed that psycho-social stress contributes to worsening of tinnitus symptoms. Interestingly, exposure to high level of stress *and* occupational noise doubles the probability of developing tinnitus. In the second study, a self-completion questionnaire was used to inquire about work- and health-related stressors and hearing problems, such as tinnitus. About one-third of working population reported hearing problems or tinnitus or both. In addition, prevalence of sleeping problems was significantly higher in subjects with tinnitus, than in the tinnitus-free subjects. Importantly, the authors found linear association between tinnitus and the magnitude and duration of stress, such as for instance occupational stress (Hasson et al., 2011). Both studies were performed with more than 10,000 subjects each, thus, providing statistical strength. Recently, we also have shown that the patients with disturbing chronic tinnitus have higher scores than patients with non-disturbing tinnitus in the subscales "worries" and "tension" measured by stress-oriented Perceived Stress Questionnaire (Seydel et al., 2010).

Interesting for the issue *tinnitus and stress* is the HPA axis, which seems to be disturbed in tinnitus patients. Hebert and Lupien have observed that the basal levels of salivary cortisol are chronically elevated in tinnitus patients, who had disturbing tinnitus on average for 5.5 years (Hebert et al., 2004). In addition, patients who had disturbing tinnitus for a longer time (on average 14.7 years) were shown to develop improper HPA responses to an experimental, psycho-social stress (Hebert and Lupien, 2007). HPA axis in tinnitus patients under stress seems to be activated later and to a lesser extend than in the healthy controls, consistent with glucocorticoid inefficiency (Yehuda et al., 1996). Such inefficiency is also found in some stress-related disorders: chronic fatigue syndrome, posttraumatic stress disorder and in burnout syndrome (Kudielka and Wust, 2010; Juster et al., 2011). Interestingly, high comorbidity of tinnitus and posttraumatic stress disorder was observed (Hinton et al., 2006; Fagelson, 2007). It is, however, possible that the observed changes in HPA axis of tinnitus patients may be a *result* and not a *cause* of tinnitus.

The link between tinnitus and negative emotional arousal was proposed many years ago by Jastreboff and Hazell to explain why is tinnitus perceived as unpleasant or even dangerous sound (Jastreboff and Hazell, 1993). Recent review of Kraus and Canlon delineates known to date anatomical connectivities between the auditory and limbic systems (reviewed in detail by Kraus and Canlon, 2012). In addition, this important work collected evidence supporting the notion of noise generating synaptic plasticity in the limbic structures. Induction of limbic plasticity is possible due to multi-level projections of the auditory system to the limbic structures. However, known projections of limbic system to the auditory system are rather limited (e.g., projections of amydala to inferior colliculus). If these projections are activated by stress and if this activation could induce plastic changes in the auditory system, remains to be determined.

Scientists in the field currently agree that tinnitus may be triggered by an injury to the inner ear causing decreased activity of the auditory nerve and lastly in plastic changes in central auditory system (Kaltenbach, 2011). Resulting plastic changes in central auditory activity are coupled with altered attention and negative emotions. Can stress induce such critical injury to the inner ear or induce plasticity in higher auditory structures? An important hint was recently delivered by a group studying mild stress model of depression in Sprague-Dawley rat with PET imaging technique. The type of stress was chronic; the stressors were of mixed types and included physical stressors (e.g., sleep deprivation, water deprivation and heat stress) and psycho-social stressors (e.g., crowding, sonic stress). After 4 weeks of random mixed stressing, brain PET analysis revealed the activation of left auditory cortex and deactivation of left inferior colliculus in stressed animals. Changes in the auditory system correlated significantly with the depressive symptoms of experimental animals (Hu et al., 2010). At the same time, no changes were detectible in the visual pathway. Interestingly, activation of left but not right auditory cortex (Brodmann areas 41 and 42) was also reported for tinnitus patients (Arnold et al., 1996; Wang et al., 2001) and could possibly be used as a tinnitus correlate for the experimental animals.

Clinical definition of stress has been improved in the recent years. Importantly, biomarkers and mechanisms are being indentified in a process of stress definition (Piazza et al., 2010). This provides the researchers and clinicians not only with more basic knowledge about stress-induced processes but also with more diagnostic power. Stress is no longer an undefined, sad state of mind but an important, distinct factor in precipitation and amplification of mental and mood disorders (Holsboer and Ising, 2010). Recent research has implicated that living in a city affects stress processing and may be responsible for increased incidence of anxiety disorders in the cities, as opposed to rural communities (Lederbogen et al., 2011). Stress may also precipitate onset of other, non-mental types of diseases, such as asthma or inflammatory bowel disease (Niess et al., 2002; Quarcoo et al., 2009), thus, stressing the role of allostatic load in non-CNS and non-neuronal organs. Including stress as factor of future investigations in the auditory, tinnitus-related research seems to be a logical consequence of above observations.

Furthermore, information collected here, indirectly implies the requirement for psychological assessment during the diagnosis of tinnitus patients, with focus on perceived stress and psychological comorbidity. Such assessment may be performed in form of a self-filled questionnaire or by a clinical psychologist.

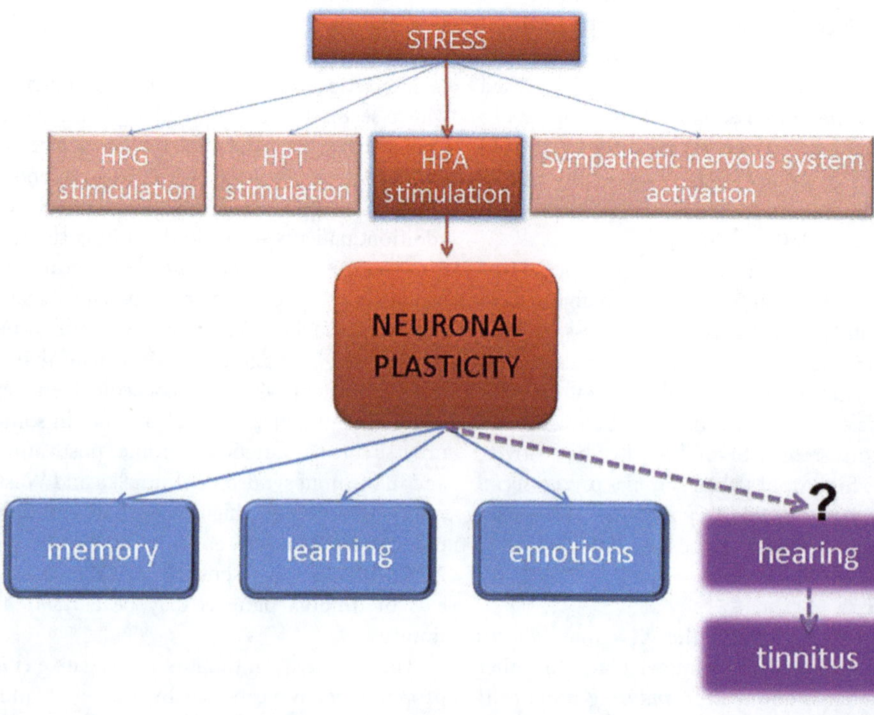

FIGURE 5 | Model of stress-induced neuronal plasticity, which has been accepted in memory, learning, and emotional systems—can it also be truth to explain the induction of auditory pathologies by stress?

Psychological intervention with a goal of stress-management strategies appears to be an indispensable element in tinnitus treatment, especially important to use in very early stages of tinnitus, before the chronification of plastic changes has taken place.

Based on the information collected here, following hypothetical models could possibly explain the causative connection of stress and tinnitus:

- First, stress may potentially activate the *local HPA axis* in the inner ear. The consequences of local overdrive in the HPA system in cochlea are so far unknown.
- Second, stress-activated HPA corticosterone release may affect *mineralcorticoid receptor function in cochlea* and possibly influence the concentration of potassium secreted by stria vascularis, resulting in tinnitus.
- Third, stress-induced activation of HPA axis and corticosteroid release could provoke *pre- or post-synaptic neuronal plasticity* of the auditory system (**Figure 5**).

Exploring the above models and obtaining a clear-cut animal model, which would combine an appropriate stress type *and* tinnitus read-out, is a challenging task. In addition, designing and conducting large epidemiological studies, where individuals would be monitored for stress parameters and followed audiometrically for decades, would be an expensive and a time-consuming mission. Nevertheless, step-by step understanding of how and to what degree the psycho-social or physical stress could affect our peripheral and central auditory system should become a goal in the basic and clinical auditory research.

REFERENCES

Amsterdam, A., and Sasson, R. (2002). The anti-inflammatory action of glucocorticoids is mediated by cell type specific regulation of apoptosis. *Mol. Cell. Endocrinol.* 189, 1–9.

Amsterdam, A., Tajima, K., and Sasson, R. (2002). Cell-specific regulation of apoptosis by glucocorticoids: implication to their anti-inflammatory action. *Biochem. Pharmacol.* 64, 843–850.

Arnold, W., Bartenstein, P., Oestreicher, E., Romer, W., and Schwaiger, M. (1996). Focal metabolic activation in the predominant left auditory cortex in patients suffering from tinnitus: a PET study with [18F]deoxyglucose. *ORL J. Otorhinolaryngol. Relat. Spec.* 58, 195–199.

Baigi, A., Oden, A., Almlid-Larsen, V., Barrenas, M. L., and Holgers, K. M. (2011). Tinnitus in the general population with a focus on noise and stress: a public health study. *Ear Hear.* 32, 787–789.

Berlucchi, G., and Buchtel, H. A. (2009). Neuronal plasticity: historical roots and evolution of meaning. *Exp. Brain Res.* 192, 307–319.

Bose, M., Munoz-Llancao, P., Roychowdhury, S., Nichols, J. A., Jakkamsetti, V., Porter, B., Byrapureddy, R., Salgado, H., Kilgard, M. P., Aboitiz, F., Dagnino-Subiabre, A., and Atzori, M. (2010). Effect of the environment on the dendritic morphology of the rat auditory cortex. *Synapse* 64, 97–110.

Calabrese, F., Molteni, R., Racagni, G., and Riva, M. A. (2009). Neuronal plasticity: a link between stress and mood disorders. *Psychoneuroendocrinology* 34(Suppl. 1), S208–S216.

Canlon, B., Erichsen, S., Nemlander, E., Chen, M., Hossain, A., Celsi, G., and Ceccatelli, S. (2003). Alterations in the intrauterine environment by glucocorticoids modifies the developmental programme of the auditory system. *Eur. J. Neurosci.* 17, 2035–2041.

Curtis, J. H. (1841). Tinnitus aurium. *Lancet* 36, 828–829.

Dagnino-Subiabre, A., Terreros, G., Carmona-Fontaine, C., Zepeda, R., Orellana, J. A., Diaz-Veliz, G., Mora, S., and Aboitiz, F. (2005). Chronic stress impairs acoustic conditioning more than visual conditioning in rats: morphological and behavioural evidence. *Neuroscience* 135, 1067–1074.

Datson, N. A., Morsink, M. C., Meijer, O. C., and de Kloet, E. R. (2008). Central corticosteroid actions: search for gene targets. *Eur. J. Pharmacol.* 583, 272–289.

de Kloet, E. R., Joels, M., and Holsboer, F. (2005). Stress and the brain: from adaptation to disease. *Nat. Rev. Neurosci.* 6, 463–475.

Fagelson, M. A. (2007). The association between tinnitus and posttraumatic stress disorder. *Am. J. Audiol.* 16, 107–117.

Funder, J. W. (1997). Glucocorticoid and mineralocorticoid receptors: biology and clinical relevance. *Annu. Rev. Med.* 48, 231–240.

Furuta, H., Mori, N., Sato, C., Hoshikawa, H., Sakai, S., Iwakura, S., and Doi, K. (1994). Mineralocorticoid type I receptor in the rat cochlea: mRNA identification by polymerase chain reaction (PCR) and *in situ* hybridization. *Hear. Res.* 78, 175–180.

Graham, C. E., Basappa, J., and Vetter, D. E. (2010). A corticotropin-releasing factor system expressed in the cochlea modulates hearing sensitivity and protects against noise-induced hearing loss. *Neurobiol. Dis.* 38, 246–258.

Graham, C. E., and Vetter, D. E. (2011). The mouse cochlea expresses a local hypothalamic-pituitary-adrenal equivalent signaling system and requires corticotropin-releasing factor receptor 1 to establish normal hair cell innervation and cochlear sensitivity. *J. Neurosci.* 31, 1267–1278.

Groeneweg, F. L., Karst, H., de Kloet, E. R., and Joels, M. (2012). Mineralocorticoid and glucocorticoid receptors at the neuronal membrane, regulators of nongenomic corticosteroid signalling. *Mol. Cell. Endocrinol.* 350, 299–309.

Hasson, D., Theorell, T., Wallen, M. B., Leineweber, C., and Canlon, B. (2011). Stress and prevalence of hearing problems in the Swedish working population. *BMC Public Health* 11, 130.

Hebert, S., and Lupien, S. J. (2007). The sound of stress: blunted cortisol reactivity to psychosocial stress in tinnitus sufferers. *Neurosci. Lett.* 411, 138–142.

Hebert, S., Paiement, P., and Lupien, S. J. (2004). A physiological correlate for the intolerance to both internal and external sounds. *Hear. Res.* 190, 1–9.

Hermida, D., Mateos, J. M., Elezgarai, I., Puente, N., Bilbao, A., Bueno-Lopez, J. L., Streit, P., and Grandes, P. (2010). Spatial compartmentalization of AMPA glutamate receptor subunits at the calyx of held synapse. *J. Comp. Neurol.* 518, 163–174.

Hildesheimer, M., Muchnik, C., Rubinstein, M., and Molho, M. (1985). Basic metabolic rate in emotional stress: its potential influence on cochlear function. *Laryngoscope* 95, 63–66.

Hinton, D. E., Chhean, D., Pich, V., Hofmann, S. G., and Barlow, D. H. (2006). Tinnitus among Cambodian refugees: relationship to PTSD severity. *J. Trauma. Stress* 19, 541–546.

Holsboer, F., and Ising, M. (2010). Stress hormone regulation: biological role and translation into therapy. *Annu. Rev. Psychol.* 61, 81–109.

Hougaard, K. S., Barrenas, M. L., Kristiansen, G. B., and Lund, S. P. (2007). No evidence for enhanced noise induced hearing loss after prenatal stress or dexamethasone. *Neurotoxicol. Teratol.* 29, 613–621.

Hu, H., Su, L., Xu, Y. Q., Zhang, H., and Wang, L. W. (2010). Behavioral and [F-18] fluorodeoxyglucose micro positron emission tomography imaging study in a rat chronic mild stress model of depression. *Neuroscience* 169, 171–181.

Iimori, K., Tanaka, M., Kohno, Y., Ida, Y., Nakagawa, R., Hoaki, Y., Tsuda, A., and Nagasaki, N. (1982). Psychological stress enhances noradrenaline turnover in specific brain regions in rats. *Pharmacol. Biochem. Behav.* 16, 637–640.

Jaggi, A. S., Bhatia, N., Kumar, N., Singh, N., Anand, P., and Dhawan, R. (2011). A review on animal models for screening potential anti-stress agents. *Neurol. Sci.* 32, 993–1005.

Jastreboff, P. J., and Hazell, J. W. (1993). A neurophysiological approach to tinnitus: clinical implications. *Br. J. Audiol.* 27, 7–17.

Joels, M., and Baram, T. Z. (2009). The neuro-symphony of stress. *Nat. Rev. Neurosci.* 10, 459–466.

Juster, R. P., Sindi, S., Marin, M. F., Perna, A., Hashemi, A., Pruessner, J. C., and Lupien, S. J. (2011). A clinical allostatic load index is associated with burnout symptoms and hypocortisolemic profiles in healthy workers. *Psychoneuroendocrinology* 36, 797–805.

Kaltenbach, J. A. (2011). Tinnitus: models and mechanisms. *Hear. Res.* 276, 52–60.

Karst, H., Berger, S., Turiault, M., Tronche, F., Schutz, G., and Joels, M. (2005). Mineralocorticoid receptors are indispensable for nongenomic modulation of hippocampal glutamate transmission by corticosterone. *Proc. Natl. Acad. Sci. U.S.A.* 102, 19204–19207.

Kraus, K. S., and Canlon, B. (2012). Neuronal connectivity and interactions between the auditory and limbic systems. Effects of noise and tinnitus. *Hear. Res.* doi: 10.1016/j.heares.2012.02.009. [Epub ahead of print].

Krugers, H. J., Hoogenraad, C. C., and Groc, L. (2010). Stress hormones and AMPA receptor trafficking in synaptic plasticity and memory. *Nat. Rev. Neurosci.* 11, 675–681.

Kudielka, B. M., Schommer, N. C., Hellhammer, D. H., and Kirschbaum, C. (2004). Acute HPA axis responses, heart rate, and mood changes to psychosocial stress (TSST) in humans at different times of day. *Psychoneuroendocrinology* 29, 983–992.

Kudielka, B. M., and Wust, S. (2010). Human models in acute and chronic stress: assessing determinants of individual hypothalamus-pituitary-adrenal axis activity and reactivity. *Stress* 13, 1–14.

Lanting, C. P., de Kleine, E., and van Dijk, P. (2009). Neural activity underlying tinnitus generation: results from PET and fMRI. *Hear. Res.* 255, 1–13.

Lederbogen, F., Kirsch, P., Haddad, L., Streit, F., Tost, H., Schuch, P., Wust, S., Pruessner, J. C., Rietschel, M., Deuschle, M., and Meyer-Lindenberg, A. (2011). City living and urban upbringing affect neural social stress processing in humans. *Nature* 474, 498–501.

Lupien, S. J., Maheu, F., Tu, M., Fiocco, A., and Schramek, T. E. (2007). The effects of stress and stress hormones on human cognition: implications for the field of brain and cognition. *Brain Cogn.* 65, 209–237.

Lupien, S. J., McEwen, B. S., Gunnar, M. R., and Heim, C. (2009). Effects of stress throughout the lifespan on the brain, behaviour and cognition. *Nat. Rev. Neurosci.* 10, 434–445.

Madrigal, J. L., Caso, J. R., de Cristóbal, J., Cardenas, A., Leza, J. C., Lizasoain, I., Lorenzo, P., and Moro, M. A. (2003). Effect of subacute and chronic immobilisation stress on the outcome of permanent focal cerebral ischaemia in rats. *Brain Res.* 979, 137–145.

Mateijsen, D. J., Kingma, C. M., de Jong, P. E., Wit, H. P., and Albers, F. W. (2001). Aldosterone assessment in patients with Meniere's disease. *ORL J. Otorhinolaryngol. Relat. Spec.* 63, 280–286.

Mazurek, B., Haupt, H., Joachim, R., Klapp, B. F., Stover, T., and Szczepek, A. J. (2010). Stress induces transient auditory hypersensitivity in rats. *Hear. Res.* 259, 55–63.

McEwen, B. S. (2003). Mood disorders and allostatic load. *Biol. Psychiatry* 54, 200–207.

McEwen, B. S., and Gianaros, P. J. (2011). Stress- and allostasis-induced brain plasticity. *Annu. Rev. Med.* 62, 431–445.

McEwen, B. S., and Wingfield, J. C. (2003). The concept of allostasis in biology and biomedicine. *Horm. Behav.* 43, 2–15.

Mebis, L., and van den Berghe, G. (2009). The hypothalamus-pituitary-thyroid axis in critical illness. *Neth. J. Med.* 67, 332–340.

Meltser, I., and Canlon, B. (2011). Protecting the auditory system with glucocorticoids. *Hear. Res.* 281, 47–55.

Muchnik, C., Hildesheimer, M., and Rubinstein, M. (1980). Effect of emotional stress on hearing. *Arch. Otorhinolaryngol.* 228, 295–298.

Nakagawa, R., Tanaka, M., Kohno, Y., Noda, Y., and Nagasaki, N. (1981). Regional responses of rat brain noradrenergic neurones to acute intense stress. *Pharmacol. Biochem. Behav.* 14, 729–732.

Nava, E., and Roder, B. (2011). Adaptation and maladaptation insights from brain plasticity. *Prog. Brain Res.* 191, 177–194.

Niess, J. H., Monnikes, H., Dignass, A. U., Klapp, B. F., and Arck, P. C. (2002). Review on the influence of stress on immune mediators, neuropeptides and hormones with relevance for inflammatory bowel disease. *Digestion* 65, 131–140.

Piazza, J. R., Almeida, D. M., Dmitrieva, N. O., and Klein, L. C. (2010). Frontiers in the use of biomarkers of health in research on stress and aging. *J. Gerontol. B Psychol. Sci. Soc. Sci.* 65, 513–525.

Popoli, M., Yan, Z., McEwen, B. S., and Sanacora, G. (2011). The stressed synapse: the impact of stress and glucocorticoids on glutamate transmission. *Nat. Rev. Neurosci.* 13, 22–37.

Quarcoo, D., Pavlovic, S., and Joachim, R. A. (2009). Stress and airway reactivity in a murine model of allergic airway inflammation. *Neuroimmunomodulation* 16, 318–324.

Ruel, J., Wang, J., Rebillard, G., Eybalin, M., Lloyd, R., Pujol, R., and Puel, J. L. (2007). Physiology, pharmacology and plasticity at the inner hair cell synaptic complex. *Hear. Res.* 227, 19–27.

Seydel, C., Haupt, H., Szczepek, A. J., Klapp, B. F., and Mazurek, B. (2010). Long-term improvement in tinnitus after modified tinnitus retraining therapy enhanced by a variety of psychological approaches. *Audiol. Neurootol.* 15, 69–80.

Thomas, W., and Harvey, B. J. (2011). Mechanisms underlying rapid aldosterone effects in the kidney. *Annu. Rev. Physiol.* 73, 335–357.

Tsigos, C., and Chrousos, G. P. (2002). Hypothalamic-pituitary-adrenal axis, neuroendocrine factors and stress. *J. Psychosom. Res.* 53, 865–871.

Ulrich-Lai, Y. M., and Herman, J. P. (2009). Neural regulation of endocrine and autonomic stress responses. *Nat. Rev. Neurosci.* 10, 397–409.

van Cruijsen, N., Dullaart, R. P., Wit, H. P., and Albers, F. W. (2005). Analysis of cortisol and other stress-related hormones in patients with Meniere's disease. *Otol. Neurotol.* 26, 1214–1219.

Vicario, M., Alonso, C., Guilarte, M., Serra, J., Martinez, C., Gonzalez-Castro, A. M., Lobo, B., Antolin, M., Andreu, A. L., Garcia-Arumi, E., Casellas, M., Saperas, E., Malagelada, J. R., Azpiroz, F., and Santos, J. (2012). Chronic psychosocial stress induces reversible mitochondrial damage and corticotropin-releasing factor receptor type-1 upregulation in the rat intestine and IBS-like gut dysfunction. *Psychoneuroendocrinology* 37, 65–77.

Wang, H., Tian, J., Yin, D., Jiang, S., Yang, W., Han, D., Yao, S., and Shao, M. (2001). Regional glucose metabolic increases in left auditory cortex in tinnitus patients: a preliminary study with positron emission tomography. *Chin. Med. J. (Engl.)* 114, 848–851.

Wang, H., Yin, G., Rogers, K., Miralles, C., de Blas, A. L., and Rubio, M. E. (2011). Monaural conductive hearing loss alters the expression of the GluA3 AMPA and glycine receptor alpha1 subunits in bushy and fusiform cells of the cochlear nucleus. *Neuroscience* 199, 438–451.

Wang, Y., and Liberman, M. C. (2002). Restraint stress and protection from acoustic injury in mice. *Hear. Res.* 165, 96–102.

Weitzman, E. D., Fukushima, D., Nogeire, C., Roffwarg, H., Gallagher, T. F., and Hellman, L. (1971). Twenty-four hour pattern of the episodic secretion of cortisol in normal subjects. *J. Clin. Endocrinol. Metab.* 33, 14–22.

Whirledge, S., and Cidlowski, J. A. (2010). Glucocorticoids, stress, and fertility. *Minerva Endocrinol.* 35, 109–125.

Yao, X., and Rarey, K. E. (1996). Localization of the mineralocorticoid receptor in rat cochlear tissue. *Acta Otolaryngol.* 116, 493–496.

Yehuda, R., Levengood, R. A., Schmeidler, J., Wilson, S., Guo, L. S., and Gerber, D. (1996). Increased pituitary activation following metyrapone administration in post-traumatic stress disorder. *Psychoneuroendocrinology* 21, 1–16.

Yoshida, N., Kristiansen, A., and Liberman, M. C. (1999). Heat stress and protection from permanent acoustic injury in mice. *J. Neurosci.* 19, 10116–10124.

Zhong, S. X., and Liu, Z. H. (2009). Expression patterns of Nedd4 isoforms and SGK1 in the rat cochlea. *Acta Otolaryngol.* 129, 935–939.

Zuo, J., Curtis, L. M., Yao, X., ten Cate, W. J., Bagger-Sjoback, D., Hultcrantz, M., and Rarey, K. E. (1995). Glucocorticoid receptor expression in the postnatal rat cochlea. *Hear. Res.* 87, 220–227.

17

Tinnitus: Network pathophysiology-network pharmacology

Ana B. Elgoyhen[1]*, Berthold Langguth[2], Sven Vanneste[3] and Dirk De Ridder[3]

[1] *Instituto de Investigaciones en Ingeniería Genética y Biología Molecular, Consejo Nacional de Investigaciones Científicas y Técnicas and Tercera Cátedra de Farmacología, Facultad de Medicina, Universidad de Buenos Aires, Buenos Aires, Argentina*
[2] *Interdisciplinary Tinnitus Clinic, Departments of Psychiatry and Psychotherapy, University of Regensburg, Regensburg, Germany*
[3] *TRI, BRAI²N and Department of Neurosurgery, University Hospital Antwerp, Edegem, Belgium*

****Correspondence:***
Ana B. Elgoyhen, Instituto de Investigaciones en Ingeniería Genética y Biología Molecular, Consejo Nacionla de Investigaciones Científicas y Técnicas, Vuelta de Obligado 2490, 1428 Buenos Aires, Argentina.
e-mail: elgoyhen@dna.uba.ar, abelgoyhen@gmail.com

Tinnitus, the phantom perception of sound, is a prevalent disorder. One in 10 adults has clinically significant subjective tinnitus, and for one in 100, tinnitus severely affects their quality of life. Despite the significant unmet clinical need for a safe and effective drug targeting tinnitus relief, there is currently not a single Food and Drug Administration (FDA)-approved drug on the market. The search for drugs that target tinnitus is hampered by the lack of a deep knowledge of the underlying neural substrates of this pathology. Recent studies are increasingly demonstrating that, as described for other central nervous system (CNS) disorders, tinnitus is a pathology of brain networks. The application of graph theoretical analysis to brain networks has recently provided new information concerning their topology, their robustness and their vulnerability to attacks. Moreover, the philosophy behind drug design and pharmacotherapy in CNS pathologies is changing from that of "magic bullets" that target individual chemoreceptors or "disease-causing genes" into that of "magic shotguns," "promiscuous" or "dirty drugs" that target "disease-causing networks," also known as network pharmacology. In the present work we provide some insight into how this knowledge could be applied to tinnitus pathophysiology and pharmacotherapy.

Keywords: graph analysis, brain networks, network pharmacology, phantom percept, tinnitus, small-world, scale-free, magic bullets

TINNITUS PHARMACOTHERAPY: WHERE DO WE STAND?

Tinnitus, the phantom perception of sound, represents a highly prevalent and distressing condition. Although most cases of tinnitus derive from deprivation of auditory input, it goes beyond the classical definition of an otologic illness, since it encompasses a range of symptoms that are likely to place a huge burden on patients and significantly impair quality of life (Jastreboff, 1990). This can include irritability, agitation, stress, insomnia, anxiety, and depression. In fact, for one in 100 adults, tinnitus affects their ability to lead a normal day-to-day life (Vio and Holme, 2005). Estimates indicate that 13 million people in Western Europe and the USA currently seek medical advice for their tinnitus (Vio and Holme, 2005).

The quest toward finding a drug that targets tinnitus has not been that fulfilling. Although a wide variety of compounds is used off-label to treat tinnitus patients, there is still no US Food and Drug Administration (FDA) or European Medicines Agency (EMA) approved drug on the market. The list of used compounds includes anticonvulsants, anxiolytic, antidepressants, NMDA antagonists, cholinergic antagonists, antihistamines, vasodilators, antipsychotics, and calcium antagonists, to name a few (Langguth et al., 2009; Elgoyhen and Langguth, 2010). In some cases, the rationale behind the use of them is to treat the co-morbidities that come along with tinnitus, like depression and anxiety (Johnson et al., 1993; Sullivan et al., 1993; Bahmad et al., 2006). In others, it is derived from the use of drugs which are effective in disorders thought to share some commonalities with tinnitus, like anticonvulsants used in epilepsy (Hoekstra et al., 2011) and the calcium antagonist gabapentin used in neuropathic pain (Bauer and Brozoski, 2007). Even further, some drugs are used based on known underlying neuronal changes thought to be a neural correlate of tinnitus. Such is the case of NMDA receptor antagonists (Azevedo and Figueiredo, 2007; Figueiredo et al., 2008; Suckfull et al., 2011) and $GABA_A$ agonists (Johnson et al., 1993; Gananca et al., 2002; Azevedo and Figueiredo, 2007), used with the hope of reversing the increased neuronal excitability observed in several regions of the auditory pathway (Eggermont and Roberts, 2004). Some drugs have been reported to provide moderate relief of symptoms in a subset of patients. However, most drugs have not proven sufficient effectiveness in randomized controlled clinical trials in order to be approved and marketed specifically for tinnitus (Langguth et al., 2009; Elgoyhen and Langguth, 2010; Langguth and Elgoyhen, 2011).

Thus, novel pharmacological approaches for treating tinnitus are required in order to address a widely recognized, yet largely underserved, and unmet, clinical need. Although early on classified as an auditory problem, recent work is indicating that tinnitus is a central nervous system (CNS) disorder, where dynamic multiple parallel overlapping brain networks are involved (Eggermont and Roberts, 2004; Schlee et al., 2009a,b; De Ridder et al., 2011a). Thus, strategies followed in the development of drugs for other CNS pathologies might give some insight into possible avenues in the design of tinnitus pharmacotherapies. In the present work we review some recent trends in the discovery of CNS acting drugs, describe new ways of analyzing brain networks in health and disease and propose how this knowledge could be extrapolated to tinnitus.

DRUG DISCOVERY IN CNS DISORDERS

Serendipity has played a major role in the initial discovery of CNS acting compounds, like the first psychotropic drugs that led to modern pharmacological treatment of psychiatric diseases (Ban, 2006). Although a detailed understanding of the pathophysiology and etiology of CNS disorders remains elusive, the last decade has witnessed a huge leap in our understanding of the basic biological processes that contribute to many human disorders. However, this has not been paralled by an increase in the number of approved new molecular entities. From 1950 to 2008, the FDA approved 1222 new drugs including biologicals (Munos, 2009). Although the investment of pharmaceutical industries in research and development has grown from US$2 to $50 billion/year from 1980 to 2005 (Conn and Roth, 2008; Paul et al., 2010), the number of approved drugs per year, about 25, is not greater than 50 years ago. Moreover, of those 25, only two were for psychiatric diseases in 2009 (Hughes, 2010). Thus, the scale of investment has not been matched by output. In addition, there has not been much innovation (Rask-Andersen et al., 2011). For example, the most widely prescribed antipsychotics olanzapine, risperidone, and quetiapine, share mechanisms of action with clozapine, discovered in the 1950s (Conn and Roth, 2008). Clozapine was developed as a chlorpromazine analog, whose antipsychotic actions were discovered serendipitously when being used as a preanesthetic agent in psychiatric patients (Delay et al., 1952). For more modern antipsychotics (with the exceptions of aripiprazole and the substituted benzamides) a major goal has been to create clozapine-like compounds, devoid of its more serious side effects (Roth et al., 2004; Conn and Roth, 2008). A similar scenario can be seen in the case of drugs used for anxiety, depression, and epilepsy. Thus, the gold standard of drug discovery as from the 1960s has been the design of more selective drugs with ideally one specific target, with the aim of reducing side effects (Roth et al., 2004; Hopkins, 2007, 2008; Conn and Roth, 2008). However, over the past decade, there has been a significant decrease in the rate by which new drug candidates translated into effective clinical therapies. Even more striking, there has been a worrying rise in late-stage phase 2 and phase 3 attrition, that is leading to a reduction in revenues and a financial shock to the pharmaceutical industry (Kola and Landis, 2004; Hopkins, 2007, 2008). This might derive from the innermost strategy behind modern drug design: drugs selective for a single molecular target, the "one gene, one drug, one disease" paradigm best known as the Paul Ehrlich's "magic bullet" concept of chemotherapy (Kaufmann, 2008), without acknowledging the network structure of the brain and the properties and behavior of real world networks as described in the following sections.

COMPLEX REAL WORLD NETWORKS

Reductionism dominated biological research during the last century and provided a wealth of information regarding the individual cellular components and their functions. However, biological functions can rarely be attributed to an individual molecule. Instead, they are the consequence of complex interactions between the cell's numerous constituents, such as proteins, DNA, RNA, small molecules, and of intercellular interactions (Kitano, 2002; Barabasi and Oltvai, 2004). Therefore, a key challenge for biology in the twenty-first century is to understand the structure and the dynamics of the complex intra- and intercellular web of interactions that contribute to the structure and function of a living cell, organ or organism (Barabasi and Oltvai, 2004). Thus, reductionism has made its way to holism and systems biology has emerged as a scientific discipline. It is based upon the notion that all the properties, function and/or behavior of a given system cannot be determined or explained by the properties and function of its component parts alone. Instead, the system as a whole determines in an important way how the parts behave and as a result new properties emerge (Kitano, 2002). These "emergent" properties cannot be predicted *a priori*, based on the properties of the individual elements. Such is the case of the mind and of mind states like consciousness, emergent properties of the brain occurring between multiple physical and functional levels (Gazzaniga, 2010; Bassett and Gazzaniga, 2011).

An important milestone over the past decade has been the understanding that the structure and evolution of networks appearing in social, technological, and natural systems over time follows a number of basic and reproducible organizing principles, which can be explained by the application of graph theoretical analysis to describe network properties (Albert and Barabasi, 2002). A graph is an abstract representation of a network where nodes or vertices are connected by links or edges (**Figure 1**). For more than 40 years scientists treated complex networks as being

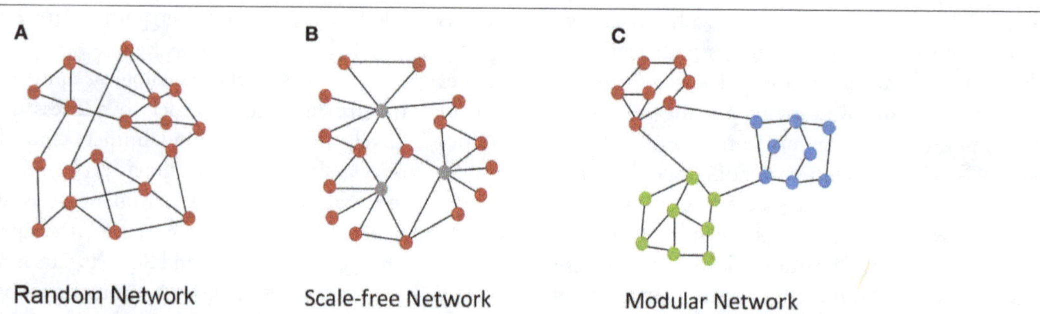

FIGURE 1 | Network topologies. (A) An example of a random network with no high degree hubs, where nodes (red circles) are connected by edges (black lines). **(B)** A scale-free network with high degree hubs (gray circles). **(C)** A modular network where nodes within a module (i.e., red, green, and blue modules) are highly connected to each other and only sparsely connected to nodes of another module.

random (Erdos and Renyi, 1959). In random graphs, connections between the network nodes are present with a fixed and equal likelihood (Erdos and Renyi, 1959). However, Watts and Strogatz (1998) demonstrated that most real world networks are not random nor regular lattices, but follow the "small-world" phenomenon, where the path length between nodes (the average of the shortest distance between pairs of nodes counted in number of edges) is small, like in random networks, but the clustering coefficient (the likelihood that neighbors of a node will also be connected) is high, unlike, random networks. Watts and Strogatz described the small-world properties of networks found in the nervous system of the nematode *Caenorhabditis elegans*, a social network of actors and the network of power plants in the United States. A second major discovery in real world network topology was presented by Barabasi and Albert (1999). They proposed a model for the growth of a network where the likelihood that newly added edges connect to a node depends upon the degree (number of edges) of this node, following a preferential attachment behavior. Thus, nodes that have a high degree (hubs) are more likely to get even more edges. This is the network equivalent of "the rich getting richer" (Barabasi and Bonabeau, 2003). Networks generated in this way maintain the short path length of small-world networks (Cohen and Havlin, 2003), but are characterized by a degree distribution described by a power law. These networks are called "scale-free" in the sense that some hubs have a seemingly unlimited number of links and no node is typical of the others (**Figure 1**). Many other small-world networks have exponential or exponentially truncated power law distributions, implying relatively reduced probabilities of huge hubs (Amaral et al., 2000; Albert and Barabasi, 2002). Determining the topology of a network is important in order to understand the system's behavior, as power laws emerge when there is a transition from disorder to order (Barabasi, 2002). The accidental failure of a number of nodes in a random network can fracture the system into non-communicating islands. In contrast, scale-free networks are resilient to change, have error tolerance and attack vulnerability: they are more robust in the face of random failures or attacks, but they are highly vulnerable to a coordinated attack against their Achilles' heel, the hubs (Albert et al., 2000). These alternate behaviors acquire utmost importance when designing pharmacotherapies for network pathologies.

Since the first description of scale-free networks, most complex networks have been described to have this topology: scientific papers linked by citations, the World Wide Web (Albert et al., 1999; Barabasi and Albert, 1999), e-mail networks (Ebel et al., 2002), epidemic spreads (Pastor-Satorras and Vespignani, 2001), airline transportation networks (Newman, 2003), metabolic, protein-protein interaction and gen interaction networks (Jeong et al., 2000; Podani et al., 2001; Ravasz et al., 2002; Wuchty et al., 2003; Almaas et al., 2004; Barabasi and Oltvai, 2004; Tong et al., 2004), to name a few. But what about brain networks?

BRAIN NETWORKS

Only recently graph theoretical analysis has been applied to the study of brain networks. These has been motivated by the idea that brain functions are not solely attributable to individual regions and connections, but are emergent features of the topology of the network as a whole, the "connectome" of the brain (Sporns, 2011a). Moreover, it has been boosted by the advancement of the analysis of brain connectivity both at the structural and functional levels (Sporns, 2011a). In this section we will only highlight some important findings and conclusions derived from the application of graph analysis to the topology of brain networks. For comprehensive reviews see Reijneveld et al. (2007), Bullmore and Sporns (2009), Bullmore and Bassett (2011), Sporns (2011a).

Magnetic resonance imaging (MRI) as well as diffusor tensor/spectrum/kurtosis imaging (DTI/DSI/DKI) and the application of graph analysis to some of these data are delivering increasingly detailed maps of large scale human brain structural connectivity and of its topology (**Figure 2**). In addition, graph analysis to functional connectivity, that is correlated activity in a network, can be applied to data derived from functional MRI (fMRI), magnetoencephalography (MEG), and electroencephalography (EEG). One important caveat to the graph-based study of functional brain organization is how to define the individual nodes that makes up a brain network. If the nodes of the graph do not accurately represent reality then the graph theoretic properties will diverge from the true properties of the system. Therefore, data acquisition and preprocessing are important issues (for review see Bullmore and Bassett, 2011). Effective

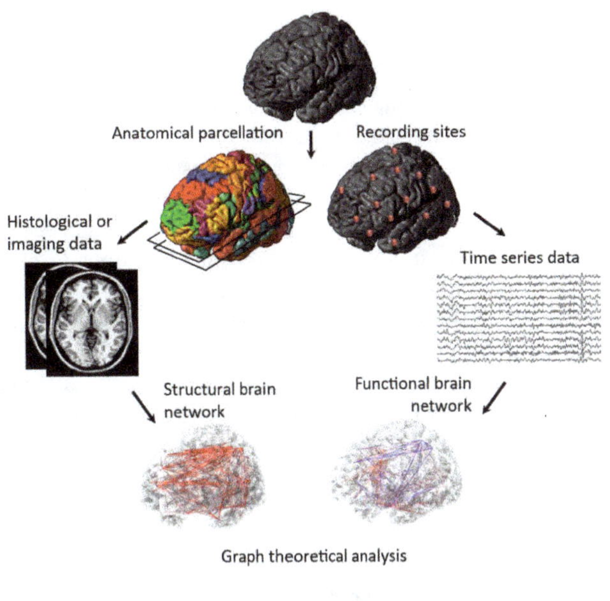

FIGURE 2 | Graph analysis to brain networks. Structural (including either gray or white matter measurements using histological or imaging data) or functional data (including resting-state fMRI, fMRI, EEG, or MEG data) is the starting point. Nodes are defined (e.g., anatomically defined regions of histological, MRI or diffusion tensor imaging data in structural networks or EEG electrodes or MEG sensors in functional networks) and an association between nodes is established (coherence, connection probability, or correlations in cortical thickness). The pairwise association between nodes is then computed, and usually thresholded to create a binary (adjacency) matrix. A brain network is then constructed from nodes (brain regions) and edges (pairwise associations that were larger than the chosen threshold).

connectivity of brain networks, which refers to information transfer in a network and has some directionality embedded in it, can be analyzed by transfer entropy, Granger causality, or partial directed coherence to generate a directed graph, which involves estimating the causal influence that each element of a system exerts on the behavior of other elements (Sporns, 2011b). However, so far, most graph analyses have been applied to structural and functional connectivity to generate undirected graphs. In addition, although most studies use simpler unweighted graphs, weighted network analysis also has been applied. In these graphs edges can have continuously variable weights indicating the strength or effectiveness of connections (Reijneveld et al., 2007).

Graph analysis of structural and functional connectivity is consistently showing characteristic non-random properties of brain networks (Reijneveld et al., 2007; Bullmore and Sporns, 2009; Bullmore and Bassett, 2011; Sporns, 2011c). At the structural level, several studies have revealed small-world attributes (Bullmore and Sporns, 2009; Sporns, 2011c). Such is the case of the analysis of human brain networks on the basis of correlations in cortical gray matter thickness measured using MRI (He et al., 2007; Chen et al., 2008), DTI, and tractography of cortical and basal brain gray matter areas (Iturria-Medina et al., 2007, 2008; Gong et al., 2009) and diffusion spectrum imaging of cortical regions (Hagmann et al., 2007). In addition, these studies demonstrate the presence of hierarchical brain modules. Modularity refers to the existence of clusters or "network communities" whose constituent brain regions are more densely connected to each other than to regions in other modules (**Figure 1**). Thus, neurons and brain regions that are spatially close have a relatively high probability of being connected forming a module, whereas connections between spatially remote neurons or brain regions are less likely. Since longer axonal projections are more expensive in terms of their material and energy costs, this layout minimizes wiring costs (Chklovskii et al., 2002). Nodes of high degree, hubs, exist within modules, and also connect to hubs in other modules, thus maintaining the short path length typical of small-world networks, providing high global efficiency of parallel information transfer (Bullmore and Sporns, 2009; Sporns, 2011c). However, structural brain networks seem to lack extremely high degree nodes characteristic of a scale-free network and rather follow an exponentially truncated power law distribution (He et al., 2007).

Additional information of brain network topology has derived from functional imaging and electrophysiology. Graph analysis from fMRI data has described small-world topology of brain networks, with a truncated power law distribution (Salvador et al., 2005; Achard et al., 2006). In contrast, scale-free topology has been also described in networks derived from fMRI recordings both during task and resting state (Eguiluz et al., 2005; van den Heuvel et al., 2008). Functional connectivity also has been analyzed using a measure of generalized synchronization and then thresholded to generate functional networks, in several studies derived from MEG data sets (Stam and van Dijk, 2002; Stam, 2004). In addition, graph analysis has been applied to wavelet correlation estimates of frequency-dependent functional connectivity between MEG sensors (Bassett et al., 2006). These studies have shown small-world properties of brain networks. Graph analysis to EEG wavelet coefficients found small-world properties in the alpha and beta band networks (Jin et al., 2011). The development of time-varying graphs with fixed nodes but evolving links derived from scalp EEG recordings reported both small-world and scale-free topology of brain networks (Dimitriadis et al., 2010). Two further studies that have used alternate analysis different from graph theory to EEG recordings, have also shown scale-free properties of brain activity: the analysis of fine temporal structures of arrhythmic brain activity by using nested-frequency EEG analysis (He et al., 2010) and EEG microstates (van de Ville et al., 2010).

From the available structural and functional studies it can be concluded that large-brain networks exhibit a similar organization, with several studies demonstrating functional clusters or modules, highly connected hub nodes, short path lengths, and high global efficiency. The general picture that arises so far from structural studies is that brain networks have small-world topologies but are not scale-free. However, at the functional level it is still a matter of debate whether they are also scale-free (Reijneveld et al., 2007). Differences might derive from the fact that different methods describe different aspects of neuronal networks. From an evolutionary perspective, it can be argued that small-world brain networks have been selected to solve the economic problem of maximizing information processing efficiency, while minimizing wiring costs (Bullmore and Sporns, 2009). Structural studies have revealed important hubs within the parietal and frontal lobes of the cerebral cortex (Iturria-Medina et al., 2008; Gong et al., 2009; van den Heuvel and Sporns, 2011). Most importantly, several independent diffusion imaging data sets have reported a high centrality for the precuneus, the posterior cingulate cortex, and neighboring regions (Hagmann et al., 2007, 2008; Iturria-Medina et al., 2007, 2008). A very recent study that applied graph analysis to DTI data showed the presence of 12 strongly interconnected bihemispheric hub regions, comprising the precuneus, superior frontal, and superior parietal cortex, as well as the subcortical hippocampus, putamen, and thalamus (van den Heuvel and Sporns, 2011). Importantly, these hub regions were not only individually central but formed a "rich club" organization, since they were found to be more densely interconnected than would be expected based only on their degree. This rich club organization of the human brain connectome might optimize global brain communication efficiency for healthy cognitive brain functioning (van den Heuvel and Sporns, 2011).

The analysis of underlying structural and functional network topologies provides a powerful tool to understand the system's behavior that cannot be attained with other approaches to complex systems. Thus, if the brain had a scale-free topology, it would be very vulnerable to hub failures or attacks (Albert et al., 2000). In their analysis of discrete wavelet transform to fMRI time series, Achard and collaborators (2006) described small-world properties of cortical and subcortical regions with a truncated power law distribution, which were as resilient to random error, but more resistant to targeted attacks than scale-free networks. Moreover, up to 40% of the most connected nodes in the brain network could be eliminated before precipitating a 50% reduction in size (and twofold increase in path length) of the largest connected cluster. Therefore, the small-world architecture of the brain may confer distinctive benefits in terms of robustness to both random elimination of nodes and selective attack on hubs (Achard et al., 2006). Thus, it increases resilience and reduces vulnerability to individual hub attacks. In addition, the rich club organization described by van den Heuvel and Sporns (2011) provides an additional level of resilience to its core, in case of malfunction of any one of its individual key hubs.

BRAIN NETWORKS IN PATHOLOGY

Only very recently graph theoretical analysis has been applied to a wide variety of CNS disorders and, therefore, the power of this approach toward understanding brain pathology is at its infancy. Changes in network topology have been analyzed in disorders such as schizophrenia, epilepsy, Alzheimer's disease, multiple sclerosis, acute depression, fronto-temporal lobe degeneration, stroke, spinal cord injury, early blindness, and attention deficit hyperactivity disorder (for reviews see Reijneveld et al., 2007; Bassett and Bullmore, 2009; Bullmore and Sporns, 2009).

Reduction in small-world properties has been described in patients with Alzheimer's disease, associated with less efficient information exchange between brain areas, supporting the disconnection hypothesis proposed for this pathology, as well as for many other neurological and psychiatric disorders (Catani and Ffytche, 2005). A loss of small-world properties has also been described in schizophrenia, again supporting the disconnection hypothesis. Network organization derived from graph analysis appears to have increased randomization (Bassett et al., 2008; Lynall et al., 2010; Rubinov and Bassett, 2011) and to be less cost-efficient (Bassett et al., 2009) when compared with healthy controls. In addition, topological abnormalities in people with schizophrenia include a reduced hierarchy of the multimodal cortex (Bassett et al., 2008) and less globally integrated brain structures, with a reduced central role for key frontal hubs, resulting in a limited structural capacity to integrate information across brain regions (Lynall et al., 2010; van den Heuvel et al., 2010). Loss of small-world organization has also been reported in depressed patients during sleep (Leistedt et al., 2009), increased randomization in frontal lobe epilepsy (van Dellen et al., 2009) and shift to more regular networks in children with attention deficit hyperactivity disorder (Wang et al., 2009).

Thus, it seems that in general, brain pathology leads to alteration in small-world network properties with a decreased global integration. Although, it is too soon to fully appreciate the power of graph analysis in CNS disorders, it undoubtedly opens new avenues toward understanding brain diseases. Changes in network topology might be used as clinically useful diagnostic markers and to monitor progression of disease states (Bullmore and Sporns, 2009). Moreover, graph theory allows identifying hubs and modeling network attacks (Albert et al., 2000), which might give hints to determine which treatment approach is the best option at the network level.

NETWORK PHARMACOLOGY

One major outcome derived from the fact that most complex biological systems are networks, either small-world and/or scale-free, very robust, and resilient to change, has been a very recent shift in the philosophy behind drug design and pharmacotherapy, which is leading to a new trend: in Andrew Hopkins' own words "*network pharmacology: the next paradigm in drug discovery*" (Hopkins, 2008). This means moving away from Ehrlich's "magic bullets" that target individual chemoreceptors or "disease-causing genes" (Kaufmann, 2008), into "magic shotguns", "promiscuous" or "dirty drugs" that target "disease-causing networks" (Roth et al., 2004; Csermely et al., 2005; Sams-Dodd, 2005; Hopkins, 2008). Following systems biology principle of emergence, combinations of compounds could be more effective than the sum of the effectiveness of the individual agents themselves (Keith et al., 2005; Kung et al., 2005). Shotguns can make a dramatic impact on disease outcome, as evidenced by the success of the multidrug antiretroviral therapy in decreasing human immunodeficiency virus mortality rates (Imaz et al., 2011). Moreover, multiple attacks have been selected in nature as defense systems and communication, therefore, magic shotguns seem as an evolutionary selected feature. Thus, snake (Bohlen et al., 2011), spider (Rash and Hodgson, 2002; Siemens et al., 2006) cone snail (Olivera and Teichert, 2007) and scorpion (Rodriguez de la Vega et al., 2010) venoms comprise multimolecules, plants employ batteries of various factors to avoid pathogenic attacks (Uma et al., 2011) and honey bee queens produce a mandibular pheromone that is a cocktail of nine interacting components required to attract worker bees, to attract drones for mating and to prevent workers from reproducing (Keeling et al., 2003).

The importance of multi-targeting pharmacology has also recently been encouraged by the observation that novel well-tolerated protein kinase drugs, such as Gleevec (Imatinib) and Sutent (SU11248), exhibit binding promiscuity for multiple kinases and therefore are less selective than initially thought (Hampton, 2004; Fabian et al., 2005). Polypharmacology is probably not a novel notion, however, what is new is the acknowledgment of its benefits for efficacy. Thus, the pleiotropic actions of clozapine are probably responsible for its exceptionally beneficial actions in schizophrenia and related disorders. Clozapine has a very complex pharmacological profile, with high affinity for a number of receptors, including dopamine (D4), serotonin (5-HT2A, 5-HT2C, 5-HT6, 5-HT7), muscarinic (M1, M2, M3, M4, M5), adrenergic (α1- and α2-subtypes), and other biogenic amine receptors (Roth et al., 2004). Moreover, many newer generation anti-psychotics might have failed in the clinics because of higher target specificity (Roth et al., 2004). Likewise, the pleiotropic actions of antidepressants on signal transduction and neuronal mitogenesis are probably required for the beneficial effects of antidepressants on mood disorders. Moreover, the "dual- and triple-action" antidepressants, which inhibit the reuptake of both 5-HT and other biogenic amines (for example, dopamine and noradrenaline), have been shown to be more effective than "single-action" antidepressants (Roth et al., 2004; Millan, 2006). In a recent study, Yildirim et al. (Yildirim et al., 2007) applied network analysis to 1178 FDA-approved drugs and drugs targets as of March 29, 2006, in order to understand drug design strategies followed by the pharmaceutical industry. To investigate the relationships between approved drugs and their targets they built a bipartite drug-target network by integrating publicly available drug data with genetic-disease associations, gene-expression information and protein-protein interaction data. If drugs acted selectively on single targets, one would expect isolated, bipartite nodes and not a network structure. Not surprisingly, the authors found a rich network of polypharmacology interactions between drugs and their targets. Moreover, drugs acting on single targets were the exception. They found a giant component, the largest connected component of the network, with 476 drugs comprising a tightly interconnected neurological drug cluster. Thus, although initially designed as magic bullets, most CNS-acting drugs are magic shotguns and this is probably the reason behind the fact that they are effective in CNS disorders.

The use of multi-targets is further supported by the work of Agoston and collaborators (Agoston et al., 2005). Most studies that have analyzed the stability of networks under failures or attacks have used a model with a complete elimination of an element from the network in order to assess network stability (Albert et al., 2000; Watts, 2002; Shargel et al., 2003; Valente et al., 2004). Agoston and collaborators (Agoston et al., 2005), however, used an alternative approach, where they studied if the partial inactivation of several targets is more efficient than the complete inactivation of a single target. This scenario most closely resembles pharmacotherapy, since at plasma concentrations attained with pharmacological doses, most drugs probably weaken targets rather completely ablate them. Moreover, if only a partial weakening of targets is needed, this could probably be attained at lower plasma concentrations, thus requiring lower doses with concomitant fewer side effects. Partial attacks also mimic other physiological scenarios and treatments, where the complete elimination of a node within a network is a rather unusual phenomenon. By analyzing the regulatory scale-free network of *E. coli* and *S. cerevisiae* Agoston and collaborators (2005) concluded that the efficacy of attenuation of targets by multi-target attacks is higher than that of a single-target knockout. In terms of pharmacology, this suggests that drugs with multiple targets or drug combinations might have a better chance to affect the complex equilibrium of the whole system than single target drugs. Moreover, it is sufficient that these multi-target drugs affect their targets only partially, which correlates with the low-affinity interactions of most drugs with several of their targets (Csermely et al., 2005).

Given that promiscuous or dirty drugs are probably more efficient than highly selective ones, can they be designed rationally? In principle, the magic shotgun approach can be attained in four ways: using a drug with multiple mechanisms of actions, prescribing a combination of drugs, the development of multicomponent drugs that contain two or more active ingredients formulated in the same delivery device, or a designer polypharmacology, e.g., a drug with two or more pharmacophores (Borisy et al., 2003; Morphy et al., 2004; Roth et al., 2004; Csermely et al., 2005; Keith et al., 2005; Hopkins, 2007, 2008). The complexity imposed by exploring dosage ranging, drug interaction, and safety studies may significantly raise the practical cost and complexity of developing combination therapies. Potential drug interactions at the pharmacokinetic and pharmacodynamic level have to be considered, since two drugs that themselves are efficient and safe when prescribed separately might not necessarily be efficient and safe when used in combination (Hopkins et al., 2006). However, these problems can be reduced with polypharmacology, since it allows combination therapies at lower doses, resulting in higher efficacy and/or reduced side-effects compared to monotherapies (Morphy et al., 2004; Keith et al., 2005). For example, low-dose combinations of calcium-channel blockers and angiotensin-receptor antagonists are effective for the treatment of hypertension (Andreadis et al., 2005) and low doses of atypical antipsychotics, such as quetiapine, olanzapine, or risperidone, can improve the antidepressant efficacy of selective serotonin reuptake inhibitors, such as fluoxetine, in the treatment of refractory depressed patients (Rasmussen, 2006). Pharmacodynamic and pharmacokinetic relationship, are substantially less complex if polypharmacological action is derived from a single agent and thus approaches to develop multifunctional drugs with more than one pharmacophore are under way (Morphy et al., 2004). An example is ladostigil (TV3326), a novel neuroprotective agent being investigated for the treatment of neurodegenerative disorders like Alzheimer's disease, Lewy body disease, and Parkinson's disease. It combines the acetylcholinesterase and monoamino oxidase (MAO)-A and -B activities in one molecule and was developed by combining the active (MAO inhibitory and neuroprotective) pharmacophore of the antiparkinsonian MAO-B inhibitor rasagiline with the carbamate cholinesterase inhibitory moiety of the anti-Alzheimer's drug rivastigmine (Weinstock et al., 2006).

Finding the right combination of targets to aim imposes a further complexity when compared to single target therapies. This is the main challenge faced at present in network pharmacology and the field is still "lost in translation" in trying to understand the meaning and the outreach of this new discipline. Following network biology principles, drug discovery approaches might involve the identification of combinations of small molecules that perturb networks in a desired fashion. Drug combinations have been used with compounds already known to be effective in the disease of interest, or where there is a clear rationale for the combination (Millan, 2006). However, such limited combination testing samples only a tiny fraction of the combinatorial pharmacological space and is unlikely to result in the selection of optimal combinations among the very large number of possibilities. A small number of compounds will provide a very large number of combinations and, therefore, efficient screening methods are needed. High-throughput based behavioral screenings which rely on the semi-automated screening of candidate drugs in broad-based behavioral assays in animals, might be used to screen libraries of compounds and find those combinations which are enriched for activity at CNS targets. These approaches that are increasingly offered by specialized companies, have the advantage that they analyze responses to drugs at the level of entire organisms and, therefore, based in their biological function, without the need of having a lead compound, as needed in *in vitro* assays (Roth et al., 2004; Millan, 2006). In addition, large scale multielectrode brain recordings in animals now offer unique opportunities to assay spatiotemporal patterns of neuronal assemblies in brain networks (Buzsaki, 2004;

Lehew and Nicolelis, 2008). Graph analysis applied to these multielectrode array approaches might aid toward defining changes in brain topology and hubs in animal models of disease and restoration of the topology during treatment. These methods can provide insights into network-level mechanisms of action of compounds, even when synapse or receptor-level mechanisms are not understood. In addition, it is likely that graph analysis to structural and functional brain networks will further broaden our understanding of treatment effects, will aid toward the design of new therapeutical approaches and help to decipher how therapeutically effective pharmacotherapeutic treatments act on topologically sub-optimal network configurations in patients (Bullmore and Sporns, 2009). Thus, the potential use of fMRI on optimizing drug development (phMRI, pharmacological MRI) is beginning to be appreciated and promises to be part of a sequence of events that could transform drug development for disorders of the CNS (Honey and Bullmore, 2004; Borsook et al., 2006).

Although the rationale behind the use of magic shotguns, promiscuous or dirty drugs is compelling, pharmaceutical industries are being very slow in conquering these approaches. This is probably due to the fact that it is still a challenge to decipher which combinatorial assembly of targets (nodes) to aim, on the one hand, and which combination of dirty drugs is needed in order to best weaken those nodes, on the other. Moreover, the balancing act of optimizing multiple activities, while minimizing unwanted off-target side effects, is a challenge (Hopkins, 2007, 2008). However, network pharmacology will probably become an essential component of drug-development strategies. Indeed, network concepts have already been applied in drug discovery studies in anti-cancer drugs for example (Azmi et al., 2010). Moreover, drug-target networks linking approved or experimental drugs to their protein targets have helped to organize and visualize the considerable knowledge that exists concerning the interplay between diseases, drug targets and drugs (Yildirim et al., 2007; Keiser et al., 2009). The analysis of these networks have indicated that many drugs can be considered palliative, since they do not target the actual disease-associated proteins but proteins in their network neighborhood (Yildirim et al., 2007) and have aided to predict new molecular targets for known drugs (Keiser et al., 2009). Interestingly, Loging and collaborators (Loging et al., 2007) have suggested a high-throughput electronic-biology approach based on *in silico* data mining of existing databases and integration of this information for drug discovery. These few examples show the power of network approaches. Examples of how these approaches might be applied to tinnitus are developed in the following section.

BACK TO TINNITUS

An increasing amount of work is supporting the proposal that tinnitus is a CNS pathology where dynamic, multiple, parallel, and overlapping brain networks are at stake (Jastreboff, 1990; Eggermont and Roberts, 2004; Weisz et al., 2007; Schlee et al., 2009a,b; De Ridder et al., 2011a; Leaver et al., 2011). Thus, results obtained in research animals (Eggermont and Roberts, 2004) and humans (Muhlnickel et al., 1998) have shown cortical map plasticity and reorganization of the primary auditory cortex, which correlates with the intensity of the perceived sound (Muhlnickel et al., 1998). Moreover, increased spontaneous activity and increased neural synchrony in cortical neurons have been reported in several regions of the CNS (Norena and Eggermont, 2003; Eggermont, 2007). In addition, MEG studies have shown that tinnitus is related to gamma band activity in the auditory cortex, along with decreased alpha and increased theta or delta activity (Llinas et al., 1999; Weisz et al., 2005, 2007) and EEG studies have further shown that gamma band activity in the auditory cortex reflects the tinnitus intensity (van der Loo et al., 2009). These map changes and cortical synchronized activity are necessary but probably not sufficient for the conscious perception of the phantom sound, which needs functional connectivity to a network of higher order brain "neuronal global workspace" areas (De Ridder et al., 2011a). In accordance, an MEG study has shown a global tinnitus network of long-range cortical connections outside the central auditory system including the right parietal cortex, the right frontal lobe and the anterior cingulate cortex, which project top-down influences on the primary auditory cortex and thus amplify neuronal activity in the sensory cortex (Schlee et al., 2008, 2009a). Moreover, tinnitus has an affective component, since in some patients it is accompanied by stress, depression, and anxiety. Therefore, in addition to the perceptual network, a distress network is activated which comprises the medial temporal lobe (amygdala and hippocampus), parahippocampal areas, insula, and the anterior cingulate cortex (Vanneste et al., 2010; De Ridder et al., 2011b). Salience and mnemonic networks are also activated, evidenced by enhanced activity of the amygdala in positron emission tomography imaging (Mirz et al., 2000), by changes in the hippocampal area and by transient tinnitus diminution after suppression of the amygdalo-hippocampal complex by amytal (De Ridder et al., 2006, 2011b). Thus, there is compelling evidence for a distributed tinnitus brain network, which includes sensory auditory areas together with cortical regions involved in perceptual, emotional, mnemonic, attentional, and salience functions (De Ridder et al., 2011a).

In spite of the above existent electrophysiological and functional imaging data derived from tinnitus patients, there is no published work describing the application of graph theoretical analysis to this data. Graph analysis to the tinnitus network might complement insight derived from the study of more localized small brain areas. Moreover, it might be worth applying graph analysis to structural networks, since structural deficits in tinnitus patients have been described in limbic and auditory pathways by structural imaging approaches (Lee et al., 2007; Landgrebe et al., 2009; Crippa et al., 2010; Husain et al., 2011; Leaver et al., 2011). A clear analogy exists between phantom pain and tinnitus and the available knowledge concerning phantom pain and neuropathic pain has advanced our understanding of the underlying pathophysiological changes in tinnitus (Moller, 2007; De Ridder et al., 2011a). However, there is no published data showing the application of graph analysis to these pathologies either, therefore, the topology of brain networks in phantom perception remains unknown. Graph theory could help to refine the topology of the tinnitus network, with the identification of nodes and high degree hubs, modules and clusters. Moreover, simulation of network attacks might aid toward the design of better treatment strategies.

The global tinnitus network of long-range cortical connections outside the central auditory pathway described by Schlee and collaborators (2008, 2009a) by MEG and phase synchronization in the gamma frequencies, speaks toward functionally integrated distributed brain regions. Synchronization of oscillatory responses in the beta- and gamma-band is involved in a variety of cognitive functions, such as routing of signals across distributed cortical networks, perceptual grouping, attention-dependent stimulus selection, sensory-motor integration, working memory and perceptual awareness (Uhlhaas and Singer, 2006). Thus, synchronization plays a crucial role in the exchange of information between cortical areas and both phase and strength of neuronal oscillations in the gamma frequency band influence the amount and speed of information transfer (Buehlmann and Deco, 2010). The global tinnitus network of long-range cortical connections resembles the global neuronal workspace model, where neurons distributed in distant cortical areas need to be accessed for conscious perception (Dehaene and Naccache, 2001; Baars, 2002, 2005). Interestingly, the topology of the global neuronal workspace has been just recently analyzed by graph theoretical analysis during a cognitive effortful task (Kitzbichler et al., 2011). Emergence of a less clustered and less modular network configuration, more globally efficient, with more long-distance synchronization between brain regions, especially in functional networks oscillating at beta and gamma frequency intervals, was reported. This indicates that entrance to the global neuronal workspace breaks modularity in order to allow human brain functional networks to transiently adopt a more efficient but less economical configuration (Kitzbichler et al., 2011). Moreover, the authors propose that, as cognitive effort increases, emergent long-range synchronization provides topological short-cuts between cortical areas that are otherwise segregated from each other in the more modular configuration of the network under cognitively non-demanding conditions and, therefore, increases the global efficiency of the network to subserve transfer of parallel information. This finding is in accordance with the dynamic model of global workspace formation, in which modular subsystems with a locally synchronized community structure during unconscious processing are suddenly replaced by the ignition of a globally synchronized network of neurons with long-range axons densely distributed in prefrontal, parieto-temporal, and cingulate cortices, in response to a consciously attended stimulus (Dehaene and Changeux, 2005, 2011). Thus, following the graph analysis of the neuronal global workspace one could predict a non-random tinnitus network with more long-distance synchronization between brain regions and shorter path lengths which increase global efficiency of information transfer. Interestingly, several independent graph analysis to structural studies in normal subjects have reported a high centrality for the precuneus, the posterior cingulate cortex and neighboring regions (Hagmann et al., 2007, 2008; Iturria-Medina et al., 2007, 2008), two regions that have been shown to be part of the tinnitus network (Schlee et al., 2009b; Vanneste et al., 2010; De Ridder et al., 2011b). Since the precuneus and the posterior cingulate cortex are both pivotal for conscious information processing (Dehaene and Changeux, 2011), it might be the case that they acquire a higher degree in the phantom percept network.

Being a complex network pathology, tinnitus treatment would best benefit from a promiscuous or multi-target drug approach. This is supported by a recent report in which deanxit, the combination of the antidepressant melitracen and the antipsychotic flupentixol, has proven superior to placebo in a cross-over trial as add-on medication to clonazepam (Meeus et al., 2011). Although there is no tinnitus approved drug on the market, one serendipitous discovery in tinnitus pharmacotherapy deserves further analysis. Beginning with the accidental discovery of the tinnitus suppressing effect of the local anesthetic procaine (Bárány, 1935), intravenous administration of local anesthetics such as lidocaine have been used in the treatment of tinnitus (for review see Trellakis et al., 2007). Available data indicate that lidocaine is able to reduce tinnitus in 60% of patients in a dose-dependent manner (Haginomori et al., 1995; Otsuka et al., 2003; Baguley et al., 2005). Because of poor biological availability after oral administration, lidocaine is not effective when taken orally. Thus, other anti-arrythmics or local anesthetics have been used without much success. This includes tocainide, flecainide, and mexiletine (Blayney et al., 1985; Hulshof and Vermeij, 1985b; Fortnum and Coles, 1991; Dobie, 1999; Trellakis et al., 2007). Moreover, based on the fact that lidocaine blocks voltage-gated sodium channels, some anticonvulsants that also act on voltage-gated sodium channels like carbamazepine have been used in tinnitus, without much success (Donaldson, 1981; Marks et al., 1981; Hulshof and Vermeij, 1985a). This accidental discovery might be further evaluated and acted upon under the light of network analysis. Two examples of network approaches to this observation are described below.

Brain imaging studies have shown changes in activity in several CNS regions after lidocaine infusion (Mirz et al., 1999; Andersson et al., 2000; Reyes et al., 2002). Graph analysis of functional brain networks might help refine the hubs that are mostly influenced by lidocaine in tinnitus-sensitive patients. This might help understand the mechanism of action of this compound and guide further developments. This type of analysis has been applied to the effect of the dopamine receptor subtype 2 antagonist sulpiride, showing that it impairs network efficiency by an effect most clearly localized to dorsal cingulate and lateral temporal cortical hubs (Achard and Bullmore, 2007). Moreoever, these findings have been correlated with changes in the topology of the aging brain (Achard and Bullmore, 2007).

Lidocaine has pleiotropic effects on several proteins aside from the well-known block of voltage-gated sodium channels (Trellakis et al., 2007). Following an e-biology approach (Loging et al., 2007), one could mine existing databases (including, but not restricted to, medline) to define the pharmacological space of lidocaine targets. Moreover, one could follow the same approach to define the pharmacological space of other local anesthetics, antiarrythmics, and anticonvulsants. A drug-target network linking drugs to their protein targets (Yildirim et al., 2007; Keiser et al., 2009) would help organize and visualize these data, define the target interplay for the different compounds and finally make predictions concerning the add-on effects that lidocaine has when compared to compounds that are non-effective in tinnitus.

These two examples are just a glimpse of how network analysis might lead us forward in our understanding of tinnitus and of its treatment. Most importantly, it will move us further away from a reductionist way of looking at tinnitus. Tinnitus cannot be seen solely as a pathology of increased excitation or decreased inhibition at different relays of the auditory pathway including the cochlea, cochlear nucleus, inferior colliculus, and sensory auditory cortex. Moreover, the notion of emergence of complex systems might guide us further in tinnitus research and pharmacotherapy. Thus, for example, although benzodiazepines are used in tinnitus patients with the aim of increasing inhibitory gabaergic pathways, recent studies have shown that $GABA_A$ receptors can be excitatory in the mature cortex depending on the excitability of the network the neuron is embedded in and on the spatiotemporal relationship to other depolarizing stimulus (Gulledge and Stuart, 2003; Szabadics et al., 2006 and references thereof). These findings imply that different brain regions might qualitative and/or quantitative respond differently to drugs. At least in part, this might be due to drug actions on emergent network properties conferred to neurons as the result of their membership in the network, rather than being solely due to the intrinsic binding of the drug to a specific receptor in the neuron.

CONCLUSIONS

In summary, graph analysis to complex networks is aiding toward understanding the behavior of the brain in health and disease. Being tinnitus a CNS disorder where multiple parallel overlapping networks are disturbed, graph analysis might aid to identify the topology of the network including its hubs. Since brain networks are best treated with multi-target drugs that attack the disease-causing network, tinnitus pharmacological treatments could benefit from dirty or promiscuous drugs. Network analysis to tinnitus pathology and treatment might help to look for the right thing, in the right place and at the right time.

ACKNOWLEDGMENTS

Ana Belén Elgoyhen, Berthold Langguth, and Dirk De Ridder are funded by the Tinnitus Research Initiative.

REFERENCES

Achard, S., and Bullmore, E. (2007). Efficiency and cost of economical brain functional networks. *PLoS Comput. Biol.* 3, e17. doi: 10.1371/journal.pcbi.0030017

Achard, S., Salvador, R., Whitcher, B., Suckling, J., and Bullmore, E. (2006). A resilient, low-frequency, small-world human brain functional network with highly connected association cortical hubs. *J. Neurosci.* 26, 63–72.

Agoston, V., Csermely, P., and Pongor, S. (2005). Multiple weak hits confuse complex systems: a transcriptional regulatory network as an example. *Phys. Rev. E Stat. Nonlin. Soft Matter Phys.* 71, 051909.

Albert, R., and Barabasi, A. L. (2002). Statistical mechanics of complex networks. *Rev. Mod. Phys.* 74, 47–98.

Albert, R., Jeong, H., and Barabasi, A. L. (1999). Internet: diameter of the world-wide web. *Nature* 401, 130–131.

Albert, R., Jeong, H., and Barabasi, A. L. (2000). Error and attack tolerance of complex networks. *Nature* 406, 378–382.

Almaas, E., Kovacs, B., Vicsek, T., Oltvai, Z. N., and Barabasi, A. L. (2004). Global organization of metabolic fluxes in the bacterium Escherichia coli. *Nature* 427, 839–843.

Amaral, L. A., Scala, A., Barthelemy, M., and Stanley, H. E. (2000). Classes of small-world networks. *Proc. Natl. Acad. Sci. U.S.A.* 97, 11149–11152.

Andersson, G., Lyttkens, L., Hirvela, C., Furmark, T., Tillfors, M., and Fredrikson, M. (2000). Regional cerebral blood flow during tinnitus: a PET case study with lidocaine and auditory stimulation. *Acta. Otolaryngol.* 120, 967–972.

Andreadis, E. A., Tsourous, G. I., Marakomichelakis, G. E., Katsanou, P. M., Fotia, M. E., Vassilopoulos, C. V., and Diamantopoulos, E. J. (2005). High-dose monotherapy vs low-dose combination therapy of calcium channel blockers and angiotensin receptor blockers in mild to moderate hypertension. *J. Hum. Hypertens.* 19, 491–496.

Azevedo, A. A., and Figueiredo, R. R. (2007). Treatment of tinnitus with acamprosate. *Prog. Brain Res.* 166, 273–277.

Azmi, A. S., Wang, Z., Philip, P. A., Mohammad, R. M., and Sarkar, F. H. (2010). Proof of concept: network and systems biology approaches aid in the discovery of potent anticancer drug combinations. *Mol. Cancer Ther.* 9, 3137–3144.

Baars, B. J. (2002). The conscious access hypothesis: origins and recent evidence. *Trends Cogn. Sci.* 6, 47–52.

Baars, B. J. (2005). Global workspace theory of consciousness: toward a cognitive neuroscience of human experience. *Prog. Brain Res.* 150, 45–53.

Baguley, D. M., Jones, S., Wilkins, I., Axon, P. R., and Moffat, D. A. (2005). The inhibitory effect of intravenous lidocaine infusion on tinnitus after translabyrinthine removal of vestibular schwannoma: a double-blind, placebo-controlled, crossover study. *Otol. Neurotol.* 26, 169–176.

Bahmad, F. M. Jr., Venosa, A. R., and Oliveira, C. A. (2006). Benzodiazepines and GABAergics in treating severe disabling tinnitus of predominantly cochlear origin. *Int. Tinnitus J.* 12, 140–144.

Ban, T. A. (2006). The role of serendipity in drug discovery. *Dialogues Clin. Neurosci.* 8, 335–344.

Barabasi, A. (ed). (2002). *Linked: The New Science of Networks.* Cambridge: Perseus Publishing.

Barabasi, A. L., and Albert, R. (1999). Emergence of scaling in random networks. *Science* 286, 509–512.

Barabasi, A. L., and Bonabeau, E. (2003). Scale-free networks. *Sci. Am.* 288, 60–69.

Barabasi, A. L., and Oltvai, Z. N. (2004). Network biology: understanding the cell's functional organization. *Nat. Rev. Genet.* 5, 101–113.

Bárány, R. (1935). Die Beeinfiussung des Ohrensausens durch intravenos injezierte Lokalanasthetika. *Acta. Otoralyngol.* 23, 201–203.

Bassett, D. S., and Bullmore, E. T. (2009). Human brain networks in health and disease. *Curr. Opin. Neurol.* 22, 340–347.

Bassett, D. S., Bullmore, E., Verchinski, B. A., Mattay, V. S., Weinberger, D. R., and Meyer-Lindenberg, A. (2008). Hierarchical organization of human cortical networks in health and schizophrenia. *J. Neurosci.* 28, 9239–9248.

Bassett, D. S., Bullmore, E. T., Meyer-Lindenberg, A., Apud, J. A., Weinberger, D. R., and Coppola, R. (2009). Cognitive fitness of cost-efficient brain functional networks. *Proc. Natl. Acad. Sci. U.S.A.* 106, 11747–11752.

Bassett, D. S., and Gazzaniga, M. S. (2011). Understanding complexity in the human brain. *Trends Cogn. Sci.* 15, 200–209.

Bassett, D. S., Meyer-Lindenberg, A., Achard, S., Duke, T., and Bullmore, E. (2006). Adaptive reconfiguration of fractal small-world human brain functional networks. *Proc. Natl. Acad. Sci. U.S.A.* 103, 19518–19523.

Bauer, C. A., and Brozoski, T. J. (2007). Gabapentin. *Prog. Brain Res.* 166, 287–301.

Blayney, A. W., Phillips, M. S., Guy, A. M., and Colman, B. H. (1985). A sequential double blind cross-over trial of tocainide hydrochloride in tinnitus. *Clin. Otolaryngol. Allied Sci.* 10, 97–101.

Bohlen, C., Chesler, A., Sharif-Naeini, R., Medzihradszky, K., Zhou, S., King, D., Sánchez, E., Burlingame, A., Basbaum, A., and Julius, D. (2011). A heteromeric Texas coral snake toxin targets acid-sensing ion channels to produce pain. *Nature* 479, 410–414.

Borisy, A. A., Elliott, P. J., Hurst, N. W., Lee, M. S., Lehar, J., Price, E. R., Serbedzija, G., Zimmermann, G. R., Foley, M. A., Stockwell, B. R., and Keith, C. T. (2003). Systematic discovery of multicomponent therapeutics. *Proc. Natl. Acad. Sci. U.S.A.* 100, 7977–7982.

Borsook, D., Becerra, L., and Hargreaves, R. (2006). A role for fMRI in optimizing CNS drug development. *Nat. Rev. Drug Discov.* 5, 411–424.

Buehlmann, A., and Deco, G. (2010). Optimal information transfer in the cortex through synchronization. *PLoS Comput. Biol.* 6. doi: 10.1371/journal.pcbi.1000934

Bullmore, E. T., and Bassett, D. S. (2011). Brain graphs: graphical models of the human brain connectome. *Annu. Rev. Clin. Psychol.* 7, 113–140.

Bullmore, E., and Sporns, O. (2009). Complex brain networks: graph theoretical analysis of structural and functional systems. *Nat. Rev. Neurosci.* 10, 186–198.

Buzsaki, G. (2004). Large-scale recording of neuronal ensembles. *Nat. Neurosci.* 7, 446–451.

Catani, M., and Ffytche, D. H. (2005). The rises and falls of disconnection syndromes. *Brain* 128, 2224–2239.

Chen, Z. J., He, Y., Rosa-Neto, P., Germann, J., and Evans, A. C. (2008). Revealing modular architecture of human brain structural networks by using cortical thickness from MRI. *Cereb. Cortex* 18, 2374–2381.

Chklovskii, D. B., Schikorski, T., and Stevens, C. F. (2002). Wiring optimization in cortical circuits. *Neuron* 34, 341–347.

Cohen, R., and Havlin, S. (2003). Scale-free networks are ultrasmall. *Phys. Rev. Lett.* 90, 058701.

Conn, P. J., and Roth, B. L. (2008). Opportunities and challenges of psychiatric drug discovery: roles for scientists in academic, industry, and government settings. *Neuropsychopharmacology* 33, 2048–2060.

Crippa, A., Lanting, C. P., Van Dijk, P., and Roerdink, J. B. (2010). A diffusion tensor imaging study on the auditory system and tinnitus. *Open Neuroimag. J.* 4, 16–25.

Csermely, P., Agoston, V., and Pongor, S. (2005). The efficiency of multi-target drugs: the network approach might help drug design. *Trends Pharmacol. Sci.* 26, 178–182.

De Ridder, D., Elgoyhen, A. B., Romo, R., and Langguth, B. (2011a). Phantom percepts: tinnitus and pain as persisting aversive memory networks. *Proc. Natl. Acad. Sci. U.S.A.* 108, 8075–8080.

De Ridder, D., Fransen, H., Francois, O., Sunaert, S., Kovacs, S., and Van De Heyning, P. (2006). Amygdalohippocampal involvement in tinnitus and auditory memory. *Acta. Otolaryngol. Suppl.* 126, 50–53.

De Ridder, D., Vanneste, S., and Congedo, M. (2011b). The distressed brain: a group blind source separation analysis on tinnitus. *PLoS One* 6, e24273. doi: 10.1371/journal.pone.0024273

Dehaene, S., and Changeux, J. P. (2005). Ongoing spontaneous activity controls access to consciousness: a neuronal model for inattentional blindness. *PLoS Biol.* 3, e141. doi: 10.1371/journal.pbio.0030141

Dehaene, S., and Changeux, J. P. (2011). Experimental and theoretical approaches to conscious processing. *Neuron* 70, 200–227.

Dehaene, S., and Naccache, L. (2001). Towards a cognitive neuroscience of consciousness: basic evidence and a workspace framework. *Cognition* 79, 1–37.

Delay, J., Deniker, P., and Harl, J. M. (1952). Therapeutic method derived from hiberno-therapy in excitation and agitation states. *Ann. Med. Psychol. (Paris)* 110, 267–273.

Dimitriadis, S. I., Laskaris, N. A., Tsirka, V., Vourkas, M., Micheloyannis, S., and Fotopoulos, S. (2010). Tracking brain dynamics via time-dependent network analysis. *J. Neurosci. Methods* 193, 145–155.

Dobie, R. A. (1999). A review of randomized clinical trials in tinnitus. *Laryngoscope* 109, 1202–1211.

Donaldson, I. (1981). Tegretol: a double blind trial in tinnitus. *J. Laryngol. Otol.* 95, 947–951.

Ebel, H., Mielsch, L. I., and Bornholdt, S. (2002). Scale-free topology of e-mail networks. *Phys. Rev. E Stat. Nonlin. Soft Matter Phys.* 66, 035103.

Eggermont, J. J. (2007). Correlated neural activity as the driving force for functional changes in auditory cortex. *Hear. Res.* 229, 69–80.

Eggermont, J. J., and Roberts, L. E. (2004). The neuroscience of tinnitus. *Trends Neurosci.* 27, 676–682.

Eguiluz, V. M., Chialvo, D. R., Cecchi, G. A., Baliki, M., and Apkarian, A. V. (2005). Scale-free brain functional networks. *Phys. Rev. Lett.* 94, 018102.

Elgoyhen, A. B., and Langguth, B. (2010). Pharmacological approaches to the treatment of tinnitus. *Drug Discov. Today* 15, 300–305.

Erdos, P., and Renyi, A. (1959). On random graphs: I. *Publ. Math.* 6, 290–297.

Fabian, M. A., Biggs, W. H. 3rd, Treiber, D. K., Atteridge, C. E., Azimioara, M. D., Benedetti, M. G., Carter, T. A., Ciceri, P., Edeen, P. T., Floyd, M., Ford, J. M., Galvin, M., Gerlach, J. L., Grotzfeld, R. M., Herrgard, S., Insko, D. E., Insko, M. A., Lai, A. G., Lelias, J. M., Mehta, S. A., Milanov, Z. V., Velasco, A. M., Wodicka, L. M., Patel, H. K., Zarrinkar, P. P., and Lockhart, D. J. (2005). A small molecule-kinase interaction map for clinical kinase inhibitors. *Nat. Biotechnol.* 23, 329–336.

Figueiredo, R. R., Langguth, B., Mello De Oliveira, P., and Aparecida De Azevedo, A. (2008). Tinnitus treatment with memantine. *Otolaryngol. Head Neck Surg.* 138, 492–496.

Fortnum, H. M., and Coles, R. R. (1991). Trial of flecainide acetate in the management of tinnitus. *Clin. Otolaryngol. Allied Sci.* 16, 93–96.

Gananca, M. M., Caovilla, H. H., Gananca, F. F., Gananca, C. F., Munhoz, M. S., Da Silva, M. L., and Serafini, F. (2002). Clonazepam in the pharmacological treatment of vertigo and tinnitus. *Int. Tinnitus J.* 8, 50–53.

Gazzaniga, M. S. (2010). Neuroscience and the correct level of explanation for understanding mind. An extraterrestrial roams through some neuroscience laboratories and concludes earthlings are not grasping how best to understand the mind-brain interface. *Trends Cogn. Sci.* 14, 291–292.

Gong, G., He, Y., Concha, L., Lebel, C., Gross, D. W., Evans, A. C., and Beaulieu, C. (2009). Mapping anatomical connectivity patterns of human cerebral cortex using *in vivo* diffusion tensor imaging tractography. *Cereb. Cortex* 19, 524–536.

Gulledge, A. T., and Stuart, G. J. (2003). Excitatory actions of GABA in the cortex. *Neuron* 37, 299–309.

Haginomori, S., Makimoto, K., Araki, M., Kawakami, M., and Takahashi, H. (1995). Effect of lidocaine injection of EOAE in patients with tinnitus. *Acta. Otolaryngol.* 115, 488–492.

Hagmann, P., Cammoun, L., Gigandet, X., Meuli, R., Honey, C. J., Wedeen, V. J., and Sporns, O. (2008). Mapping the structural core of human cerebral cortex. *PLoS Biol.* 6, e159. doi: 10.1371/journal.pbio.0060159

Hagmann, P., Kurant, M., Gigandet, X., Thiran, P., Wedeen, V. J., Meuli, R., and Thiran, J. P. (2007). Mapping human whole-brain structural networks with diffusion MRI. *PLoS One* 2, e597. doi: 10.1371/journal.pone.0000597

Hampton, T. (2004). "Promiscuous" anticancer drugs that hit multiple targets may thwart resistance. *JAMA* 292, 419–422.

He, B. J., Zempel, J. M., Snyder, A. Z., and Raichle, M. E. (2010). The temporal structures and functional significance of scale-free brain activity. *Neuron* 66, 353–369.

He, Y., Chen, Z. J., and Evans, A. C. (2007). Small-world anatomical networks in the human brain revealed by cortical thickness from MRI. *Cereb. Cortex* 17, 2407–2419.

Hoekstra, C. E., Rynja, S. P., Van Zanten, G. A., and Rovers, M. M. (2011). Anticonvulsants for tinnitus. *Cochrane Database Syst. Rev.* CD007960.

Honey, G., and Bullmore, E. (2004). Human pharmacological MRI. *Trends Pharmacol. Sci.* 25, 366–374.

Hopkins, A. L. (2007). Network pharmacology. *Nat. Biotechnol.* 25, 1110–1111.

Hopkins, A. L. (2008). Network pharmacology: the next paradigm in drug discovery. *Nat. Chem. Biol.* 4, 682–690.

Hopkins, A. L., Mason, J. S., and Overington, J. P. (2006). Can we rationally design promiscuous drugs? *Curr. Opin. Struct. Biol.* 16, 127–136.

Hughes, B. (2010). 2009 FDA drug approvals. *Nat. Rev. Drug Discov.* 9, 89–92.

Hulshof, J. H., and Vermeij, P. (1985a). The value of carbamazepine in the treatment of tinnitus. *ORL J. Otorhinolaryngol. Relat. Spec.* 47, 262–266.

Hulshof, J. H., and Vermeij, P. (1985b). The value of tocainide in the treatment of tinnitus. A double-blind controlled study. *Arch. Otorhinolaryngol.* 241, 279–283.

Husain, F. T., Medina, R. E., Davis, C. W., Szymko-Bennett, Y., Simonyan, K., Pajor, N. M., and Horwitz, B. (2011). Neuroanatomical changes due to hearing loss and chronic tinnitus: a combined VBM and DTI study. *Brain Res.* 1369, 74–88.

Imaz, A., Falco, V., and Ribera, E. (2011). Antiretroviral salvage therapy for multiclass drug-resistant HIV-1-infected patients: from clinical trials to daily clinical practice. *AIDS Rev.* 13, 180–193.

Iturria-Medina, Y., Canales-Rodriguez, E. J., Melie-Garcia, L., Valdes-Hernandez, P. A., Martinez-Montes, E., Aleman-Gomez, Y., and Sanchez-Bornot, J. M. (2007). Characterizing brain anatomical connections using diffusion weighted MRI and graph theory. *Neuroimage* 36, 645–660.

Iturria-Medina, Y., Sotero, R. C., Canales-Rodriguez, E. J., Aleman-Gomez, Y., and Melie-Garcia, L. (2008). Studying the human brain anatomical network via diffusion-weighted MRI and Graph Theory. *Neuroimage* 40, 1064–1076.

Jastreboff, P. J. (1990). Phantom auditory perception (tinnitus): mechanisms of generation and perception. *Neurosci. Res.* 8, 221–254.

Jeong, H., Tombor, B., Albert, R., Oltvai, Z. N., and Barabasi, A. L. (2000). The large-scale organization of metabolic networks. *Nature* 407, 651–654.

Jin, S. H., Lin, P., and Hallett, M. (2011). Reorganization of brain functional small-world networks during finger movements. *Hum. Brain Mapp.*

Johnson, R. M., Brummett, R., and Schleuning, A. (1993). Use of alprazolam for relief of tinnitus. A double-blind study. *Arch. Otolaryngol. Head Neck Surg.* 119, 842–845.

Kaufmann, S. H. (2008). Paul Ehrlich: founder of chemotherapy. *Nat. Rev. Drug Discov.* 7, 373.

Keeling, C. I., Slessor, K. N., Higo, H. A., and Winston, M. L. (2003). New components of the honey bee (Apis mellifera L.) queen retinue pheromone. *Proc. Natl. Acad. Sci. U.S.A.* 100, 4486–4491.

Keiser, M. J., Setola, V., Irwin, J. J., Laggner, C., Abbas, A. I., Hufeisen, S. J., Jensen, N. H., Kuijer, M. B., Matos, R. C., Tran, T. B., Whaley, R., Glennon, R. A., Hert, J., Thomas, K. L., Edwards, D. D., Shoichet, B. K., and Roth, B. L. (2009). Predicting new molecular targets for known drugs. *Nature* 462, 175–181.

Keith, C. T., Borisy, A. A., and Stockwell, B. R. (2005). Multicomponent therapeutics for networked systems. *Nat. Rev. Drug Discov.* 4, 71–78.

Kitano, H. (2002). Systems biology: a brief overview. *Science* 295, 1662–1664.

Kitzbichler, M. G., Henson, R. N., Smith, M. L., Nathan, P. J., and Bullmore, E. T. (2011). Cognitive effort drives workspace configuration of human brain functional networks. *J. Neurosci.* 31, 8259–8270.

Kola, I., and Landis, J. (2004). Can the pharmaceutical industry reduce attrition rates? *Nat. Rev. Drug Discov.* 3, 711–715.

Kung, C., Kenski, D. M., Dickerson, S. H., Howson, R. W., Kuyper, L. F., Madhani, H. D., and Shokat, K. M. (2005). Chemical genomic profiling to identify intracellular targets of a multiplex kinase inhibitor. *Proc. Natl. Acad. Sci. U.S.A.* 102, 3587–3592.

Landgrebe, M., Langguth, B., Rosengarth, K., Braun, S., Koch, A., Kleinjung, T., May, A., De Ridder, D., and Hajak, G. (2009). Structural brain changes in tinnitus: grey matter decrease in auditory and non-auditory brain areas. *Neuroimage* 46, 213–218.

Langguth, B., and Elgoyhen, A. (2011). Emerging pharmacotherapy of tinnitus. *Expert Opin. Emerg. Drugs* 16, 603–606.

Langguth, B., Salvi, R., and Elgoyhen, A. B. (2009). Emerging pharmacotherapy of tinnitus. *Expert Opin. Emerg. Drugs* 14, 687–702.

Leaver, A. M., Renier, L., Chevillet, M. A., Morgan, S., Kim, H. J., and Rauschecker, J. P. (2011). Dysregulation of limbic and auditory networks in tinnitus. *Neuron* 69, 33–43.

Lee, Y. J., Bae, S. J., Lee, S. H., Lee, J. J., Lee, K. Y., Kim, M. N., Kim, Y. S., Baik, S. K., Woo, S., and Chang, Y. (2007). Evaluation of white matter structures in patients with tinnitus using diffusion tensor imaging. *J. Clin. Neurosci.* 14, 515–519.

Lehew, G., and Nicolelis, M. A. L. (2008). "State-of-the-art microwire array design for chronic neural recordings in behaving animals," in *Methods for Neural Ensemble Recordings*, 2nd Edn, ed M. A. L. Nicolelis (Boca Raton, FL: CRC Press) Chapter 1.

Leistedt, S. J., Coumans, N., Dumont, M., Lanquart, J. P., Stam, C. J., and Linkowski, P. (2009). Altered sleep brain functional connectivity in acutely depressed patients. *Hum. Brain Mapp.* 30, 2207–2219.

Llinas, R. R., Ribary, U., Jeanmonod, D., Kronberg, E., and Mitra, P. P. (1999). Thalamocortical dysrhythmia: a neurological and neuropsychiatric syndrome characterized by magnetoencephalography. *Proc. Natl. Acad. Sci. U.S.A.* 96, 15222–15227.

Loging, W., Harland, L., and Williams-Jones, B. (2007). High-throughput electronic biology: mining information for drug discovery. *Nat. Rev. Drug Discov.* 6, 220–230.

Lynall, M. E., Bassett, D. S., Kerwin, R., Mckenna, P. J., Kitzbichler, M., Muller, U., and Bullmore, E. (2010). Functional connectivity and brain networks in schizophrenia. *J. Neurosci.* 30, 9477–9487.

Marks, N. J., Onisiphorou, C., and Trounce, J. R. (1981). The effect of single doses of amylobarbitone sodium and carbamazepine in tinnitus. *J. Laryngol. Otol.* 95, 941–945.

Meeus, O., De Ridder, D., and Van De Heyning, P. (2011). Administration of the combination clonazepam-Deanxit as treatment for tinnitus. *Otol. Neurotol.* 32, 701–709.

Millan, M. J. (2006). Multi-target strategies for the improved treatment of depressive states: conceptual foundations and neuronal substrates, drug discovery and therapeutic application. *Pharmacol. Ther.* 110, 135–370.

Mirz, F., Gjedde, A., Ishizu, K., and Pedersen, C. B. (2000). Cortical networks subserving the perception of tinnitus–a PET study. *Acta. Otolaryngol. Suppl.* 543, 241–243.

Mirz, F., Pedersen, B., Ishizu, K., Johannsen, P., Ovesen, T., Stodkilde-Jorgensen, H., and Gjedde, A. (1999). Positron emission tomography of cortical centers of tinnitus. *Hear. Res.* 134, 133–144.

Moller, A. R. (2007). Tinnitus and pain. *Prog. Brain Res.* 166, 47–53.

Morphy, R., Kay, C., and Rankovic, Z. (2004). From magic bullets to designed multiple ligands. *Drug Discov. Today* 9, 641–651.

Muhlnickel, W., Elbert, T., Taub, E., and Flor, H. (1998). Reorganization of auditory cortex in tinnitus. *Proc. Natl. Acad. Sci. U.S.A.* 95, 10340–10343.

Munos, B. (2009). Lessons from 60 years of pharmaceutical innovation. *Nat. Rev. Drug Discov.* 8, 959–968.

Newman, M. (2003). The structure and function of complex networks. *SIAM Rev.* 45, 167–256.

Norena, A. J., and Eggermont, J. J. (2003). Changes in spontaneous neural activity immediately after an acoustic trauma: implications for neural correlates of tinnitus. *Hear. Res.* 183, 137–153.

Olivera, B. M., and Teichert, R. W. (2007). Diversity of the neurotoxic Conus peptides: a model for concerted pharmacological discovery. *Mol. Interv.* 7, 251–260.

Otsuka, K., Pulec, J. L., and Suzuki, M. (2003). Assessment of intravenous lidocaine for the treatment of subjective tinnitus. *Ear Nose Throat J.* 82, 781–784.

Pastor-Satorras, R., and Vespignani, A. (2001). Epidemic dynamics and endemic states in complex networks. *Phys. Rev. E Stat. Nonlin. Soft Matter Phys.* 63, 066117.

Paul, S. M., Mytelka, D. S., Dunwiddie, C. T., Persinger, C. C., Munos, B. H., Lindborg, S. R., and Schacht, A. L. (2010). How to improve R&D productivity: the pharmaceutical industry's grand challenge. *Nat. Rev. Drug Discov.* 9, 203–214.

Podani, J., Oltvai, Z. N., Jeong, H., Tombor, B., Barabasi, A. L., and Szathmary, E. (2001). Comparable system-level organization of Archaea and Eukaryotes. *Nat. Genet.* 29, 54–56.

Rash, L. D., and Hodgson, W. C. (2002). Pharmacology and biochemistry of spider venoms. *Toxicon* 40, 225–254.

Rask-Andersen, M., Almen, M. S., and Schioth, H. B. (2011). Trends in the exploitation of novel drug targets. *Nat. Rev. Drug Discov.* 10, 579–590.

Rasmussen, K. (2006). Creating more effective antidepressants: clues from the clinic. *Drug Discov. Today* 11, 623–631.

Ravasz, E., Somera, A. L., Mongru, D. A., Oltvai, Z. N., and Barabasi, A. L. (2002). Hierarchical organization of modularity in metabolic networks. *Science* 297, 1551–1555.

Reijneveld, J. C., Ponten, S. C., Berendse, H. W., and Stam, C. J. (2007). The application of graph theoretical analysis to complex networks in the brain. *Clin. Neurophysiol.* 118, 2317–2331.

Reyes, S. A., Salvi, R. J., Burkard, R. F., Coad, M. L., Wack, D. S., Galantowicz, P. J., and Lockwood, A. H. (2002). Brain imaging of the effects of lidocaine on tinnitus. *Hear. Res.* 171, 43–50.

Rodriguez de la Vega, R. C., Schwartz, E. F., and Possani, L. D. (2010). Mining on scorpion venom biodiversity. *Toxicon* 56, 1155–1161.

Roth, B. L., Sheffler, D. J., and Kroeze, W. K. (2004). Magic shotguns versus magic bullets: selectively non-selective drugs for mood disorders and schizophrenia. *Nat. Rev. Drug Discov.* 3, 353–359.

Rubinov, M., and Bassett, D. S. (2011). Emerging evidence of connectomic abnormalities in schizophrenia. *J. Neurosci.* 31, 6263–6265.

Salvador, R., Suckling, J., Coleman, M. R., Pickard, J. D., Menon, D., and Bullmore, E. (2005). Neurophysiological architecture of functional magnetic resonance images of human brain. *Cereb. Cortex* 15, 1332–1342.

Sams-Dodd, F. (2005). Target-based drug discovery: is something wrong? *Drug Discov. Today* 10, 139–147.

Schlee, W., Hartmann, T., Langguth, B., and Weisz, N. (2009a). Abnormal resting-state cortical coupling in chronic tinnitus. *BMC Neurosci.* 10, 11.

Schlee, W., Mueller, N., Hartmann, T., Keil, J., Lorenz, I., and Weisz, N. (2009b). Mapping cortical hubs in tinnitus. *BMC Biol.* 7, 80.

Schlee, W., Weisz, N., Bertrand, O., Hartmann, T., and Elbert, T. (2008). Using auditory steady state responses to outline the functional connectivity in the tinnitus brain. *PLoS One* 3, e3720. doi: 10.1371/journal.pone.0003720

Shargel, B., Sayama, H., Epstein, I. R., and Bar-Yam, Y. (2003). Optimization of robustness and connectivity in complex networks. *Phys. Rev. Lett.* 90, 068701.

Siemens, J., Zhou, S., Piskorowski, R., Nikai, T., Lumpkin, E. A., Basbaum, A. I., King, D., and Julius, D. (2006). Spider toxins activate the capsaicin receptor to produce inflammatory pain. *Nature* 444, 208–212.

Sporns, O. (2011a). The human connectome: a complex network. *Ann. N.Y. Acad. Sci.* 1224, 109–125.

Sporns, O. (ed). (2011b). *Networks of the Brain.* Cambridge, MA: MIT Press.

Sporns, O. (2011c). The non-random brain: efficiency, economy, and complex dynamics. *Front. Comput. Neurosci.* 5, 5. doi: 10.3389/fncom.2011.00005

Stam, C., and van Dijk, B. (2002). Synchronization likelihood: an unbiased measure of generalized synchronization in multivariate data sets. *Physica. D* 163, 236–251.

Stam, C. J. (2004). Functional connectivity patterns of human magnetoencephalographic recordings: a 'small-world' network? *Neurosci. Lett* 355, 25–28.

Suckfull, M., Althaus, M., Ellers-Lenz, B., Gebauer, A., Gortelmeyer, R., Jastreboff, P. J., Moebius, H. J., Rosenberg, T., Russ, H., Wirth, Y., and Krueger, H. (2011). A randomized, double-blind, placebo-controlled clinical trial to evaluate the efficacy and safety of neramexane in patients with moderate to severe subjective tinnitus. *BMC Ear Nose Throat Disord.* 11, 1.

Sullivan, M., Katon, W., Russo, J., Dobie, R., and Sakai, C. (1993). A randomized trial of nortriptyline for severe chronic tinnitus. Effects on depression, disability, and tinnitus symptoms. *Arch. Intern. Med.* 153, 2251–2259.

Szabadics, J., Varga, C., Molnar, G., Olah, S., Barzo, P., and Tamas, G. (2006). Excitatory effect of GABAergic axo-axonic cells in cortical microcircuits. *Science* 311, 233–235.

Tong, A. H., Lesage, G., Bader, G. D., Ding, H., Xu, H., Xin, X., Young, J., Berriz, G. F., Brost, R. L., Chang, M., Chen, Y., Cheng, X., Chua, G., Friesen, H., Goldberg, D. S., Haynes, J., Humphries, C., He, G., Hussein, S., Ke, L., Krogan, N., Li, Z., Levinson, J. N., Lu, H., Menard, P., Munyana, C., Parsons, A. B., Ryan, O., Tonikian, R., Roberts, T., Sdicu, A. M., Shapiro, J., Sheikh, B., Suter, B., Wong, S. L., Zhang, L. V., Zhu, H., Burd, C. G., Munro, S., Sander, C., Rine, J., Greenblatt, J., Peter, M., Bretscher, A., Bell, G., Roth, F. P., Brown, G. W., Andrews, B., Bussey, H., and Boone, C. (2004). Global mapping of the yeast genetic interaction network. *Science* 303, 808–813.

Trellakis, S., Lautermann, J., and Lehnerdt, G. (2007). Lidocaine: neurobiological targets and effects on the auditory system. *Prog. Brain Res.* 166, 303–322.

Uhlhaas, P. J., and Singer, W. (2006). Neural synchrony in brain disorders: relevance for cognitive dysfunctions and pathophysiology. *Neuron* 52, 155–168.

Uma, B., Swaroopa Rani, T., and Podile, A. R. (2011). Warriors at the gate that never sleep: non-host resistance in plants. *J. Plant Physiol.* 168, 2141–2152.

Valente, A. X., Sarkar, A., and Stone, H. A. (2004). Two-peak and three-peak optimal complex networks. *Phys. Rev. Lett.* 92, 118702.

van de Ville, D., Britz, J., and Michel, C. M. (2010). EEG microstate sequences in healthy humans at rest reveal scale-free dynamics. *Proc. Natl. Acad. Sci. U.S.A.* 107, 18179–18184.

van Dellen, E., Douw, L., Baayen, J. C., Heimans, J. J., Ponten, S. C., Vandertop, W. P., Velis, D. N., Stam, C. J., and Reijneveld, J. C. (2009). Long-term effects of temporal lobe epilepsy on local neural networks: a graph theoretical analysis of corticography recordings. *PLoS One* 4, e8081. doi: 10.1371/journal.pone.0008081

van den Heuvel, M. P., Mandl, R. C., Stam, C. J., Kahn, R. S., and Hulshoff Pol, H. E. (2010). Aberrant frontal and temporal complex network structure in schizophrenia: a graph theoretical analysis. *J. Neurosci.* 30, 15915–15926.

van den Heuvel, M. P., and Sporns, O. (2011). Rich-club organization of the human connectome. *J. Neurosci.* 31, 15775–15786.

van den Heuvel, M. P., Stam, C. J., Boersma, M., and Hulshoff Pol, H. E. (2008). Small-world and scale-free organization of voxel-based resting-state functional connectivity in the human brain. *Neuroimage* 43, 528–539.

van der Loo, E., Gais, S., Congedo, M., Vanneste, S., Plazier, M., Menovsky, T., Van De Heyning, P., and De Ridder, D. (2009). Tinnitus intensity dependent gamma oscillations of the contralateral auditory cortex. *PLoS One* 4, e7396. doi: 10.1371/journal.pone.0007396

Vanneste, S., Plazier, M., Der Loo, E., De Heyning, P. V., Congedo, M., and De Ridder, D. (2010). The neural correlates of tinnitus-related distress. *Neuroimage* 52, 470–480.

Vio, M. M., and Holme, R. H. (2005). Hearing loss and tinnitus: 250 million people and a US$10 billion potential market. *Drug Discov. Today* 10, 1263–1265.

Wang, L., Zhu, C., He, Y., Zang, Y., Cao, Q., Zhang, H., Zhong, Q., and Wang, Y. (2009). Altered small-world brain functional networks in children with attention-deficit/hyperactivity disorder. *Hum. Brain Mapp.* 30, 638–649.

Watts, D. J. (2002). A simple model of global cascades on random networks. *Proc. Natl. Acad. Sci. U.S.A.* 99, 5766–5771.

Watts, D. J., and Strogatz, S. H. (1998). Collective dynamics of 'small-world' networks. *Nature* 393, 440–442.

Weinstock, M., Luques, L., Bejar, C., and Shoham, S. (2006). Ladostigil, a novel multifunctional drug for the treatment of dementia co-morbid with depression. *J. Neural Transm. Suppl.* 70, 443–446.

Weisz, N., Moratti, S., Meinzer, M., Dohrmann, K., and Elbert, T. (2005). Tinnitus perception and distress is related to abnormal spontaneous brain activity as measured by magnetoencephalography. *PLoS Med.* 2, e153. doi: 10.1371/journal.pmed.0020153

Weisz, N., Muller, S., Schlee, W., Dohrmann, K., Hartmann, T., and Elbert, T. (2007). The neural code of auditory phantom perception. *J. Neurosci.* 27, 1479–1484.

Wuchty, S., Oltvai, Z. N., and Barabasi, A. L. (2003). Evolutionary conservation of motif constituents in the yeast protein interaction network. *Nat. Genet.* 35, 176–179.

Yildirim, M. A., Goh, K. I., Cusick, M. E., Barabasi, A. L., and Vidal, M. (2007). Drug-target network. *Nat. Biotechnol.* 25, 1119–1126.

18

Structural changes of the corpus callosum in tinnitus

***Eugen Diesch*[1]*, Verena Schummer*[2]*, Martin Kramer*[2] *and Andre Rupp*[3]**

[1] *Department of Clinical and Cognitive Neuroscience, Central Institute of Mental Health, Medical Faculty Mannheim, Heidelberg University, Mannheim, Germany*
[2] *Small Animal Clinic, Department of Veterinary Clinical Sciences, University of Gießen, Gießen, Germany*
[3] *Section of Biomagnetism, Department of Neurology, University Hospital Heidelberg, Heidelberg, Germany*

Correspondence:
Eugen Diesch, Department of Clinical and Cognitive Neuroscience, Central Institute of Mental Health, Medical Faculty Mannheim, Heidelberg University, Square J5, D-68159 Mannheim, Germany.
e-mail: eugen.diesch@zi-mannheim.de

Objectives: In tinnitus, several brain regions seem to be structurally altered, including the medial partition of Heschl's gyrus (mHG), the site of the primary auditory cortex. The mHG is smaller in tinnitus patients than in healthy controls. The corpus callosum (CC) is the main interhemispheric commissure of the brain connecting the auditory areas of the left and the right hemisphere. Here, we investigate whether tinnitus status is associated with CC volume. **Methods:** The midsagittal cross-sectional area of the CC was examined in tinnitus patients and healthy controls in which an examination of the mHG had been carried out earlier. The CC was extracted and segmented into subregions which were defined according to the most common CC morphometry schemes introduced by Witelson (1989) and Hofer and Frahm (2006). **Results**: For both CC segmentation schemes, the CC posterior midbody was smaller in male patients than in male healthy controls and the isthmus, the anterior midbody, and the genou were larger in female patients than in female controls. With CC size normalized relative to mHG volume, the normalized CC splenium was larger in male patients than male controls and the normalized CC splenium, the isthmus and the genou were larger in female patients than female controls. Normalized CC segment size expresses callosal interconnectivity relative to auditory cortex volume. **Conclusion**: It may be argued that the predominant function of the CC is excitatory. The stronger callosal interconnectivity in tinnitus patients, compared to healthy controls, may facilitate the emergence and maintenance of a positive feedback loop between tinnitus generators located in the two hemispheres.

Keywords: tinnitus, auditory cortex, corpus callosum, MRI volumetry

INTRODUCTION

Tinnitus is an auditory phantom sensation that is experienced in the absence of adequate acoustic stimulation. Affected individuals often describe it as kind of ringing, hissing, or buzzing, most often continuous, sometimes intermittent. Tinnitus affects a considerable proportion of the general population, with a minority experiencing considerable distress (Hazell, 1990; Feldmann, 1998; Baguley and McFerran, 2002; Lockwood et al., 2002; Eggermont and Roberts, 2004; Shargorodsky et al., 2010). Often, but not always, tinnitus is associated with a certain measure of hearing loss mostly of the upper part of the range of hearing (Henry et al., 1999). Hearing loss represents the most prevalent risk factor for tinnitus (Sindhusake et al., 2003; Moller, 2007).

The pathophysiological mechanisms underlying tinnitus are largely unknown. The disorder is characterized by hyperexcitability resulting from a reduction of inhibitory processes and gain increase at various stages of the afferent auditory pathway including the auditory cortex (Salvi et al., 2000; Syka, 2002; Diesch et al., 2004; Eggermont and Roberts, 2004; Parra and Pearlmutter, 2007; Sun et al., 2009; Norena, 2011). Maladaptive plastic changes of the functional organization of the auditory system and the auditory cortex in particular seem to be implicated (Mühlnickel et al., 1998; Wienbruch et al., 2006). Several brain regions of tinnitus patients appear to be structurally altered, among them the thalamus and the nucleus accumbens (Mühlau et al., 2006), the inferior colliculus and the hippocampus (Landgrebe et al., 2009), and the medial partition of Heschl's gyrus (mHG), the anatomical site of the primary auditory cortex (Schneider et al., 2009).

Schneider et al. (2009) found smaller gray matter volumes of the medial partition of mHG in tinnitus patients than in healthy controls. Compared to hearing-impaired controls without tinnitus, patients with bilateral tinnitus showed mHG volume reduction in both hemispheres. Patients with unilateral tinnitus also showed mHG volume reduction. However, in these patients the reduction occurred almost exclusively on the side ipsilateral to the affected ear. To make sense of these volumetric reduction and lateralization effects the interconnection via the corpus callosum (CC) of the auditory cortices of the left and the right hemisphere may have to be considered.

Audition assumes a special status with regard to callosal connection. While in vision and somatosensation only the midline zone features callosal fiber connections, in audition callosal projections are distributed across the full extent of the auditory cortex (Bamiou et al., 2007). The CC fully connects homotopic and heterotopic auditory cortical areas of the two hemispheres. The callosal input to either hemisphere is characterized by a particular balance of excitatory and inhibitory processes. At the single unit level, the callosal fibers originating from cortical pyramidal cells are neurochemically excitatory. However, as they may terminate on inhibitory interneurons of the contralateral side, callosal projections are both excitatory and inhibitory functionally (Bloom and Hynd, 2005; Karayannis et al., 2007; Tang et al., 2007).

The CC is smaller in smaller brains (Jancke et al., 1997). More specifically, a smaller auditory cortex presumably gives rise to a smaller number of callosal fibers crossing to the contralateral side. In tinnitus, as long as the callosal volume reduction were proportional to the volume reduction of the auditory cortex, nothing would be expected to change. However, if the reduction in the number of callosal fibers were proportionally larger than the reduction of auditory cortex volume, the transcallosal influence would be weakened. In this case, if the default transcallosal influence were mainly inhibitory, the reduction in interhemispheric inhibition might be hypothesized to facilitate the emergence and maintenance of tinnitus. Conversely, if the reduction in the number of callosal fibers were proportionally smaller than the reduction of auditory cortex volume or if reduction of auditory cortex volume was accompanied by an increase of the number of callosal fibers, the transcallosal influence would be amplified. If the default transcallosal influence were largely excitatory, the increase in interhemispheric excitation likely would facilitate the development and persistence of tinnitus.

Apart from cortical volume, hemisphere asymmetry of cortical volume may also be important. On the basis of findings in rats, Galaburda et al. (1990) and Rosen et al. (1989) have proposed the existence of an inverse relationship between callosal connectivity and the magnitude of cortical hemisphere asymmetry. In humans, this inverse relationship has been confirmed by Aboitiz et al. (1992b,c), and Dorion et al. (2000), and with some caveats relating to the influence of gender and handedness, Luders et al. (2003). Luders et al. reported an inverse relationship between midsagittal callosal area and perisylvian asymmetries for males, but not for females. In the sample studied by Schneider et al. (2009), the mHG ipsilateral to the ear affected by tinnitus was smaller and the interhemispheric mHG asymmetry index was larger in patients with unilateral tinnitus than in healthy controls. Given the relationship between hemisphere asymmetry and CC size, it may be hypothesized that the Schneider et al. hemisphere asymmetry index is correlated with CC size, with gender eventually modulating the relationship. Furthermore, under the assumption that the default transcallosal influence were predominantly inhibitory, reduced CC size would mean reduced inhibition and potentially facilitate the development and maintenance of tinnitus.

MATERIALS AND METHODS

STUDY PARTICIPANTS

In the current study, the midsagittal cross-sectional surface area of the CC was determined for T1-weighted structural MR images (Siemens TRIO, 3 T, MPRAGE, matrix 256 × 256 mm^2, 176 sagittal slices, slice thickness 1 mm, TR 1930 ms, TE 4.38 ms) obtained from 105 subjects. Of these, 99 had been acquired in a prior volumetric study of the medial part (mHG) of Heschl's gyrus (Schneider et al., 2009) [1]. Six additional structural scans were available for the present study. Thus, CC volumetric scores were determined for 105 subjects and cross-correlations between CC and mHG volumetric scores for 99 subjects. Given the composition of the sample, the distribution of subjects across tinnitus status, musicality, and sex was almost the same as in the Schneider et al. (2009) study. As in Schneider et al. (2009), tinnitus patients were accepted to the study if they presented with chronic tonal or quasi-tonal tinnitus with a tinnitus frequency above 1 kHz. Tinnitus was considered chronic if its onset dated back 6 months or more. Individuals with noisiform or pulsatile tinnitus, Ménière's disease, otosclerosis, chronic headache, neurological disorders such as brain tumors, and individuals being treated for mental disorders were excluded from the study. Tinnitus was defined as chronic if it had lasted for more than 6 months. Controls did not present with tinnitus. Participants were assigned to the musician group if they worked as professional musicians, earned a score of at least 25 on the Advanced Measures of Music Audiation (AMMA) test, a standardized test of musicality which is independent of musical expertise (Gordon, 1989, 1998), or both. There were 25 musicians with tinnitus, 10 of them female, 38 non-musicians with tinnitus, 10 of them female, 31 musicians (13 female) without tinnitus, and 11 non-musicians (7 female) without tinnitus (**Table 1**). Pure-tone audiograms were obtained for 12 tonal frequencies between 125 Hz and 15 kHz to document the extent of hearing loss (**Figure 1**).

Summary indices of hearing loss were determined by computing averages across frequencies, i.e., across right and left ear low frequency (125 Hz–746 Hz) and high frequency (1.183 kHz–15 kHz) hearing loss scores. For patients, hearing loss at the tinnitus frequency was computed both for the left and the right ear by interpolating between the respective hearing loss values that were closest to the tinnitus frequency on the frequency axis. The equivalent tonal frequency and the minimum masking level of the tinnitus were determined using the methods described in Schneider et al. (2009). There was no significant difference between musicians with tinnitus and non-musicians with tinnitus with regard to the tinnitus frequency ($t_{(60)} = 1.13$, n.s.) or the tinnitus minimum masking level ($t_{(41)} = 1.14$, n.s.). Patients were also asked to complete the German version of the Tinnitus Questionnaire (TQ, Hallam et al., 1988; Hallam, 1996) published by Goebel and Hiller (Goebel and Hiller, 1994, 1998). Musicians with tinnitus attained significantly lower scores than non-musicians with tinnitus on the TQ ($t_{(46)} = 4.16$, $p < 0.0005$) and its subscales (tinnitus intrusiveness: $t_{(57)} = 5.23$, $p < 0.0005$, cognitive and emotional distress: $t_{(46)} = 3.78$, $p < 0.0005$, somatic complaints: $t_{(46)} = 2.12$, $p < 0.05$, auditory and perceptual difficulties: $t_{(46)} = 2.33$, $p < 0.025$, sleep disturbances: $t_{(46)} = 2.41$, $p < 0.02$).

CORPUS CALLOSUM SEGMENTATION

Morphological analysis of the CC was done in analogy to the procedure described by Luders et al. (2003). The midline sagittal cross-sectional surface area of the CC was reconstructed from the T1-weighted MRI data with the software program MRIcro (Ver. 1.40). Midsagittal sections were identified relative to the interhemispheric fissure in sagittal, horizontal, and coronal views. They were confirmed by the presence of the cerebral falx. The

[1] The data of seven of the 106 subjects that were examined in the Schneider et al. (2009) study could not be retrieved from backup media.

Table 1 | Subject characteristics, psychoacoustic test results, and TQ tinnitus questionnaire scores.

	NN	MN	NT	MT
SUBJECT CHARACTERISTICS/GROUP				
N [all (female)]	11 (7)	31 (13)	38 (10)	25 (10)
Age in years [mean (SEM)]	39.3 (3.6)	38.9 (1.8)	49.0 (1.8)	39.2 (2.6)
Handedness [N left-handed]	1	0	4	1
Tinnitus onset [years (SEM)]	–	–	10.1 (1.5)	10.9 (2.7)
PSYCHOACOUSTICS				
Tinnitus frequency [kHz (SEM)]	–	–	7.5 (0.5)	8.7 (1.1)
Tinnitus minimum masking level [dB]	–	–	17.2 (4.3)	26.1 (6.9)
AMMA tonal score	21.8 (0.64)	31.2 (0.89)	20.7 (0.5)	29.4 (0.7)
GOEBEL HILLER QUESTIONNAIRE				
Total score [mean (SEM)]	–	–	32.2 (3.7)	14.2 (2.1)
Tinnitus intrusiveness	–	–	9.1 (0.7)	4.1 (0.5)
Cognitive and emotional distress	–	–	15.2 (2.0)	6.2 (1.2)
Somatic complaints	–	–	1.2 (0.3)	0.5 (0.2)
Auditory and perceptual difficulties	–	–	4.6 (0.7)	2.4 (0.6)
Sleep disturbances	–	–	2.0 (0.3)	1.0 (0.3)

*In parentheses: number of females in line 1, SEM otherwise. **NN**, non-musicians without tinnitus; **MN**, musicians without tinnitus; **NT**, non-musicians with tinnitus; **MT**, musicians with tinnitus; **LE**, left ear; **RE**, right ear; **BE**, both ears; **LH**, left hemisphere; **RH**, right hemisphere. For some subjects, psychoacoustic and questionnaire data were not available. AMMA test results were available for nine subjects in group NN, 22 subjects in group MN, 24 subjects in group NT, and 24 subjects in group MT, tinnitus frequency for 38 subjects in group NT and 24 subjects in group MT, and tinnitus minimum masking level for 25 subjects in group NT and 18 subjects in group MT. Tinnitus questionnaire scores were available for 25 subjects in group NT with the exception of tinnitus intrusiveness for which there were scores from 35 subjects. The corresponding numbers for group MT were 23 and 24.*

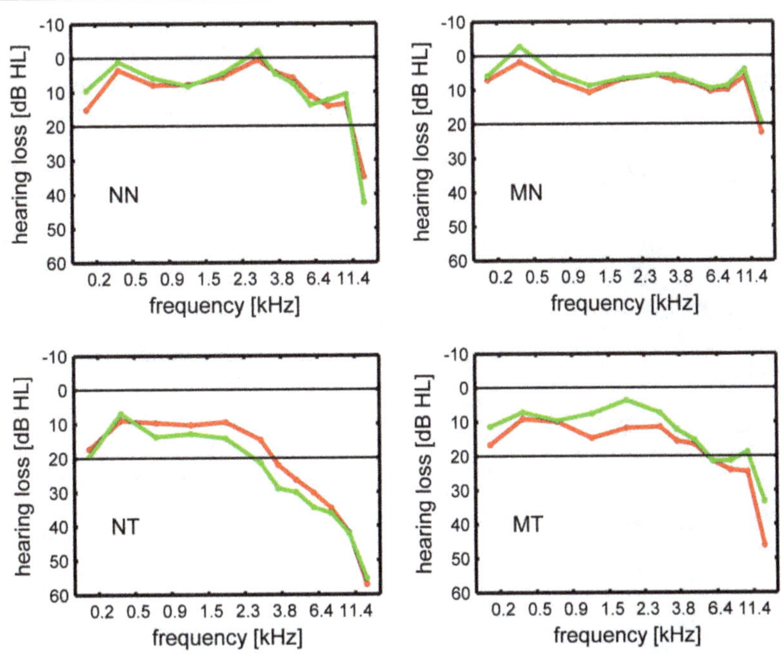

FIGURE 1 | Hearing loss in dB HL in the left ear (green line) and the right ear (red line). NN, non-musicians without tinnitus; MN, musicians without tinnitus; NT, non-musicians with tinnitus; MT, musicians with tinnitus.

original sagittal slices were reorientated to maximize apparent extent of the CC in the sagittal view. Using MRIcro's free rotation function, the whole brain was resliced such that the longitudinal fissure ran parallel to the sagittal slices. A tissue intensity contrast-based region-of-interest (ROI) comprising the CC was defined in the slice that included the longitudinal fissure and the two neighboring slices to the left and the right using the MRIcro "image intensity defined 3D ROI" function. Tissue intensity thresholds were manually adjusted on an individual basis to optimally capture and extract the CC. If the CC and neighboring structures like the fornix did not differ in intensity or else were not segregated by an intensity-marked boundary, the automatic segmentation was corrected manually. The CC surface area image thus delineated was extracted from each of the three selected slices and saved for further processing. The segmentation was performed blindly, i.e., without knowledge on the side of the segmenter of the participant group the brain originated from.

Using procedures written in matlab and functions of the matlab image processing toolbox, the extracted CC images were segmented into subregions defined by the segmentation schemes put forward by Witelson (1989) and Hofer and Frahm (2006). The CC segmentation proposed by Witelson (1989) is the one most frequently used. As the Witelson scheme has been derived from non-human primates, the human diffusion tensor imaging-derived scheme proposed by Hofer and Frahm (2006) was used as an alternative. **Figure 2** illustrates the 2 segmentation schemes. The Witelson scheme employs four coronal subdivisions located at, from anterior to posterior, 1/3, 1/2, 2/3, and 4/5 of the total length of the CC. These subdivisions section the CC into five partitions representing the genu, the anterior part of the midbody, the posterior part of the midbody, the isthmus, and the splenium. The Hofer and Frahm scheme places the subdivisions somewhat differently, at 1/6, 1/2, 2/3, and 3/4. Relative to the Witelson scheme, the Hofer and Frahm scheme reduces segments 1 and 4 in size, increases segments 2 and 5, and leaves segment 3 unchanged.

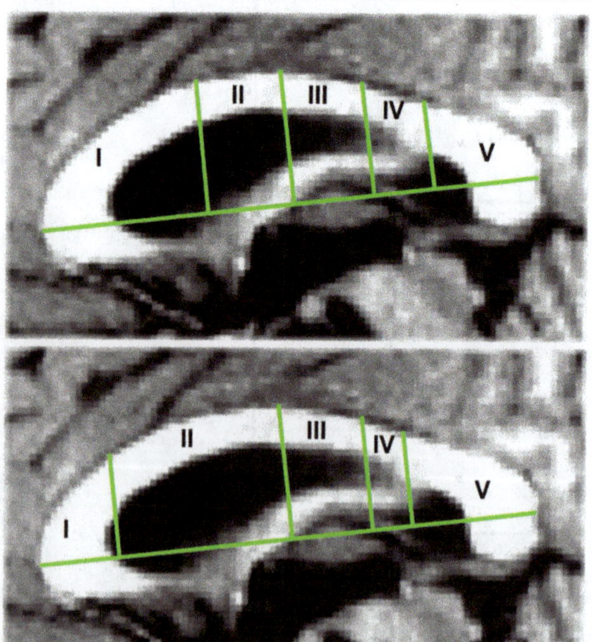

FIGURE 2 | (Top) The Witelson (1989) segmentation of the corpus callosum with four coronal subdivisions at, from anterior to posterior, 1/3, 1/2, 2/3, and 4/5 of the corpus callosum total length. **(Bottom)** The Hofer and Frahm (2006) segmentation with subdivisions at 1/6, 1/2, 2/3, and 3/4 of the total length.

Area measurements for the entire CC surface area and the surface area of each of the segments were obtained in mm^2 and pooled across the three sagittal slices selected. For a subset of 10 brains both intra- and inter-rater reliability coefficients were determined. For the entire CC surface area the intra-rater reliability was $r = 0.97$ and the inter-rater reliability $r = 0.98$. Intra-rater reliability ranged from 0.94 and inter-rater reliability from 0.96 to 0.99 for the Witelson and the Hofer and Frahm segments.

DATA ANALYSIS

The Witelson CC segment surface area scores and, separately, the Hofer and Frahm scores were submitted to a multivariate analysis of covariance (SPSS procedures GLM and MANOVA) with the CC segment scores as dependent variables, musicality and tinnitus status as grouping factors, and with whole intracranial brain size as a covariate. Intracranial brain size was determined using the Brainsuite software package (Shattuck and Leahy, 2002). The whole brain size covariate was used to normalize the CC segment scores. Simple effects analyses were run with sex as parameter. In analogy to Schneider et al. (2009), the analysis was rerun with age, handedness, and the four summary hearing loss indices as additional covariates. Because univariate analysis, but not multivariate analysis, offers the possibility to localize effects to particular CC segments, both multivariate and univariate contrasts were considered.

In the Schneider et al. (2009) study, the gray matter volumes of the mHG of both hemispheres were computed. The mHG was partitioned in eight successive cross-sectional 3 mm-slices orientated perpendicularly to the major axis of the respective individual mHG. For each of the eight homologous segment pairs, an index of volumetric (a) symmetry was computed in terms of the standardized difference between the right and the left hemisphere volume: $\delta S = (VRH - VLH)/(VRH + VLH)$. This index assumes positive values if the right hemisphere volume is larger than the left hemisphere volume and negative values if the left hemisphere volume is larger than the right hemisphere volume. For the present study, bilateral compound mHG segment volumes comprising homologous mHG segment pairs were computed and submitted to multivariate analysis of covariance with whole brain size as a covariate. The maximum of the absolute volumetric asymmetry, $\max(\text{abs}(\delta S))$, was calculated and the segment index score of the segment where the asymmetry attained its maximum was determined.

Presumably, any putative alterations of CC size in tinnitus would be closely related to the alterations in the auditory cortex. However, a smaller CC in tinnitus patients, compared with healthy controls, could represent an epiphenomenon of the smaller auditory cortex rather than a structural factor that might be related to tinnitus in its own right. To disentangle these alternatives, normalized CC segment surface scores, i.e., CC segment scores divided by the total bilateral compound mHG volume to the power of 2/3, i.e., normalized CCsurface = $\text{CCsurface}/\text{mHGvolume}^{(2/3)}$, were computed and submitted to analysis of variance. For tinnitus patients, correlations were computed between the normalized CC segment surface scores and the Goebel and Hiller (1994, 1998) tinnitus questionnaire total score as well as the "tinnitus intrusiveness" subscale score.

When they were computed across all study participants, Schneider et al. (2009) found significant negative correlations between three of the four summary indices of hearing loss and left and right hemisphere mHG volume. These correlations were recomputed for the present sample, both without and with age as a covariate. In addition, (partial) correlations were computed between the hearing loss indices and total CC surface area, the surface area of the anterior CC (Witelson/Hofer and Frahm segments I and II), and the surface area of the posterior CC (Witelson/Hofer and Frahm segments III, IV, and V) surface area. Again in correspondence with Schneider et al. (2009), in order to more closely examine the relationship between CC surface area and hearing loss, the partial correlations of these CC surface area indices and the hearing loss indices were also determined separately for the four groups of subjects. In the tinnitus groups, the partial correlations with left and right ear hearing loss estimated for the tinnitus frequency was also determined.

The maximum absolute mHG segment asymmetry and its segmental location were also submitted to analyses of variance with tinnitus status and musicality as grouping factors and sex as the parameter in simple effects analyses. To assess the hypothesis of a negative correlation between hemispheric asymmetry and CC size, partial correlations, with whole brain size as a covariate, between the maximum absolute volumetric asymmetry score and the CC segment surface area scores were computed.

RESULTS

Table 2 summarizes the corpus callosum (CC) segmentation results. Tinnitus status did not show a significant multivariate effect on CC segment size (Witelson: $T^2_{(5,96)} = 0.11$, n.s.; Hofer and Frahm: $T^2_{(5,96)} = 0.10$, n.s.). However, there were significant univariate effects. For both segmentation schemes the third segment was significantly smaller in tinnitus patients than in healthy controls (Witelson/Hofer and Frahm segment III: $F_{(1,100)} = 5.56$, $p < 0.02$). For musicality results differed between the segmentation schemes both with regard to multivariate (Witelson: $T^2_{(5,96)} = 0.09$, n.s.; Hofer and Frahm: $T^2_{(5,96)} = 0.13$, $p < 0.05$) and univariate effects (Witelson segment II: $F_{(1,100)} = 5.98$, $p < 0.02$; Hofer segment I: $F_{(1,100)} = 5.48$, $p < 0.025$; Hofer segment II: $F_{(1,100)} = 5.35$, $p < 0.025$; Hofer segment IV: $F_{(1,100)} = 5.81$, $p < 0.02$). The Witelson segment II and the Hofer segments I and IV were smaller in musicians than non-musicians. The Hofer segment II was larger in musicians than in non-musicians. There were no other significant multivariate or univariate effects.

In the simple effect analyses, the multivariate effect of tinnitus status onto CC segment size was significant in males (Witelson: $T^2_{(5,96)} = 0.12$, $p < 0.05$; Hofer and Frahm: $T^2_{(5,96)} = 0.12$, $p < 0.05$), but not in females (Witelson: $T^2_{(5,96)} = 0.08$, n.s.; Hofer and Frahm: $T^2_{(5,96)} = 0.09$, n.s.). There were no significant multivariate effects of musicality and the musicality-by-tinnitus status interaction in either group. As to univariate tests, CC segment III was significantly smaller in male tinnitus patients than male healthy controls (Witelson, Hofer and Frahm: $F_{(1,100)} = 10.00$, $p < 0.002$). In males there were no significant univariate effects of musicality and of the musicality-by-tinnitus status interaction. In female tinnitus patients, the segments Witelson II and Hofer and Frahm I and IV were significantly larger than in female

Table 2 | Corpus callosum segment sagittal surface area in mm^2 (standard deviation in parentheses) according to (a) Witelson (1989) and (b) Hofer and Frahm (2006) subdivided by sex (1: male, 0: female), musicality (1: musician, 0: non-musician), and tinnitus status (1: with tinnitus, 0: without tinnitus).

(a) WITELSON

Sex	Mus	Tin	W1	W2	W3	W4	W5
1	1	1	269.5 (45.7)	78.3 (11.2)	69.1 (9.2)	62.0 (12.7)	192.7 (28.4)
		0	282.2 (29.3)	88.9 (20.8)	78.7 (11.6)	65.6 (15.2)	208.5 (24.1)
	0	1	234.1 (49.3)	96.5 (35.9)	69.1 (9.5)	54.5 (18.2)	198.1 (36.3)
		0	259.8 (82.3)	98.5 (33.4)	79.0 (8.6)	58.5 (16.0)	194.3 (13.2)
0	1	1	249.9 (49.8)	84.8 (31.8)	69.2 (9.3)	58.7 (10.6)	190.0 (29.3)
		0	240.6 (41.5)	74.4 (11.4)	68.2 (9.1)	57.1 (11.9)	177.6 (27.5)
	0	1	217.1 (58.4)	117.6 (47.2)	74.7 (18.0)	56.0 (21.8)	196.7 (43.2)
		0	240.0 (60.6)	85.1 (22.4)	73.4 (11.1)	56.6 (15.4)	184.7 (28.5)

(b) HOFER

Sex	Mus	Tin	H1	H2	H3	H4	H5
1	1	1	181.1 (33.0)	166.7 (28.4)	69.1 (9.2)	35.1 (6.8)	219.5 (33.4)
		0	197.8 (33.5)	173.3 (33.5)	78.7 (11.6)	40.0 (6.9)	234.1 (27.0)
	0	1	197.3 (50.0)	133.2 (45.4)	69.1 (9.5)	42.9 (13.5)	209.8 (40.2)
		0	209.8 (39.6)	148.5 (55.8)	79.0 (8.6)	45.3 (11.0)	207.3 (33.7)
0	1	1	184.4 (43.9)	150.4 (32.6)	69.2 (9.3)	39.7 (14.3)	209.4 (26.7)
		0	159.4 (35.3)	155.5 (22.4)	68.2 (9.1)	33.5 (6.9)	201.2 (31.9)
	0	1	215.7 (59.6)	119.1 (50.5)	74.7 (18.0)	54.9 (24.0)	198.1 (41.3)
		0	178.7 (38.1)	146.4 (46.2)	73.4 (11.1)	39.1 (8.6)	201.9 (26.3)

healthy controls (Witelson II: $F_{(1, 100)} = 5.48$, $p < 0.025$; Hofer and Frahm I: $F_{(1, 100)} = 6.26$, $p < 0.02$; Hofer and Frahm IV: $F_{(1, 100)} = 7.60$, $p < 0.01$). In females, the same segments were smaller in musicians than non-musicians (Witelson II: $F_{(1, 100)} = 5.81$, $p < 0.02$; Hofer and Frahm I: $F_{(1, 100)} = 5.52$, $p < 0.025$; Hofer and Frahm IV: $F_{(1, 100)} = 6.51$, $p < 0.02$).

These results were essentially preserved in the extended covariate analysis with intracranial brain size, age, handedness, and the four summary hearing loss indices as covariates both in males (tinnitus status: Witelson: $T^2_{(5, 79)} = 0.15$, $p < 0.05$; Hofer and Frahm: $T^2_{(5, 79)} = 0.14$, $p < 0.06$; Witelson/Hofer and Frahm segment III: $F_{(1, 83)} = 8.56$, $p < 0.005$) and females (tinnitus status: segment Witelson II: $F_{(1, 83)} = 3.82$, $p < 0.06$; segment Hofer and Frahm I: $F_{(1, 83)} = 4.59$, $p < 0.05$; segment Hofer and Frahm IV: $F_{(1, 83)} = 6.65$, $p < 0.02$; musicality: segment Witelson II: $F_{(1, 83)} = 5.98$, $p < 0.02$; segment Hofer and Frahm I: $F_{(1, 83)} = 5.92$, $p < 0.02$; segment Hofer and Frahm IV: $F_{(1, 83)} = 6.81$, $p < 0.02$).

There were significant multivariate and univariate effects both of tinnitus status and musicality on bilateral compound mHG segment volume (tinnitus status: $T^2_{(8, 86)} = 0.23$, $p < 0.02$, $F_{(1, 93)} = 10.5–13.1$, $p < 0.002–0.0005$; musicality: $T^2_{(8, 86)} = 0.65$, $p < 0.0005$, $F_{(1, 93)} = 24.7–48.6$, $p < 0.0005$). There were no significant effects of the interaction. All eight bilateral compound mHG segments were smaller in tinnitus patients than in healthy controls and larger in musicians than in non-musicians. In the simple effects analyses, the multivariate effects of tinnitus status and the interaction of tinnitus status and musicality were not significant either for males or females. However, in the univariate analysis all eight bilateral compound mHG segments were significantly smaller in male tinnitus patients than in male healthy controls ($F_{(1, 93)} = 4.6–8.3$, $p < 0.05–0.005$). For all bilateral compound mHG segments, the difference went into the same direction in females, but without attaining significance ($F_{(1, 93)} = 0.9–3.6$, $p < 0.40–0.07$). For musicality, multivariate and univariate effects were significant in males and in females. In both groups, each of the segments was significantly larger in musicians than in non-musicians (males: $T^2_{(8, 86)} = 0.33$, $p < 0.001$, $F_{(1, 93)} = 4.1–24.1$, $p < 0.05–0.0005$; females: $T^2_{(8, 86)} = 0.21$, $p < 0.05$, $F_{(1, 93)} = 7.6–12.9$, $p < 0.01–0.001$).

Normalized CC segment size showed significant multivariate effects of tinnitus status (Witelson: $T^2_{(5, 90)} = 0.17$, $p < 0.02$; Hofer and Frahm: $T^2_{(5, 90)} = 0.16$, $p < 0.02$). In the univariate analysis, the Witelson segments II ($F_{(1, 94)} = 5.9$, $p < 0.02$) and V ($F_{(1, 94)} = 10.8$, $p < 0.001$) and the Hofer and Frahm segments I ($F_{(1, 94)} = 8.1$, $p < 0.005$), IV ($F_{(1, 94)} = 5.9$, $p < 0.02$), and V ($F_{(1, 94)} = 8.5$, $p < 0.005$) were significant. Musicality also featured significant multi- and univariate effects (Witelson: $T^2_{(5, 90)} = 0.51$, $p < 0.0005$, $F_{(1, 94)} = 13.9–45.4$, $p < 0.0005–0.00005$; Hofer: $T^2_{(5, 90)} = 0.54$, $p < 0.0005$, $F_{(1, 94)} = 9.5–45.4$, $p < 0.005–0.00005$), with each of the segments individually attaining significance. Normalized CC segment size was larger for tinnitus patients than for healthy controls and larger for non-musicians than for musicians (**Figure 3**). There were no significant multi- or univariate effects of the tinnitus status-by-musicality interaction.

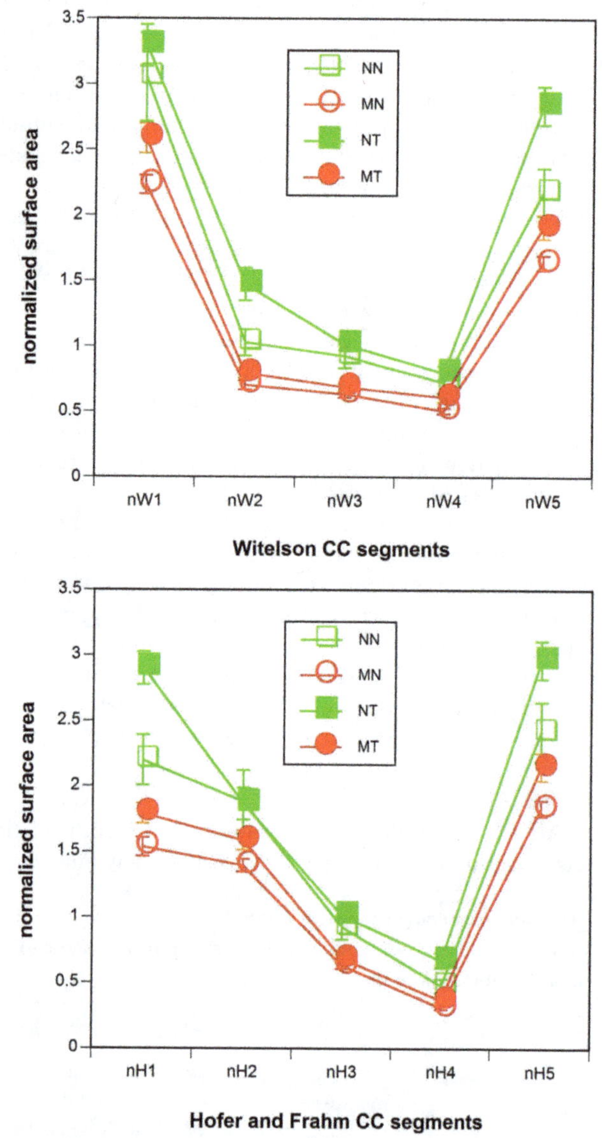

FIGURE 3 | Normalized (top) Witelson (1989) and (bottom) Hofer and Frahm (2006) CC segment size. Red: musicians. Green: non-musicians. Filled symbols: tinnitus patients. Open symbols: healthy controls. NN, non-musicians without tinnitus; MN, musicians without tinnitus; NT, non-musicians with tinnitus; MT, musicians with tinnitus.

In simple effects analyses with sex as parameter the multivariate effects of musicality and, with the exception of the Hofer and Frahm segment II, all univariate effects of musicality were preserved both for males (Witelson: $T^2_{(5, 90)} = 0.20$, $p < 0.005$, $F_{(1, 94)} = 5.5–17.7$, $p < 0.05–0.0005$; Hofer: $T^2_{(5, 90)} = 0.21$, $p < 0.005$, $F_{(1, 94)} = 3.3–17.7$, $p < 0.08–0.0005$) and females (Witelson: $T^2_{(5, 90)} = 0.17$, $p < 0.02$, $F_{(1, 94)} = 5.5–15.1$, $p < 0.025–0.0005$; Hofer: $T^2_{(5, 90)} = 0.16$, $p < 0.02$, $F_{(1, 94)} = 2.8–15.1$, $p < 0.10–0.0005$). However, the multivariate effects of tinnitus status were not preserved in the simple effects analysis either for males or females. Of the tinnitus status univariate effects only a few survived both for males (Witelson V: $F_{(1,94)} = 4.2$, $p < 0.05$; Hofer and Frahm segment V: $F_{(1,94)} = 5.6$, $p < 0.02$) and females (Witelson segment II: $F_{(1,94)} = 7.3$, $p < 0.01$; Witelson segment V: $F_{(1,94)} = 4.1$, $p < 0.05$; Hofer and Frahm segment I: $F_{(1,94)} = 6.5$, $p < 0.02$; Hofer and Frahm segment IV: $F_{(1,94)} = 7.8$, $p < 0.01$).

The correlations of normalized CC segment size with the total score of the Goebel and Hiller (1994, 1998) tinnitus questionnaire were positive throughout ($r = 0.12$–0.47) and attained significance at the $p < 0.05$ level or better in the Witelson segments I, III, IV, and V and the Hofer and Frahm segments II, III, and V. For tinnitus intrusiveness the range of correlations was $r = 0.22$–0.46, with the Witelson segments I, III, IV, and V and the Hofer and Frahm segments I, II, III, and V being significant, again at $p < 0.05$ or better. The correlations with 'normalized total CC size were $r = 0.36$, df $= 46$, $p < 0.02$ (Goebel and Hiller total score) and $r = 0.43$, df $= 46$, $p < 0.001$ (Goebel and Hiller intrusiveness score). By comparison, the total bilateral compound mHG volume was correlated negatively with the Goebel and Hiller total score ($r = -0.44$, df $= 46$, $p < 0.002$) and the Goebel and Hiller intrusiveness score ($r = -0.48$, df $= 46$, $p < 0.0005$) (**Figure 4**).

Several of the correlations of bilateral compound, left hemisphere, and right hemisphere mHG volume with left and right ear low and high frequency hearing loss were statistically significant (**Table 3**, lines 1–3). The mHG volume indices were also significantly correlated with age, but the relationship of mHG volume and hearing loss was not completely accounted for by the age confound. When age was partialled out, the significance of the correlations of high frequency hearing loss in the left ear with bilateral compound and with right hemisphere mHG volume was preserved. By comparison, all correlations and partial correlations of total, anterior, and posterior CC surface area with the hearing loss indices were close to zero and statistically not significant (**Table 3**, lines 4–6). This picture did not change when the correlations and partial correlations were computed separately for males and females. The groupwise examination of the relationship of CC surface area and hearing loss resulted in a range of partial correlation coefficients, again with age as the covariate, of (-0.61 to -0.02) for non-musicians without tinnitus, of (-0.01–0.18) for musicians without tinnitus, and of (-0.13–0.19) for non-musicians with tinnitus, none of them statistically significant. However, for musicians with tinnitus the 12 partial correlation coefficients computed ranged from $r_{part} = 0.01$ to $r_{part} = 0.66$, 8 of them attained statistical significance, and 3 of them—the correlations between right ear high frequency hearing loss and anterior CC surface area ($r_{part} = 0.58$, $p < 0.004$), left ear hearing loss at the tinnitus frequency and anterior CC surface area ($r_{part} = 0.66$, $p < 0.001$), and left ear hearing loss at the tinnitus frequency and total CC surface area ($r_{part} = 0.66$, $p < 0.001$)—survived Bonferroni-Holmes correction. When male and female musicians with tinnitus were considered separately, the correlations of left ear hearing loss at the tinnitus frequency with total CC surface area ($r_{part} = 0.73$, $p < 0.003$) and anterior CC surface area ($r_{part} = 0.76$, $p < 0.002$) in males and of left ear high frequency loss with total CC surface area ($r_{part} = 0.87$, $p < 0.005$) and right ear low frequency loss with anterior CC surface area ($r_{part} = 0.93$, $p < 0.001$) in females survived Bonferroni-Holmes correction.

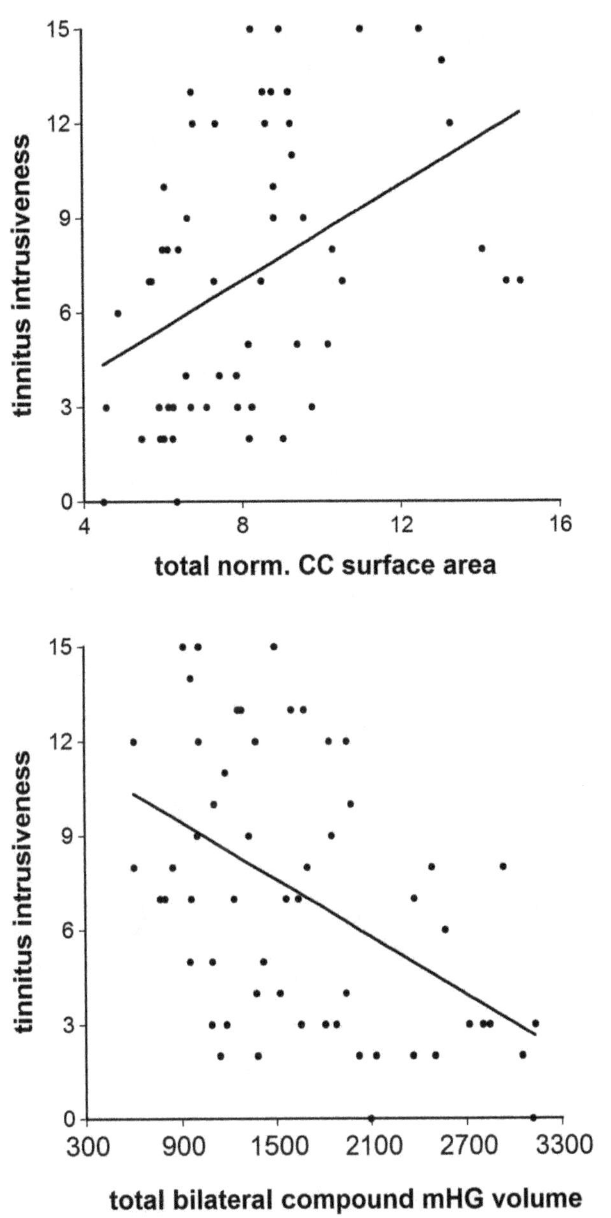

FIGURE 4 | The correlation between the Goebel and Hiller (1994, 1998) tinnitus questionnaire "tinnitus intrusiveness" subscale and (top) total normalized corpus callosum midsagittal surface area and (bottom) total bilateral compound mHG volume.

The distribution of the segmental location of the mHG asymmetry maximum is displayed in **Figure 5**. The most frequent segmental location of the maximum asymmetry differed between tinnitus patients and controls ($F_{(1,95)} = 10.30$, $p < 0.002$). In tinnitus patients, the asymmetry maximum was located most frequently in the medial segment S1. In healthy controls, the most frequent location of this maximum was a

Table 3 | Correlations of total bilateral mHG volume, total mHG volume of the left (LH) and the right hemisphere (RH), total corpus callosum (CC) volume, anterior CC surface area, and posterior CC surface area with chronological age, left ear low frequency loss (LE LF loss), right ear low frequency loss (RE LF loss), left ear high frequency loss (LE HF loss), and right ear high frequency loss (RE HF loss).

Correlation	Age	LE LF loss	RE LF loss	LE HF loss	RE HF loss
Bilateral mHG	−0.42**	−0.30*/−0.16	−0.18/−0.04	−0.51**/−0.31*	−0.42**/−0.13
LH mHG mHG volume [mm^3] (SEM)	−0.39**	−0.28*/−0.16	−0.16/−0.04	−0.45**/−0.25	−0.34**/−0.03
RH mHG mHG volume [mm^3] (SEM)	−0.39**	−0.28*/−0.14	−0.17/−0.03	−0.51**/−0.33*	−0.47**/−0.23
CC	−0.16	−0.11/−0.08	−0.12/−0.10	−0.05/0.03	−0.07/0.01
CC anterior	−0.19	−0.10/−0.06	−0.08/−0.05	−0.06/0.05	−0.08/0.04
CC posterior	−0.10	−0.10/−0.09	−0.14/−0.15	−0.03/−0.01	−0.04/−0.02

For the four hearing loss indices, the corresponding partial correlations, with age as a covariate, are also presented. Correlations and partial correlations marked by an asterisk are significant at the 0.01 level, correlations marked by two asterisks at the 0.0005 level.

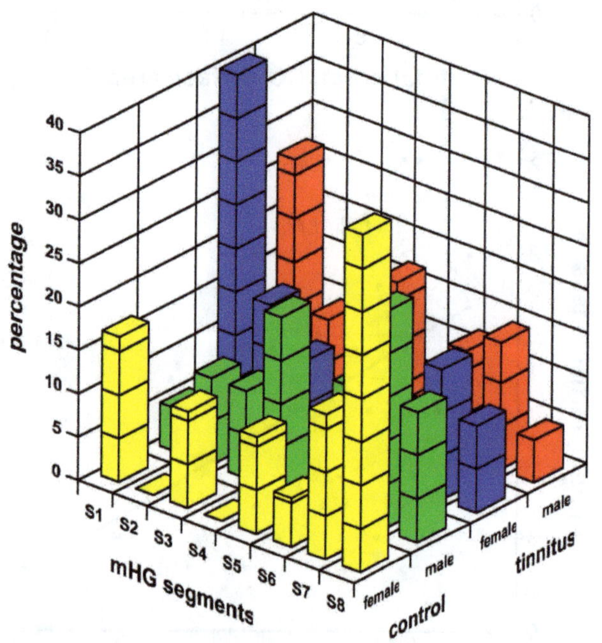

FIGURE 5 | The segmental location of the mHG asymmetry maximum in male and female tinnitus patients and healthy controls. The mHG segments are numbered from most medial (S1) to most lateral (S8).

lateral one, in segment S7 (males) or S8 (females). The effect was statistically marginal for males ($F_{(1,95)} = 3.15$, $p < 0.08$), but significant for females ($F_{(1,95)} = 7.14$, $p < 0.01$). Musicality and the musicality-by-tinnitus status interaction were not significant.

Because of the difference between tinnitus patients and controls in the segmental location of the mHG asymmetry maximum, maximum medial (segments 1–4) and maximum lateral (segments 5–8) segment asymmetry were determined separately. The maximum medial mHG segment asymmetry was larger for tinnitus patients than healthy controls ($F_{(1,95)} = 7.74, p < 0.01$). Simple effect analyses showed that this contrast was significant for males ($F_{(1,95)} = 8.21$, $p < 0.005$), but not for females ($F_{(1,95)} = 1.68$, n.s). Musicality and the musicality-by-tinnitus status interaction were not significant. There were no significant effects of tinnitus status, musicality, or their interaction on maximum lateral mHG segment asymmetry.

However, for the maximum medial mHG segment asymmetry, none of the partial correlations with CC segment size, with whole brain size as a covariate, was statistically significant. Significant partial correlations were obtained for male musicians between maximum lateral mHG segment asymmetry and the size of the third Witelson/the third Hofer and Frahm CC segment ($r_{part} = -0.43$, df = 29, $p < 0.02$) and the second Hofer and Frahm CC segment ($r_{part} = -0.38$, df = 29, $p < 0.05$). With tinnitus status as an additional covariate, these correlations were hardly affected (third Witelson/third Hofer and Frahm CC segment: $r_{part} = -0.40$, df = 28, $p < 0.05$; second Hofer and Frahm CC segment: $r_{part} = -0.37$, df = 28, $p < 0.05$).

DISCUSSION

The present study revealed effects of tinnitus status on CC midsagittal segment surface area that were dependent on sex and, for females, on the segmentation scheme used, Witelson (1989) or Hofer and Frahm (2006). In males, when the size of the entire brain was taken into account, the posterior midbody of the CC, i.e., the Witelson and Hofer and Frahm segment III, was smaller in tinnitus patients than in healthy controls. In female tinnitus patients, the Witelson segment II and the Hofer and Frahm segments I and IV were larger than they were in female healthy controls. The results were not appreciably altered when age, handedness, and indices of hearing loss were added as covariates. This pattern of findings does not lend itself to a straightforward interpretation. Fibers interconnecting the primary and association auditory cortical fields of both sides have been located in the posterior midbody, corresponding to the Witelson/Hofer and Frahm segment III (Aboitiz et al., 1992a; Chance et al., 2006), but also in the isthmus, corresponding to the Witelson/Hofer and Frahm segment IV (Cipolloni and Pandya, 1985; Witelson, 1989; Aboitiz et al., 1992a; Hofer and Frahm, 2006), and in the splenium, corresponding to the Witelson/Hofer and Frahm segment V (Sugishita et al., 1995; Pollmann et al., 2002; Fujimoto et al., 2006). The role in females of the Witelson segment II which carries premotor and supplementary motor fibers (Witelson, 1989; Hofer and Frahm, 2006) and of the Hofer and Frahm segment I which carries prefrontal fibers (Hofer and Frahm, 2006) suggests that attentional factors may be involved.

It seems difficult to make sense of the difference between males and females in the effect of tinnitus on CC segment size, decrease of the posterior midbody in males and increase of the isthmus and the genou in females. As the relationship of CC surface area to hearing loss was small and statistically insignificant, both for the sample as a whole and for males and females taken separately, the difference cannot be accounted for in terms of hearing loss or the effect of hearing loss on CC size varying between the sexes. Tinnitus might eventually be facilitated by CC size decrease, if CC function were predominantly inhibitory, and by CC size increase, if its function were predominantly excitatory. There is not much reason to assume that the CC functions in a predominantly inhibitory fashion in males and a predominantly excitatory fashion in females. While some researchers have claimed that the female CC, if scaled relative to whole brain size, is larger and thus facilitates transfer of information between the hemispheres (Oka et al., 1999; Mitchell et al., 2003), others have not found a difference (Bishop and Wahlsten, 1997; Luders et al., 2006; Zarei et al., 2006). Thus, there is little reason to speculate on the possibility of males and females differing with regard to the relation of tinnitus to callosal structure and function. Most probably then, CC segment surface area, even if related to whole brain size, does not provide a structural measure that lends itself to a functional interpretation.

When it came to the analysis of normalized CC segment surface area with normalization relative to the size of the auditory cortex, the pattern of results was more homogeneous and lent itself to a more straightforward interpretation. Both tinnitus status and musicality were significant in the multivariate analysis. In the univariate analysis, the Witelson segments II and V and the Hofer and Frahm segments I, II, and V were significantly larger in tinnitus patients than they were in healthy controls. The direction of the effect was the same in the remaining segments, although without attaining significance. Furthermore, all normalized Witelson and Hofer and Frahm segments were significantly larger in non-musicians than in musicians. The simple effects analyses largely reproduced the main analysis. In males, the Witelson and the Hofer and Frahm segment V and in females, the Witelson segments II and V and the Hofer and Frahm segments I and IV were significantly larger in patients than in healthy controls. Both for males and females the difference went into the same direction for the segments where the effect fell short of significance. Within the tinnitus group, subjective ratings of tinnitus intrusiveness were correlated positively with the normalized size of the majority of both Witelson and Hofer and Frahm segments and negatively with total bilateral compound mHG volume. The effect of tinnitus on Witelson segment V and the Hofer and Frahm segments IV and V is to be expected, as these segments carry fibers projecting from primary and association auditory cortex.

As normalized CC segments represent a ratio of absolute CC segment size to mHG size, the effect of larger normalized CC segments in tinnitus could be the result of larger absolute CC segment size, smaller mHG size, or both. In males with tinnitus, absolute CC segment size was smaller or equal and in females with tinnitus, it was larger or equal to what it was in controls. In males, smaller mHG size seems to be the predominant factor, while in females both factors seem to be involved. However, the tinnitus-related increase of normalized CC segment size in males shows that the reduction in the absolute size of CC segments was not proportionate to the mHG size reduction. Thus, both in male and female tinnitus patients certain segments of the CC are disproportionately large relative to the auditory cortex and may, therefore, be hypothesized to provide an enhanced connection between the hemispheres, possibly including a wider spatial range of convergent and divergent fiber projections.

The surface area of the midsagittal CC may mirror the number of axons interconnecting the two hemispheres (Aboitiz et al., 1992a) or a decrease in fiber density resulting from an increase in the diameter of or the distance between fibers (LaMantia and Rakic, 1990). Be that as it may, in either case the callosal transmission of information, of functionally excitatory and inhibitory influences, would be facilitated. Functionally, callosal projections are both excitatory and inhibitory (Bloom and Hynd, 2005; Karayannis et al., 2007; Tang et al., 2007). Findings in patients that underwent callosotomy as a treatment of otherwise intractable epilepsy suggest that the excitatory influence is the dominant one. Section of the CC disrupts the spread of seizures between the hemispheres (Ojemann, 1987). Although cases of a disruption of seizure inhibition by callosotomy have also been reported (Spencer et al., 1984; Ferbert et al., 1992; Netz et al., 1995), this effect is not as profound as the disruption of the interhemispheric spread of seizures (Bloom and Hynd, 2005). Assuming that it is hypersynchronous firing of neurons in the auditory cortex that represents the neurophysiological correlate of tinnitus (Eggermont and Roberts, 2004; Eggermont, 2007) and that the default transcallosal influence is mainly excitatory, the CC may well facilitate the development and maintenance of tinnitus. The synchronous activity of a population of single units in one hemisphere may be facilitated by the excitatory transcallosal inputs it receives and may in turn facilitate the emergence of one or more descendant synchronized populations via its callosal projection onto the auditory cortex of the respective contralateral hemisphere. And this maladaptive facilitatory function would necessarily be enhanced in subjects whose CC were disproportionally large and thus provided a particularly strong interhemispheric connection with a wider spatial range of convergent and divergent projections. Even if a putative tinnitus generator was originally restricted to one hemisphere, the establishment over time of such a positive feedback loop may facilitate the emergence of one or more mirror generators on the respective contralateral side. While most patients (85.0%) included in the dataset of the Oregon tinnitus archive (http://www.tinnitusarchive.org/) did not remember any kind of change in perceived tinnitus localization since the onset of their tinnitus, it is fitting that the by far most frequent kind of change (10.9%) was "Started on one side, now on both." This percentage is not small given that the majority of answers indicated a bilateral tinnitus location ("both ears": 63.0%, "fills head": 11.4%). Unfortunately, there is little information on whether and how the location of the hearing impairment and the duration of the tinnitus since its onset and the interaction of these factors affect the distribution of perceived tinnitus location.

The anterior CC carries premotor, supplementary motor, and prefrontal fiber projections (Witelson, 1989; Hofer and Frahm, 2006). As a result of training and practice, it is larger in musicians than in non-musicians (Schlaug et al., 1995, 2009). The finding in the present study of positive correlations in both male and female musicians with tinnitus between some of the indicators of hearing loss and anterior CC surface area may be taken to suggest that, in musicians, hearing loss may lead to an increase in anterior CC size. A potentially related positive correlation, between postero-medial left hemisphere mHG volume and right ear hearing loss, was found in musicians with tinnitus by Schneider et al. (2009). These findings invite some more speculative considerations. In the present study, while musicians with tinnitus did not differ in the tinnitus minimum masking level from non-musicians without tinnitus, they earned significantly lower scores on the tinnitus questionnaire and its subscales. This may indicate that musical training and practice may serve a protective function. The hypothetical mechanism underlying a putative protective function may relate to the fact that the playing of an instrument generates regularly patterned and correlated reafferent input streams to the auditory and the somatosensory system. There are multiple somatosensory entries into the auditory system that are capable of modulating auditory cortex activity (Schroeder et al., 2001; Lakatos et al., 2007). Increase of auditory cortex size and enhancement of fiber projections through the anterior CC may represent components of a protective auditory-motor-somatosensory-auditory loop.

The second hypothesis investigated, that tinnitus patients, on the average, exhibit a larger degree of interhemispheric mHG asymmetry than healthy controls and that mHG asymmetry is negatively correlated with the size of the posterior CC segments that transmit auditory information, was rejected by the data of this study. The segmental location of the maximum mHG asymmetry differed between tinnitus patients and healthy controls. For patients, the location of the mHG asymmetry maximum was extremely medial, for controls, it was extremely lateral. For males, but not females, the maximum medial asymmetry was larger for patients than for controls. However, it was the lateral, not the medial maximum asymmetry that was correlated negatively with the surface area of the posterior midbody segment of the CC, and this correlation was hardly at all affected by tinnitus status.

ACKNOWLEDGMENTS

Parts of this research were supported by a grant of the Deutsche Forschungsgemeinschaft to E. Diesch and A. Rupp (Di497/3-2). We would like to thank the reviewers of an earlier version of this paper for their insightful and constructive comments. Please address correspondence to Eugen Diesch. (e-mail: eugen.diesch@zi-mannheim.de).

REFERENCES

Aboitiz, F., Scheibel, A. B., Fisher, R. S., and Zaidel, E. (1992a). Fiber composition of the human corpus callosum. *Brain Res.* 598, 143–153.

Aboitiz, F., Scheibel, A. B., Fisher, R. S., and Zaidel, E. (1992b). Individual differences in brain asymmetries and fiber composition in the human corpus callosum. *Brain Res.* 598, 154–161.

Aboitiz, F., Scheibel, A. B., and Zaidel, E. (1992c). Morphometry of the Sylvian fissure and the corpus callosum, with emphasis on sex differences. *Brain* 115(Pt 5), 1521–1541.

Baguley, D. M., and McFerran, D. J. (2002). Current perspectives on tinnitus. *Arch. Dis. Child* 86, 141–143.

Bamiou, D. E., Sisodiya, S., Musiek, F. E., and Luxon, L. M. (2007). The role of the interhemispheric pathway in hearing. *Brain Res. Rev.* 56, 170–182.

Bishop, K. M., and Wahlsten, D. (1997). Sex differences in the human corpus callosum: myth or reality? *Neurosci. Biobehav. Rev.* 21, 581–601.

Bloom, J. S., and Hynd, G. W. (2005). The role of the corpus callosum in interhemispheric transfer of information: excitation or inhibition? *Neuropsychol. Rev.* 15, 59–71.

Chance, S. A., Casanova, M. F., Switala, A. E., and Crow, T. J. (2006). Minicolumnar structure in Heschl's gyrus and planum temporale: asymmetries in relation to sex and callosal fiber number. *Neuroscience* 143, 1041–1050.

Cipolloni, P. B., and Pandya, D. N. (1985). Topography and trajectories of commissural fibers of the superior temporal region in the rhesus monkey. *Exp. Brain Res.* 57, 381–389.

Diesch, E., Struve, M., Rupp, A., Ritter, S., Hulse, M., and Flor, H. (2004). Enhancement of steady-state auditory evoked magnetic fields in tinnitus. *Eur. J. Neurosci.* 19, 1093–1104.

Dorion, A. A., Chantome, M., Hasboun, D., Zouaoui, A., Marsault, C., Capron, C., and Duyme, M. (2000). Hemispheric asymmetry and corpus callosum morphometry: a magnetic resonance imaging study. *Neurosci. Res.* 36, 9–13.

Eggermont, J. J. (2007). Correlated neural activity as the driving force for functional changes in auditory cortex. *Hear. Res.* 229, 69–80.

Eggermont, J. J., and Roberts, L. E. (2004). The neuroscience of tinnitus. *Trends Neurosci.* 27, 676–682.

Feldmann, H. (1998). *Tinnitus: Grundlagen einer rationalen Diagnostk und Therapie*, 2. Auflage. Stuttgart, New York, NY: Thieme.

Ferbert, A., Priori, A., Rothwell, J. C., Day, B. L., Colebatch, J. G., and Marsden, C. D. (1992). Interhemispheric inhibition of the human motor cortex. *J. Physiol.* 453, 525–546.

Fujimoto, C., Ito, K., Iwasaki, S., Nakao, K., and Sugasawa, M. (2006). Reversible impairment of auditory callosal pathway in 5-fluorouracil-induced leukoencephalopathy: parallel changes in function and imaging. *Otol. Neurotol.* 27, 716–719.

Galaburda, A. M., Rosen, G. D., and Sherman, G. F. (1990). Individual variability in cortical organization: its relationship to brain laterality and implications to function. *Neuropsychologia* 28, 529–546.

Goebel, G., and Hiller, W. (1994). The tinnitus questionnaire. A standard instrument for grading the degree of tinnitus. Results of a multicenter study with the tinnitus questionnaire. *HNO* 42, 166–172.

Goebel, G., and Hiller, W. (1998). *Der Tinnitus-Fragebogen.* Göttingen: Hogrefe.

Gordon, E. (1989). *Advanced Measures of Music Audiation.* Chikago: GIA Publications.

Gordon, E. (1998). *Introduction to Research and the Psychology of Music.* Chikago: GIA Publications.

Hallam, R. S. (1996). *Manual of the Tinnitus Questionnaire (TQ).* London: Psychological Corporation.

Hallam, R. S., Jakes, S. C., and Hinchcliffe, R. (1988). Cognitive variables in tinnitus annoyance. *Br. J. Clin. Psychol.* 27(Pt 3), 213–222.

Hazell, J. (1990). Tinnitus and disability with ageing: adaptation and management. *Acta Otolaryngol. Suppl.* 476, 202–208.

Henry, J. A., Meikle, M., and Gilbert, A. (1999). "Audiometric correlates of tinnitus pitch: insights from the Tinnitus Data Registry," in *Proceedings of the Sixth International Tinnitus Seminar*, ed J. W. P. Hazell (London: The Tinnitus and Hyperacusis Centre), 51–57.

Hofer, S., and Frahm, J. (2006). Topography of the human corpus callosum revisited–comprehensive fiber tractography using diffusion tensor magnetic resonance imaging. *Neuroimage* 32, 989–994.

Jancke, L., Staiger, J. F., Schlaug, G., Huang, Y., and Steinmetz, H. (1997). The relationship between corpus callosum size and forebrain volume. *Cereb. Cortex* 7, 48–56.

Karayannis, T., Huerta-Ocampo, I., and Capogna, M. (2007). GABAergic and pyramidal neurons of deep cortical layers directly receive and differently integrate callosal input. *Cereb. Cortex* 17, 1213–1226.

Lakatos, P., Chen, C. M., O'Connell, M. N., Mills, A., and Schroeder, C. E. (2007). Neuronal oscillations and multisensory interaction in primary auditory cortex. *Neuron* 53, 279–292.

LaMantia, A. S., and Rakic, P. (1990). Cytological and quantitative characteristics of four cerebral commissures in the rhesus monkey. *J. Comp Neurol.* 291, 520–537.

Landgrebe, M., Langguth, B., Rosengarth, K., Braun, S., Koch, A., Kleinjung, T., May, A., De Ridder, R. D., and Hajak, G. (2009). Structural brain changes in tinnitus: grey matter decrease in auditory and non-auditory brain areas. *Neuroimage* 46, 213–218.

Lockwood, A. H., Salvi, R. J., and Burkard, R. F. (2002). Tinnitus. *N. Engl. J. Med.* 347, 904–910.

Luders, E., Narr, K. L., Zaidel, E., Thompson, P. M., and Toga, A. W. (2006). Gender effects on callosal thickness in scaled and unscaled space. *Neuroreport* 17, 1103–1106.

Luders, E., Rex, D. E., Narr, K. L., Woods, R. P., Jancke, L., Thompson, P. M., Mazziotta, J. C., and Toga, A. W. (2003). Relationships between sulcal asymmetries and corpus callosum size: gender and handedness effects. *Cereb. Cortex* 13, 1084–1093.

Mitchell, T. N., Free, S. L., Merschhemke, M., Lemieux, L., Sisodiya, S. M., and Shorvon, S. D. (2003). Reliable callosal measurement: population normative data confirm sex-related differences. *AJNR Am. J. Neuroradiol.* 24, 410–418.

Moller, A. R. (2007). Tinnitus: presence and future. *Prog. Brain Res.* 166, 3–16.

Mühlau, M., Rauschecker, J. P., Oestreicher, E., Gaser, C., Röttinger, M., Wohlschläger, A. M., Simon, F., Etgen, T., Conrad, B., and Sander, D. (2006). Structural brain changes in tinnitus. *Cereb. Cortex* 16, 1283–1288.

Mühlnickel, W., Elbert, T., Taub, E., and Flor, H. (1998). Reorganization of auditory cortex in tinnitus. *Proc. Natl. Acad. Sci. U.S.A.* 95, 10340–10343.

Netz, J., Ziemann, U., and Homberg, V. (1995). Hemispheric asymmetry of transcallosal inhibition in man. *Exp. Brain Res.* 104, 527–533.

Norena, A. J. (2011). An integrative model of tinnitus based on a central gain controlling neural sensitivity. *Neurosci. Biobehav. Rev.* 35, 1089–1109.

Ojemann, G. A. (1987). Surgical therapy for medically intractable epilepsy. *J. Neurosurg.* 66, 489–499.

Oka, S., Miyamoto, O., Janjua, N. A., Honjo-Fujiwara, N., Ohkawa, M., Nagao, S., Kondo, H., Minami, T., Toyoshima, T., and Itano, T. (1999). Re-evaluation of sexual dimorphism in human corpus callosum. *Neuroreport* 10, 937–940.

Parra, L. C., and Pearlmutter, B. A. (2007). Illusory percepts from auditory adaptation. *J. Acoust. Soc. Am.* 121, 1632–1641.

Pollmann, S., Maertens, M., Von Cramon, D. Y., Lepsien, J., and Hugdahl, K. (2002). Dichotic listening in patients with splenial and nonsplenial callosal lesions. *Neuropsychology* 16, 56–64.

Rosen, G. D., Sherman, G. F., and Galaburda, A. M. (1989). Interhemispheric connections differ between symmetrical and asymmetrical brain regions. *Neuroscience* 33, 525–533.

Salvi, R. J., Wang, J., and Ding, D. (2000). Auditory plasticity and hyperactivity following cochlear damage. *Hear. Res.* 147, 261–274.

Schlaug, G., Forgeard, M., Zhu, L., Norton, A., Norton, A., and Winner, E. (2009). Training-induced neuroplasticity in young children. *Ann. N.Y. Acad. Sci.* 1169, 205–208.

Schlaug, G., Jancke, L., Huang, Y., and Steinmetz, H. (1995). *In vivo* evidence of structural brain asymmetry in musicians. *Science* 267, 699–701.

Schneider, P., Andermann, M., Wengenroth, M., Goebel, R., Flor, H., Rupp, A., and Diesch, E. (2009). Reduced volume of Heschl's gyrus in tinnitus. *Neuroimage* 45, 927–939.

Schroeder, C. E., Lindsley, R. W., Specht, C., Marcovici, A., Smiley, J. F., and Javitt, D. C. (2001). Somatosensory input to auditory association cortex in the macaque monkey. *J. Neurophysiol.* 85, 1322–1327.

Shargorodsky, J., Curhan, G. C., and Farwell, W. R. (2010). Prevalence and characteristics of tinnitus among US adults. *Am. J. Med.* 123, 711–718.

Shattuck, D. W., and Leahy, R. M. (2002). BrainSuite: an automated cortical surface identification tool. *Med. Image Anal.* 6, 129–142.

Sindhusake, D., Golding, M., Newall, P., Rubin, G., Jakobsen, K., and Mitchell, P. (2003). Risk factors for tinnitus in a population of older adults: the blue mountains hearing study. *Ear Hear.* 24, 501–507.

Spencer, S. S., Spencer, D. D., Glaser, G. H., Williamson, P. D., and Mattson, R. H. (1984). More intense focal seizure types after callosal section: the role of inhibition. *Ann. Neurol.* 16, 686–693.

Sugishita, M., Otomo, K., Yamazaki, K., Shimizu, H., Yoshioka, M., and Shinohara, A. (1995). Dichotic listening in patients with partial section of the corpus callosum. *Brain* 118(Pt 2), 417–427.

Sun, W., Lu, J., Stolzberg, D., Gray, L., Deng, A., Lobarinas, E., and Salvi, R. J. (2009). Salicylate increases the gain of the central auditory system. *Neuroscience* 159, 325–334.

Syka, J. (2002). Plastic changes in the central auditory system after hearing loss, restoration of function, and during learning. *Physiol. Rev.* 82, 601–636.

Tang, J., Xiao, Z., and Suga, N. (2007). Bilateral cortical interaction: modulation of delay-tuned neurons in the contralateral auditory cortex. *J. Neurosci.* 27, 8405–8413.

Wienbruch, C., Paul, I., Weisz, N., Elbert, T., and Roberts, L. E. (2006). Frequency organization of the 40-Hz auditory steady-state response in normal hearing and in tinnitus. *Neuroimage* 33, 180–194.

Witelson, S. F. (1989). Hand and sex differences in the isthmus and genu of the human corpus callosum. A postmortem morphological study. *Brain* 112(Pt 3), 799–835.

Zarei, M., Johansen-Berg, H., Smith, S., Ciccarelli, O., Thompson, A. J., and Matthews, P. M. (2006). Functional anatomy of interhemispheric cortical connections in the human brain. *J. Anat.* 209, 311–320.

19

Music-induced cortical plasticity and lateral inhibition in the human auditory cortex as foundations for tonal tinnitus treatment

Christo Pantev[1]*, Hidehiko Okamoto[1,2] and Henning Teismann[1]

[1] Institute for Biomagnetism and Biosignalanalysis, University of Münster, Münster, Germany
[2] Department of Integrative Physiology, National Institute for Physiological Sciences, Okazaki, Japan

Correspondence:
Christo Pantev, Institute for Biomagnetism and Biosignalanalysis, University of Münster, Malmedyweg 15, 48129 Muenster, Germany.
e-mail: pantev@uni-muenster.de

Over the past 15 years, we have studied plasticity in the human auditory cortex by means of magnetoencephalography (MEG). Two main topics nurtured our curiosity: the effects of musical training on plasticity in the auditory system, and the effects of lateral inhibition. One of our plasticity studies found that listening to notched music for 3 h inhibited the neuronal activity in the auditory cortex that corresponded to the center-frequency of the notch, suggesting suppression of neural activity by lateral inhibition. Subsequent research on this topic found that suppression was notably dependent upon the notch width employed, that the lower notch-edge induced stronger attenuation of neural activity than the higher notch-edge, and that auditory focused attention strengthened the inhibitory networks. Crucially, the overall effects of lateral inhibition on human auditory cortical activity were stronger than the habituation effects. Based on these results we developed a novel treatment strategy for tonal tinnitus—tailor-made notched music training (TMNMT). By notching the music energy spectrum around the individual tinnitus frequency, we intended to attract lateral inhibition to auditory neurons involved in tinnitus perception. So far, the training strategy has been evaluated in two studies. The results of the initial long-term controlled study (12 months) supported the validity of the treatment concept: subjective tinnitus loudness and annoyance were significantly reduced after TMNMT but not when notching spared the tinnitus frequencies. Correspondingly, tinnitus-related auditory evoked fields (AEFs) were significantly reduced after training. The subsequent short-term (5 days) training study indicated that training was more effective in the case of tinnitus frequencies $\leq$8 kHz compared to tinnitus frequencies >8 kHz, and that training should be employed over a long-term in order to induce more persistent effects. Further development and evaluation of TMNMT therapy are planned. A goal is to transfer this novel, completely non-invasive and low-cost treatment approach for tonal tinnitus into routine clinical practice.

Keywords: human auditory cortex, lateral inhibition, music-induced cortical plasticity, tonal tinnitus treatment, tailor-made notched music training

INTRODUCTION

Chronic tinnitus is a prevalent symptom/syndrome that can severely affect a patient's ability to lead a normal life and can induce psychiatric distress, which may even be associated with the risk of suicide (Coles, 1984). Chronic tinnitus is one of the most common auditory disorders, currently affecting 10–15% of the general adult population (Heller, 2003). In Germany, for instance, there are about 3 Million tinnitus sufferers in need of medical help, and about 1 Million people with tinnitus fail to cope with or compensate for their tinnitus.

The contemporary view on tinnitus biology is that, although tinnitus may be triggered by injury to the inner ear, the neural generators are most readily found centrally. While the neural generators may be primarily auditory, non-auditory centers often participate. Studies of noise-induced tinnitus have given rise to the general theory that tinnitus is triggered by injury to inner ear hair-cell populations. One consequence of such injury is a loss of lateral inhibition in the cortical frequency areas which map to those areas which have been primarily damaged in the periphery; this leads, in turn, to augmented excitation in the regions spectrally neighboring the lesion. This change projects to plastic adjustments in the central auditory system, culminating in altered cortical activity. The theory also holds that central auditory system plasticity is the main centerpiece of these adjustments, whereby reduced auditory nerve input triggers a shift in the balance of excitation and inhibition centrally. This shift leads to the emergence of a tripartite complex of changes that includes hyperactivity, increased bursting activity, and increased synchrony. Such changes reflect a loss of inhibitory drive to neurons, particularly of glycinergic and GABAergic systems, however, increases in excitation via upregulations of glutamatergic and cholinergic systems may also be involved. Such changes are found at multiple levels of the auditory pathway and even in some non-auditory centers, including somatosensory and limbic regions (Martin et al., 1993; Ochi and Eggermont, 1997; Cazals et al., 1998; Norena and Eggermont, 2005; Bauer et al., 2008). This view is consistent with the three-sided nature of tinnitus, which includes auditory, attentional, and emotional components.

To date, there is no standard cure for tinnitus (Rauschecker et al., 2010). One major problem is that there are several different treatment target candidates in the brain (e.g., auditory cortex, thalamus, dorsal/ventral cochlear nuclei, inferior colliculus, cochlear nerve, and the limbic system (Langguth et al., 2010). However, it appears plausible to assume that the auditory cortex should be a treatment target because changes in the auditory cortex must exist when tinnitus is consciously perceived.

During recent years, music has been intensively used as a tool for human brain investigations. Music relates to many human brain functions, such as perception, action, cognition, emotion, learning, and memory, and is therefore an ideal tool to investigate how the human brain works and how different brain functions interact. The positive effects which music, in its various forms, has on the human brain, are not only important in the framework of basic neuroscience but they also have considerable neuro-rehabilitative potential (Pantev and Herholz, 2011).

One of the key features in the processing of auditory information in central auditory structures is lateral inhibition. The afferent auditory pathway is not only formed by excitatory neural connections but also by inhibitory networks. A central auditory pathway neuron is characterized by its tuning curve. Each neuron has a characteristic frequency (CF) to which it is most responsive and is surrounded by other neurons, so that, together, they tonotopically span a range of CFs. If the neuron is excited from a lower level, it not only projects excitation to higher levels but also distributes inhibition laterally via interneuron collaterals to adjacent neurons with higher or lower CFs. This inhibition effect depends on the firing rate of the neuron and on the number of collaterals.

Based on two major foundations—music-induced plasticity and lateral inhibition of the human auditory cortex (which will be discussed in more detail in subsequent sections)—we have developed and evaluated a novel, individualized music training procedure capable of significantly alleviating the perceived loudness of tinnitus. The strategy is based on the notion that circumscribed, hyper-synchronous neuronal activity in the auditory cortex is critical for the emergence of tinnitus perception and it is motivated by neuro-scientific data indicating that maladaptive cortical reorganization processes are associated with tinnitus generation and maintenance. The treatment regimen consists of regularly listening to so-called "tailor-made notched music training (TMNMT)," which is characterized by a suppressed frequency band centered at the individual tinnitus frequency. By having patients listen to this modified music, we intend to decrease tinnitus-related hyper-synchronous auditory cortical activity through the attraction of lateral inhibition. As a consequence, the tinnitus would be perceived as becoming less loud and less distressing. Cumulative tinnitus alleviation would indicate long-term plasticity effects that could be expressed in both primary and secondary auditory cortical structures. A crucial aspect of the TMNMT is that patients are motivated to, and able to, select and listen to their favorite music. Listening to enjoyable music is likely to activate cortical attention networks and also the reward mechanisms of the brain, both of which would promote long-term plasticity. Moreover, in our TMNMT evaluation studies we have not relied solely on behavioral outcome measures; we also recorded tinnitus-related primary and non-primary auditory cortical neuronal activity by means of magnetoencephalography (MEG). We hypothesized that behavioral markers of tinnitus alleviation would correlate positively with electrophysiological markers of tinnitus-related change in auditory cortical neural activity.

MUSIC-INDUCED PLASTICITY IN THE HUMAN AUDITORY CORTEX

In higher mammals including humans, neurons as well as some of their interconnections are formed prenatally into neural networks. For many years, the prevailing opinion was that network connections between neurons are generated primarily during cerebral maturation processes and that they would not change later. However, humans respond with considerable flexibility to new challenges throughout their entire life. Over the last three decades, experimental evidence has demonstrated that the connectivity of the adult brain is only partially determined by genetics and development during the childhood, and may be substantially modified through sensory experiences during adulthood. Thus, the functional organization of the adult brain adjusts in response to the alteration of behaviorally relevant input and processing. This was first demonstrated in a series of classical animal studies (Merzenich et al., 1983a,b; Jenkins et al., 1990; Kaas et al., 1990; Gilbert and Wiesel, 1992; Recanzone et al., 1993; Irvine and Rajan, 1995; Rauschecker et al., 1995, 1997).

The development of new, non-invasive techniques for recording brain activity has enabled neuroscientists to prove the existence of plasticity in functional neuronal networks in humans. One of these techniques, MEG [the magnetic counterpart of electroencephalography (EEG)], has become an established method for the non-invasive study of the spontaneous and evoked activity of the human cortex (Hari, 1990). The main sources of this activity are the pyramidal cells, which generate currents that flow tangentially to the surface of the head. Although MEG measurements provide only a macroscopic view of brain function, the spatial and, especially, the temporal-resolution achieved with this technique is sufficient to give indications of the functional organization and reorganizational plasticity of the human cortex by localizing the sources of evoked magnetic fields, which are elicited by different peripheral stimulation. Thus, using MEG, which allows non-invasive measurement in human subjects, changes in the cortical maps similar to those observed in the primate cortex can be demonstrated.

AUDITORY PLASTICITY IN MUSICIANS

Music relates to many brain functions and is therefore an ideal tool to investigate how the human brain works. Zatorre et al. (Zatorre et al., 2007) showed that playing a musical instrument, for example the violin, is a highly complex task (cf. **Figure 1**). The

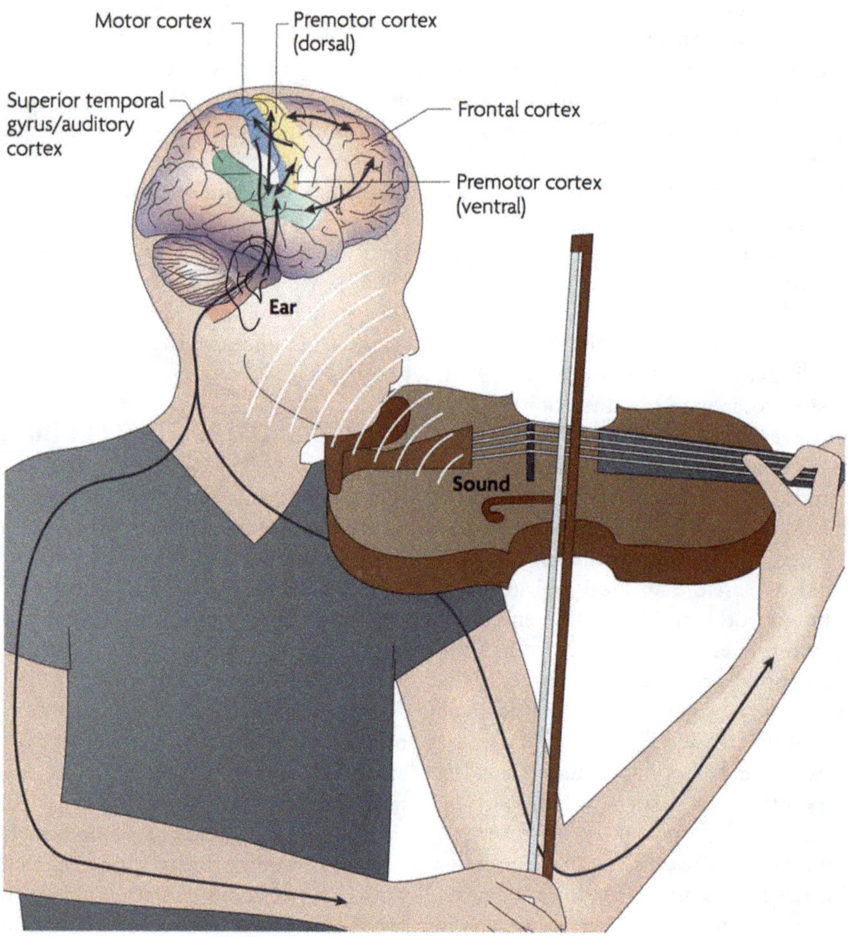

FIGURE 1 | (*From Zatorre et al., 2007*) The figure illustrates the feedback and the feedforward interactions that occur during music performance. As a musician plays an instrument, motor systems control the fine movements needed to produce sound. The sound is processed by auditory circuitry, which, in turn, is used to adjust motor output to achieve the desired effect. Output signals from premotor cortices are also thought to influence responses within the auditory cortex, even in the absence of sound, or prior to sound; conversely, motor representations are thought to be active on hearing sound, even in the absence of movement. There is, therefore, a tight linkage between sensory and production mechanisms.

whole body, including almost all sensory systems, is involved in the performance process and has to be coordinated to high degree of synchrony and accuracy. As the arms support the violin and move the bow, and the hand fingers the strings, feedback from the somatosensory perception of the body posture and fingertips is constantly integrated to fine-tune each and every movement. The auditory system has the major control function in this process, analyzing the musical correctness of the sounds produced by the violin, and using this auditory feedback to fine-tune the motor functions and therefore improve the sounds produced. Apart from the motor and sensory systems, memory and attentional, as well as emotional, systems are also involved. Because of this complex interaction, music has developed, over the last 10 years, as a tool for studying brain plasticity in different sensory modalities and as an effective way of changing the brain's functional organization and interaction between brain areas for the purpose of neuro-rehabilitation. It has been demonstrated, in a series of experiments, that musical training has pronounced effects on functional and structural human brain plasticity.

On the structural level, larger brain volume has been demonstrated in musicians compared to non-musicians in several brain areas; (auditory processing; Schlaug et al., 1995a,b; Schneider et al., 2002; Gaser and Schlaug, 2003; Bermudez et al., 2009); (visuo-spatial processing; Gaser and Schlaug, 2003; Bermudez et al., 2009); motor control: corpus callosum and precentral gyrus (Schlaug et al., 1995a; Gaser and Schlaug, 2003; Bangert and Schlaug, 2006); and cerebellum (Hutchinson et al., 2003). Such differences not only apply to gray matter: differences in white matter, between musicians and non-musicians, have also been found (Oechslin et al., 2010).

On the functional level, fundamental differences between musicians and non-musicians regarding the processing of sounds, were found not only in the auditory (Pantev et al., 1998; Tervaniemi et al., 2001; Koelsch et al., 2002; Shahin et al., 2003; Fujioka et al., 2004, 2005; Van Zuijen et al., 2004, 2005; Besson et al., 2007), but also in the somatosensory and the motor cortices (Elbert et al., 1995; Lotze et al., 2003). Therefore, in addition to the main modality, neural interactions between modalities are also enhanced in musically trained people (Schulz et al., 2003). The interplay and integration of several modalities are key elements of musical training and performance, and the multimodal integration and co-activation of the cortical areas involved during training might be an important mechanism supporting the training effects within each modality. Generally, the conditions which are most important for cortical reorganization to occur are: (1) the expansion of cortical representation through the increased use, or behaviorally relevant stimulation, of the respective receptor pool and (2) a heavy training schedule, coupled with high-levels of motivation, in a behaviorally relevant context. The results of these different studies performed on musicians confirm that extensive training has a specific and profound effect on the functional organization of the auditory cortex.

LABORATORY DEMONSTRATIONS OF AUDITORY PLASTICITY

Most studies of musically induced plasticity of the auditory cortex have been based on musicians with years of extensive training. However, training musically naive subjects for a short time in a laboratory environment is even better suited to the direct evaluation of short-term training effects and the possibility of inducing short-term plastic changes.

In one study we investigated this question by having adults, in the laboratory, learning to discriminate spectral versus virtual modes of pitch perception in ambiguous "virtual" melodies (Schulte et al., 2002). A clear change in perception was accompanied by a distinct increase in the transient gamma band response that has been found to be associated with integrative cognitive functions, such as the binding process during object recognition. An independent component analysis, which was performed on the MEG data, indicated greater synchronization of the cortical networks involved in the generation of the evoked gamma band activity after participants had achieved the ability to perceive the virtual melody. In a further study (Menning et al., 2000), we found that frequency discrimination training over the course of 3 weeks led to rapid behavioral improvements that were accompanied by enhanced N1m and mismatch responses to pitch deviations, therefore demonstrating rapid, short-term training-induced plastic changes in the human auditory cortex. In a similar fMRI study, two randomly assigned groups were compared, one of which received auditory discrimination training over the course of 1 week (Jancke et al., 2001). The results showed a differential pattern. Subjects, who improved over the course of the training and also showed improved auditory acuity, had decreased neural activity in auditory areas (planum temporale and superior temporal sulcus) on fMRI testing. Subjects who did not improve over the course of the training, and subjects in the control group (no training), did not have changes in their auditory cortical activity on fMRI measurements before and after 1 week. These results demonstrate that short-term auditory training leads, in general, to plastic changes within the human auditory cortex for the task that is trained, however, these also depend upon the effectiveness of the training for the individual concerned.

As described in **Figure 1**, playing music is all about the multimodal integration of different sensory modalities and motor functions. We, therefore, asked the following question: is it this multimodal integration that makes musical training so effective in promoting plasticity in the human auditory cortex? Multisensory integration was defined by Meredith and Stein (Meredith and Stein, 1983) as a greater neuronal response to a stimulus consisting of a combination of modalities, compared with the sum of neuronal responses to each stimulus modality separately. The different sensory modalities interact, functionally reorganize, and contribute to new qualities of perception that convey information not inherent in each single modality. We, therefore, put the hypothesis forward that the strong effects of musical training on cortical reorganization might be due to the multimodal nature of musical training. Specifically, we hypothesized that sensorimotor-auditory training, in the context of piano playing, leads to greater plasticity in the human auditory cortex than mere auditory training. This hypothesis was tested in a study of twenty-three non-musicians with no formal musical training, who were assigned randomly to either sensorimotor-auditory or to auditory experimental groups (Lappe et al., 2008). Training-induced plasticity was evaluated by comparing the mismatch negativity responses (MMN) and the performance in an auditory melody discrimination test before and after training.

For the MEG measurements before and after training, we used three- and six-tone piano sequences (**Figure 2A**). Deviant sequences differed from the standard sequence in that the last tone of the sequence was three semitones lower. During a 2 week training period, the sensorimotor-auditory group learned to play the I–IV–V–I chord progression (**Figure 2B**) in broken chords, using both hands, from a visual template that was easy to read for musical novices (**Figure 2C**).

In contrast, subjects in the auditory group merely listened to all of the training sessions of one randomly assigned subject from the sensorimotor-auditory group and had to judge the correctness of the heard sequences. As expected, auditory discrimination of short melodies improved more strongly in the group that received the piano training, compared to the listening group, as assessed by both the behavioral test and the electro-physiological MMN data, which are displayed in **Figure 3**. The source waveforms and statistical analysis clearly showed that the training effect, as seen in the increase from pre- to post-training sessions, was much larger in the sensorimotor-auditory group than in the auditory group. The multimodal sensorimotor-auditory training in non-musicians therefore resulted in greater plastic changes in the auditory cortex than auditory-only training, and this indicates the strength of the effect of sensory-motor practice on auditory representations. In this study we manipulated the subjects' experiences in a well-controlled laboratory setting, randomly assigned them to different groups, and the auditory input was identical for both the sensorimotor-auditory and the auditory group. The study, therefore, enabled us to conclude that musical instrument training which involves both the sensorimotor and the auditory system leads to stronger functional changes in auditory cortical areas than mere auditory training.

PLASTICITY INDUCED BY FUNCTIONAL DEAFFERENTATION

The experiments describe above show the influence of long-term (musical) and short-term (laboratory) training on the processes of cortical reorganization within the human auditory

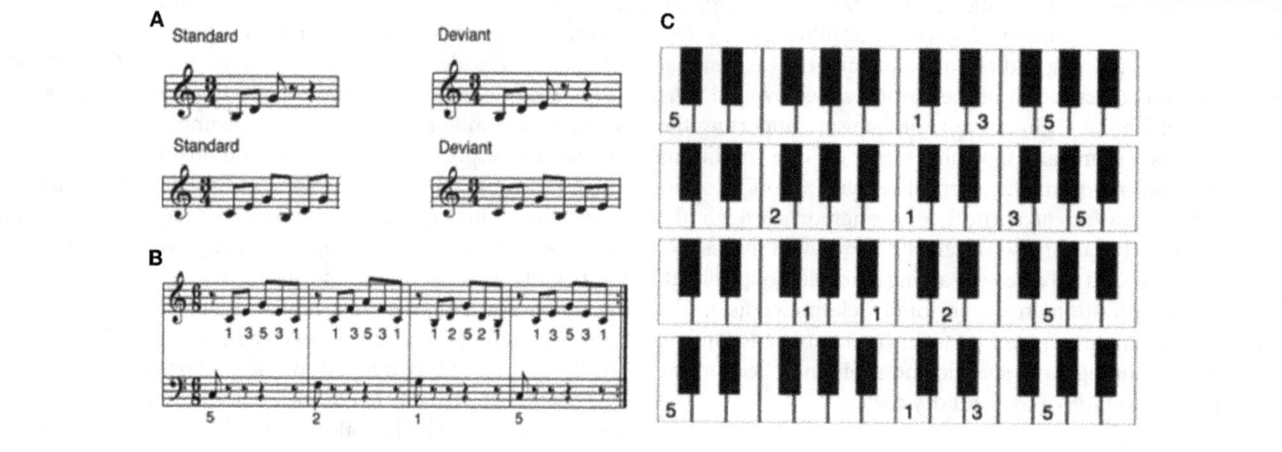

FIGURE 2 | (*From Lappe et al., 2008*). (A) Tone sequences for the standard and deviant stimuli that were used in the MEG measurements before and after training. **(B)** Musical score of the I–IV–V–I chord progression in c-major in broken chords that was used as a training sequence for SA and A training. **(C)** Visual templates for the SA training for each broken chord of the training sequence. Numbers represent the fingers (thumb, 1; index finger, 2; etc.) with which the subjects were supposed to press the corresponding piano keys. On each template, the image of the piano keyboard was depicted and the finger placement was marked. For each chord, the notes were to be played in ascending order first, and then descending again (compare score in **B**).

cortex. A complementary approach to investigating plasticity is to remove a band of frequencies from familiar sounds such as music, and determine how brain responses to the eliminated sounds are affected (a functional deafferentation approach).

In a study following this approach (Pantev et al., 1999), normal-hearing subjects listened attentively, for 3 h on 3 consecutive days, to music of their choice from which a narrow frequency band centered at 1 kHz had been removed (notching). Immediately before and after listening to the notched music, MEG measurements of auditory cortical representations were measured for a "test" stimulus (band-passed noise centered at the notched region) and a "control" stimulus (band-passed noise centered one octave below the notched region). The music had been manipulated in such a way that a notch between 0.7 and 1.3 kHz, centered on 1 kHz, was produced using a band rejection filter. It was presented binaurally through earphones at a moderate loudness (about 60–70 dB SPL). The presence of the notch ensured that, during this period of music listening, there was practically no afferent input to cortical neurons tuned to frequencies around 1 kHz. After listening to notched music, the root-mean-square (RMS) values and strength of the corresponding N1m cortical source were decreased in the case of the test stimulus, whereas they remained almost unchanged for the control stimulus. This demonstrated that the notching-out of a band of frequency-specific auditory input decreased the cortical representation of these same frequencies in just a short time period.

These results provide evidence that different organizational structures of cortical representational maps can occur or develop within a time frame as short as a few hours, in this case following functional deafferentation of the adult human auditory cortex. The time course of this notching effect is consistent with animal studies in which selected regions of the cochlea have been deafferented by electrolytic lesions (Robertson and Irvine, 1989). While the reduction in responsiveness at the functionally deafferented cortical region cannot be explained by a habituation effect, lateral inhibition is a very likely explanation (cf. Kadner et al., 2002; Pantev et al., 2004). In this case the neurons with CFs within the notched area of the music were inhibited by their neighboring neurons with CFs outside of the notch, which were stimulated by the music. This short-term plasticity effect, however, reversed within 24 h. An important question is whether longer exposure would extend the duration of this effect. We will return to this question later, where the method of notching is applied to the treatment of tonal tinnitus. That research was based on foundation studies of lateral inhibition in the human auditory cortex, to which we turn next.

LATERAL INHIBITION OF THE HUMAN AUDITORY CORTEX

Lateral inhibition plays an important role in the functioning of our sensory modalities. In 1865, Ernst Mach described the "Mach bands" in the visual modality, which are explained by lateral inhibition (Mach, 1865). The model of lateral inhibition within the auditory system was derived from the classic visual lateral inhibition scheme (Von Békésy, 1967). The afferent auditory pathway is formed not only from excitatory neural connections; inhibitory networks also play an important role (as described in the Introduction section). On the basis of one of our previous studies (Pantev et al., 2004), we proposed that inhibition in the human auditory cortex, as mediated by lateral connections, is an active mechanism that innervates inhibitory neurons and causes the attenuation of the auditory evoked response.

Habituation, in contrast, is a neural mechanism that suppresses the activity of neurons, which are repeatedly activated. Habituation seems to play an important role both in suppressing irrelevant neural activity and in enhancing the neural activity elicited by irregular sensory inputs. The "tinnitus retraining therapy" (Jastreboff and Hazell, 1993) focuses on this habituation mechanism. In our first study (Pantev et al., 2004) we compared the decrease in auditory cortical activity induced by habituation

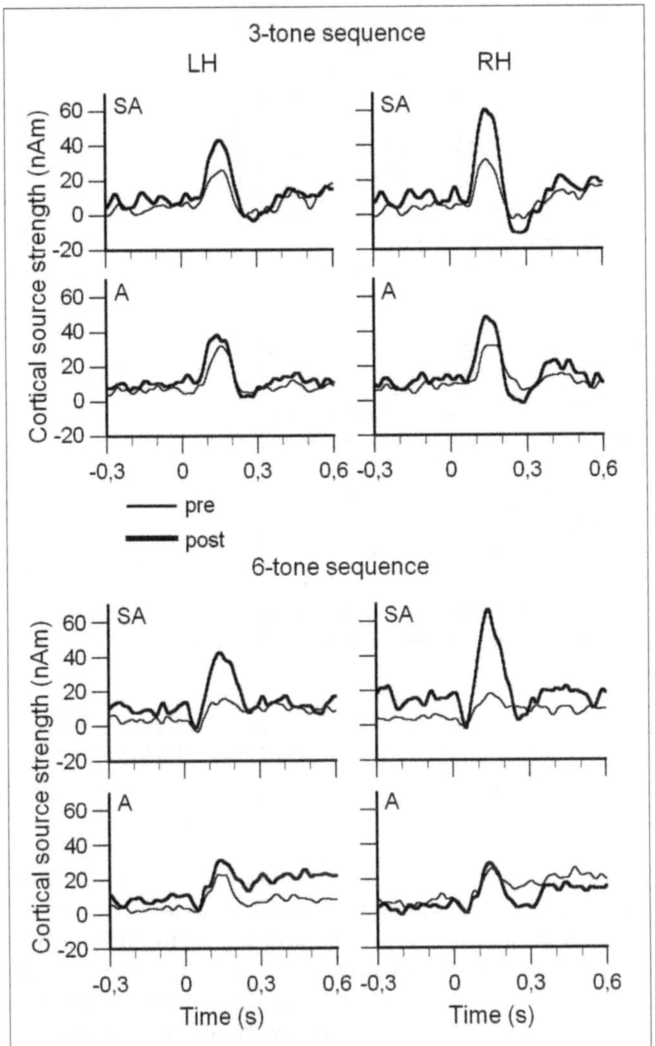

FIGURE 3 | (*Modified from Lappe et al., 2008*) Group averages of the source waveforms which were obtained after performing source space projection before and after training for both groups (SA = *Sensorimotor-Auditory*; A = *Auditory*), stimulus conditions, and hemispheres. Data for the three-tone sequences are shown in the top four panels and data for the six-tone sequences in the bottom four panels. Within each set of four panels, SA group data are shown in the top row, and A group data are shown in the bottom row. Data from the left hemisphere (LH) are presented on the left and those of the right hemisphere (RH) on the right. Thin lines indicate pre-training (pre) data and thick lines post-training (post) data.

vs. lateral inhibition within the same experiment and within the same subjects.

LATERAL INHIBITION AND HABITUATION

In this study we used a forward masking paradigm and examined the effects of white noise (WN) and comb filtered noise (CFN) maskers. The amplitude spectrum of the CFN consisted of a series of pass and eliminated-band sections with identical widths on the logarithmic frequency scale (**Figure 4**).

Each complex sound contained five spectral components corresponding either to the pass-band sections of the CFN pass-band stimulus (PB stimulus) or to the eliminated-band sections of the CFN eliminated-band stimulus (EB stimulus). The PB- and EB- stimuli evoked N1m responses originating mainly from non-primary auditory structures (Pantev et al., 1995) and, in both cases, this response was reduced in amplitude following a preceding masker (CFN or WN) The main finding, however, was that when a preceding CFN masker was used, the source strengths of the N1m responses elicited by the EB stimuli were significantly lower than those responses that were elicited by the PB stimuli. In contrast, the N1m amplitudes elicited by the both stimuli were not significantly different following the WN masker. Thus, the neural mechanisms causing the N1m decrements depended on the combination of the masking sound and the test sound. The PB stimulus was composed of frequencies corresponding to the pass-bands of the CFN, meaning that those frequencies occurring within the pass-bands were stimulated throughout the presentation of the masker and PB stimulus. Consequently, in this case, the habituation effect must have played a major role in decreasing the N1m response following the CFN masker. On the other hand, the EB stimulus was composed of frequencies corresponding to the eliminated-bands of the CFN and thus only contained the frequency bands neighboring the CFN spectral components. This meant that the neurons responding to the EB stimulus had not been excited during the preceding CFN masker, the consequence of which was that lateral inhibition must have caused the main N1m decrement. In summary, these results indicated that the inhibitory effect mediated by the lateral connections (EB condition) was stronger than the habituation effect (PB condition).

We have also investigated the amount to which the lateral inhibition effect may be dependent on the inter-stimulus interval. Using CFN forward-maskers of 3 s duration and the same test stimuli (TS) (PB and EB) as in the previously described experiment, we then varied the inter-stimulus interval between them (0.5, 1, and 2 s). In this experiment (Okamoto et al., 2004), we demonstrated again that the lateral inhibition effect on the N1m evoked response was significantly larger than the corresponding habituation effect. The N1m decrement was maximal when the time interval between the CFN and the TS was short (0.5 s) but was still detectable at intervals up to 2 s. From this experiment we concluded that stimulating the auditory system for several seconds with a sound containing sharply defined spectral contrasts (CFN) results in a temporal change in the responsiveness of the auditory cortex to complex spectral pattern sounds. Cortical responses corresponding to the non-stimulated frequency bands were more strongly reduced than those responses corresponding to the TS. Thus, the lateral inhibition effect at the level of the auditory cortex was a reasonable explanation, and the experimental results we obtained provided evidence that the effect of inhibition decayed over several seconds.

Several electroencephalographic studies on habituation of the auditory cortex showed that the amplitude of the N1 response was most strongly attenuated when the preceding and subsequent sound stimuli had the same frequency as the test frequency (Butler, 1968; Picton et al., 1974; Pantev et al., 1975; Näätänen and Picton, 1987; Näätänen et al., 1988). However, in addition to this effect upon the neural group with the same receptive field, neural

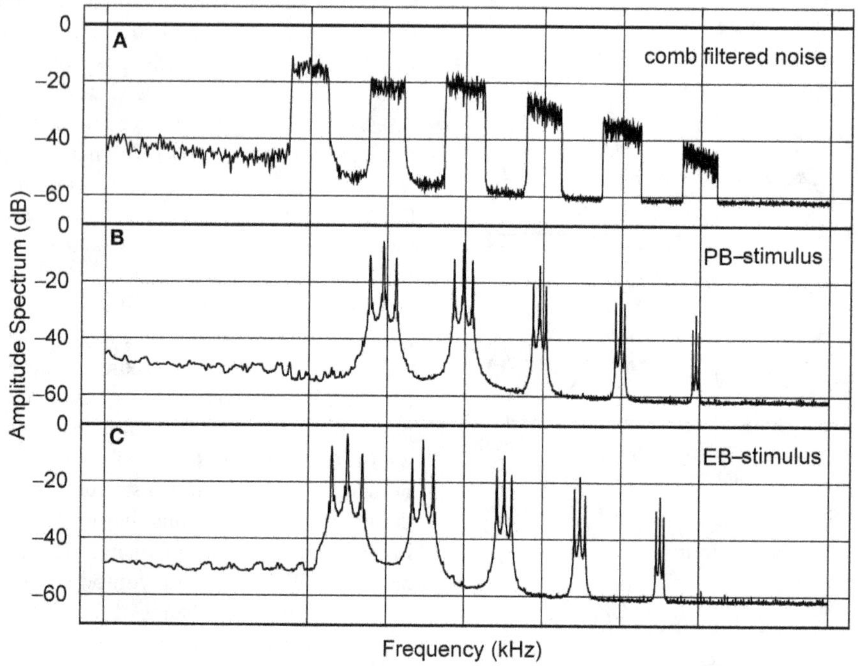

FIGURE 4 | (*Modified from Pantev et al., 2004*) Amplitude spectra of the comb filtered noise (CFN), the pass-band stimulus (PB), and the eliminated-band stimulus (EB) (rows a, b, and c, respectively). The frequency components of the PB-stimulus correspond to pass-band sections of the CFN, whereas those of the EB-stimulus correspond to eliminated-band sections of the CFN.

activity corresponding to frequencies adjacent to the test stimulus might play an important role for the neural response (Sutter and Loftus, 2003; Jääskeläinen et al., 2004; Okamoto et al., 2004; Pantev et al., 2004). In the previous experiments the eliminated bandwidths of the CFN were always the same (i.e., 1/4 octave) and so the effect of the width of the eliminated-band itself on the test stimulus remained unknown. We devised a further study to investigate whether an explanation in terms of lateral inhibition in the region of the eliminated-band frequency could be experimentally proved. Therefore, interfering masking sounds, which differed in the frequency domain, were presented between two successive 1 kHz pure tone TS. The masking sounds were WN and various band-eliminated noises (BENs) (1/8, 1/4, 1/2, and 1 octave bandwidths) centered at 1 kHz. The main finding here was that the N1m amplitude corresponding to the 1 kHz test tone was most strongly reduced when the preceding BEN had a 1/4 octave eliminated bandwidth. These experimental results can be explained mainly by the effect of lateral inhibition (Von Békésy, 1967; Ehret and Merzenich, 1988; Burrows and Barry, 1990; Rhode and Greenberg, 1994; Suga, 1995; Sutter et al., 1999) because, in this case, the eliminated bandwidth corresponds to one critical band (CB).

SIMULTANEOUS NARROW-BAND NOISE

The aforementioned studies used forward masking paradigms to investigate lateral inhibitory effects in the human auditory cortex. However, inhibitory neural interactions within human cortical tonotopic maps elicited by complex sounds continue to be poorly understood. A well-known concept in this context is the "CB" introduced by Fletcher (Fletcher, 1940). This concept describes neural groups with similar receptive fields as being part of the same CB and assumes only slight interactions between frequency-distant neuronal populations. However, neural activities elicited by distinct frequencies can influence each other. Jääskeläinen et al. (Jääskeläinen et al., 2004) observed a significant decrease in N1m-induced by a preceding masker despite the TS and masker differing by two octaves. Single cell recording studies applying simultaneous masking paradigms also demonstrated that the frequency tuning curves of auditory cortical neurons had lower and upper inhibitory side bands (Sutter et al., 1999; Sutter and Loftus, 2003; O'Connor et al., 2005). These results indicated that when sounds are presented simultaneously their interaction has non-linear frequency characteristics.

We investigated this aspect of neural interaction further using two simultaneously presented narrow-band noises (NBNs). TS1 consisted of one single NBN with a 40 Hz bandwidth centered at 1000 Hz. The five other TS consisted of two simultaneously presented NBNs each with a 20 Hz bandwidth and center frequencies set equally apart from 1000 Hz. The center-frequency differences between the two NBNs were 1/4 (TS2), 1/2 (TS3), one (TS4), two (TS5), and four (TS6) CBs, respectively. The N1m amplitude was maximal in the case of TS4 (1 CB) and minimal in the case of TS1 (single NBN). The N1m source strength increased gradually until the frequency difference between NBNs matched the CB (from TS1 to TS4) and then decreased with further increment of the frequency difference (Okamoto et al., 2005).

Two simultaneously presented sound stimuli normally activate two distinct neural groups with receptive fields corresponding to the frequency characteristics of these stimuli. However, if the stimulating sounds have very similar frequencies, the receptive fields might overlap, meaning that, within this overlapping region, a single neural group may be excited by the separate stimuli. The frequency overlap gradient between conditions might have caused a gradient in N1m source strength (TS1 > TS2 > TS3 > TS4). However, the receptive field organization of the auditory system alone cannot explain the results we obtained (TS4 > TS5; TS4 > TS6). Auditory neurons corresponding to the frequency components of one of the NBNs of TS5 or TS6 not only receive excitatory ascending inputs from that NBN, but also receive lateral inhibitory inputs from the other NBN, which was separated by more than one CB. Our finding that the N1m amplitude again reduced in response to these stimuli, which were separated by more than one CB, indicates that lateral inhibition mainly works between separate neural groups, which are activated through different peripheral band-pass filters. The results also provide some new insights into these mechanisms, which cause non-linear interactions between excitatory and inhibitory neurons when activated by sounds of different frequencies.

ASYMMETRIC LATERAL INHIBITION

In summary, lateral inhibition in the auditory system seems to contribute to improving the perceptual contrast by enhancing the spectral edge of the sound stimuli, as we have demonstrated in the human auditory cortex. However, it is not so well-known whether the lateral inhibitory effects of neural connections from the lower and higher spectral regions are similar or different. The auditory peripheral organ, the cochlea, has an asymmetric anatomical composition (Kiang and Moxon, 1974), however, the frequency tuning curve asymmetry becomes less evident in the central auditory neurons (Katsuki et al., 1958; Suga, 1995).

We hypothesized that lateral inhibition in the central auditory pathway might also be asymmetric in order to compensate for the frequency tuning curve asymmetry originating in the cochlea. To test this hypothesis, we measured auditory evoked fields (AEFs) elicited by a TS following exposure to various maskers with single-octave bandwidths eliminated and center frequencies differing in 1/6 octave steps. The goal was to investigate lateral inhibitory effects of the lower and higher spectral edges of BENs on the auditory evoked responses to a subsequent TS. We used a 1000 Hz TS throughout this experiment. The differences in the frequency domain between the TS at 1000 Hz and the lower spectral edges of the BENs were 1/6 octave (BEN1), 2/6 octave (BEN2), 3/6 octave (BEN3), 4/6 octave (BEN4), and 5/6 octave (BEN5). The smallest N1m response occurred after exposure to BEN1 and the largest after exposure to BEN3. The N1m response was also smaller following BEN4 and BEN5 than BEN3, however, the decrease was not symmetric, and was more pronounced for the lower-frequency spectral edge than the higher edge.

This result (Okamoto et al., 2007a) implied that the lower spectral edge of the BEN caused a larger decrease in N1m than the higher spectral edge. We therefore conclude that the asymmetric lateral inhibition in the central auditory pathway contributes by adjusting the asymmetric neural activities originating in the cochlea. This adjustment results in sharper frequency contrasts and better auditory performance.

EFFECTS OF ATTENTION ON LATERAL INHIBITION

Another very important issue is the relationship between lateral inhibition and attention. In most day-to-day situations we are exposed to many different types of sound signals simultaneously, yet we can easily perceive selected sounds simply by paying attention to them. This process can be tuned by the enhancement of neural responses corresponding to task-relevant stimuli (gain), by suppression of task-irrelevant neural activities via lateral inhibition (sharpening), or by both.

Previous EEG (Hillyard et al., 1973; Picton et al., 1974) and MEG (Woldorff et al., 1993) studies observed that focused auditory attention increased the N1 auditory response. The sharpening effect of attention, however, had not been demonstrated. We therefore investigated the sharpening effects of focused auditory attention on the population-level frequency tuning in the human auditory cortex by means of MEG. We posited that attention might strengthen not only the excitatory neural connections but also the inhibitory networks (cf. **Figure 5**), which would contribute to finer frequency tuning and better auditory performance.

In this experiment, we used a TS that was presented either independently or simultaneously with four different BENs queued in a random sequence. Neuronal activities evoked by BEN and TS could be divided into three categories: activity evoked exclusively by BEN, activity evoked exclusively by TS, or activity evoked by both BEN and TS (**Figures 6B1–B4**, light gray, dark gray, black areas, respectively). As shown in **Figure 6**, the activity of auditory neurons, which can be activated by both BEN and TS decreases as BEN becomes wider and/or frequency tuning becomes sharper. Thus, the diminution of overlapping areas (**Figure 6**, black areas) and the enlargement of areas activated solely by TS (**Figure 6**, dark gray areas) illustrate improved population-level frequency tuning. The TS was a 1000 Hz amplitude-modulated tone (40 Hz), and the BENs were prepared as follows: spectral frequency bands with widths of 20 Hz (BEN20), 40 Hz (BEN40), 80 Hz (BEN80), or 160 Hz (BEN160) centered on the 1000 Hz TS carrier frequency were eliminated from WN. To investigate the effects of attention, we contrasted two different attentional conditions: active listening and distracted listening. The results indicated that the population-level frequency tuning became sharper when attention was directed to the auditory domain (Okamoto et al., 2007b).

Previous studies have shown that lateral inhibition in the auditory system (Von Békésy, 1967; Suga, 1995; Pantev et al., 2004; Okamoto et al., 2005, 2007a) can sharpen frequency tuning in the auditory cortex. The inhibitory system, intensified by focused auditory attention, might have sharpened the population-level frequency tuning via the top-down auditory pathway. Therefore, focused auditory attention cannot only amplify excitatory neural activity (gain effect) but also inhibitory neural activity, leading to the sharpening of population-level frequency tuning in the human auditory cortex.

Although top-down auditory focused attention can amplify and sharpen neural activity in the human auditory cortex, the question is still unsettled about whether these attentional effects depend upon the specific location of neurons within

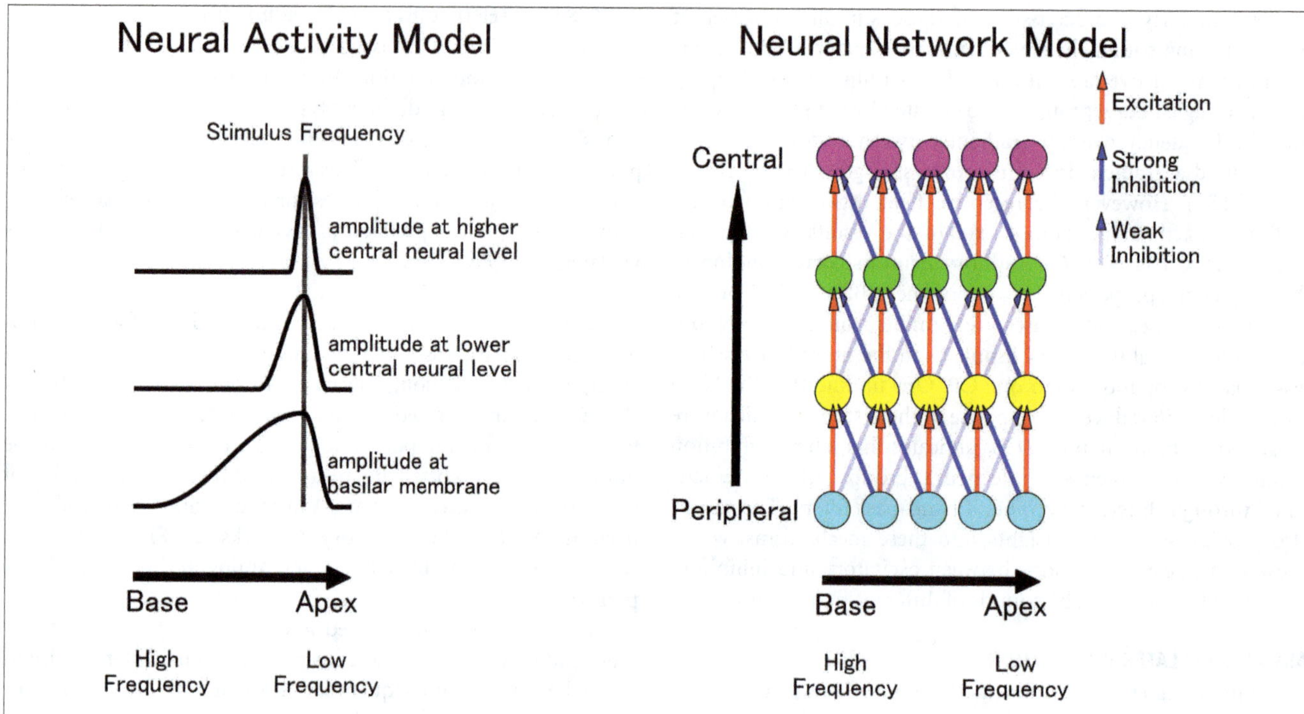

FIGURE 5 | (*Modified from Okamoto et al., 2007a,b*) A hypothesized neural network in the human auditory system. *Left*: a schematic diagram of hypothesized neural activity corresponding to a stimulus frequency from the peripheral to the central auditory pathway. Neural activity becomes sharper at more central levels, especially in the high-frequency range. *Right*: a hypothetical excitatory and inhibitory neural network from the peripheral to the central auditory pathway. Red lines indicate excitatory neural connections and blue lines indicate inhibitory connections. Solid blue lines projecting from lower to higher frequencies have stronger inhibitory effects than the dashed blue lines projecting from higher to lower frequencies.

the tonotopic maps. Psychoacoustic studies have indicated that frequency-specific auditory attention sharpens the tuning for an attended relative to an unattended frequency. This was reflected in a detection advantage for the former compared to the latter (Hafter et al., 1993; Hubner and Hafter, 1995).

Spectral cues are definitely important for neural processing in noisy environments. Based on the results described previously, we investigated whether population-level frequency tuning can be modulated by differential stimulus sequencing under auditory focused attention in awake humans (Okamoto et al., 2010a). We presented various pure tones of different frequencies (TS) simultaneously with BENs. BENs were notched with widths of one quarter (1/4 CB), one half (1/2 CB), or one CB (1 CB), centered at the frequency of the simultaneously presented TS (**Figure 7**). We contrasted two different attentional conditions within subjects: "constant sequencing" and "random sequencing." In the constant sequencing session, identical frequency TS were presented successively, with simultaneous presentation of either the 1/4, 1/2, or the 1 CB BEN. In the random sequencing session, TS with different frequencies were randomly presented. Crucially, the overall bottom-up auditory input was identical between constant sequencing and random sequencing conditions. During all conditions, subjects were instructed to focus their attention on the auditory stimuli.

The N1m responses were larger when the TS had a constant frequency, compared to random TS frequencies, particularly when BENs with narrow eliminated-bands were simultaneously presented. Moreover, while there was no sequencing effect in the wide BEN condition, the narrow BENs showed an enhanced N1m source strength for the constant sequencing as compared to the random sequencing condition.

These results suggest that constant stimulus sequencing under focused auditory attention may cause sharper and larger neural activity at the attended (constantly presented) frequency, and broader and smaller neural responses at the other frequencies, compared to the random sequencing condition. Our findings further suggest that constant stimulus sequencing during auditory focused attention can improve population-level frequency tuning in humans in a frequency-specific manner by enhancing lateral inhibition around the attended frequency.

UNANSWERED QUESTIONS

The results discussed above support the hypothesis that N1m amplitude evoked by test tones centered in the notch of BEN stimuli is reduced compared to control conditions by the distribution of lateral inhibition into the notch region from the activated side band regions. A question raised by the findings is how they relate with the results of other studies investigating the effects of BEN stimuli on brain activity and with studies investigating the effect of BEN stimuli on auditory perception. Norena and Eggermont (2003) reported that the spontaneous firing rates of neurons coding the eliminated-band frequencies increased during an interval of BEN in the primary auditory cortex of ketamine-anesthetized cats, compared to an unnotched noise condition.

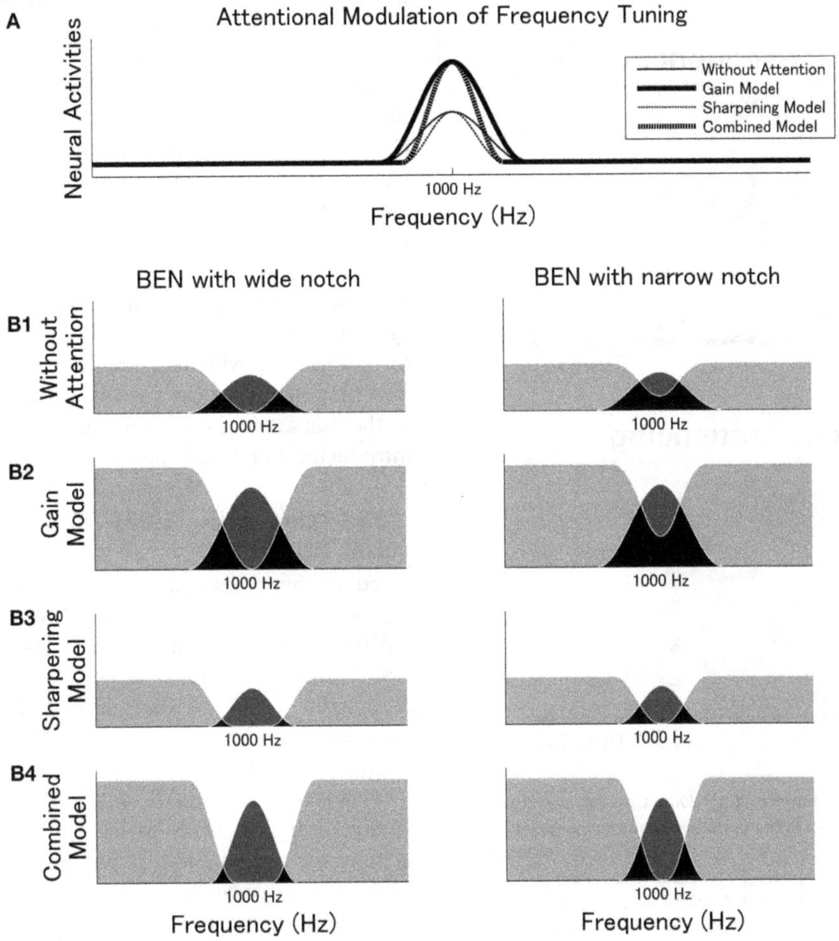

FIGURE 6 | (*Modified from Okamoto et al., 2007a,b*) Attentional modulation of frequency tuning. (A) Different effects of attention (gain, sharpening, and combined (gain plus sharpening) models) modulate the population-level neural activities corresponding to the 1000 Hz test stimulus. (B1–B4) The relationship between neural activities elicited by BEN and TS as predicted by the different attention models. Light gray areas represent neural activities exclusively elicited by BEN and dark gray areas represent neural activities exclusively elicited by TS. Black areas indicate overlap: neurons in these areas had already been activated by BEN when TS appeared. Dark gray areas represent N1m source strength reflecting TS onset. **B1** displays neural activities evoked without focused auditory attention. **B2**, **B3**, and **B4** illustrate the gain model, the sharpening model, and the combined (gain plus sharpening) model, respectively. Diagrams on the left illustrate BENs with broad spectral notches; diagrams on the right illustrate BENs with narrow spectral notches. It is notable that the size ratios of the dark gray areas between the narrow BEN and the wide BEN differ between models: **B3** and **B4** have ratios much closer to one than **B1** and **B2**, reflecting the sharpening effect of attention on population-level frequency tuning.

Further, detection thresholds for the band-eliminated frequencies are decreased (improved) in human subjects following notched compared to broadband noise (Wiegrebe et al., 1996; Norena et al., 2000). Norena and Eggermont (2003) suggested that a shift of the balance of excitation and inhibition toward reduced inhibition in the notched region could explain an increase in spontaneous firing rates in this region and lead to an increase in driven activity accounting for threshold improvement. However, this interpretation is not favored by our findings, which point to an increase in lateral inhibition distributed into the notched region. Alternatively it could be proposed that enhanced spontaneous activity or Zwicker tones experienced in the notched region reduce N1m responses by a forward masking mechanism. However, this account does not appear to explain the scope of our findings as efficiently as does the simple hypothesis of lateral inhibition distributed to the notched region. It may be relevant that the cortical sources of the N1m localize predominantly to the auditory belt area and may be modulated "top-down" by attention as well as by changes in the response properties of neurons in primary auditory cortex that have been investigated in anesthetized animals.

THE BRIDGE BETWEEN CORTICAL PLASTICITY, LATERAL INHIBITION AND THE TREATMENT OF TONAL TINNITUS

In general, adaptive plasticity in the auditory cortices of musicians as well as non-musicians, based on and induced by musical training, is a very positive phenomenon. Training-induced alterations in the cortical map correspond to perceptual correlates, which indicate superior performance. These changes are excellent examples of the "bright side" of auditory cortical plasticity,

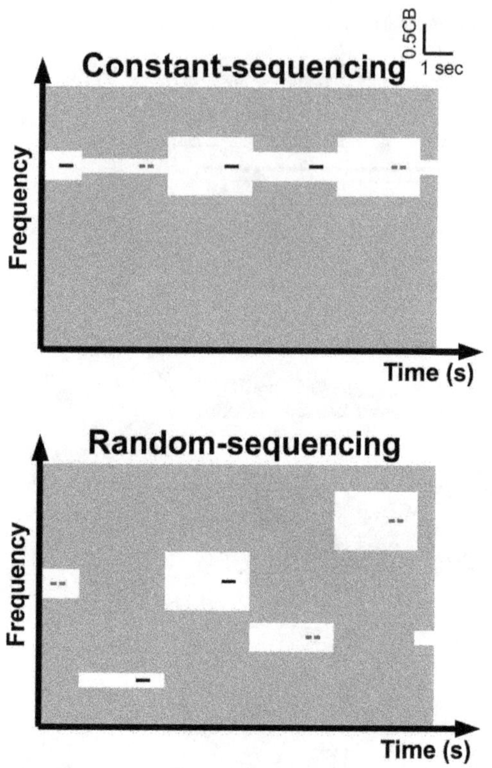

FIGURE 7 | (*Modified from Okamoto et al., 2009*) Concept and time course of auditory stimulation in the constant sequencing and random sequencing conditions. Pass-bands and stop-bands of the band-eliminated noises (BENs) are represented by the light gray and white areas, respectively. The notch-bandwidth of a BEN (white area) is either 1/4, 1/2, or 1 critical band. Target and non-target test stimuli (TS) are represented as red lines with gap (target TS, requiring a button press) and black lines without gap (non-target TS), respectively. During the constant sequencing condition (*upper graph*), the TS is a series of identical frequencies, whereas during the random sequencing condition (*lower graph*) the TS has different frequencies. The TS frequencies differed between constant sequencing blocks. In total, identical bottom-up auditory inputs are provided during the constant sequencing and random sequencing conditions.

which can enable extraordinary proficiencies. However, cortical plasticity also has "dark sides" (Elbert and Heim, 2001). When auditory cortical plasticity goes wrong, serious symptoms and pathologies can result, for example, if a peripheral lesion, which is normally by itself manageable, is influenced by an intense and stressful experience, such as the fear of serious disease, in conjunction with particular limbic system activation. In such a case, maladaptive auditory cortical reorganization, such as that which underlies tinnitus, can be triggered.

When auditory cortical plasticity has negative effects, such as tinnitus, this is, fortunately, not completely irreversible; the process of plasticity itself can be utilized in order to reverse or reduce these maladaptive changes. Such rehabilitative plasticity functions by reestablishing normal cortical functional organization to a certain degree. In order to accomplish this goal in tinnitus patients, we use the phenomenon of lateral inhibition. As demonstrated in Chapter 2, lateral inhibition can suppress interfering neural activity in the human auditory cortex. Subjective tinnitus is among the most prevalent symptoms likely to be caused by aberrant and interfering neuronal activity.

Recent auditory neuroscience research has suggested that an imbalance of excitatory and inhibitory neural interactions within the auditory cortex could lead to the perception of tinnitus (Eggermont and Roberts, 2004), however, neurophysiological tinnitus treatment has so far focused mainly on habituation mechanisms. We suggest that making use of lateral inhibition within the auditory cortex could be a valuable alternative strategy for suppressing tinnitus perception (Pantev et al., 1999, 2004). Our goal was to develop a highly specific auditory treatment strategy using an acoustic carrier (music) that could be listened to for a long time with pleasure and attention, and which would have the potential to specifically enhance lateral inhibitory impact in the human auditory cortex. In the following section, we are introducing and describing our treatment approach in detail.

"LONG-TERM" AND "SHORT-TERM" TMNMT FOR TONAL TINNITUS

Based on hypotheses derived from previous findings regarding tinnitus [e.g., Eggermont and Roberts (2004); Roberts et al. (2010)], music-induced cortical plasticity [e.g., Pantev et al. (1999)], and lateral inhibition [e.g., Pantev et al. (2004); Okamoto et al. (2005, 2007a,b)], we developed a novel tinnitus treatment strategy which specifically targets tonal tinnitus, the most frequent tinnitus subtype (http://www.tinnitusarchive.org).

This section will briefly introduce our treatment rationale. Firstly, tinnitus is likely to be the result of maladaptive plasticity in the central auditory pathway (Eggermont and Roberts, 2004). It is reasonable to assume that maladaptive changes in the auditory cortex must exist if tinnitus is present, because the tinnitus perception arises here (Eggermont, 2006). More specifically, neuronal populations in the auditory cortex which code external sounds with similar acoustic properties to the tinnitus frequency reported by patients with tonal tinnitus, are very likely to be involved in tinnitus perception (Muhlnickel et al., 1998; Diesch et al., 2004). These neuronal populations are presumably characterized by hyperactivity and hyper synchronicity (Rauschecker et al., 2010) and are, obviously, potential treatment targets but we require a non-invasive method of working specifically with them. An acoustic input with specific properties would allow us to target those particular neural populations in a non-invasive way. Secondly, maladaptive plastic changes are generally reversible (Flor et al., 1995; Candia et al., 1999; Giraux et al., 2001) and behavioral (re-)training may be one way to achieve this. Thirdly, music is a powerful agent that can be used as a neuro-rehabilitative strategy to induce adaptive cortical plasticity and reverse maladaptive plasticity (Wan and Schlaug, 2010). Music itself is not only a dynamic broadband acoustic stimulus but can also capture the attention of the listener and trigger positive emotional responses. Finally, the attenuation effects of lateral inhibition on the amplitude and synchronicity of neuronal activity in the human auditory cortex appear to be stronger than the attenuation effects of habituation (Okamoto et al., 2004; Pantev et al., 2004).

On the basis of these core assumptions and the series of experimental results reviewed in the previous sections, we developed

TMNMT. This training strategy focuses on tonal tinnitus, which patients usually describe as sounding "beep"-like or "whistle"-like. In our experience the individual tinnitus frequency, in most cases of tonal tinnitus, can be matched psycho-acoustically. We assume that neuronal populations in the auditory cortex that code the tinnitus frequency are involved in tinnitus perception (Muhlnickel et al., 1998; Diesch et al., 2004; Roberts et al., 2010), and it is thus the goal of TMNMT to specifically target these neurons in the individual tinnitus patient.

From our perspective, based on the previously outlined knowledge about functional cortical reorganization and plasticity, we feel it is reasonable to assume that the maladaptively reorganized auditory cortex of a tinnitus patient can be retrained to certain degree by frequent stimulation using specifically and individually tailored, attractive and behaviorally relevant auditory input (her/his favorite music).

We believed that regular training over the course of several months was necessary because many examples from the literature on human cortical plasticity [e.g., Candia et al. (1999)] indicate that training is most effective and its effects are most persistent if the training is performed intensively and with perseverance.

Regarding the auditory input for the treatment, we are convinced that music is an excellent choice for several reasons. Firstly, music is enjoyable: almost everyone can name songs or musical works that he or she likes to listen to. Positive emotions are experienced during musical listening (Salimpoor et al., 2011) and this implies that attention is attracted to preferred music. Various evidence shows that focused attention promotes cortical plasticity [e.g., Polley et al. (2006)] and this suggests to us that if the listener really enjoys the training by, for example, being able to choose to listen to their favorite music, they will be most open to attention-induced plasticity.

Secondly, most types of contemporary music, e.g., pop or rock music, cover a broad frequency spectrum, with considerable amounts of energy in the higher-frequency range. With such music it is therefore possible to target typical tinnitus frequencies, which are usually high (http://www.tinnitusarchive.org). The aim of modifying the music is to reduce the activity/synchronicity of neuronal populations involved in tinnitus perception. One feasible way to achieve this would be to stimulate these neurons less than all other auditory neurons. In practice we believe this can be achieved by removing part of the energy spectrum from the training music, specifically the spectrum of energy corresponding to the tinnitus frequency range. The result is literally "notched" music, exposure to which would deprive the specific neuronal population that codes the tinnitus frequency, relative to the populations responsible for coding other frequencies. We thus hypothesize that TMNMT would induce a circumscribed auditory functional deafferentation (Pantev et al., 1999) and transient sensory input deprivation. This deprivation would lead to a reduction in the level of excitation of auditory cortical neurons coding the notched frequencies, among them the tinnitus frequency. This reduction in excitation level may be caused by the (transient) strengthening of locally weakened inhibitory impact in the auditory cortex. The consequence for sufferers of chronic tinnitus should be reduction in tinnitus loudness.

TMNMT EVALUATION

To date, we have completed two major studies by means of which we evaluated the efficacy of TMNMT. The first study (Okamoto et al., 2010b; Stracke et al., 2010) was a proof-of-concept trial. The second study (Teismann et al., 2011, for details see below) was conducted in order to extend the results of the initial study, to advance the training strategy and to gain further insight regarding potential patient characteristics that may modulate the training outcome. From our perspective, the strength of both studies was that we not only evaluated tinnitus perception behaviorally but we also analyzed and evaluated tinnitus-related auditory cortical neuronal activity electrophysiologically, by means of MEG.

LONG-TERM TMNMT

For the proof-of-concept trial (Okamoto et al., 2010b; Stracke et al., 2010), we recruited a relatively small, but homogeneous with respect to their tinnitus, group of 39 patients. The participants, aged between 18 and 60 years, suffered from chronic (>12 months duration), unilateral, tonal tinnitus, with tinnitus frequencies $\leq$ 8000 Hz. The patients exhibited neither severe hearing loss nor neurological or psychiatric diseases. Before beginning training, the patients were assigned to one of three groups: target, placebo or monitoring. The assignment to target or placebo was executed pseudo-randomly and was double-blinded. Patients selected the music they most enjoyed. The target group received the real TMNMT: from their music, the frequency band of one octave width surrounding the individual tinnitus frequency was removed. The placebo group received placebo notched music therapy: the frequency band of one octave width around the tinnitus frequency remained unfiltered and, instead, the frequency range above and below this band was notched with a slowly moving filter of one octave width. The moving notch did not change the music more than the constant notch thus it was not possible to differentiate between the target and placebo music. The patients of the monitoring group were just listening to their usual music.

The TMNMT was performed over the course of 12 consecutive months. During this time period, the patients listened to their notched music for 1–2 h every day, using closed headphones supplied by us and characterized by an appropriate frequency response. The patients were instructed to listen to their notched music in a quiet environment, selecting their own moderate loudness. It was not mandatory to focus on the training music, however, if one is listening to his/her favorite music, it is very likely that attention will be directed to it. Once per week, following a strict routine, the patients assessed their perceived tinnitus loudness (as well as tinnitus-related annoyance, awareness, and handicapping) by means of a visual analogue scale. Every 6 months, tinnitus-related auditory cortical evoked activity was measured by means of MEG.

The results of this proof-of-concept study demonstrated the specific efficacy of TMNMT. After completing their training, the perceived tinnitus loudness (**Figure 8**), as well as tinnitus-related primary and non-primary auditory cortical evoked activity (**Figure 9**), was significantly reduced for patients in the target group, compared to their pre-training baseline. In contrast, in both the placebo and monitoring groups, no significant changes from the baseline were found. One interesting finding

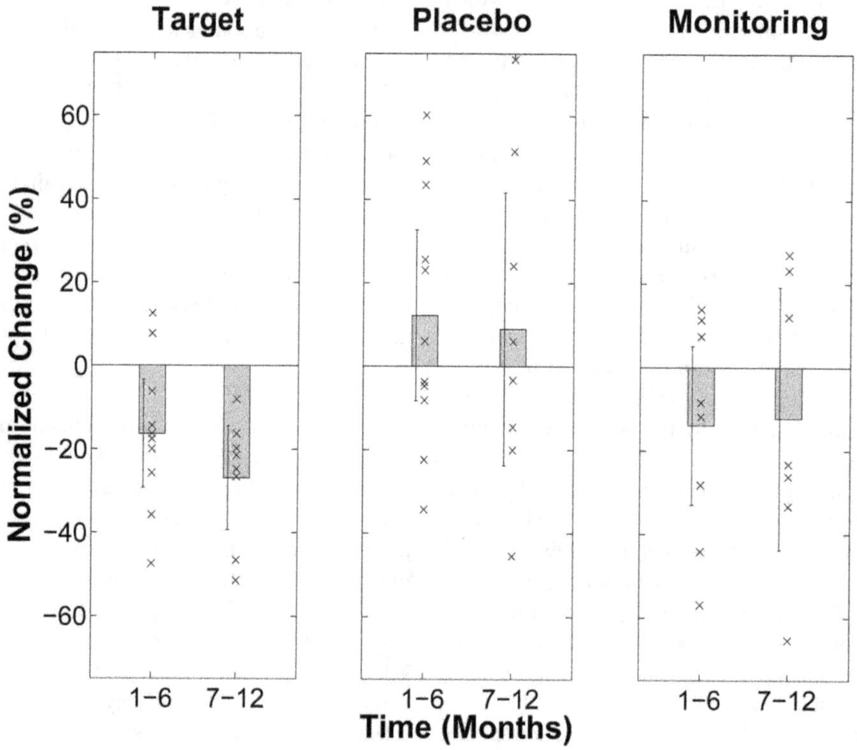

FIGURE 8 | (*Modified from Okamoto et al., 2010a,b*) Normalized tinnitus loudness change after 6 and 12 months of treatment (or monitoring) relative to baseline (=0) for the three patient groups (target TMNMT, placebo TMNMT, and monitoring). Positive change values reflect impairment; negative change values reflect improvement. The bars indicate group averages and each "×" indicates an individual data point. The error bars denote confidence intervals. As indicated by the confidence interval bars, only the changes in the target group were statistically significant.

was the significant positive correlation between tinnitus loudness change and change in primary auditory cortical evoked activity. Those patients who showed more pronounced tinnitus loudness reductions demonstrated the stronger ASSR source strength ratio reductions. Approximately 80% of patients in the target group experienced loudness alleviation to some degree, and the average reduction in tinnitus loudness in this group was approximately 25%.

SHORT-TERM INTENSIVE TMNMT

Motivated by the findings of the proof-of-concept trial, we ran a second study (Teismann et al., 2011) in order to further develop and evaluate TMNMT. In the previous study, based on theoretical and practical considerations, we had included only patients with tinnitus frequencies ≤ 8000 Hz. This time, we also included patients with tinnitus frequencies > 8000 Hz. In order to better target these patients with notched music, we "flattened" the energy spectrum of the training music, i.e., we digitally redistributed energy from lower to higher-frequency ranges and thus enriched the energy spectrum in the higher-frequency range (**Figure 10**).

To investigate whether tinnitus frequency modulates TMNMT efficacy, we divided the patients into two groups on the basis of their tinnitus frequency, with 8000 Hz as the grouping criterion. We also shortened and intensified the TMNMT considerably. In the previous study, the patients had listened to approximately 720 h of notched music over the course of 12 months. In contrast, in the second study, the patients listened to 24 h of notched music over the course of 5 consecutive days. In order to study the temporal dynamics of the training effects, we assessed tinnitus perception in the second study quite intensively. Finally, to investigate the persistency of the training effects, we applied a post training observation phase of 31 days.

In the second study we did not apply a placebo TMNMT. All patients received the target TMNMT, including the selection of their most enjoyable music and the removal of the frequency band of one octave width centered at the individual tinnitus frequency. However, to minimize potential placebo effects, patients were told, prior to the onset of the study, that they would receive either the target or a placebo TMNMT. After the completion of the study, the patients were debriefed.

The results of this study demonstrated that the short and intense TMNMT had been effective, though only for the patient group characterized by tinnitus frequencies ≤ 8000 Hz. TMNMT efficacy was reflected by reduction in perceived tinnitus loudness and tinnitus-related distress, as well as by a reduction in tinnitus-related non-primary auditory cortical evoked neuronal activity. Furthermore, the results indicated that the reductions in tinnitus loudness and evoked cortical activity achieved in this very short TMNMT scenario persisted for no longer than 2 weeks. The tinnitus-related distress alleviation, however, appeared to be longer lasting.

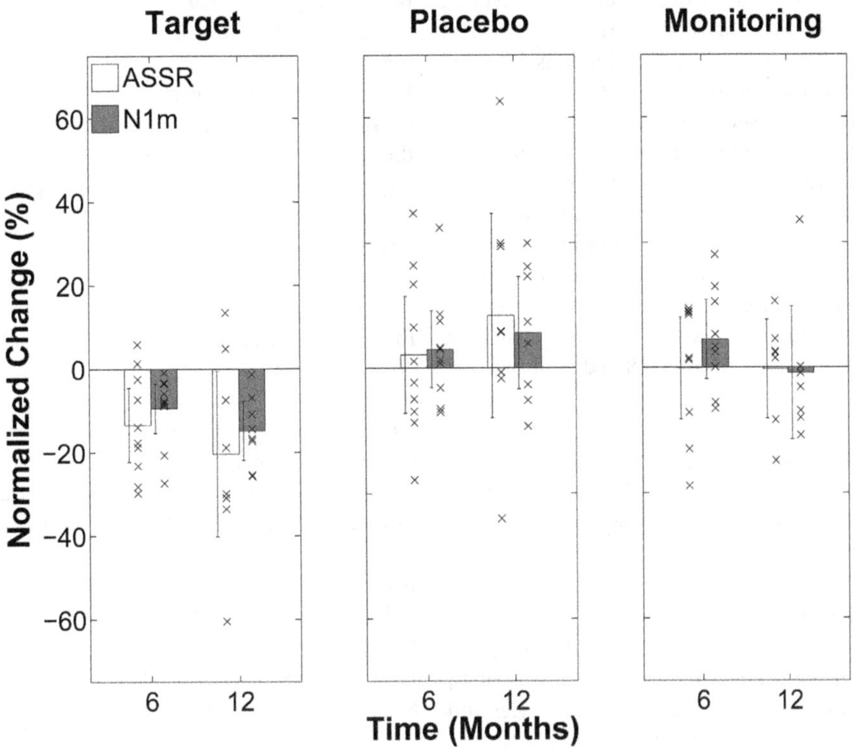

FIGURE 9 | (*Modified from Okamoto et al., 2010a,b*) Change in normalized tinnitus-related auditory cortical evoked activity after 6 and 12 months of treatment (or monitoring) relative to baseline (=0) for the three patient groups (target TMNMT, placebo TMNMT, and monitoring). Positive change values reflect increase in activity; negative change values reflect decrease in activity. The bars indicate group averages and each "×" indicates an individual data point. The error bars denote confidence intervals. Auditory steady state response (ASSR) change values are reflected by white bars and N1m change values are reflected by gray bars. As indicated by the confidence interval bars, only the changes in the target group were statistically significant.

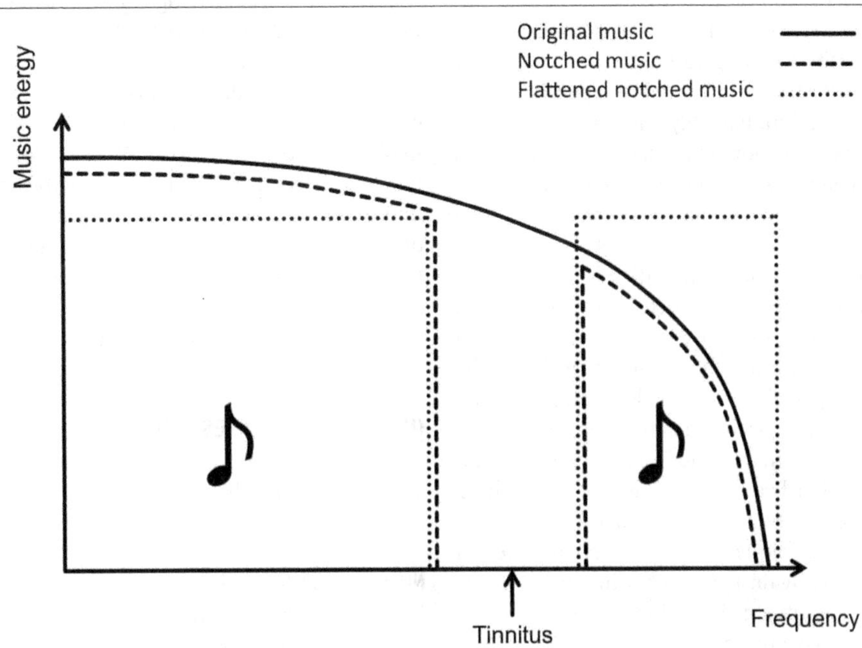

FIGURE 10 | Schematic illustration of the energy spectra of original (i.e., unmodified) music (black line), notched music (green line), and flattened notched music (blue line). The red arrow indicates the tinnitus frequency, at which the notches are centered.

On the basis of these two studies, it can currently be concluded that TMNMT is effective in reducing reported tinnitus loudness by an average of about 20% (with greater reductions in some cases), specifically for patients who suffer from chronic tonal tinnitus and who do not exhibit a greater than moderate hearing loss. Importantly, TMNMT efficacy could be demonstrated on different time scales and with varied training intensities. There are hints from pertinent literature on training-induced cortical reorganization, however, that longer-term training would probably induce more persistent and possibly permanent effects. In addition, there are hints that certain patient prerequisites, such as a very high tinnitus frequency, could counteract TMNMT efficacy. Crucially, TMNMT can specifically influence tinnitus-related auditory cortical activity.

KNOWN TMNMT RELATED ISSUES

There are several issues associated with the application of TMNMT. In the following section we will discuss some of the most relevant challenges.

Tinnitus frequency determination

Obviously, the success of TMNMT will stand and fall by the reliable determination of the tinnitus frequency. Unfortunately, identifying the tinnitus frequency is not a trivial task (Tyler and Conrad-Armes, 1983; Moore et al., 2010). Firstly, the tinnitus frequency cannot be measured objectively, but has to be matched subjectively by the patient who has to compare test tones of different frequencies to his tinnitus percept. Secondly, depending upon certain prerequisites, like the actual tonal quality of the tinnitus percept (for example, rather clear tone vs. "dirty" tone, ringing, or chirping) or hearing loss [which is often associated with frequency selectivity impairment (Okamoto et al., 2011)], it is more or less difficult for patients to compare the frequency of their tinnitus to the frequency of a test tone. Thirdly, in our experience, patients vary in their ability to compare the frequency of their tinnitus to the frequency of a test tone, probably depending upon factors such as musical education. Fourthly, there are certain typical pitfalls, such as octave confusion, that need to be considered (Moore et al., 2010). Finally, it is also our experience that tinnitus frequency matches become more reliable (i.e., vary less) with training.

In our studies, in order to match the patient's tinnitus frequency we use a high-frequency audiometer (up to 16 kHz), testing with a frequency resolution of 1/24th octave. In cases of bilateral tinnitus, we perform tinnitus matching according to the ear in which the tinnitus is perceived as being loudest. In the case of unilateral tinnitus, we use the ear in which tinnitus is perceived. If tinnitus is perceived as being "in the head," or if it is equally loud in both ears, we use the better hearing ear. During the matching procedure we start at different frequencies in order to first collect a number of potential tinnitus frequency "candidates." In a second step, we test these candidates against each other in a two-forced-choice procedure. After identifying the "winner" candidate, we test this winner against all its octaves between 1000 and 16000 Hz, again applying a two-forced choice procedure. We usually repeat this procedure on different days before the tinnitus frequency is finally determined.

Music energy spectrum

The energy spectrum of the acoustic stimulus is one critical factor that would influence TMNMT efficacy. Unfortunately, unlike WN, for example, music does not contain an equal amount of energy evenly distributed over the whole frequency range. Rather, the amount of energy generally drops considerably with increasing frequency. Thus, in terms of energy distribution, music is a more appropriate training stimulus for patients with a rather low tinnitus frequency than those with rather high tinnitus frequencies. Fortunately, from our experience, music is surprisingly "robust" against alterations of its energy spectrum so that, even though modifications like the removal of a whole octave or the "flattening" of the energy spectrum may appear to be aggressive manipulations of the music, the results most often still sound like enjoyable music to which we are able to pay attention for a considerable time.

Worthy of note is our observation that the energy distribution across frequency differs markedly between different types of music. While rock or pop music usually already contains a relatively flat spectrum, including a comparatively significant amount of high-frequency energy, this does not hold true for other music types, such as vocal music or single instruments. Even the spectrum of classical orchestral music is, from our experience, less suitable compared to common, contemporary popular music because of having less evenly distributed energy.

Equipment

The equipment used for TMNMT also appears to be a critical factor in the efficacy of the treatment. Ideally, the carefully, individually tailored acoustic input should be transmitted through the ear-canal, middle-ear, and cochlea into the central auditory pathway with as little distortion as possible. The frequency responses and transferring characteristics of the devices used to play and transduce the notched music are, therefore, critical. This includes the music player, the amplifier, the headphones, and specific device configurations such as the equalizer settings. The goal would be to achieve true-to-the original, authentic tailor-made notched music replay. We therefore use headphones with maximally linear and flat frequency response. In addition, it is important to ensure that ambient noises, which are usually of broadband type and, of course, not specifically notched, would not interact with the music modification in an unwanted manner. Thus, in addition to instructing the patients to perform the TMNMT in a preferably quiet environment, we also have recommendations regarding the necessary equipment.

OUTSTANDING QUESTIONS

Several important TMNMT-related questions remain to be answered. In the following sections we will focus on three of these questions.

NON-TONAL TINNITUS

It remains to be determined whether TMNMT could be effective in the case of non-tonal tinnitus types. For instance, a substantial number of patients report that their tinnitus sounds in some way "noise-like" (http://www.tinnitusarchive.org). From attempts at tinnitus matching it is known that, in such cases, the tinnitus percept can be compared to narrowband or broadband noise stimuli. It is usually far more difficult to match noise-like compared to tonal tinnitus percepts, and this implies that matches that are obtained in the former case would be less reliable. Moreover, a practical problem associated with the notched music treatment of noise-like tinnitus would be that rather wide frequency bands (e.g., two or three octaves) would have to be removed from the training music, which may result in qualitatively changed, distorted and less enjoyable music.

SEVERE HEARING LOSS

Obviously, TMNMT can only be effective if the acting frequencies of the stimulus are actually perceived by the patient. Unfortunately, almost all tinnitus patients have hearing loss to a certain degree (Eggermont and Roberts, 2004). In our TMNMT evaluation studies, we have so far focused on patients with no greater than moderate hearing loss (i.e., ≤ 35 dB HL in study one and ≤ 50 dB HL in study two). Many patients with tinnitus, however, have severe hearing losses, especially older patients, and this usually affects the frequencies that need to be perceived in order for TMNMT to be effective. It therefore appears unlikely that music modification alone could be enough to effectively treat such patients. From our perspective, it would be important to think about strategies for making TMNMT available for tinnitus patients with more severe hearing losses.

HOW DOES TMNMT WORK?

We have argued that the beneficial effects of TMNMT are due to the suppression of tinnitus-related neural activity by lateral inhibition distributed into the notched region. Unlike our initial 3 day study of notched sounds described earlier (Pantev et al., 1999) in which brain responses reverted to their pre-listening levels over 24 h, TMNMT was experienced daily for 12 months (Okamoto et al., 2010a,b), and the effect on brain responses persisted after period of 6 and 12 months (cf. **Figure 9**) implying persisting changes in auditory cortex. Noteworthy, there are other treatment studies, which have reported improvements in tinnitus (Davis et al., 2007; Tass et al., 2012) and reductions in loudness growth in individuals with hyperacusis (Norena and Chery-Croze, 2007). Davis et al. (2007) report reduction of tinnitus loudness after exposure to complex sounds covering the hearing loss regions where tinnitus frequencies localize, whereas Tass et al. (2012) demonstrate tinnitus loudness reduction to sequential presentation of four pure tones (coordinated reset) with a distance of one or two octaves to the tinnitus frequency (for reviews see Hoare et al., 2011; Roberts and Bosnyak, 2011). Because the sounds used in these studies covered a considerable frequency range, our results with TMNMT raise the possibility that notching out the specific tinnitus frequencies in cases of tonal tinnitus may confer added benefit. Additional research will be needed to assess this question. It should also be noted that listening to background sound for extended periods (which our subjects did) could rescale auditory sensitivity (Formby et al., 2003; Norena and Chery-Croze, 2007). Thus, listening to notched music could reduce the perceived loudness of sound in the notched frequency region, which could have been reflected in our brain measurements. Several models of tinnitus suggest that enhanced sensitivity to sound and tinnitus go together, and that procedures that benefit one will also benefit the other. Therefore, further evaluations of the different approaches are necessary in order to be able to make a final decision, which are most important factors contributing to the outcome of customized sound treatment of tonal tinnitus.

A further question concerns the effect of long-term exposure to background sound on auditory neural representations. Until recently it was believed that passive auditory experience did not change auditory representations in the mature brain unless the sounds possessed behavioral relevance (Polley et al., 2006). However, recent animal studies (Pienkowski and Eggermont, 2011, 2012; Zhou and Merzenich, 2012) have demonstrated that long-term stimulation with band-pass noise or multi-frequency stimuli resulted in reduced spontaneous firing rates and reduced responsiveness of primary auditory cortex neurons corresponding to the stimulated frequencies. At the low- or high-frequency edge region (about one octave wide) enhanced neural activity was found. At first glance, these results appear to be contradictory to our own results where reductions in neural activity were observed in the band-eliminated regions of the listened to sound. However, there are many differences between the two experimental approaches. In the aforementioned animal studies neither hearing loss nor tinnitus was present, whereas in our experiments tinnitus was present and hearing loss as well. The effect of exposure to environmental sounds could be different depending on the level of background neural activity, which is likely elevated in tinnitus. In our study we used favorite music, a behaviorally and emotionally relevant sound stimulus for the subjects that may have elevated neural activity in the band-pass regions but suppressed it in the band-eliminated regions. In contrast, the above-mentioned animal studies used irrelevant noises as sound stimuli. In order to perceive behaviorally relevant environmental sound signals through the noise, the animals may have needed to increase the sensitivity of neurons, whose characteristic frequencies were not covered by the spectrum of the TS. Clearly, understanding the neural effects of long-term sound exposure is important not only for the prevention of hearing disorders but also for treating tinnitus (Okamoto et al., 2010b, 2011; Pienkowski and Eggermont, 2012).

LOOKING AHEAD

We strive for two important goals. The first is the further optimization of the TMNMT strategy. This includes, among other things, examining the effectiveness of the tinnitus treatment as a function of the width of the spectral notch in TMNMT and experimentally testing the combination of TMNMT with complementary strategies, including tinnitus counseling. We assume that the enrichment of TMNMT with further effective strategies should induce a significant increase in the effects of rehabilitative reorganizational cortical plasticity in the tinnitus networks, and might potentially prolong the alleviation of the tinnitus percept.

The second goal is to transfer the optimized TMNMT strategy into clinical practice. This step involves evaluating the treatment efficacy in a large sample of tinnitus patients. The applicability of TMNMT depends substantially on its practicability, an important aspect of which is the quality and usability of the tools, which provide the treatment to patients. The goal is to develop professional and high-quality "state of the art" hard- and software-solutions, which are easy for the tinnitus patients to use and would win their acceptance. We plan to carefully evaluate the efficacy of the optimized TMNMT in a large sample of patients with tonal tinnitus [about 65% of tinnitus patients suffer from tonal tinnitus (Stouffer and Tyler, 1990)]. The clinical trial will involve regular audiological, psychophysical, neuroimaging, and psychometric outcome evaluations, and the optimized treatment is expected to induce significant reductions of tinnitus loudness, distress, and handicap.

In summary, the TMNMT approach can be considered as an enjoyable, low-cost, and presumably causal treatment that is capable of specifically alleviating tinnitus perception. In these times of restricted resources within the health system, it is of paramount importance to develop cost-efficient rehabilitation programs. Another important potential advantage of TMNMT is that, by being taught to perform the training on their own, patients are educated to carry the responsibility for their own future well-being. This is in line with current trends in healthcare systems, to treat the patient as a responsible partner able to undertake shared decision-making. The expected results will be of great interest for the community of oto-rhino-laryngologists, audiologists, neurologists, and psychotherapists far beyond the current research environment.

ACKNOWLEDGMENTS

We thank Bernhard Ross and Andreas Wollbrink for technical support, Karin Berning for organizing the data acquisition, Ross Parfitt for valuable discussions and proof-reading, and our test subjects for their diligent collaboration. This work has been supported by IZKF CRA05, Deutsche Forschungsgemeinschaft (Pa 392/10-2, Pa 392/10-3, Pa 392/14-1, Pa 392/13-1), TRI Pantev, CIHR 2001–2003 "MEG studies of the auditory cortex," Pantev, Canada Research Chair "Human Cortical Plasticity," 2001–2003; CIHR "Understanding, treating and preventing tinnitus"; Japan Society for the Promotion of Science for Young Scientists (23689070), and "Strategic Research Program for Brain Sciences" (Development of biomarker candidates for social behavior).

REFERENCES

Bangert, M., and Schlaug, G. (2006). Specialization of the specialized in features of external human brain morphology. *Eur. J. Neurosci.* 24, 1832–1834.

Bauer, C. A., Turner, J. G., Caspary, D. M., Myers, K. S., and Brozoski, T. J. (2008). Tinnitus and inferior colliculus activity in chinchillas related to three distinct patterns of cochlear trauma. *J. Neurosci. Res.* 86, 2564–2578.

Bermudez, P., Lerch, J. P., Evans, A. C., and Zatorre, R. J. (2009). Neuroanatomical correlates of musicianship as revealed by cortical thickness and voxel-based morphometry. *Cereb. Cortex* 19, 1583–1596.

Besson, M., Schon, D., Moreno, S., Santos, A., and Magne, C. (2007). Influence of musical expertise and musical training on pitch processing in music and language. *Restor. Neurol. Neurosci.* 25, 399–410.

Burrows, D. L., and Barry, S. J. (1990). Electrophysiological evidence for the critical band in humans: middle-latency responses. *J. Acoust. Soc. Am.* 88, 180–184.

Butler, R. A. (1968). Effect of changes in stimulus frequency and intensity on habituation of the human vertex potential. *J. Acoust. Soc. Am.* 44, 945–950.

Candia, V., Elbert, T., Altenmuller, E., Rau, H., Schafer, T., and Taub, E. (1999). Constraint-induced movement therapy for focal hand dystonia in musicians. *Lancet* 353, 42–42.

Cazals, K., Horner, C., and Huang, Z. W. (1998). Alterations in average spectrum of cochleoneural activity by long-term salicylate treatment in the guinea pig, a plausible index of tinnitus. *J. Neurophysiol.* 80, 2113–2120.

Coles, R. (1984). Epidemiology of tinnitus: (1) prevalence. *J. Laryngol. Otol. Suppl.* 9, 7–15.

Davis, P. B., Paki, B., and Hanley, P. J. (2007). Neuromonics tinnitus treatment: third clinical trial. *Ear Hear.* 28, 242–259.

Diesch, E., Struve, M., Rupp, A., Ritter, S., Hulse, M., and Flor, H. (2004). Enhancement of steady-state auditory evoked magnetic fields in tinnitus. *Eur. J. Neurosci.* 19, 1093–1104.

Eggermont, J. J. (2006). Cortical tonotopic map reorganization and its implications for treatment of tinnitus. *Acta Otolaryngol. Suppl.* 556, 9–12.

Eggermont, J. J., and Roberts, L. E. (2004). The neuroscience of tinnitus. *Trends Neurosci.* 27, 676–682.

Ehret, G., and Merzenich, M. M. (1988). Complex sound analysis (frequency resolution, filtering and spectral integration) by single units of the inferior colliculus of the cat. *Brain Res.* 472, 139–163.

Elbert, T., Pantev, C., Wienbruch, C., Rockstroh, B., and Taub, E. (1995). Increased cortical representation of the fingers of the left hand in string players. *Science* 270, 305–307.

Elbert, T., and Heim, S. (2001). A light and a dark side. *Nature* 411, 139.

Fletcher, H. (1940). Auditory patterns. *Rev. Mod. Phys.* 12, 47–65.

Flor, H., Elbert, T., Knecht, S., Wienbruch, C., Pantev, C., Birbaumer, N., Larbig, W., and Taub, E. (1995). Phantom-limb pain as a perceptual correlate of cortical reorganization following arm amputation. *Nature* 375, 482–484.

Formby, C., Sherlock, L. P., and Gold, S. L. (2003). Adaptive plasticity of loudness induced by chronic attenuation and enhancement of the acoustic background. *J. Acoust. Soc. Am.* 114, 55–58.

Fujioka, T., Trainor, L. J., Ross, B., Kakigi, R., and Pantev, C. (2004). Musical training enhances automatic encoding of melodic contour and interval structure. *J. Cogn. Neurosci.* 16, 1010–1021.

Fujioka, T., Trainor, L. J., Ross, B., Kakigi, R., and Pantev, C. (2005). Automatic encoding of polyphonic melodies in musicians and non-musicians. *J. Cogn. Neurosci.* 17, 1578–1592.

Gaser, C., and Schlaug, G. (2003). Brain structures differ between musicians and non-musicians. *J. Neurosci.* 23, 9240–9245.

Gilbert, C. D., and Wiesel, T. N. (1992). Receptive field dynamics in adult primary visual cortex. *Nature* 356, 150–152.

Giraux, P., Sirigu, A., Schneider, F., and Dubernard, J. M. (2001). Cortical reorganization in motor cortex after graft of both hands. *Nat. Neurosci.* 4, 691–692.

Hafter, E. R., Schlauch, R. S., and Tang, J. (1993). Attending to auditory filters that were not stimulated directly. *J. Acoust. Soc. Am.* 94, 743–747.

Hari, R. (1990). Magnetic evoked fields of the human brain: basic principles and applications. *Electroencephalogr. Clin. Neurophysiol. Suppl.* 41, 3–12.

Heller, A. (2003). Classification and epidemiology of tinnitus. *Otolaryngol. Clin. North Am.* 36, 239.

Hillyard, S. A., Hink, R. F., Schwent, V. L., and Picton, T. W. (1973). Electrical signs of selective attention in the human brain. *Science* 182, 177–180.

Hoare, D. J., Kowalkowski, V. L., Kang, S., and Hall, D. A. (2011). Systematic review and meta-analyses of randomized controlled trials examining tinnitus management. *Laryngoscope* 121, 1555–1564.

Hubner, R., and Hafter, E. R. (1995). Cuing mechanisms in auditory signal detection. *Percept. psychophys.* 57, 197–202.

Hutchinson, S., Lee, L. H., Gaab, N., and Schlaug, G. (2003). Cerebellar volume of musicians. *Cereb. Cortex* 13, 943–949.

Irvine, D. R. F., and Rajan, R. (1995). "Plasticity in the mature auditory system," in *Advances in Hearing Research*, eds G. A. Manley, G. M. Klump, C. Köppl, H. Fastl, and H. Oeckinhaus (Singapore: World Scientific Publishing Co.), 3–23.

Jancke, L., Gaab, N., Wustenberg, T., Scheich, H., and Heinze, H. J. (2001). Short-term functional plasticity in the human auditory cortex: an fMRI study. *Cogn. Brain Res.* 12, 479–485.

Jastreboff, P. J., and Hazell, J. W. (1993). A neurophysiological approach to tinnitus: clinical implications. *Br. J. Audiol.* 27, 7–17.

Jenkins, W. M., Merzenich, M. M., Ochs, M. T., Allard, T., and Guic-Robles, E. (1990).

Functional reorganization of primary somatosensory cortex in adult owl monkeys after behaviorally controlled tactile stimulation. *J. Neurophysiol.* 63, 82–104.

Jääskeläinen, I. P., Ahveninen, J., Bonmassar, G., Dale, A. M., Ilmoniemi, R. J., Levanen, S., Lin, F. H., May, P., Melcher, J., Stufflebeam, S., Tiitinen, H., and Belliveau, J. W. (2004). Human posterior auditory cortex gates novel sounds to consciousness. *Proc. Natl. Acad. Sci. U.S.A.* 101, 6809–6814.

Kaas, J. H., Krubitzer, L. A., Chino, Y. M., Langston, A. L., Polley, E. H., and Blair, N. (1990). Reorganization of retinotopic cortical maps in adult mammals after lesions of the retina. *Science* 248, 229–231.

Kadner, A., Viirre, E., Wester, D. C., Walsh, S. F., Hestenes, J., Vankov, A., and Pineda, J. A. (2002). Lateral inhibition in the auditory cortex: an EEG index of tinnitus? *Neuroreport* 13, 443–446.

Katsuki, Y., Sumi, T., Uchiyama, H., and Watanabe, T. (1958). Electric responses of auditory neurons in cat to sound stimulation. *J. Neurophysiol.* 21, 569–588.

Kiang, N. Y., and Moxon, E. C. (1974). Tails of tuning curves of auditory-nerve fibers. *J. Acoust. Soc. Am.* 55, 620–630.

Koelsch, S., Schmidt, B. H., and Kansok, J. (2002). Effects of musical expertise on the early right anterior negativity: an event-related brain potential study. *Psychophysiology* 39, 657–663.

Langguth, B., Kleinjung, T., Landgrebe, M., De Ridder, D., and Hajak, G. (2010). rTMS for the treatment of tinnitus: the role of neuronavigation for coil positioning. *Neurophysiol. Clin.* 40, 45–58.

Lappe, C., Herholz, S. C., Trainor, L. J., and Pantev, C. (2008). Cortical plasticity induced by short-term unimodal and multimodal musical training. *J. Neurosci.* 28, 9632–9639.

Lotze, M., Scheler, G., Tan, H. R., Braun, C., and Birbaumer, N. (2003). The musician's brain: functional imaging of amateurs and professionals during performance and imagery. *Neuroimage* 20, 1817–1829.

Mach, E. (1865). Über die Wirkung der räumlichen Vertheilung des Lichtreizes auf die Netzhaut. *Akademie der Wissenschaften in Wien, Sitzungberichte, math.-nat. Cl.* 52, 303–322.

Martin, W. H., Schwegler, J. W., Scheibelhoffer, J., and Ronis, M. L. (1993). Salicylate-induced changes in cat auditory nerve activity. *Laryngoscope* 103, 600–604.

Menning, H., Roberts, L. E., and Pantev, C. (2000). Plastic changes in the auditory cortex induced by intensive frequency discrimination training. *Neuroreport* 11, 817–822.

Meredith, M. A., and Stein, B. E. (1983). Interactions among converging sensory inputs in the superior colliculus. *Science* 221, 389–391.

Merzenich, M. M., Kaas, J. H., Wall, J., Nelson, R. J., Sur, M., and Felleman, D. (1983a). Topographic reorganization of somatosensory cortical areas 3b and 1 in adult monkeys following restricted deafferentation. *Neuroscience* 8, 33–55.

Merzenich, M. M., Kaas, J. H., Wall, J. T., Sur, M., Nelson, R. J., and Felleman, D. J. (1983b). Progression of change following median nerve section in the cortical representation of the hand in areas 3b and 1 in adult owl and squirrel monkeys. *Neuroscience* 10, 639–665.

Moore, B. C., Vinay, and Sandhya. (2010). The relationship between tinnitus pitch and the edge frequency of the audiogram in individuals with hearing impairment and tonal tinnitus. *Hear. Res.* 261, 51–56.

Muhlnickel, W., Elbert, T., Taub, E., and Flor, H. (1998). Reorganization of auditory cortex in tinnitus. *Proc. Natl. Acad. Sci. U.S.A.* 95, 10340–10343.

Norena, A. J., and Chery-Croze, S. (2007). Enriched acoustic environment rescales auditory sensitivity. *Neuroreport* 18, 1251–1255.

Norena, A., Micheyl, C., and Chery-Croze, S. (2000). An auditory negative after-image as a human model of tinnitus. *Hear. Res.* 149, 24–32.

Norena, A. J., and Eggermont, J. J. (2003). Neural correlates of an auditory afterimage in prmary auditory cortex. *J. Assoc. Res. Otolaryngol.* 4, 312–328.

Norena, A. J., and Eggermont, J. J. (2005). Enriched acoustic environment after noise trauma reduces hearing loss and prevents cortical map reorganization. *J. Neurosci.* 25, 699–705.

Näätänen, R., and Picton, T. (1987). The N1 wave of the human electric and magnetic response to sound: a review and an analysis of the component structure. *Psychophysiology* 24, 375–425.

Näätänen, R., Sams, M., Alho, K., Paavilainen, P., Reinikainen, K., and Sokolov, E. N. (1988). Frequency and location specificity of the human vertex n1-wave. *Electroencephalogr. Clin. Neurophysiol.* 69, 523–531.

O'Connor, K. N., Petkov, C. I., and Sutter, M. L. (2005). Adaptive stimulus optimization for auditory cortical neurons. *J. Neurophysiol.* 94, 4051–4067.

Ochi, K., and Eggermont, J. J. (1997). Effects of quinine on neural activity in cat primary auditory cortex. *Hear. Res.* 105, 105–118.

Oechslin, M. S., Imfeld, A., Loenneker, T., Meyer, M., and Jancke, L. (2010). The plasticity of the superior longitudinal fasciculus as a function of musical expertise: a diffusion tensor imaging study. *Front. Hum. Neurosci.* 3:76. doi: 10.3389/neuro.09.076.2009

Okamoto, H., Kakigi, R., Gunji, A., Kubo, T., and Pantev, C. (2005). The dependence of the auditory evoked N1m decrement on the bandwidth of preceding notch-filtered noise. *Eur. J. Neurosci.* 21, 1957–1961.

Okamoto, H., Kakigi, R., Gunji, A., and Pantev, C. (2007a). Asymmetric lateral inhibitory neural activity in the auditory system: a magnetoencephalographic study. *BMC Neurosci.* 8, 33.

Okamoto, H., Stracke, H., Wolters, C. H., Schmael, F., and Pantev, C. (2007b). Attention improves population-level frequency tuning in human auditory cortex. *J. Neurosci.* 27, 10383–10390.

Okamoto, H., Ross, B., Kakigi, R., Kubo, T., and Pantev, C. (2004). N1m recovery from decline after exposure to noise with strong spectral contrasts. *Hear. Res.* 196, 77–86.

Okamoto, H., Stracke, H., Lagemann, L., and Pantev, C. (2010a). Bottom-up driven involuntary auditory evoked field change: constant sound sequencing amplifies but does not sharpen neural activity. *J. Neurophysiol.* 103, 244–249.

Okamoto, H., Stracke, H., Stoll, W., and Pantev, C. (2010b). Listening to tailor-made notched music reduces tinnitus loudness and tinnitus-related auditory cortex activity. *Proc. Natl. Acad. Sci. U.S.A.* 107, 1207–1210.

Okamoto, H., Stracke, H., Zwitserlood, P., Roberts, L. E., and Pantev, C. (2009). Frequency-specific modulation of population-level frequency tuning in human auditory cortex. *BMC Neurosci.* 10, 1.

Okamoto, H., Teismann, H., Kakigi, R., and Pantev, C. (2011). Broadened population-level frequency tuning in human auditory cortex of portable music player users. *PLoS ONE* 6:e17022. doi: 10.1371/journal.pone.0017022

Pantev, C., Bertrand, O., Eulitz, C., Verkindt, C., Hampson, S., Schuierer, G., and Elbert, T. (1995). Specific tonotopic organizations of different areas of the human auditory cortex revealed by simultaneous magnetic and electric recordings. *Electroencephalogr. Clin. Neurophysiol.* 94, 26–40.

Pantev, C., Kevanishvili, Z. S., Galle, E., and Khachidze, O. (1975). ERA-stimulation with free-programable frequency and intensity sequence – a method to reduce the examination time. *Arch. Otorhinolaryngol.* 211, 43–49.

Pantev, C., Okamoto, H., Ross, B., Stoll, W., Ciurlia-Guy, E., Kakigi, R., and Kubo, T. (2004). Lateral inhibition and habituation of the human auditory cortex. *Eur. J. Neurosci.* 19, 2337–2344.

Pantev, C., Oostenveld, R., Engelien, A., Ross, B., Roberts, L. E., and Hoke, M. (1998). Increased auditory cortical representation in musicians. *Nature* 392, 811–814.

Pantev, C., Wollbrink, A., Roberts, L. E., Engelien, A., and Lutkenhoner, B. (1999). Short-term plasticity of the human auditory cortex. *Brain Res.* 842, 192–199.

Pantev, C., and Herholz, S. C. (2011). Plasticity of the human auditory cortex related to musical training. *Neurosci. Biobehav. Rev.* 35, 2140–2154.

Picton, T. W., Hillyard, S. A., Krausz, H. I., and Galambos, R. (1974). Human auditory evoked potentials. I. Evaluation of components. *Electroencephalogr. Clin. Neurophysiol.* 36, 179–190.

Pienkowski, M., and Eggermont, J. J. (2011). Cortical tonotopic map plasticity and behavior. *Neurosci. Biobehav. Rev.* 35, 2117–2128.

Pienkowski, M., and Eggermont, J. J. (2012). Reversible long-term changes in auditory processing in mature auditory cortex in the absence of hearing loss induced by passive, moderate-level sound exposure. *Ear Hear.* 33, 305–314.

Polley, D. B., Steinberg, E. E., and Merzenich, M. M. (2006). Perceptual learning directs auditory cortical map reorganization through top-down influences. *J. Neurosci.* 26, 4970–4982.

Rauschecker, J. P., Leaver, A. M., and Muhlau, M. (2010). Tuning out the noise: limbic-auditory interactions in tinnitus. *Neuron* 66, 819–826.

Rauschecker, J. P., Tian, B., Pons, T., and Mishkin, M. (1997). Serial and parallel processing in rhesus monkey auditory cortex. *J. Comp. Neurol.* 382, 89–103.

Rauschecker, J. P., Tian, B., and Hauser, M. (1995). Processing of complex sounds in the macaque nonprimary auditory cortex. *Science* 268, 111–114.

Recanzone, G., Schreiner, C., and Merzenich, M. (1993). Plasticity in the frequency representation of primary auditory cortex following discrimination training in adult owl monkeys. *J. Neurosci.* 13, 87–103.

Rhode, W. S., and Greenberg, S. (1994). Lateral suppression and inhibition in the cochlear nucleus of the cat. *J. Neurophysiol.* 71, 493–514.

Roberts, L. E., and Bosnyak, D. J. (2011). "Auditory training in tinnitus," in *Textbook of Tinnitus*, eds A. Møller, T. Kleinjung, B. Langguth, and D. De Ridder (New York, NY: Springer), 563–573.

Roberts, L. E., Eggermont, J. J., Caspary, D. M., Shore, S. E., Melcher, J. R., and Kaltenbach, J. A. (2010). Ringing ears: the neuroscience of tinnitus. *J. Neurosci.* 30, 14972–14979.

Robertson, D., and Irvine, D. R. (1989). Plasticity of frequency organization in auditory cortex of guinea pigs with partial unilateral deafness. *J. Comp. Neurol.* 282, 456–471.

Salimpoor, V. N., Benovoy, M., Larcher, K., Dagher, A., and Zatorre, R. J. (2011). Anatomically distinct dopamine release during anticipation and experience of peak emotion to music. *Nat. Neurosci.* 14, 257–262.

Schlaug, G., Jäncke, L., Huang, Y., Staiger, J. F., and Steinmetz, H. (1995a). Increased corpus callosum size in musicians. *Neuropsychologia* 33, 1047–1055.

Schlaug, G., Jancke, L., Huang, Y., and Steinmetz, H. (1995b). *In vivo* evidence of structural brain asymmetry in musicians. *Science* 267, 699–701.

Schneider, P., Scherg, M., Dosch, H. G., Specht, H. J., Gutschalk, A., and Rupp, A. (2002). Morphology of Heschl's gyrus reflects enhanced activation in the auditory cortex of musicians. *Nat. Neurosci.* 5, 688–694.

Schulte, M., Knief, A., Seither-Preisler, A., and Pantev, C. (2002). Different modes of pitch perception and learning-induced neuronal plasticity of the human auditory cortex. *Neural Plast.* 9, 161–175.

Schulz, M., Ross, B., and Pantev, C. (2003). Evidence for training-induced crossmodal reorganization of cortical functions in trumpet players. *Neuroreport* 14, 157–161.

Shahin, A. J., Bosnyak, D. J., Trainor, L. J., and Roberts, L. E. (2003). Enhancement of neuroplastic P2 and N1c auditory evoked potentials in musicians. *J. Neurosci.* 23, 5545–5552.

Stouffer, J. L., and Tyler, R. S. (1990). Characterization of tinnitus by tinnitus patients. *J. Speech Hear. Disord.* 55, 439–453.

Stracke, H., Okamoto, H., and Pantev, C. (2010). Customized notched music training reduces tinnitus loudness. *Commun. Integr. Biol.* 3, 274–277.

Suga, N. (1995). Sharpening of frequency tuning by inhibition in the central auditory system: tribute to Yasuji Katsuki. *Neurosci. Res.* 21, 287–299.

Sutter, M. L., Schreiner, C. E., Mclean, M., O'connor, K. N., and Loftus, W. C. (1999). Organization of inhibitory frequency receptive fields in cat primary auditory cortex. *J. Neurophysiol.* 82, 2358–2371.

Sutter, M. L., and Loftus, W. C. (2003). Excitatory and inhibitory intensity tuning in auditory cortex: evidence for multiple inhibitory mechanisms. *J. Neurophysiol.* 90, 2629–2647.

Tass, P. A., Adamchic, I., Freund, H.-J., von Stackelberg, T., and Hauptmann, C. (2012). Counteracting tinnitus by acoustic coordinated reset neuromodulation. *Restor. Neurol. Neurosci.* 30, 135–159.

Teismann, H., Okamoto, H., and Pantev, C. (2011). Short and intense tailor-made notched music training against tinnitus: the tinnitus frequency matters. *PLoS ONE* 6:e24685. doi: 10.1371/journal.pone.0024685

Tervaniemi, M., Rytkonen, M., Schroger, E., Ilmoniemi, R. J., and Naatanen, R. (2001). Superior formation of cortical memory traces for melodic patterns in musicians. *Learn. Mem.* 8, 295–300.

Tyler, R. S., and Conrad-Armes, D. (1983). Tinnitus pitch: a comparison of three measurement methods. *Br. J. Audiol.* 17, 101–107.

Van Zuijen, T. L., Sussman, E., Winkler, I., Näätänen, R., and Tervaniemi, M. (2004). Grouping of sequential sounds–an event-related potential study comparing musicians and nonmusicians. *J. Cogn. Neurosci.* 16, 331–338.

Van Zuijen, T. L., Sussman, E., Winkler, I., Näätänen, R., and Tervaniemi, M. (2005). Auditory organization of sound sequences by a temporal or numerical regularity–a mismatch negativity study comparing musicians and non-musicians. *Brain Res. Cogn. Brain Res.* 23, 270–276.

Von Békésy, G. (1967). *Sensory Inhibition.* Princeton, NJ: Princeton University Press.

Wan, C. Y., and Schlaug, G. (2010). Music making as a tool for promoting brain plasticity across the life span. *Neuroscientist* 16, 566–577.

Wiegrebe, L., Kossl, M., and Schmidt, S. (1996). Auditory enhancement at the absolute threshold of hearing and its relationship to the Zwicker tone. *Hear. Res.* 100, 171–180.

Woldorff, M. G., Gallen, C. C., Hampson, S. A., Hillyard, S. A., Pantev, C., Sobel, D., and Bloom, F. E. (1993). Modulation of early sensory processing in human auditory cortex during auditory selective attention. *Proc. Natl. Acad. Sci. U.S.A.* 90, 8722–8726.

Zatorre, R. J., Chen, J. L., and Penhune, V. B. (2007). When the brain plays music: auditory-motor interactions in music perception and production. *Nat. Rev. Neurosci.* 8, 547–558.

Zhou, X., and Merzenich, M. M. (2012). Environmental noise exposure degrades normal listening processes. *Nat. Commun.* 3, 843.

20

Computational models of neurophysiological correlates of tinnitus

Roland Schaette[1]* and Richard Kempter[2]

[1] Ear Institute, University College London, London, UK
[2] Institute for Theoretical Biology, Humboldt-Universität zu Berlin and Bernstein Center for Computational Neuroscience, Berlin, Germany

Correspondence:
Roland Schaette, Ear Institute, University College London, 332 Gray's Inn Road, London WC1X 8EE, UK.
e-mail: r.schaette@ucl.ac.uk

The understanding of tinnitus has progressed considerably in the past decade, but the details of the mechanisms that give rise to this phantom perception of sound without a corresponding acoustic stimulus have not yet been pinpointed. It is now clear that tinnitus is generated in the brain, not in the ear, and that it is correlated with pathologically altered spontaneous activity of neurons in the central auditory system. Both increased spontaneous firing rates and increased neuronal synchrony have been identified as putative neuronal correlates of phantom sounds in animal models, and both phenomena can be triggered by damage to the cochlea. Various mechanisms could underlie the generation of such aberrant activity. At the cellular level, decreased synaptic inhibition and increased neuronal excitability, which may be related to homeostatic plasticity, could lead to an over-amplification of natural spontaneous activity. At the network level, lateral inhibition could amplify differences in spontaneous activity, and structural changes such as reorganization of tonotopic maps could lead to self-sustained activity in recurrently connected neurons. However, it is difficult to disentangle the contributions of different mechanisms in experiments, especially since not all changes observed in animal models of tinnitus are necessarily related to tinnitus. Computational modeling presents an opportunity of evaluating these mechanisms and their relation to tinnitus. Here we review the computational models for the generation of neurophysiological correlates of tinnitus that have been proposed so far, and evaluate predictions and compare them to available data. We also assess the limits of their explanatory power, thus demonstrating where an understanding is still lacking and where further research may be needed. Identifying appropriate models is important for finding therapies, and we therefore, also summarize the implications of the models for approaches to treat tinnitus.

Keywords: tinnitus, computational model, hearing loss, homeostatic plasticity, lateral inhibition, gain adaptation

INTRODUCTION

Over the last two decades, our understanding of tinnitus has increased greatly through the results of animal models of tinnitus. As tinnitus can often be related to cochlear damage, animal models have used acoustic trauma or ototoxic drugs to induce hearing loss and to study changes in the central auditory system. After hearing loss, a variety of changes that could contribute to tinnitus have been observed; most notably, increased spontaneous neuronal activity throughout the central auditory system (see Kaltenbach, 2011, for a review), but not at the level of the auditory nerve (AN) (Liberman and Dodds, 1984; Heinz and Young, 2004). Importantly, increases in spontaneous firing rates were correlated to behavioral signs of tinnitus in animals (Brozoski et al., 2002; Kaltenbach et al., 2004; Middleton et al., 2011), and they have been linked to decreases in inhibition (Dong et al., 2009; Middleton et al., 2011). Also an increase in the synchrony of the neuronal discharge has been observed in the auditory cortex after noise trauma (Norena and Eggermont, 2003). Furthermore, a reorganization of the tonotopic map in the auditory cortex has also been found after hearing loss (Rajan and Irvine, 1998; Rauschecker, 1999; Irvine et al., 2000; Komiya and Eggermont, 2000).

Human neuroimaging studies on tinnitus have also shown changes in spontaneous neuronal activity (Weisz et al., 2005, 2007; Lorenz et al., 2009) where spontaneous rhythmic brain activity displayed a decrease in power in the alpha band and increases in power in the delta and gamma frequency bands. Moreover, an association between tinnitus and reorganization of the tonotopic map in the auditory cortex has been reported (Mühlnickel et al., 1998). These studies in humans and animals show that tinnitus is not generated in the ear, but in the brain itself (Eggermont and Roberts, 2004; Roberts et al., 2010). However, the exact mechanisms that lead to the development of this phantom sensation have still remained elusive.

Further progress in understanding tinnitus has been made using computational models, which are the main topic of this review. Such models, also called "theories" or "hypotheses," provide a motivational and interpretational framework for possibly diverse sets of data, and, ideally explain how the data fit together to yield a more complete understanding of tinnitus. Because the data on which models are based are from different levels, i.e., from the microscopic molecular and single-neuron level to the macroscopic levels of large-scale brain signals and behavior, computational models must capture these different levels to be in line with salient features of the respective data. Therefore, modeling at different levels is justified, but one also needs models that bridge across levels. Such models could also link research across different fields, for example research on humans and animals or research *in vivo* and *in vitro*.

However, not all models are equally valuable. To outline some basic criteria for "good" models, let us summarize some general principles, which might help to justify our selection of models in this review. Regardless of the level of modeling, a model should always be as simple as possible and be based on as few reasonable assumptions as is feasible. This rule determines the predictive power of a model, i.e., its ability to generate testable predictions on the outcome of future experiments. One such example could be how a specific type of hearing loss determines the tinnitus pitch or the tinnitus spectrum. Good models are falsifiable, and progress in understanding is closely related to ruling out models. Therefore, models should be quantitative and tell us how large a new effect should be, for example, what the loudness of the tinnitus is. Because of this need for verifiability, we have excluded qualitative models from this review. Quantitative or "computational" models also might permit a mathematical analysis and facilitate numerical simulations on a computer. In the following, we will evaluate each reviewed model based on these criteria.

The appropriate level of detail for a model is, in general, a highly controversial issue. An oversimplified or abstract model may ignore many experimental details and could provide misleading results; on the other hand, an excessively complex model can reproduce many experimental results but may lack predictive power because of too many unconstrained or "free" parameters and too many *ad-hoc* assumptions. The adequate detail of modeling, therefore, strongly depends on available data, i.e., on the physiology of the auditory system in general, and on tinnitus in particular. Interestingly, the available computational models on tinnitus, which are all described below, are rather more abstract than detailed.

In summary, a computational model of tinnitus should (1) explain how neural correlates of tinnitus could arise, (2) outline which mechanisms might be involved, and (3) predict how the processes that give rise to tinnitus can be suppressed or reversed. Before we summarize the available computational models of tinnitus, let us briefly introduce the basic mechanisms employed by these models.

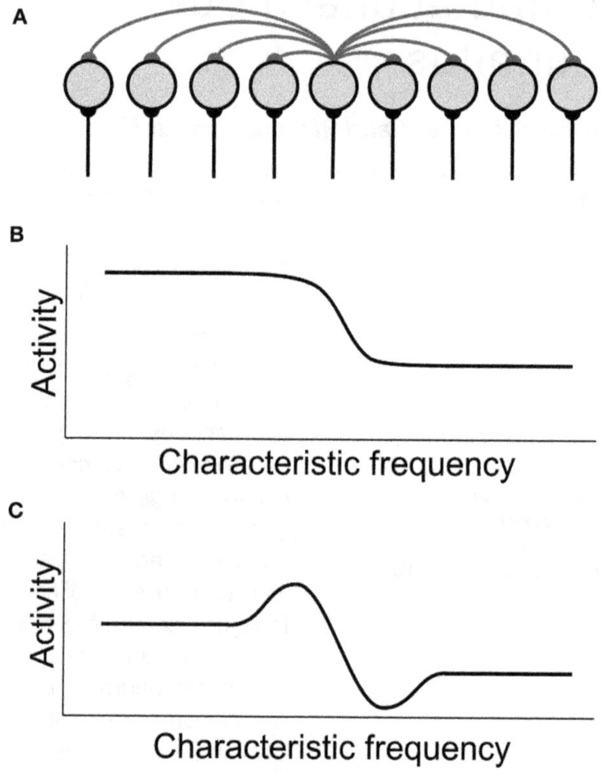

FIGURE 1 | Schematic illustration of lateral-inhibition models. **(A)** Depiction of a layer of neurons with lateral inhibition. Neurons are represented by gray circles, lateral inhibitory connections by gray lines (only the inhibitory projections from the central neuron to its neighbors are shown), and excitatory afferents by black lines. **(B)** Hypothetical auditory activity pattern with a drop toward high frequencies, as it could for example occur in the spontaneous activity of the auditory nerve after noise-induced hearing loss. **(C)** Activity pattern in the lateral-inhibition network driven by the input shown in **(B)**. An activity peak is generated at the edge of the input pattern but below the region of hearing loss.

BASIC MECHANISMS EXPLORED IN COMPUTATIONAL MODELS OF TINNITUS

Three main mechanisms have been explored in computational models of tinnitus: lateral inhibition, homeostatic plasticity, and gain adaptation.

Lateral inhibition is inhibition between neighboring neurons in a neuronal structure (**Figure 1A**). Functionally, in the auditory system it also means inhibition between frequency channels, i.e., inhibition between neurons whose characteristic frequency (CF) is close, but not identical. Lateral inhibition is ubiquitous in the brain, and it is assumed to be a basic mechanism of information processing in neural circuits. Lateral inhibition also plays a role in keeping neural networks balanced, and it can enhance the activity difference between neurons with high and low levels of activity in a neuronal network (**Figures 1B,C**). One example of lateral inhibition in the auditory system is its involvement in the sharpening of receptive fields. Lateral inhibition has been found at all central processing stages from the cochlear nucleus (Roberts and Trussell, 2010) to the auditory cortex (de la Rocha et al., 2008).

Homeostatic plasticity is a plasticity mechanism that stabilizes the mean activity of neurons on time scales of hours to days (Turrigiano et al., 1998; Turrigiano, 1999). This mechanism sets the basic operating point of neurons and ensures that neurons are neither inactive nor too active when averaged over time windows of hours to days. In cell culture, homeostatic plasticity in response to activity deprivation has been shown to scale up the strength of excitatory synapses (Turrigiano et al., 1998) and increase intrinsic neuronal excitability (Desai et al., 1999), while the strength of inhibitory synapses was scaled down (Kilman et al., 2002). On the other hand, when activity was pathologically increased by blocking inhibition, excitatory synapses were scaled down, neuronal excitability was decreased, and inhibition was scaled up, which restored circuit activity back to a normal level (Turrigiano et al., 1998; Rannals and Kapur, 2011). Similar changes have also been observed in the auditory system *in vivo* after hearing loss, cochlear damage, or auditory deprivation (Suneja et al., 1998a,b; Oleskevich and Walmsley, 2002; Vale and Sanes, 2002; Muly et al., 2004; Vale et al., 2004; Caspary et al., 2005; Kotak et al., 2005; Whiting et al., 2009).

Gain adaptation adjusts the responses of single-neurons or neuronal circuits to their input, thus enabling neurons to cope with the wide dynamic range of natural signals. Gain adaptation occurs at various stages of the auditory pathway. Fast gain adaptation on the time scale of seconds has been observed for example in the AN (Wen et al., 2009) and the inferior colliculus (IC) (Dean et al., 2005, 2008). Such fast adaptation phenomena are usually caused by the activation of adaptation currents (Benda and Herz, 2003). Slower adaptation mechanisms on a time scale of minutes can involve modulation of ion channels (van Welie et al., 2004). On longer time scales of hours to days, gain adaptation can be seen as functionally equivalent to homeostatic plasticity.

OVERVIEW OF COMPUTATIONAL MODELS OF NEUROPHYSIOLOGICAL CORRELATES OF TINNITUS

In the following section, we present the main features of the computational models of neurophysiological correlates of tinnitus that have been proposed so far. As already mentioned, we have excluded qualitative models because they do not give rise to detailed predictions, which makes them hard to falsify. The remaining quantitative models are grouped by mechanisms and then presented in chronological order, to highlight the development of the different concepts.

The first computational model that addressed the question of how a neural correlate of tinnitus could arise in the central auditory system after noise-induced damage to structures of the inner ear was the auditory brainstem model proposed by Gerken (1996). In this model, lateral inhibition was the key mechanism responsible for generating a tinnitus-related pattern of neuronal activity. Another basic model assumption was that after noise-induced cochlear damage, the spontaneous activity of AN fibers is reduced in the high-frequency range, creating a drop in the profile of spontaneous activity along the tonotopic axis. The drop starts at CFs corresponding to the audiogram edge. When such a pattern of activity is processed by a neuronal structure with lateral inhibition, the neurons just below and at the edge receive less lateral inhibition than their counterparts at lower frequencies. In contrast, the neurons just above the edge receive more lateral inhibition than the other neurons with higher CFs. As a consequence, the edge in the activity profile is amplified, leading to a peak in the profile of spontaneous activity (**Figure 1C**). When this activity peak is interpreted by higher stages of the auditory system as sound-evoked activity, a tinnitus sensation is created. In the Gerken-model, lateral inhibition was assumed to occur at the level of the IC, and the model employed a feed-forward architecture. However, as the circuit of the IC was not explicitly modeled, the model can rather be seen as a generic demonstration of the effects of lateral inhibition. Moreover, Gerken did not assume plastic changes to take place in the auditory system after hearing loss. The model's achievement was to demonstrate that even though there is no direct indication of a neural correlate of tinnitus at the level of the AN, central processing of distorted AN output could give rise to tinnitus-related patterns of spontaneous activity. The basic prediction following from this and all other lateral inhibition models is that tinnitus will emerge almost instantaneously when the profile of spontaneous activity is changed by hearing loss, as no plastic changes are required. The resulting tinnitus pitch will be associated with the audiogram edge.

Also in 1996, lateral inhibition was proposed as a key factor to explain why most people start hearing phantom sounds after spending some time in a sound-proof booth (Kral and Majernik, 1996). Kral and Majernik used a neural network model with several layers, each with lateral inhibition, and they assumed stochastic spontaneous activity, such as the spontaneous activity of AN fibers, as an input to the network. Processing of this spontaneous activity by the feed-forward network with lateral inhibition resulted in several distinct activity peaks along the tonotopic axis, and the peaks occurred at random locations. Kral and Majernik proposed that these activity peaks could underlie the perception of tinnitus in absolute silence, and that in normal acoustic environments, the spontaneous activity is masked by ambient noise. Whether this mechanism could also account for the emergence of tinnitus after hearing loss was not investigated, but in principle the predictions of this model should match those of the Gerken-model.

Lateral inhibition was combined with plasticity in the central auditory system by Langner and Wallhäusser-Franke (1999). The model was set up as a multi-layer feed-forward network with lateral inhibition representing processing in the auditory brainstem and midbrain, with additional modulatory inputs representing feedback from the auditory cortex and amygdala. Specific details of the auditory brainstem and midbrain circuitry were omitted for simplicity. Their model was inspired by c-fos labeling data showing increased activity correlations between the auditory and the limbic system after salicylate administration. In the model, lateral inhibition in the first processing stages amplified unevenness in the tonotopic profile of spontaneous activity, which was caused by cochlear damage. As to be expected for a lateral inhibition model, the resulting activity peaks were located close to the edge of hearing loss, as it was there that the contrast between the output of the undamaged and the damaged parts of the cochlea produced the greatest unevenness in the spontaneous activity. The activity peaks were then further amplified by positive feedback at higher stages, which was attributed to the action of the auditory cortex and the amygdala. This feedback elevated the activity peaks substantially above the level of spontaneous activity, possibly generating a highly salient tinnitus percept.

The putative role of lateral inhibition in generating tinnitus-related patterns of neural activity was further explored by Bruce et al. (2003). They showed that also in a recurrent network of spiking model neurons, lateral inhibition could generate an activity peak at the edge of hearing loss. However, they also found that the generation of such a peak depended not only on the contrast between the levels of spontaneous activity in the healthy and the damaged region, but also on the overall level of input received by the network, and the time constants of excitation and inhibition. The time constants needed to be long enough, and the input rates high enough, so that an interaction between excitatory and inhibitory postsynaptic potentials could take place. For low input rates to the network, the enhancement of the edge was not significant.

The development of neural correlates of tinnitus at the level of the auditory cortex has been explored in a model by Dominguez et al. (2006). This model comprised a network of spiking model neurons with pyramidal cells and inhibitory interneurons. The thalamic stage was modeled through a network with lateral inhibition as employed by Bruce et al. (2003), and the network received random afferent input. Hearing loss was modeled by decreasing the firing rate of the inputs to the thalamus stage. After simultaneously increasing the strength of lateral excitatory connections and decreasing the strength of lateral inhibitory connections in the cortical network model in the region affected by the hearing loss, pyramidal neurons displayed increased spontaneous firing rates and increased synchrony. Additionally, the network displayed an activity peak in the region of hearing loss. Without this plasticity, the peak was located below the edge of hearing loss. Thus, the model by Dominguez et al. (2006) demonstrated that decreases in inhibition and increases in excitation, as observed in animals after the induction of hearing loss, can lead to the development of a neural correlate of tinnitus in a recurrent neuronal network. Moreover, if the peak in the profile of spontaneous activity was interpreted as the dominant tinnitus pitch, the model would predict a tinnitus pitch in the region of hearing loss.

How gain adaptation in the auditory system might give rise to the perception of phantom sounds was addressed by Parra and Pearlmutter (2007). They considered an abstract model organized in frequency channels. Gain adaptation was implemented by calculating a running average of input activity for each channel, which was then used as a normalization factor to scale the channel's output. If a channel did not receive input, for example due to hearing loss, its average input activity was close to the neuronal noise level (i.e., spontaneous activity), and the normalization factor was low. As a consequence, the output of this channel was scaled-up. Because also the spontaneous input activity was scaled by the low normalization factor, it was effectively amplified, leading to increased spontaneous activity in the output, which was interpreted as tinnitus. In addition to gain adaptation, Parra and Pearlmutter also analyzed the effects of lateral inhibition in their model. They showed that lateral inhibition combined with a steep audiogram slope could lead to a pronounced "tinnitus" peak in the profile of spontaneous activity. However, shallow audiogram slopes did not produce such peaks, which matched the experimental finding that for noise-induced hearing loss, tinnitus is associated with steep audiogram slopes (König et al., 2006). The pitch of the model tinnitus was then located in the region of hearing loss, at the "elbow" of the audiogram where hearing loss has reached a plateau.

Functional mechanisms to explain changes in excitation and inhibition after hearing loss and how these changes are connected to the development of tinnitus were studied by Schaette and Kempter (2006, 2008, 2009) in a model based on the physiology of the AN and the cochlear nucleus. This computational model showed that activity stabilization through homeostatic plasticity after hearing loss could account for changes in excitation and inhibition as well as for the development of increased spontaneous firing rates. The model assumed that hearing loss reduces AN activity with a concomitant reduction in excitatory drive to the central auditory system (**Figure 2A**). In order to stabilize mean neuronal activity, homeostatic plasticity then generated increased excitatory gain and reduced inhibitory gain in neurons downstream of the AN, restoring average neuronal activity to normal levels. However, as neurons became more excitable, spontaneous activity was amplified, leading to neuronal hyperactivity, which was interpreted as a tinnitus percept (**Figure 2B**). The model thus suggested that tinnitus could be an unwanted side-effect of a stabilization of neuronal activity levels in the central auditory system after hearing loss. Tinnitus pitch predicted from the audiograms of patients with noise-induced hearing loss was located in the region of hearing loss (Schaette and Kempter, 2009). Interestingly, in the model not all types and degrees of cochlear damage increased central spontaneous activity to comparable degrees. Loss of outer hair cells and moderate noise damage led to the greatest increases in spontaneous firing rates whereas inner hair cell loss and severe noise damage could even cause spontaneous firing rates to decrease (Schaette and Kempter, 2006, 2008). Moreover, different response types of model DCN projection neurons differed in their disposition for hyperactivity (Schaette and Kempter, 2008), indicating that not all central neurons might necessarily develop increased spontaneous firing rates after hearing loss.

The effects of homeostatic plasticity were also studied in the cortex-based model of Chrostowski et al. (2011), which built up on the model of Dominguez et al. (2006). As in the earlier model, they considered a network of spiking model neurons based on features of the auditory cortex, but only a simplified thalamic stage without lateral inhibition. The activity of the pyramidal cells of the cortical network was stabilized by homeostatic plasticity. When hearing loss was induced in the model by decreasing the activity of thalamic afferents, homeostatic plasticity increased the strength of excitatory projections onto the pyramidal neurons and decreased the strength of the inhibitory synapses. These changes lead to a combination of increased spontaneous firing rates and increased synchrony of the neuronal discharge in the pyramidal neurons of the model network. Interestingly, while the increase in spontaneous firing rates was rather uniform across the range of hearing loss, the greatest increase in synchrony occurred near the audiogram edge. This synchrony maximum was restricted to a relatively narrow range of CFs, and could thus be interpreted as giving rise to a tone-like tinnitus sensation, even though the hearing loss and the increases in spontaneous activity spanned a large frequency range. Moreover, the model also displayed traveling waves of excitation, which confirmed another study on homeostatic plasticity in cortical network models (Houweling et al., 2005).

DIFFERENCES AND SIMILARITIES OF THE COMPUTATIONAL MODELS OF TINNITUS

The majority of the computational models of tinnitus employed firing-rate-based frameworks. Spiking neurons can be considered to represent a higher degree of biological realism, but it should be noted that in all studies the choice of model neurons corresponded to the type of neuronal data that was to be modeled: changes in the synchrony of the spontaneous neuronal activity, i.e., a measure where the timing of action potentials is important, have only been investigated in the auditory cortex, whereas the putative neuronal correlates of tinnitus in subcortical stages have only been reported in terms of average firing rates. Consequently, all models based on the auditory brainstem are firing-rate models (Gerken, 1996; Schaette and Kempter, 2006, 2008, 2009), and the cortex-based models employ spiking neurons (Dominguez et al., 2006; Chrostowski et al., 2011).

Models based on firing rates and on spikes provided similar results regarding the role of lateral inhibition, which basically amplifies edges. However, the spiking neuronal network by Bruce et al. (2003) highlighted an additional potential dependence on neuronal properties, i.e., the interplay between the effects of lateral inhibition and synaptic time constants, which was not apparent in the firing-rate models. For homeostatic plasticity, on the other hand, qualitatively similar results were obtained for feed-forward firing-rate and recurrent spiking models, demonstrating the robustness of the mechanism.

The models that refer to specific brain structures are phenomenological models that only contain simplified versions of the neuronal circuits they are representing (Dominguez et al., 2006; Schaette and Kempter, 2006, 2008, 2009; Chrostowski et al., 2011). The remaining more generic models are not based on a specific brain structure in the first place (Gerken, 1996; Kral and Majernik, 1996; Bruce et al., 2003; Parra and Pearlmutter, 2007). An evaluation of the effects of different kinds of cochlear damage beyond a mere threshold increase or simple activity reduction was only performed by Schaette and Kempter (2006, 2008, 2009). Thus, we can safely conclude that none of the models contains unnecessary detail. Moreover, all models are simple enough to be fully tractable, and they are also specific enough in their structure, assumptions, and predictions to be testable and falsifiable. In the following, we will discuss the implications of the models for putative mechanisms of tinnitus generation by comparing their predictions to experimental findings. We will assess the limitations of the current modeling approaches, and finally give an outlook for future directions.

EVALUATION OF THE MODELS AND THEIR IMPLICATIONS FOR PUTATIVE MECHANISMS UNDERLYING THE GENERATION OF TINNITUS

The computational models that we have reviewed demonstrate that lateral inhibition, homeostatic plasticity, and gain adaptation could all in principle be involved in generating tinnitus-related neuronal activity patterns. Interestingly, all models focussed on how auditory input that was altered by hearing loss, induces changes in subsequent stages of the auditory system. This model feature indicates that not the process of cochlear damage as such, but rather the effects of the input signal to the auditory brain might generate tinnitus. This view could also explain how tinnitus is related to the kind and degree of hearing loss.

Computational models of tinnitus offer an explanation for the plastic changes that were observed in the central auditory system in animal models of tinnitus. Decreases in inhibition, for example, were found all along the auditory pathway, and this decrease can be explained through homeostatic plasticity or gain adaptation. In that respect, gain adaptation models (Parra and Pearlmutter, 2007) and homeostatic plasticity models (Schaette and Kempter, 2006, 2008, 2009; Chrostowski et al., 2011) suggest that tinnitus might not be the result of abnormal or aberrant plasticity, but rather that phantom sounds could arise as a side-effect of plasticity mechanisms that normally ensure proper function of the auditory brain. Plasticity triggered by hearing loss might simply produce unwanted effects when AN activity is pathologically altered, i.e., in a way that the plasticity mechanism is not designed to cope with.

Computational models of tinnitus must account for basic experimental findings. For example, in tonal tinnitus, a basic feature is its pitch, which is related to the shape of the audiogram. For noise-induced hearing loss, models based on lateral inhibition as the main mechanism (Gerken, 1996; Kral and Majernik, 1996) predict tinnitus pitch at the audiogram edge (Schaette and Kempter, 2009). Even though this relation between tinnitus pitch and the audiogram edge is supported by a recent study (Moore and Vinay, 2010), other studies report tinnitus pitch to be above the audiogram edge, i.e., within the region of hearing loss (Norena et al., 2002; König et al., 2006; Roberts et al., 2008; Pan et al., 2009; Sereda et al., 2011). Models based on homeostatic plasticity predict tinnitus pitch to be within the region of hearing loss (Schaette and Kempter, 2009) because activity stabilization through homeostatic plasticity leads to an elevation of central spontaneous activity in the frequency range that is affected by hearing loss (**Figure 2B**).

In general, lateral-inhibition models of tinnitus produce a "tinnitus" activity peak at a discontinuity or edge in the profile of spontaneous activity along the tonotopic axis (**Figures 1B,C**). However, not all kinds of cochlear damage produce such an edge. Pure loss of outer hair cells through ototoxic drugs like gentamycin or cisplatin, for example, increases the hearing thresholds but does not change the spontaneous firing rates of AN fibers (Dallos and Harris, 1978), yet tinnitus is a common side-effect of cisplatin chemotherapy (Sprauten et al., 2011). In that case, a model relying on lateral inhibition only, i.e., without additional plasticity, would not predict the occurrence of tinnitus. A homeostatic plasticity model or gain adaptation model, on the other hand, would predict the occurrence of a neural correlate of tinnitus also for pure loss of outer hair cells (Schaette and Kempter, 2006, 2008; Parra and Pearlmutter, 2007).

Evaluating model predictions in a new experimental setting is a particularly challenging test for any model. For example, plasticity models predict that tinnitus only occur when hearing is impaired, yet a significant fraction of tinnitus patients present with a normal audiogram (Barnea et al., 1990; Sanchez et al., 2005). This subgroup of tinnitus patients thus presents a considerable challenge for the hypotheses of tinnitus generation that have been formalized in the computational models summarized above. However, normal hearing thresholds do not necessarily indicate the absence of cochlear damage. In fact, it has been shown in mice that noise trauma that only leads to a temporary increase in the hearing thresholds still causes permanent damage to the synaptic contacts between inner hair cells and AN fibers (Kujawa

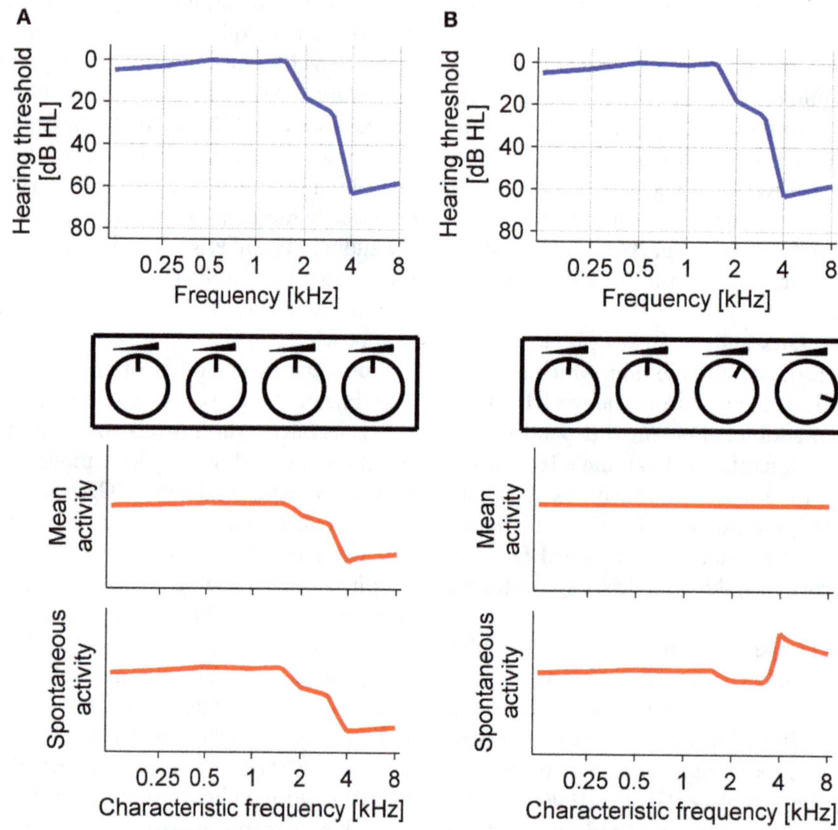

FIGURE 2 | Schematic illustration of homeostatic plasticity models. The "knobs" represent the effective response gain of neurons in the central auditory system, determined by the strength of excitatory and inhibitory synapses as well as intrinsic neuronal excitability. **(A)** Before homeostatic plasticity: noise-induced hearing loss (example audiogram in the top panel) has reduced mean and spontaneous activity in the central auditory system (bottom panels). **(B)** After homeostatic plasticity: the response gain has been increased to restore the mean activity of central auditory neurons back to its target level. However, spontaneous activity is amplified through the increased gain, giving rise to increased spontaneous firing rates in the region of hearing loss.

and Liberman, 2009). When the AN stage of the homeostasis-hyperactivity model by Schaette and Kempter was adjusted to reflect this deafferentation of AN fibers, the model predicted the development of a neural correlate of tinnitus in response to the decrease in overall AN input (Schaette and McAlpine, 2011). This model result is supported by auditory brainstem response (ABR) data of tinnitus patients with normal audiograms, where a significant reduction of the amplitude of wave I of the ABR in conjunction with normal amplitudes of the centrally generated wave V was found, suggesting the presence of "hidden hearing loss" together with increased central gain (Schaette and McAlpine, 2011). Homeostasis models further predict that non-traumatic but prolonged reduction of auditory input, for example through an earplug, should lead to the occurrence of phantom sounds. This was tested experimentally in a study where participants with normal hearing and no tinnitus continuously wore an earplug for seven days. Eleven out of 18 participants perceived phantom sounds after seven days of wearing the earplug, and the phantom sounds disappeared after removing the earplug (Schaette et al., 2012).

We can conclude that a large body of evidence suggests that plasticity is a necessary ingredient of computational models of tinnitus, whereas models based on lateral inhibition only are not able to explain basic features of the data on tinnitus.

LIMITATIONS OF CURRENT MODELS AND FUTURE DIRECTIONS

The computational models of tinnitus that have been proposed so far are almost exclusively focussed on the ascending auditory pathway. Feedback connections were omitted, and the extralemniscal pathway was not considered. Moreover, information processing and plasticity were mostly considered in a bottom-up fashion only. Top-down influences and modulation were addressed only by Langner and Wallhäusser-Franke (1999). The focus on bottom-up models can be explained by the fact that computational models need to be constrained by experimental data. The physiology of the classical ascending auditory pathway has been studied extensively whereas information about the function of feedback connections and also the extralemniscal pathways is still relatively scarce. Moreover, while a computational model needs to be as complex as necessary, ideally it should not be any more complex than required. If a phenomenon of interest can be accounted for by a simple model that captures the standard aspects of physiology, it is not necessary to include further structures and/or mechanisms that are not known well enough because such a model extension would introduce more and possibly unconstrained parameters.

In line with the idea of adequate simplicity, most models either focussed on a small part of the auditory pathway, such as the brainstem (Gerken, 1996; Schaette and Kempter, 2006, 2008, 2009) or the thalamus and cortex (Dominguez et al., 2006; Chrostowski et al., 2011), or models were not related to a particular brain region (Kral and Majernik, 1996; Parra and Pearlmutter, 2007). A unifying model that combines the aspects of these model classes could now be attempted. It would be especially interesting to see how increased spontaneous activity and activity stabilization in brainstem structures might interact with plasticity at the level of the auditory cortex. It is conceivable that less drastic changes in excitation and inhibition might be required to stabilize cortical activity when homeostatic mechanisms also increase activity in the sub-cortical processing stages. To study the interaction of subcortical and cortical levels, the respective time scales of changes are important. In any case, a combined model of brainstem, thalamus, and cortex could potentially also incorporate thalamic gating mechanisms, which have recently been implied to play a role in tinnitus (Rauschecker et al., 2010). Such unifying models might help to understand why hearing loss not always leads to tinnitus. This puzzling fact is especially important as animal studies have shown a direct relation between the degree of hearing loss and the development of putative neuronal correlates of tinnitus (Mulders et al., 2011).

At the cortical level, it might be an interesting future directive to quantitatively explore the reorganization of tonotopic maps and the relation of this phenomenon to tinnitus. Cortical reorganization can be induced by hearing loss (Irvine et al., 2000) and it was implicated as a contributor to tinnitus (Mühlnickel et al., 1998; Engineer et al., 2011), but it has not yet been explored in a computational model. Modeling studies not related to the auditory system showed that spike-timing-dependent plasticity could be the driving force for such reorganization (Song and Abbott, 2001; Young et al., 2007). An analysis of the interplay of reorganization and homeostatic plasticity could be especially interesting since recent experimental studies have reported different roles for reorganization, from promoting (Engineer et al., 2011) to reducing tinnitus (Yang et al., 2011).

So far, computational models of tinnitus have looked at neuronal activity at a microscopic level, as measured for example with microelectrodes. Another interesting aspect for future modeling studies would be to consider macroscopic signals like EEG and MEG and to include cortical rhythms. MEG studies in tinnitus patients showed that tinnitus is associated with a decrease in the power of the alpha rhythm and an increase in power in the delta frequency band (Weisz et al., 2005, 2007). Moreover, an increase in gamma power accompanied temporary tinnitus after noise exposure (Ortmann et al., 2011). Building up on models of the generation of cortical rhythms (Freyer et al., 2011) and on models that relate neuronal spiking activity to field potentials (Kuokkanen et al., 2010), future modeling studies on tinnitus could explore which parameter changes generate the observed changes in cortical rhythms, and then try to relate parameter changes to microscopic models of changes in spiking activity of neurons. Potentially, such an approach might help to bridge the gaps between animal models of tinnitus and human studies.

IMPLICATIONS AND PREDICTIONS OF THE MODELS FOR TINNITUS TREATMENTS

Before we provide an assessment of the predictions of the model for tinnitus treatments, we point out that all models we have discussed are basically bottom-up. Therefore, model predictions for tinnitus treatments also concern bottom-up approaches, and the models are not applicable to treatments employing top-down influences, like cognitive behavioral therapy.

The models based on homeostatic plasticity (Schaette and Kempter, 2006, 2008, 2009; Chrostowski et al., 2011) and gain control (Parra and Pearlmutter, 2007) make specific predictions for treatments employing acoustic or electric stimulation. These models predict that a stimulation strategy that succeeds in restoring normal AN activity should completely abolish tinnitus. For acoustic stimulation, this would correspond to the "perfect hearing aid," and its effects would be similar to the disappearance of earplug-induced phantom sounds after removing the earplug (Schaette et al., 2012). However, the perfect hearing aid has not been invented yet. If AN activity cannot be restored, the concept of homeostatic plasticity suggests that a certain increase in AN activity should be sufficient to dampen the increased central gain and thus to reduce tinnitus. This dampening could be achieved by acoustic stimulation with noise that is spectrally matched to the hearing loss (Schaette and Kempter, 2006, 2008). Alternatively, for steeply sloping hearing loss, an amplification strategy could also try to smooth the transition from good to impaired hearing and thus to reduce the effective slope of the audiogram. This would lead to a spontaneous activity pattern with less pronounced peaks (Parra and Pearlmutter, 2007; Schaette and Kempter, 2009), corresponding to a reduction of the tinnitus salience.

In general, hearing aids and noise devices provide a certain degree of tinnitus relief (Trotter and Donaldson, 2008). However, on average the treatment success is quite limited. A prerequisite for all acoustic stimulation treatments is evoked activity in AN fibers and central auditory neurons. Further the stimulation device needs to be able to drive all frequency channels of the auditory system that are required for the treatment. However, both these assumptions might not be justified. One direct caveat for acoustic treatments is the limited frequency range of behind-the-ear devices that are commonly used to deliver the acoustic stimulation. Most behind-the-ear hearing aids and noise generators have an upper cut-off frequency in the range of 5–6 kHz, and tinnitus patients with a higher tinnitus pitch do in fact show less benefit from these devices, possibly because they do not receive adequate stimulation in their tinnitus frequency range (Schaette et al., 2010). In that case, the tinnitus models based on plasticity and gain control predict that treatment will not be effective. Furthermore, certain kinds of cochlear damage could also be major obstacles for acoustic stimulation strategies aimed at re-normalizing or at least increasing AN activity. A recent study found evidence for cochlear dead regions in 16 out of 20 participants with chronic tinnitus (Kiani et al., unpublished results). Tinnitus pitch was either at the dead region's edge frequency or inside the dead region. A cochlear dead region occurs when a stretch of the cochlea is devoid of functioning inner hair cells, and, as a consequence, the corresponding frequency channels of the auditory system cannot be stimulated acoustically. Moreover, "hidden hearing loss," i.e., the deafferentation of AN fibers in tinnitus patients with a normal audiogram (Schaette and McAlpine, 2011), might also complicate a re-normalization of AN activity through acoustic stimulation.

In case of severe cochlear damage, electric stimulation of AN fibers, for example by means of a cochlear implant, could be another option. As long as a sufficient number of AN fibers can be stimulated, homeostatic plasticity and gain control models would also predict a reduction of tinnitus. This prediction is in line with the observation that cochlear implants can strongly reduce tinnitus (Punte et al., 2011), even generating long-lasting after-effects after the stimulation has been turned off (van de Heyning et al., 2008).

Computational models of tinnitus could be especially valuable as tools for understanding, evaluating and predicting the effects of drug treatments against tinnitus. Most of the drugs that have been recently tested for tinnitus increase inhibition in the brain. This treatment is motivated by animal studies that identified a correlation between reduced inhibition and increased spontaneous neuronal activity and tinnitus. At this point it is essential to determine whether decreased inhibition is truly the underlying cause for the development of tinnitus. The experimental data and predictions of computational models are consistent with the underlying cause being the average level of activity in the auditory system, which controls homeostatic plasticity, and thus also regulates inhibition. When inhibition is increased after hearing loss, for example by administering a drug like gabapentin, activity in the auditory system is reduced to an even greater degree than before. In that case, homeostatic plasticity would decrease the efficacy of inhibitory synapses further and also strengthen excitation, thus counterbalancing the effects of the drug. After the drug treatment has been ceased, there might even be an overshoot of activity if the drug is metabolized faster than the time constant of homeostatic plasticity. Such model-based considerations could help to explain why drugs like gabapentin are not more effective than placebo (Aazh et al., 2011).

CONCLUSIONS

Computational models of tinnitus opened up a functional view on plastic changes in the auditory system after hearing loss and their relation to tinnitus. Moreover, the quantitative approach used in computational modeling contributed to an assessment of different candidate mechanisms for the development of tinnitus, inspiring new experiments in order to test model predictions. In the future, a combination of brainstem and cortex models and an inclusion of feedback mechanisms could be important steps toward a more comprehensive model of tinnitus generation. Such theoretical approaches will complement and motivate further experimental studies, and a combined theoretical and experimental approach will contribute to the development of targeted tinnitus therapies in the future.

ACKNOWLEDGMENTS

We would like to thank Warren Bakay for helpful comments on this manuscript. This work was supported by the British Tinnitus Association, by the Deutsche Forschungsgemeinschaft (DFG) through the SFB 618 "Theoretical Biology", and the Bundesministerium für Bildung und Forschung (BMBF) through the Bernstein Center for Computational Neuroscience Berlin (01GQ1001A) and through the Bernstein Focus: Neuronal Basis of Learning (01GQ0972).

REFERENCES

Aazh, H., El Refaie, A., and Humphriss, R. (2011). Gabapentin for tinnitus: a systematic review. *Am. J. Audiol.* 20, 151–158.

Barnea, G., Attias, J., Gold, S., and Shahar, A. (1990). Tinnitus with normal hearing sensitivity: extended high-frequency audiometry and auditory-nerve brain-stem-evoked responses. *Audiology* 29, 36–45.

Benda, J., and Herz, A. V. (2003). A universal model for spike-frequency adaptation. *Neural Comput.* 15, 2523–2564.

Brozoski, T. J., Bauer, C. A., and Caspary, D. M. (2002). Elevated fusiform cell activity in the dorsal cochlear nucleus of chinchillas with psychophysical evidence of tinnitus. *J. Neurosci.* 22, 2383–2390.

Bruce, I. C., Bajaj, H. S., and Ko, J. (2003). "Lateral-inhibitory-network models of tinnitus," in *5th IFAC Symposium on Modelling and Control in Biomedical Systems.* (Melbourne, Australia).

Caspary, D. M., Schatteman, T. A., and Hughes, L. F. (2005). Age-related changes in the inhibitory response properties of dorsal cochlear nucleus output neurons: role of inhibitory inputs. *J. Neurosci.* 25, 10952–10959.

Chrostowski, M., Yang, L., Wilson, H. R., Bruce, I. C., and Becker, S. (2011). Can homeostatic plasticity in deafferented primary auditory cortex lead to travelling waves of excitation? *J. Comput. Neurosci.* 30, 279–299.

Dallos, P., and Harris, D. (1978). Properties of auditory nerve responses in absence of outer hair cells. *J. Neurophysiol.* 41, 365–383.

de la Rocha, J., Marchetti, C., Schiff, M., and Reyes, A. D. (2008). Linking the response properties of cells in auditory cortex with network architecture: cotuning versus lateral inhibition. *J. Neurosci.* 28, 9151–9163.

Dean, I., Harper, N. S., and McAlpine, D. (2005). Neural population coding of sound level adapts to stimulus statistics. *Nat. Neurosci.* 8, 1684–1689.

Dean, I., Robinson, B. L., Harper, N. S., and McAlpine, D. (2008). Rapid neural adaptation to sound level statistics. *J. Neurosci.* 28, 6430–6438.

Desai, N. S., Rutherford, L. C., and Turrigiano, G. G. (1999). Plasticity in the intrinsic excitability of cortical pyramidal neurons. *Nat. Neurosci.* 2, 515–520.

Dominguez, M., Becker, S., Bruce, I., and Read, H. (2006). A spiking neuron model of cortical correlates of sensorineural hearing loss: spontaneous firing, synchrony, and tinnitus. *Neural Comput.* 18, 2942–2958.

Dong, S., Mulders, W. H., Rodger, J., and Robertson, D. (2009). Changes in neuronal activity and gene expression in guinea-pig auditory brainstem after unilateral partial hearing loss. *Neuroscience* 159, 1164–1174.

Eggermont, J. J., and Roberts, L. E. (2004). The neuroscience of tinnitus. *Trends Neurosci.* 27, 676–682.

Engineer, N. D., Riley, J. R., Seale, J. D., Vrana, W. A., Shetake, J. A., Sudanagunta, S. P., Borland, M. S., and Kilgard, M. P. (2011). Reversing pathological neural activity using targeted plasticity. *Nature* 470, 101–104.

Freyer, F., Roberts, J. A., Becker, R., Robinson, P. A., Ritter, P., and Breakspear, M. (2011). Biophysical mechanisms of multistability in resting-state cortical rhythms. *J. Neurosci.* 31, 6353–6361.

Gerken, G. M. (1996). Central tinnitus and lateral inhibition: an auditory brainstem model. *Hear. Res.* 97, 75–83.

Heinz, M. G., and Young, E. D. (2004). Response growth with sound level in auditory-nerve fibers after noise-induced hearing loss. *J. Neurophysiol.* 91, 784–795.

Houweling, A. R., Bazhenov, M., Timofeev, I., Steriade, M., and Sejnowski, T. J. (2005). Homeostatic synaptic plasticity can explain post-traumatic epileptogenesis in chronically isolated neocortex. *Cereb. Cortex* 15, 834–845.

Irvine, D. R., Rajan, R., and McDermott, H. J. (2000). Injury-induced reorganization in adult auditory cortex and its perceptual consequences. *Hear. Res.* 147, 188–199.

Kaltenbach, J. A. (2011). Tinnitus: models and mechanisms. *Hear. Res.* 276, 52–60.

Kaltenbach, J. A., Zacharek, M. A., Zhang, J., and Frederick, S. (2004). Activity in the dorsal cochlear nucleus of hamsters previously tested for tinnitus following intense tone exposure. *Neurosci. Lett.* 355, 121–125.

Kilman, V., van Rossum, M. C., and Turrigiano, G. G. (2002). Activity deprivation reduces miniature IPSC amplitude by decreasing the number of postsynaptic GABA(A) receptors clustered at neocortical synapses. *J. Neurosci.* 22, 1328–1337.

Komiya, H., and Eggermont, J. J. (2000). Spontaneous firing activity of cortical neurons in adult cats with reorganized tonotopic map following pure-tone trauma. *Acta Otolaryngol.* 120, 750–756.

König, O., Schaette, R., Kempter, R., and Gross, M. (2006). Course of hearing loss and occurrence of tinnitus. *Hear. Res.* 221, 59–64.

Kotak, V. C., Fujisawa, S., Lee, F. A., Karthikeyan, O., Aoki, C., and Sanes, D. H. (2005). Hearing loss raises excitability in the auditory cortex. *J. Neurosci.* 25, 3908–3918.

Kral, A., and Majernik, V. (1996). On lateral inhibition in the auditory system. *Gen. Physiol. Biophys.* 15, 109–127.

Kujawa, S. G., and Liberman, M. C. (2009). Adding insult to injury: cochlear nerve degeneration after "temporary" noise-induced hearing loss. *J. Neurosci.* 29, 14077–14085.

Kuokkanen, P. T., Wagner, H., Ashida, G., Carr, C. E., and Kempter, R. (2010). On the origin of the extracellular field potential in the nucleus laminaris of the barn owl (*Tyto alba*). *J. Neurophysiol.* 104, 2274–2290.

Langner, G., and Wallhäusser-Franke, E. (1999). "Computer simulation of a tinnitus model based on tinnitus activity in the auditory cortex," in *Sixth International Tinnitus Seminar,* ed J. W. P. Hazell (Cambridge, UK: The Tinnitus and Hyperacusis Centre).

Liberman, M. C., and Dodds, L. W. (1984). Single-neuron labeling and chronic cochlear pathology. II. Stereocilia damage and alterations of spontaneous discharge rates. *Hear. Res.* 16, 43–53.

Lorenz, I., Muller, N., Schlee, W., Hartmann, T., and Weisz, N. (2009). Loss of alpha power is related to increased gamma synchronization-A marker of reduced inhibition in tinnitus? *Neurosci. Lett.* 453, 225–228.

Middleton, J. W., Kiritani, T., Pedersen, C., Turner, J. G., Shepherd, G. M., and Tzounopoulos, T. (2011). Mice with behavioral evidence of tinnitus exhibit dorsal cochlear nucleus hyperactivity because of decreased GABAergic inhibition. *Proc. Natl. Acad. Sci. U.S.A.* 108, 7601–7606.

Moore, B. C., and Vinay, S. (2010). The relationship between tinnitus pitch and the edge frequency of the audiogram in individuals with hearing impairment and tonal tinnitus. *Hear. Res.* 261, 51–56.

Mühlnickel, W., Elbert, T., Taub, E., and Flor, H. (1998). Reorganization of auditory cortex in tinnitus. *Proc. Natl. Acad. Sci. U.S.A.* 95, 10340–10343.

Mulders, W. H., Ding, D., Salvi, R., and Robertson, D. (2011). Relationship between auditory thresholds, central spontaneous activity, and hair cell loss after acoustic trauma. *J. Comp. Neurol.* 519, 2637–2647.

Muly, S. M., Gross, J. S., and Potashner, S. J. (2004). Noise trauma alters D-[3H]aspartate release and AMPA binding in chinchilla cochlear nucleus. *J. Neurosci. Res.* 75, 585–596.

Norena, A., Micheyl, C., Chery-Croze, S., and Collet, L. (2002). Psychoacoustic characterization of the tinnitus spectrum: implications for the underlying mechanisms of tinnitus. *Audiol. Neurootol.* 7, 358–369.

Norena, A. J., and Eggermont, J. J. (2003). Changes in spontaneous neural activity immediately after an acoustic trauma: implications for neural correlates of tinnitus. *Hear. Res.* 183, 137–153.

Oleskevich, S., and Walmsley, B. (2002). Synaptic transmission in the auditory brainstem of normal and congenitally deaf mice. *J. Physiol.* 540, 447–455.

Ortmann, M., Muller, N., Schlee, W., and Weisz, N. (2011). Rapid increases of gamma power in the auditory cortex following noise trauma in humans. *Eur. J. Neurosci.* 33, 568–575.

Pan, T., Tyler, R. S., Ji, H., Coelho, C., Gehringer, A. K., and Gogel, S. A. (2009). The relationship between tinnitus pitch and the audiogram. *Int. J. Audiol.* 48, 277–294.

Parra, L. C., and Pearlmutter, B. A. (2007). Illusory percepts from auditory adaptation. *J. Acoust. Soc. Am.* 121, 1632–1641.

Punte, A. K., Vermeire, K., Hofkens, A., De Bodt, M., De Ridder, D., and van de Heyning, P. (2011). Cochlear implantation as a durable tinnitus treatment in single-sided deafness. *Cochlear Implants Int.* 12(Suppl. 1), S26–S29.

Rajan, R., and Irvine, D. R. (1998). Neuronal responses across cortical field A1 in plasticity induced by peripheral auditory organ damage. *Audiol. Neurootol.* 3, 123–144.

Rannals, M. D., and Kapur, J. (2011). Homeostatic strengthening of inhibitory synapses is mediated by the accumulation of $GABA_A$ receptors. *J. Neurosci.* 31, 17701–17712.

Rauschecker, J. P. (1999). Auditory cortical plasticity: a comparison with other sensory systems. *Trends Neurosci.* 22, 74–80.

Rauschecker, J. P., Leaver, A. M., and Muhlau, M. (2010). Tuning out the noise: limbic-auditory interactions in tinnitus. *Neuron* 66, 819–826.

Roberts, L. E., Eggermont, J. J., Caspary, D. M., Shore, S. E., Melcher, J. R., and Kaltenbach, J. A. (2010). Ringing ears: the neuroscience of tinnitus. *J. Neurosci.* 30, 14972–14979.

Roberts, L. E., Moffat, G., Baumann, M., Ward, L. M., and Bosnyak, D. J. (2008). Residual inhibition functions overlap tinnitus spectra and the region of auditory threshold shift. *J. Assoc. Res. Otolaryngol.* 9, 417–435.

Roberts, M. T., and Trussell, L. O. (2010). Molecular layer inhibitory interneurons provide feedforward and lateral inhibition in the dorsal cochlear nucleus. *J. Neurophysiol.* 104, 2462–2473.

Sanchez, T. G., Medeiros, I. R., Levy, C. P., Ramalho Jda, R., and Bento, R. F. (2005). Tinnitus in normally hearing patients: clinical aspects and repercussions. *Br. J. Otorhinolaryngol.* 71, 427–431.

Schaette, R., and Kempter, R. (2006). Development of tinnitus-related neuronal hyperactivity through homeostatic plasticity after hearing loss: a computational model. *Eur. J. Neurosci.* 23, 3124–3138.

Schaette, R., and Kempter, R. (2008). Development of hyperactivity after hearing loss in a computational model of the dorsal cochlear nucleus depends on neuron response type. *Hear. Res.* 240, 57–72.

Schaette, R., and Kempter, R. (2009). Predicting tinnitus pitch from patients' audiograms with a computational model for the development of neuronal hyperactivity. *J. Neurophysiol.* 101, 3042–3052.

Schaette, R., König, O., Hornig, D., Gross, M., and Kempter, R. (2010). Acoustic stimulation treatments against tinnitus could be most effective when tinnitus pitch is within the stimulated frequency range. *Hear. Res.* 269, 95–101.

Schaette, R., and McAlpine, D. (2011). Tinnitus with a normal audiogram: physiological evidence for hidden hearing loss and computational model. *J. Neurosci.* 31, 13452–13457.

Schaette, R., Turtle, C., and Munro, K. J. (2012). Reversible induction of phantom auditory sensations through simulated unilateral hearing loss. *PLoS One.* doi: 10.1371/journal.pone.0035238

Sereda, M., Hall, D. A., Bosnyak, D. J., Edmondson-Jones, M., Roberts, L. E., Adjamian, P., and Palmer, A. R. (2011). Re-examining the relationship between audiometric profile and tinnitus pitch. *Int. J. Audiol.* 50, 303–312.

Song, S., and Abbott, L. F. (2001). Cortical development and remapping through spike timing-dependent plasticity. *Neuron* 32, 339–350.

Sprauten, M., Darrah, T. H., Peterson, D. R., Campbell, M. E., Hannigan, R. E., Cvancarova, M., Beard, C., Haugnes, H. S., Fossa, S. D., Oldenburg, J., and Travis, L. B. (2011). Impact of long-term serum platinum concentrations on neuro- and ototoxicity in cisplatin-treated survivors of testicular cancer. *J. Clin. Oncol.* 30, 300–307.

Suneja, S. K., Benson, C. G., and Potashner, S. J. (1998a). Glycine receptors in adult guinea pig brain stem auditory nuclei: regulation after unilateral cochlear ablation. *Exp. Neurol.* 154, 473–488.

Suneja, S. K., Potashner, S. J., and Benson, C. G. (1998b). Plastic changes in glycine and GABA release and uptake in adult brain stem auditory nuclei after unilateral middle ear ossicle removal and cochlear ablation. *Exp. Neurol.* 151, 273–288.

Trotter, M. I., and Donaldson, I. (2008). Hearing aids and tinnitus therapy: a 25-year experience. *J. Laryngol. Otol.* 122, 1052–1056.

Turrigiano, G. G. (1999). Homeostatic plasticity in neuronal networks: the more things change, the more they stay the same. *Trends Neurosci.* 22, 221–227.

Turrigiano, G. G., Leslie, K. R., Desai, N. S., Rutherford, L. C., and Nelson, S. B. (1998). Activity-dependent scaling of quantal amplitude in neocortical neurons. *Nature* 391, 892–896.

Vale, C., and Sanes, D. H. (2002). The effect of bilateral deafness on excitatory and inhibitory synaptic strength in the inferior colliculus. *Eur. J. Neurosci.* 16, 2394–2404.

Vale, C., Juiz, J. M., Moore, D. R., and Sanes, D. H. (2004). Unilateral cochlear ablation produces greater loss of inhibition in the contralateral inferior colliculus. *Eur. J. Neurosci.* 20, 2133–2140.

van de Heyning, P., Vermeire, K., Diebl, M., Nopp, P., Anderson, I., and De Ridder, D. (2008). Incapacitating unilateral tinnitus in single-sided deafness treated by cochlear implantation. *Ann. Otol. Rhinol. Laryngol.* 117, 645–652.

van Welie, I., van Hooft, J. A., and Wadman, W. J. (2004). Homeostatic scaling of neuronal excitability by synaptic modulation of so-matic hyperpolarization-activated Ih channels. *Proc. Natl. Acad. Sci. U.S.A.* 101, 5123–5128.

Weisz, N., Moratti, S., Meinzer, M., Dohrmann, K., and Elbert, T. (2005). Tinnitus perception and distress is related to abnormal spontaneous brain activity as measured by magnetoencephalography. *PLoS Med.* 2:e153. doi: 10.1371/journal.pmed.0020153

Weisz, N., Muller, S., Schlee, W., Dohrmann, K., Hartmann, T., and Elbert, T. (2007). The neural code of auditory phantom perception. *J. Neurosci.* 27, 1479–1484.

Wen, B., Wang, G. I., Dean, I., and Delgutte, B. (2009). Dynamic range adaptation to sound level statistics in the auditory nerve. *J. Neurosci.* 29, 13797–13808.

Whiting, B., Moiseff, A., and Rubio, M. E. (2009). Cochlear nucleus neurons redistribute synaptic AMPA and glycine receptors in response to monaural conductive hearing loss. *Neuroscience* 163, 1264–1276.

Yang, S., Weiner, B. D., Zhang, L. S., Cho, S. J., and Bao, S. (2011). Homeostatic plasticity drives tinnitus perception in an animal model. *Proc. Natl. Acad. Sci. U.S.A.* 108, 14974–14979.

Young, J. M., Waleszczyk, W. J., Wang, C., Calford, M. B., Dreher, B., and Obermayer, K. (2007). Cortical reorganization consistent with spike timing-but not correlation-dependent plasticity. *Nat. Neurosci.* 10, 887–895.

Permissions

All chapters in this book were first published by Frontiers; hereby published with permission under the Creative Commons Attribution License or equivalent. Every chapter published in this book has been scrutinized by our experts. Their significance has been extensively debated. The topics covered herein carry significant findings which will fuel the growth of the discipline. They may even be implemented as practical applications or may be referred to as a beginning point for another development.

The contributors of this book come from diverse backgrounds, making this book a truly international effort. This book will bring forth new frontiers with its revolutionizing research information and detailed analysis of the nascent developments around the world.

We would like to thank all the contributing authors for lending their expertise to make the book truly unique. They have played a crucial role in the development of this book. Without their invaluable contributions this book wouldn't have been possible. They have made vital efforts to compile up to date information on the varied aspects of this subject to make this book a valuable addition to the collection of many professionals and students.

This book was conceptualized with the vision of imparting up-to-date information and advanced data in this field. To ensure the same, a matchless editorial board was set up. Every individual on the board went through rigorous rounds of assessment to prove their worth. After which they invested a large part of their time researching and compiling the most relevant data for our readers.

The editorial board has been involved in producing this book since its inception. They have spent rigorous hours researching and exploring the diverse topics which have resulted in the successful publishing of this book. They have passed on their knowledge of decades through this book. To expedite this challenging task, the publisher supported the team at every step. A small team of assistant editors was also appointed to further simplify the editing procedure and attain best results for the readers.

Apart from the editorial board, the designing team has also invested a significant amount of their time in understanding the subject and creating the most relevant covers. They scrutinized every image to scout for the most suitable representation of the subject and create an appropriate cover for the book.

The publishing team has been an ardent support to the editorial, designing and production team. Their endless efforts to recruit the best for this project, has resulted in the accomplishment of this book. They are a veteran in the field of academics and their pool of knowledge is as vast as their experience in printing. Their expertise and guidance has proved useful at every step. Their uncompromising quality standards have made this book an exceptional effort. Their encouragement from time to time has been an inspiration for everyone.

The publisher and the editorial board hope that this book will prove to be a valuable piece of knowledge for researchers, students, practitioners and scholars across the globe.

List of Contributors

Eugen Diesch
Department of Clinical and Cognitive Neuroscience, Central Institute of Mental Health, Medical Faculty Mannheim, Heidelberg University, Mannheim, Germany

Martin Andermann and Andre Rupp
Department of Neurology, Section of Biomagnetism, University Hospital Heidelberg, Heidelberg, Germany

Peter Michael Kreuzer, Martin Schecklmann and Timm B. Poeppl
Department of Psychiatry and Psychotherapy, University of Regensburg, Regensburg, Germany

Veronika Vielsmeier
Department of Otolaryngology, University of Regensburg, Regensburg, Germany

Goeran Hajak
Department of Psychiatry and Psychotherapy, University of Regensburg, Regensburg, Germany
Department of Psychiatry, Psychosomatic Medicine and Psychotherapy, Bezirkskrankenhaus Bamberg, Bamberg, Germany

Tobias Kleinjung
Department of Otolaryngology, University of Regensburg, Regensburg, Germany
Department of Otolaryngology, University of Zurich, Zurich, Switzerland

Amber M. Leaver, Anna Seydell-Greenwald, Ted K. Turesky and Josef P. Rauschecker
Department of Neuroscience, Georgetown University Medical Center, Washington, DC, USA

Susan Morgan
Division of Audiology, Georgetown University Hospital, Washington, DC, USA

Hung J. Kim
Department of Otolaryngology, Georgetown University Hospital, Washington, DC, USA

P. G. Sand and B. Langguth
Department of Psychiatry, University of Regensburg, Regensburg, Germany

J. Itzhacki, A. Bauer, S. Geis, Z. E. Cárdenas-Conejo and V. Pimentel
Experimental and Clinical Neurosciences Graduate Program, University of Regensburg, Regensburg, Germany

T. Kleinjung
Department of Otorhinolaryngology, University of Regensburg, Regensburg, Germany
Department of Otorhinolaryngology, University of Zurich, Zurich, Switzerland

Daniel Stolzberg, Richard J. Salvi and Brian L. Allman
Center for Hearing and Deafness, University at Buffalo, The State University of New York, Buffalo, NY, USA

Sven Vanneste and Dirk De Ridder
Brai2n, TRI and Department of Neurosurgery, University Hospital Antwerp, Antwerp, Belgium

Ilya Adamchic and Christian Hauptmann
Institute of Neuroscience and Medicine - Neuromodulation, Research Center Jülich, Jülich, Germany

Peter A. Tass
Institute of Neuroscience and Medicine - Neuromodulation, Research Center Jülich, Jülich, Germany
Department of Stereotactic and Functional Neurosurgery, University of Cologne, Cologne, Germany

Thomas Brozoski and Carol Bauer
Division of Otolaryngology, Southern Illinois University School of Medicine, Springfield, IL, USA

Boris Odintsov
Biomedical Imaging Center, Beckman Institute for Advanced Science and Technology, University of Illinois, Urbana Champaign, Urbana, IL, USA

Astrid Lehner, Michael Landgrebe, Timm Benjamin Poeppl and Peter Michal Kreuzer
Department of Psychiatry and Psychotherapy, University of Regensburg, Regensburg, Germany
Tinnitus Center, University of Regensburg, Regensburg, Germany

Winfried Schlee
OBOB Laboratory, Department of Psychology, University of Konstanz, Konstanz, Germany and University of Trento, Trento, Italy

Nathan Weisz
Clinical and Biological Psychology, Institute of Psychology and Education, University of Ulm, Ulm, Germany

Janice E. Chang
Department of Anatomy and Neurobiology, University of California Irvine, Irvine, CA, USA

Fan-Gang Zeng
Department of Anatomy and Neurobiology, University of California Irvine, Irvine, CA, USA
Department of Otolaryngology – Head and Neck Surgery, University of California Irvine, Orange, CA, USA

Susanne Dehmel and Daniel Eisinger
Department of Otolaryngology, Kresge Hearing Research Institute, University of Michigan, Ann Arbor, MI, USA

Susan E. Shore
Department of Otolaryngology, Kresge Hearing Research Institute, University of Michigan, Ann Arbor, MI, USA
Department of Molecular and Integrative Physiology, University of Michigan, Ann Arbor, MI, USA

Dave R. M. Langers, Emile de Kleine and Pim van Dijk
Department of Otorhinolaryngology/Head and Neck Surgery, University Medical Center Groningen, University of Groningen, Groningen, Netherlands
Graduate School of Medical Sciences (Research School of Behavioural and Cognitive Neurosciences), University of Groningen, Groningen, Netherlands

Larry E. Roberts, Daniel J. Bosnyak and David C. Thompson
Department of Psychology, Neuroscience, and Behaviour, McMaster University, Hamilton, ON, Canada

Astrid Lehner, Peter M. Kreuzer, Elmar Frank and Rainer Rupprecht
Department of Psychiatry and Psychotherapy, University of Regensburg, Regensburg, Germany

Jason W. Middleton and Thanos Tzounopoulos
Department of Otolaryngology, University of Pittsburgh, Pittsburgh, PA, USA
Department of Neurobiology, University of Pittsburgh, Pittsburgh, PA, USA
Center for the Neural Basis of Cognition, University of Pittsburgh, Pittsburgh, PA, USA

Birgit Mazurek and Agnieszka J. Szczepek
Molecular Biology Research Laboratory, Department of Otorhinolaryngology, Charité - Universitätsmedizin Berlin, Campus Charité Mitte, Berlin, Germany
Tinnitus Center, Charité - Universitätsmedizin Berlin, Campus Charité Mitte, Berlin, Germany

Heidemarie Haupt
Molecular Biology Research Laboratory, Department of Otorhinolaryngology, Charité - Universitätsmedizin Berlin, Campus Charité Mitte, Berlin, Germany

Heidi Olze
Tinnitus Center, Charité - Universitätsmedizin Berlin, Campus Charité Mitte, Berlin, Germany
Department of Otorhinolaryngology, Charité - Universitätsmedizin Berlin, Campus Virchow Klinikum, Berlin, Germany

Ana B. Elgoyhen
Instituto de Investigaciones en Ingeniería Genética y Biología Molecular, Consejo Nacional de Investigaciones Científicas y Técnicas and Tercera Cátedra de Farmacología, Facultad de Medicina, Universidad de Buenos Aires, Buenos Aires, Argentina

Berthold Langguth
Interdisciplinary Tinnitus Clinic, Departments of Psychiatry and Psychotherapy, University of Regensburg, Regensburg, Germany

Verena Schummer and Martin Kramer
Small Animal Clinic, Department of Veterinary Clinical Sciences, University of Gießen, Gießen, Germany

Andre Rupp
Section of Biomagnetism, Department of Neurology, University Hospital Heidelberg, Heidelberg, Germany

Christo Pantev and Henning Teismann
Institute for Biomagnetism and Biosignalanalysis, University of Münster, Münster, Germany

Hidehiko Okamoto
Institute for Biomagnetism and Biosignalanalysis, University of Münster, Münster, Germany
Department of Integrative Physiology, National Institute for Physiological Sciences, Okazaki, Japan

Roland Schaette
Ear Institute, University College London, London, UK

Richard Kempter
Institute for Theoretical Biology, Humboldt-Universität zu Berlin and Bernstein Center for Computational Neuroscience, Berlin, Germany

Index

Printed in the USA
CPSIA information can be obtained
at www.ICGtesting.com
LVHW080051211023
761596LV00010BA/2014